Autophagy and Metabolic Syndrome: From Molecular Mechanisms to Clinical Consequences

Autophagy and Metabolic Syndrome: From Molecular Mechanisms to Clinical Consequences

Editor: Esther Bennett

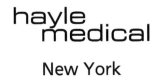

New York

Hayle Medical,
750 Third Avenue, 9th Floor,
New York, NY 10017, USA

Visit us on the World Wide Web at:
www.haylemedical.com

ISBN 978-1-64647-559-9 (Hardback)

Cataloging-in-Publication Data

Autophagy and metabolic syndrome : from molecular mechanisms to
clinical consequences / edited by Esther Bennett.
    p. cm.
Includes bibliographical references and index.
ISBN 978-1-64647-559-9
1. Metabolic syndrome. 2. Autophagic vacuoles. 3. Lysosomal storage diseases.
4. Metabolism--Disorders. 5. Molecular biology. 6. Metabolic syndrome--Treatment.
I. Bennett, Esther.
RC662.4 .A88 2023
616.399--dc23

Contents

Preface

In my initial years as a student, I used to run to the library at every possible instance to grab a book and learn something new. Books were my primary source of knowledge and I would not have come such a long way without all that I learnt from them. Thus, when I was approached to edit this book; I became understandably nostalgic. It was an absolute honor to be considered worthy of guiding the current generation as well as those to come. I put all my knowledge and hard work into making this book most beneficial for its readers.

Autophagy is a process in which cells capture their own cytoplasm and organelles and consume them in lysosomes. This mechanism preserves the health of cells and tissues through the replacement of damaged and outdated cellular components with new ones. The breakdown products serve as inputs to cellular metabolism. Autophagy prevents degenerative diseases as it is a powerful promoter of metabolic homeostasis at both the cellular and whole animal level. It reduces ubiquitinated protein accumulation in the brain, disposes-off the aggregation-prone proteins and damaged organelles that cause Huntington's disease and Parkinson's disease. The metabolic syndrome refers to a group of medical conditions which increase the likelihood of heart disease, diabetes and stroke. It encompasses high blood sugar, hypertension, high cholesterol levels and excess fat around the waist. The process of autophagy has an effect on the development of metabolic syndrome since the metabolic syndrome is caused due to the accumulation of damaged cellular constituents. This book includes some of the vital pieces of works being conducted across the world, on various topics related to autophagy and metabolic syndrome. It is appropriate for students seeking detailed information in this area of medicine as well as for experts.

I wish to thank my publisher for supporting me at every step. I would also like to thank all the authors who have contributed their researches in this book. I hope this book will be a valuable contribution to the progress of the field.

Editor

Phytochemicals: Targeting Mitophagy to Treat Metabolic Disorders

Zuqing Su[1†], Yanru Guo[1,2†], Xiufang Huang[1,3†], Bing Feng[1], Lipeng Tang[1], Guangjuan Zheng[1]* and Ying Zhu[1]*

[1] Guangdong Provincial Hospital of Chinese Medicine, The Second Clinical College of Guangzhou University of Chinese Medicine, Guangzhou, China, [2] Guizhou University of Traditional Chinese Medicine, Guiyang, China, [3] The First Affiliated Hospital of Guangzhou University of Chinese Medicine, Guangzhou, China

*Correspondence:
Guangjuan Zheng
zhengguangjuan@gzucm.edu.cn
Ying Zhu
zhuying3340@gzucm.edu.cn

[†] These authors have contributed equally to this work

Metabolic disorders include metabolic syndrome, obesity, type 2 diabetes mellitus, non-alcoholic fatty liver disease and cardiovascular diseases. Due to unhealthy lifestyles such as high-calorie diet, sedentary and physical inactivity, the prevalence of metabolic disorders poses a huge challenge to global human health, which is the leading cause of global human death. Mitochondrion is the major site of adenosine triphosphate synthesis, fatty acid β−oxidation and ROS production. Accumulating evidence suggests that mitochondrial dysfunction-related oxidative stress and inflammation is involved in the development of metabolic disorders. Mitophagy, a catabolic process, selectively degrades damaged or superfluous mitochondria to reverse mitochondrial dysfunction and preserve mitochondrial function. It is considered to be one of the major mechanisms responsible for mitochondrial quality control. Growing evidence shows that mitophagy can prevent and treat metabolic disorders through suppressing mitochondrial dysfunction-induced oxidative stress and inflammation. In the past decade, in order to expand the range of pharmaceutical options, more and more phytochemicals have been proven to have therapeutic effects on metabolic disorders. Many of these phytochemicals have been proved to activate mitophagy to ameliorate metabolic disorders. Given the ongoing epidemic of metabolic disorders, it is of great significance to explore the contribution and underlying mechanisms of mitophagy in metabolic disorders, and to understand the effects and molecular mechanisms of phytochemicals on the treatment of metabolic disorders. Here, we investigate the mechanism of mitochondrial dysfunction in metabolic disorders and discuss the potential of targeting mitophagy with phytochemicals for the treatment of metabolic disorders, with a view to providing a direction for finding phytochemicals that target mitophagy to prevent or treat metabolic disorders.

Keywords: phytochemicals, metabolic disorders, mitophagy, mitochondrial dysfunction, oxidative stress, inflammatory response

INTRODUCTION

Autophagy, an evolutionarily conserved catabolic process, degrades intracellular constituents including lipid, glycogen and protein to maintain cellular energy homeostasis in the absence of nutrients (Vargas et al., 2017). In this process, double-membrane vesicles (autophagosomes) will enfold intracellular constituents and then transfer to lysosomes to form autolysosomes where the lysosomal enzyme can degrade the enveloped cargoes. According to the different methods of delivering cytoplasmic components to lysosomes, autophagy can be divided into three different types: macroautophagy (hereafter referred to as autophagy), microautophagy and chaperone-mediated autophagy. Moreover, according to the specificity of the degradation substrate, autophagy can be classified into mitophagy, pexophagy, reticulophagy, ribophagy and xenophagy.

About 50 years ago, autophagy was first described to be triggered to maintain cellular energy balance and cell survival under nutrition-deprived conditions. In the past 10 years, due to the in-depth understanding of the role of autophagy, accumulating study has indicated that autophagy plays a vital role in the physiology and pathology of many diseases, such as metabolic disorders, cancer, Alzheimer's disease and Parkinson's disease. Nowadays, it is commonly accepted that autophagy, especially mitophagy, plays a crucial role in the pathology of metabolic disorders such as non-alcoholic fatty liver, type 2 diabetes and metabolic syndrome (Vásquez-Trincado et al., 2016; Sarparanta et al., 2017; Dombi et al., 2018).

Phytochemicals extracted from natural plants have been widely used to treat metabolic diseases including metabolic syndrome (Cicero and Colletti, 2016), type 2 diabetes (Moreno-Valdespino et al., 2020), obesity (Li et al., 2019), insulin resistance (Mahdavi et al., 2021) and cardiovascular diseases (Pop et al., 2018) due to relative safety and multiple beneficial effects. According to an estimation issued by the World Health Organization in 2008, about 80% of diabetic patients rely on herbal medicine (Bacanli et al., 2019).

In view of the fact that more and more phytochemicals are applied to the treatment of metabolic diseases, it is necessary to have a more comprehensive understanding of the effects and potential mechanisms of phytochemicals on metabolic diseases. Therefore, this review will focus on the regulatory mechanisms of mitophagy in metabolic disorders and further explore the potential of targeting mitophagy with phytochemicals for the prevention or treatment of metabolic disorders.

MITOCHONDRIAL DYSFUNCTION AND OXIDATIVE STRESS

Mitochondrion regulates many physiological functions such as adenosine triphosphate (ATP) synthesis, free radicals generation, fatty acid β—oxidation, calcium homeostasis, and cell survival and death (Liu L. et al., 2020; Kirtonia et al., 2021). Mitochondria are dynamic organelles that can fleetly adapt to changes in cellular energy metabolism by regulating mitochondrial biogenesis, mitochondrial fission, mitochondrial fusion and removal of damaged mitochondria (Vásquez-Trincado et al., 2016; Mills et al., 2017; Keenan et al., 2020). Of note, the uppermost physiological function of mitochondria is to produce ATP via oxidative phosphorylation (OXPHOS) (Bhatti et al., 2017). During OXPHOS, mitochondria will inevitably produce by-product superoxide anions, which can be further converted into reactive oxygen species (ROS) or reactive nitrogen species (RNS) (Kalyanaraman et al., 2018). Under physiological conditions, ROS and RNS act as the regulatory mechanism for cellular redox homeostasis (Liu and Butow, 2006). Mitochondrial ROS, one of the major sources of cellular ROS, consists of hydrogen peroxide (H_2O_2), superoxide (O^-_2), and hydroxyl (OH), which can impair lipids, proteins and DNA, resulting in mitochondrial dysfunction and cell apoptosis (Kirtonia et al., 2020; Tan et al., 2021). There are various defense systems to counter ROS-induced oxidative stress, such as catalase (CAT), superoxide dismutase (SOD) and glutathione peroxidase (GSH-PX). However, high levels of ROS will unduly oxidize lipids, DNA and proteins, thereby destroying cell membranes and other cellular structures. In general, mitochondrial ROS can damage mitochondrial DNA to disturb the physiological functions of mitochondria. And the accumulation of damaged mitochondria and the overexpression of mitochondrial ROS will reinforce each other, forming a vicious cycle, and eventually lead to mitochondrial dysfunction. Accumulating evidence has shown that oxidative stress is involved in various pathological conditions including insulin resistance, type 2 diabetes and metabolic syndrome (Yaribeygi et al., 2019). Therefore, the regulation of mitochondrial ROS is of key relevance for cellular homeostasis (Kirtonia et al., 2020).

MITOCHONDRION: STRUCTURE AND FUNCTION

Mitochondrial dysfunction is responsible for various metabolic diseases. Therefore, targeting mitochondrial dysfunction will be a promising therapeutic strategy for metabolic disorders. Nevertheless, due to the high complexity of mitochondrial structure and function, targeting mitochondria for the treatment of metabolic disorders will be an arduous and challenging task. Mitochondrion is a double-membrane organelle with its own unique genome, containing 800 to 1000 copies of mitochondrial DNA (mtDNA) (Chen and Butow, 2005). The mitochondrion is constituted by the outer mitochondrial membrane (OMM), the intermembrane space (IMS), inner mitochondrial membrane (IMM) and mitochondrial matrix (Iacobazzi et al., 2017). Although the outer mitochondrial membrane is more permeable than the inner mitochondrial membrane, only molecules with a molecular weight of 5 kDa or less can cross the outer mitochondrial membrane due to the existence of the voltage-dependent anion channel (VDAC). The IMM and mitochondrial matrix contain various enzymes responsible for electron transport chain (ETC) and ATP generation. The tricarboxylic acid (TCA) cycle, one of the hallmark pathways in metabolism, plays an important role in the oxidation of respiratory substrates for ATP synthesis in the mitochondrial matrix (Sweetlove et al., 2010). During this process, electrons will be released and are absorbed by the ETC to produce ATP, which is the major source of cellular energy (Bhatti et al., 2017).

In IMM, complexes I (NADH ubiquinone reductase), II (Succinate dehydrogenase), III (Ubiquinol-cytochrome c reductase), and IV (Cytochrome c oxidase) constitute the ETC, and complex V is an ATP synthase (Shamsi et al., 2008). The hydrogen atoms released during the TCA cycle and fatty acid β-oxidation processes will be transferred to NAD + or FAD + to form NADH or $FADH_2$ (St John et al., 2005). Then the electrons provided by NADH and FADH2 will be transferred to complex I and complex II, respectively, and then to complex III and complex IV. Meanwhile, ETC can generate electrochemical gradient by transporting protons into the intermembrane space. The electrochemical gradient serves as a source of potential energy for generating ATP in the complex V (Shamsi et al., 2008). Under physiological conditions, 0.4 to 4% of oxygen consumed by mitochondria is incompletely reduced, which will lead to the generation of ROS, and other reactive species such as nitric oxide (NO) and RNS (Bhatti et al., 2017; Marí and Colell, 2021). Despite there being multiple enzymatic and non-enzymatic antioxidant defense mechanisms in eukaryotic cells, excessive reactive species will inevitably damage mitochondrial proteins/enzymes, mitochondrial membranes and mtDNA, thereby impairing ATP generation (Bhatti et al., 2017).

MITOCHONDRIAL QUALITY CONTROL

Mitophagy-Mediated Mitochondrial Quality Control

Considering the crucial role of mitochondria in cellular homeostasis, monitoring the quality of mitochondrial is important to avoid adverse effects (Ni et al., 2015; Pickles et al., 2018; Chan, 2020). Mitochondrial quality control can be acted in many forms including molecular, organellar and cellular levels. It's worth noting that CAT, SOD and GSH-PX, as molecular-level oxidative stress defense mechanisms, can effectively decelerate the pace of oxidative damage to mitochondria (Naraki et al., 2021). However, the ROS-scavenging system cannot completely prevent excessive ROS-mediated damage to mitochondria. Accordingly, inhibiting the excessive production of ROS is gradually considered as a more effective way to prevent oxidative damage (Simona et al., 2019).

It is known that the clearance mechanism of damaged mitochondria, an important source of mitochondrial ROS, will be the potent therapeutic strategy for oxidative stress (Angajala et al., 2018; Wang R. et al., 2019). It is now generally accepted that damaged and dysfunctional mitochondria will be removed through mitophagy. In this process, damaged and dysfunctional mitochondria will be captured by autophagic membranes and further delivered to lysosomes, in which mitochondria will be degraded and the degradation products will be used as energy source for metabolism (**Figure 1**). With the deepening of the understanding of the physiological and pathological role of mitophagy, impaired mitophagy has been proved to be related to the development of various diseases including insulin resistance,

type 2 diabetes, metabolic syndrome and non-alcoholic fatty liver disease (Su et al., 2019).

Other Mitochondrial Quality Control Mechanisms

In addition to mitophagy-dependent mitochondrial quality control, mitochondrion also has its own regulatory mechanisms for mitochondrial quality control, such as the mitochondrial unfolded protein response (UPRmt) and mitochondrial fusion and fission (Roque et al., 2020).

The mitochondrial unfolded protein response (UPRmt) is a stress response pathway that can be activated by multiple stress conditions including mitochondrial DNA defects, decreased mitochondrial membrane potential, accumulated unfolded mitochondrial proteins and ROS detoxification (Hernando-Rodríguez and Artal-Sanz, 2018; Roque et al., 2020). At present, the molecular mechanism of UPRmt in *Caenorhabditis elegans* (*C. elegans*) is better understood than in mammals. Activating transcription factor associated with stress (ATFS-1), a key regulatory factor for UPRmt in *Caenorhabditis elegans*, has an N-terminal mitochondrial targeting sequence. Normally, ATFS-1 is imported into mitochondria and is degraded by the matrix-localized protease LON. However, in the case of mitochondrial stress such as respiratory chain dysfunction and ROS, a portion of ATFS-1 will be transferred to the nucleus to activate UPRmt to regulate the abundance of mitochondrial chaperones and proteases to preserve mitochondrial homeostasis (Wrobel et al., 2015; Melber and Haynes, 2018). It's worth noting that if mitochondrial dysfunction continues to worsen, other mitochondrial quality control mechanisms, such as mitophagy, will be activated to clear away those dysfunctional mitochondria (Ma X. et al., 2020).

Mitochondria are dynamic organelles that continuously undergo fission and fusion to maintain the balance of small fragmented mitochondria and long interconnected mitochondrial network, which is essential for cell growth, division, and distribution of mitochondria during differentiation (van der Bliek et al., 2013; Roque et al., 2020). Mitochondrial fission will split a mitochondrion into a healthy mitochondrion with increased mitochondrial membrane potential and a dysfunctional one containing diminished mitochondrial membrane potential, damaged proteins and damaged mtDNA. And then the dysfunctional mitochondrion will be targeted and degraded by mitochondrial quality control mechanisms such as mitophagy (Tahrir et al., 2019). Various regulatory factors involved in mitochondrial fission include dynamin-related protein 1 (DRP1), fission 1 (Fis1), mitochondria fission factor (Mff), mitochondrial dynamics protein of 49 kDa (MID49) and MID51 (Ni et al., 2015). When mitochondrial fission occurs, DRP1 will translocate to the outer mitochondrial membrane from cytoplasm via actin and microtubule mechanisms, and then interacts with Fis1, MFF, MID49 and MID51 to cleave mitochondrion (Anzell et al., 2018). On the other hand, mitochondrial fusion allows damaged mitochondria to fuse with healthy mitochondria to facilitate the equilibration of mitochondrial components, such as mtDNA, proteins and

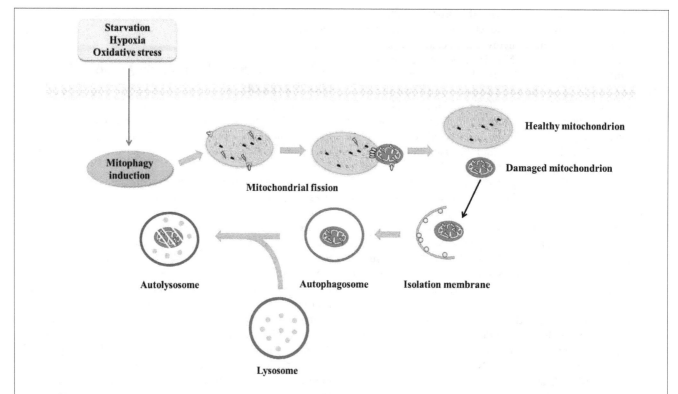

FIGURE 1 | Diagram illustrates the mechanisms of mitophagy. Damaged and dysfunctional mitochondria will be segregated by autophagic membranes. And the autophagosome fuses with lysosome to form autophagolysosome, in which mitochondria will be degraded by lysosomal enzyme and the degradation products will be used as substrates for energy metabolism.

metabolites, thereby enhancing respiratory chain activity and maintaining mitochondrial homeostasis (Baker et al., 2011). Mitochondrial fusion is regulated by dynamin-related GTPase proteins mitofusin 1 (MFN1), mitofusin 2 (MFN2) and optic atrophy 1 (OPA1). MFN1 and MFN2 are responsible for the fusion of the outer mitochondrial membranes, and OPA1 is responsible for the fusion of the inner mitochondrial membranes (Ni et al., 2015). Therefore, outer mitochondrial membrane fusion is carried out in an MFN1/MFN2-dependent manner and inner mitochondrial membrane fusion is performed in an OPA1-dependent manner, and GTP hydrolysis provides energy for the process (Roque et al., 2020). However, when the stimulation severely interferes with mitochondria and causes the mitochondrial membrane potential to dissipate, mitochondrial fusion will be halted to prevent those mitochondria from fusing with the healthy network, thereby limiting the damage caused by dysfunctional mitochondria (Baker et al., 2011).

MITOCHONDRIAL DYSFUNCTION AND INSULIN RESISTANCE

Insulin resistance is a pathological state in which target cells including hepatic cells, adipose cells and skeletal muscle cells are insensitive to the physiological level of insulin (Vazirani et al., 2016; Archer et al., 2018; Nishida et al., 2021). Mounting evidence reveals that insulin resistance is a common risk factor for various

metabolic diseases such as metabolic syndrome, obesity, type 2 diabetes, non-alcoholic fatty liver disease and cardiovascular diseases (Patel et al., 2016; Gluvic et al., 2017; Yazıcı and Sezer, 2017; Czech, 2020; Fujii et al., 2020). Of note, a growing number of studies have established the causal relationship between mitochondrial dysfunction and insulin resistance (Ba Razzoni et al., 2012; Yazıcı and Sezer, 2017; Yaribeygi et al., 2019). Now, the complexity of mitochondrial function and the complicated relationship between mitochondrial dysfunction and the pathogenesis of insulin resistance have led to the development of many theories describing the mechanism connecting mitochondrial dysfunction and insulin resistance.

Ectopic Lipid Accumulation and Insulin Resistance

When the causal relationship between mitochondrial dysfunction and insulin resistance was first confirmed, more and more theories describing the relationship between mitochondrial dysfunction and insulin resistance were proposed. Mitochondria are the main sites of fatty acid β-oxidation, which is the main degradation mechanism of fatty acids in cells (Su et al., 2019). Therefore, mitochondrial dysfunction will cause inefficient fatty acid oxidation, which will lead to ectopic lipid accumulation in non-adipose tissues including liver, muscle and pancreas (Martin and McGee, 2014). Ectopic lipid accumulation will result in the remarkable increase in lipid metabolites such as ceramide and diacylglycerol, which are verified to impair insulin signaling pathway and cause insulin resistance (Montgomery et al., 2019). Now, many theories describing the potential mechanism of ceramide-induced insulin resistance have been put forward (Petersen and Shulman, 2017). First, evidence shows that ceramide induces insulin resistance via suppressing ATK activation through two mechanisms: increases proteinphosphatase-2A (PP2A) and PKCζ activities, thereby disturbing AKT translocation (Petersen and Shulman, 2017). Moreover, the connection among ceramide, adipose inflammation and NLRP3 inflammasome also provides another evidence for ceramide-induced insulin resistance (Turpin et al., 2014; Xia et al., 2015; Petersen and Shulman, 2017). One putative mechanism is that diacylglycerol promotes the membrane translocation of PKCε, which in turn phosphorylates insulin receptor Thr1160 to impair insulin receptor kinase (IRK) activity, thereby inducing insulin resistance (Petersen et al., 2016). In conclusion, mitochondrial dysfunction will cause ectopic lipid accumulation, thereby resulting in the significant increase of ceramide and diacylglycerol, which will directly or indirectly suppress insulin signaling pathway to induce insulin resistance.

Mitochondrial ROS and Insulin Resistance

Mitochondrial ROS has been recognized as the leading cause of insulin resistance. Bloch-Damti and Bashan (2005) brought forward a viewpoint that mitochondrial ROS should be accepted as a possible cause of insulin resistance in animal models of diabetes. However, these initial evidence don't specify whether ROS that induces insulin resistance originates from mitochondria. Since mitochondria are the major sources of cellular ROS, it is necessary to explore the role of mitochondrial ROS in insulin resistance. Indeed, subsequent studies verified the causal relationship of mitochondrial ROS and insulin resistance (Anderson et al., 2009). Anderson et al. believe that mitochondrial ROS is not only an indicator of energy balance, but also a regulator of cellular redox environment, linking cellular metabolic balance with the control of insulin sensitivity (Anderson et al., 2009). There are several potential mechanisms linking mitochondrial ROS and insulin resistance. First, mitochondrial ROS activates various serine kinases that phosphorylate IRS protein and suppresses serine/threonine phosphatase activity to inhibit insulin signaling pathway (Kim et al., 2008; Fisher-Wellman and Neufer, 2012). Furthermore, mitochondrial ROS activates apoptosis signal-regulating kinase 1 (ASK1) and c-jun NH2-terminal kinases (JNK), increases serine phosphorylation of IRS-1, and decreases insulin-stimulated tyrosine phosphorylation of IRS-1, resulting in insulin resistance (Nishikawa and Araki, 2007). However, the only available experimental data has just begun to support those mechanisms, and the detailed mechanism of mitochondrial ROS-induced insulin resistance still needs further exploration.

MITOPHAGY SIGNALING PATHWAYS

Mitophagy, a mitochondrial quality control mechanism, selectively removes dysfunctional mitochondria to preserve mitochondrial function and maintain cellular energy homeostasis. In mammalian cells, there are three main signaling pathways that regulate mitophagy: PINK1/Parkin-dependent mitophagy, BNIP3/NIX- dependent mitophagy and FUNDC1-dependent mitophagy.

PINK1/Parkin-Dependent Mitophagy

Lemasters et al. (1998) discovered that dysfunctional mitochondria were engulfed into autophagosome and then fused with lysosome, in which the dysfunctional mitochondria were degraded. Then Lemasters (2005) further proposed the concept "mitophagy" for the first time to describe the process of eliminating damaged mitochondria. Narendra et al. (2009) confirmed that PTEN-induced putative kinase 1 (PINK1) and the E3 ubiquitin ligase Parkin are two crucial mediators regulating mitophagy in mammalian cells. In general, PINK1 is located in the outer mitochondrial membrane, but PINK1 cannot be detected in healthy mitochondria. Because, after being located into the mitochondrial matrix, PINK1 is cleaved by intramembrane-cleaving protease PARL and then the truncated form of PINK1 is released into the cytoplasm, in which PINK1 is further degraded by the ubiquitin proteasome system to remain at a low basal level (Wu et al., 2015; Wang H. et al., 2019). However, in dysfunctional mitochondria, PINK1 cannot be transported into the inner mitochondrial membrane, thereby avoiding cleavage by intramembrane-cleaving protease PARL. Subsequently, PINK1 located in the outer mitochondrial membrane will recruit autophagy receptors including SQSTM1/p62, nuclear dot protein 52 (NDP52) and optineurin (OPTN), which can bind to LC3 to combine the dysfunctional mitochondria and autophagosomes, eventually dysfunctional mitochondria will be degraded in autolysosome (Moreira et al., 2017). To further activate mitophagy, PINK1 also phosphorylates Ser65 in the ubiquitin and ubiquitin-like domain of Parkin, and further facilitates Parkin localization from the cytosol to the outer mitochondrial membrane of dysfunctional mitochondria (Wang H. et al., 2019; Ma X. et al., 2020).

Additionally, Parkin can also promote the ubiquitination of the mitochondrial fusion proteins mitofusin 1 (MFN1) and mitofusin 2 (MFN2), the mitochondrial adapter protein Miro1, translocase of outer mitochondrial membrane 20 (TOM20), and voltage-dependent anion channel (VDAC) to induce mitophagy (Nardin et al., 2016; Bradshaw et al., 2020). Normally, there are two major mechanisms involved in Parkin-dependent mitophagy: the first mechanism is that Parkin ubiquitinates MFN1 and MFN2, and further degraded by the proteasome, resulting in mitochondrial fission. Mitochondrial fission contributes to the separation of dysfunctional mitochondria from healthy network, and then dysfunctional mitochondria will be engulfed by autophagosomes and further degraded in autolysosomes (Eid et al., 2016; Ma X. et al., 2020). Additionally, Parkin-mediated the ubiquitination of mitochondrial outer membrane proteins VDAC will promote the recognition of VDAC by autophagy receptors such as histone deacetylase 6 (HDAC6) and p62. Subsequently, p62 will bind to LC3 positive autophagosomes to promote dysfunctional mitochondria to be captured by autophagosomes and then be degraded in autolysosomes (**Figure 2**; Moreira et al., 2017).

BNIP3/NIX-Dependent Mitophagy

In order to cope with hostile environments such as hypoxia and nutritional deficiencies, mitochondrial fission will enhance and mitophagy activation will also increase to degrade excessive mitochondria, and finally adaptively reducing mitochondrial quantity and maintaining cellular energy homeostasis. Generally speaking, this kind of stress-induced mitophagy is mediated by BCL-2/adenovirus E1B interacting protein 3 (BNIP3) and Nip-like protein X (NIX) (Lampert et al., 2019; Xu et al., 2020). Of note, contrary to PINK1/Parkin-mediated indirect connection between damaged mitochondria and autophagosomes, BNIP3 and NIX induce mitophagy by direct connecting damaged mitochondria to autophagosomes (Moreira et al., 2017). The phosphorylation of Ser17 and Ser24 on BNIP3 can promote the affinity of BNIP3 and LC3, thereby activating mitophagy (Zhu et al., 2013). Furthermore, Beclin1 induces mitophagy in the form of Beclin1-Vps34 -Vps15 complexes (Ma et al., 2014; Wang et al., 2017). However, Bcl-2 and Bcl-XL can bind to the BH3 domain of Beclin1 to form Beclin1-Bcl-2-Bcl-XL complexes to inhibit mitophagy. It is interesting to note that BNIP3 and NIX are easier to bind to Bcl-2 and Bcl-XL than Beclin1, which release Beclin1 from Beclin1-Bcl-2-Bcl-XL complexes and subsequently induces mitophagy (M Chiara et al., 2014; Chiang et al., 2018). What's more, rashomolog enriched in brain (Rheb) can activate the mammalian target of rapamycin (mTOR) to inhibit mitophagy, but BNIP3 can suppress Rheb/mTOR activation (Gong et al., 2018). Similar to BNIP3, NIX also can directly interact with LC3, and the phosphorylation of Ser34 and Ser35 on NIX further promotes this interaction. Moreover, Parkin-mediated NIX ubiquitination will recruit NBR1, an autophagy cargo receptor, to enhance mitophagy-mediated degradation of dysfunctional mitochondria.

Glick et al. (2012) have confirmed that elevated lipid synthesis, reduced fatty acids β-oxidation, impaired glucose tolerance, and elevated ROS levels, inflammation response and steatohepatitis are found in liver-specific BNIP3 gene knockout mice. Further research finds that elevated numbers of mitochondria but impaired mitochondrial function are also found in liver-specific BNIP3 gene knockout mice, which is characterized by loss of mitochondrial membrane potential, dysfunctional oxidative phosphorylation and reduced fatty acids β-oxidation (Glick et al., 2012; Boland et al., 2014). These results confirm the critical role of BNIP3 in maintaining mitochondrial integrity, which contributes to the prevention and treatment of metabolic diseases (**Figure 2**).

FUNDC1-Dependent Mitophagy

FUN14 domain-containing 1 (FUNDC1) contains a conserved LC3-interacting region (LIR). Accumulating study confirms that FUNDC1 is a crucial hypoxia-mediated mitophagy regulator (Chen et al., 2017; Li et al., 2018; Zhang, 2020). Similar to BNIP3/NIX, FUNDC1 directly interacts with LC3 through its LIR under hypoxic conditions (Kuang et al., 2016). However, under normal conditions, protein kinase Src and CK2 will phosphorylate Tyr18 and Ser13 of FUNDC1 to disturb its

interaction with LC3 (Kuang et al., 2016). Nevertheless, the serine/threonine kinase UNC-51 like kinase 1 (ULK1) can phosphorylate FUNDC1 at Ser17 to activate mitophagy under hypoxic conditions. Moreover, mitochondrial fission and fusion mediators including PGAM5, OPA1 and DRP1 can interact with FUNDC1 to regulate mitophagy. Under hypoxic conditions, the mitochondrial phosphatase PGAM5 dephosphorylates the Ser13 of FUNDC1 to promote its interaction with LC3 (Ma K. et al., 2020). PGAM5-mediated dephosphorylation of FUNDC1 also disrupts its association with mitochondrial fusion protein OPA1, thereby inhibiting mitochondrial fusion (Ma K. et al., 2020).

Under normoxic conditions, FUNDC1 is located in the endoplasmic reticulum-mitochondria contact sites. In order to cope with hypoxic stress, FUNDC1 associates with the endoplasmic reticulum (ER) protein calnexin (CANX) in mitochondria-associated ER membranes and then recruits DRP1 to promote mitochondrial fission and further activates mitophagy (Palikaras et al., 2018). Although FUNDC1, BNIP3 and NIX can directly interact with LC3 to activate mitophagy, the interaction among FUNDC1, BNIP3 and NIX is still not well explained, and their synergy is very important for mitophagy-mediated mitochondrial quality control (**Figure 2**).

PHYTOCHEMICALS

Phytochemicals derived from natural plants are often used to prevent and/or treat metabolic disorders due to their unique therapeutic properties and safety (Bacanli et al., 2019). Plentiful medicinal and non-medicinal natural plants have been used to treat diseases from time immemorial in the world on account of the accessibility and low cost. Studies have shown that phytochemicals such as akebia saponin D, quercetin, cyanidin-3-O-glucoside, corilagin, notoginsenoside R1, scutellarin, salvianolic acid B, resveratrol and curcumin show protective effects against metabolic diseases, and their plant origins, effects and molecular mechanisms on metabolic diseases are provided in **Table 1**.

PHYTOCHEMICAL-MEDIATED MITOPHAGY IN METABOLIC DISORDERS

Non-alcoholic Fatty Liver Disease

Non-alcoholic fatty liver disease (NAFLD) refers to the accumulation of fat in the liver of an individual, which is not caused by excessive alcohol consumption (Younossi et al., 2016; Geng et al., 2021). There is a consensus that NAFLD is the risk factor of non-alcoholic steatohepatitis, cirrhosis and hepatocellular carcinoma. Currently, more and more phytochemicals have been found to target mitophagy to prevent/treat metabolic diseases. For example, akebia saponin D, the major active component of *Dipsacus asper* Wall. ex Henry, activates BNIP3-mediated mitophagy to alleviate hepatic steatosis in oleic acid-induced buffalo rat liver cells. Liu et al. have observed that quercetin, the most common flavonoid from

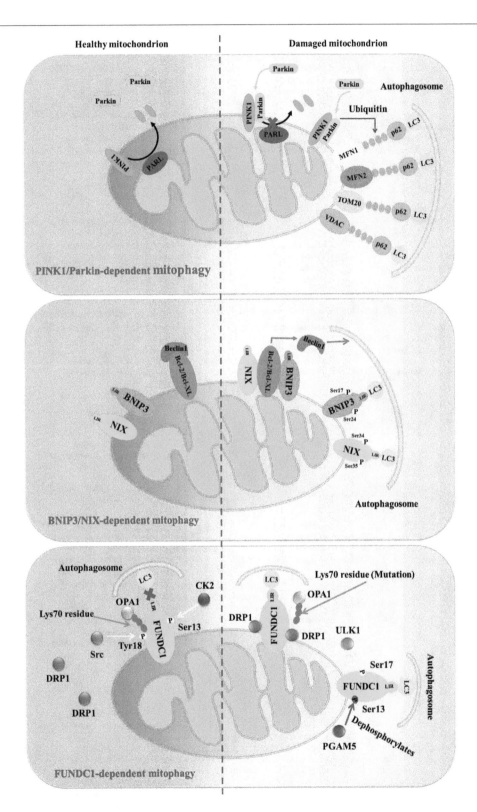

FIGURE 2 | Diagram illustrates the signaling pathway regulating mitophagy. In damaged mitochondria, PINK1 located in the outer mitochondrial membrane, can phosphorylate Ser65 in the ubiquitin and ubiquitin-like domain of Parkin and further facilitates its localization from the cytosol to the outer mitochondrial membrane. Moreover, Parkin can also promote the ubiquitination of MFN1, MFN2, TOM20 and VDAC to further induce mitophagy. In response to hypoxia and nutritional deprivation, BNIP3 and NIX-mediated mitophagy is induced. In this process, BNIP3 and NIX directly interact with LC3 to enhance mitophagy. And BNIP3 and NIX also bind to the BH3 domain of Beclin1 to activate mitophagy. What's more, similar to BNIP3/NIX, FUNDC1 interacts with LC3 through its LIR to activate mitophagy under hypoxic conditions.

TABLE 1 | The plant origins, protective effects and mechanisms of phytochemicals on metabolic disorders.

Phytochemical	Plant origin	Health effect	Molecular mechanism	References
Akebia saponin D	*Dipsacus asper* Wall. ex Henry; *Lonicera rupicola* Hook. f. et Thoms. var. *syringantha* (Maxim.) Zabel; *Dioscorea futschauensis* Uline ex R.Kunth; *Anemone rupestris* Hook. f. et Thoms. subsp. *gelida* (Maxim.) Lauener.	● Atherosclerosis; ● Hyperlipidemia; ● Hepatic steatosis; ● Metabolic syndrome; ● Acute myocardial infarction.	● Suppressing oxidative stress; ● Enhancing autophagy; ● Regulating intestinal microbiota; ● Enhancing mitophagy; ● Suppressing intestinal barrier injury; ● Scavenging lipid peroxidation and preventing mitochondrial damage.	Li et al., 2010; Gong et al., 2018; Yang S. et al., 2019; Zhou et al., 2019b; Yang et al., 2021
Quercetin	*Astragalus membranaceus(Fisch.)*Bge.; *Sophora japonica* L.; *Platycladus orientalis* (L.) Franco; *Panax notoginseng* (Burk.) F. H. Chen; *Solanum tuberosum* L.; *Hippophae rhamnoides* L.	● Type 2 diabetes mellitus; ● Cardiovascular; ● Non-alcoholic fatty liver disease; ● Obesity; ● Alcohol-induced liver injury; ● Ethanol-induced liver steatosis.	● Suppressing insulin resistance; ● Suppressing inflammation response and oxidative stress; ● Enhancing lipid metabolism; ● Enhancing hepatic VLDL assembly and lipophagy; ● Suppressing chronic inflammation.	Eid and Haddad, 2017; Patel et al., 2018; Zhu et al., 2018; Yang H. et al., 2019
Cyanidin-3-O-glucoside	Black rice; Black soya bean; *Ipomoea batatas (L.)* Lam; *Lagerstroemia indica* L.; *Begonia fimbristipula* Hance.	● Diabetic nephropathy; ● Non-alcoholic fatty liver disease; ● Hypercholesterolemia; ● Obesity; ● Metabolic syndrome.	● Enhancing glutathione pool; ● Regulating the secretion of adipokines from brown adipose tissue; ● Enhancing LXRα-CYP7A1-bile acid excretion pathway; ● Suppressing the expression of lipoprotein lipase; ● Suppressing inflammation response.	Wang et al., 2012; Bhaswant et al., 2015; Pei et al., 2018; Qin et al., 2018; Li X. et al., 2020
Corilagin	*Phyllanthus urinaria* L.; *Phyllanthus emblica* L.; *Phyllanthus ussuriensis* Rupr. et Maxim.; *Phyllanthus niruri* Linn.; *Geranium wilfordii* Maxim.	● Acetaminophen-induced hepatotoxicity; ● Hepatic fibrosis; ● Non-alcoholic fatty liver disease; ● Atherosclerosis; ● Type 2 diabetes mellitus.	● Enhancing AMPK/GSK3β-Nrf2 signaling pathway; ● Suppressing miR-21-regulated TGF-β1/Smad signaling pathway; ● Suppressing oxidative stress and restoring autophagic flux; ● Suppressing toll-like receptor-4 signaling pathway.	Lv et al., 2019; Zhang R. et al., 2019; Zhou et al., 2019c; Li Y. et al., 2020
Notoginsenoside R1	*Panax notoginseng* (Burk.) F. H. Chen.	● Diabetic retinopathy; ● Chronic atrophic gastritis; ● Type 2 diabetes mellitus; ● Cardiac hypertrophy; ● Atherosclerosis.	● Enhancing PINK1-dependent mitophagy; ● Suppressing oxidative stress; ● Suppressing inflammation response; ● Suppressing proinflammatory monocytes; ● Suppressing TLR4/NF-κB pathway; ● Enhancing Nrf2-mediated HO-1 expression.	Chen et al., 2019; Luo et al., 2019; Zhang B. et al., 2019; Liu H. et al., 2020
Scutellarin	*Erigeron breviscapus* (Vant.) Hand. - Mazz.; *Scutellaria altissima* L.; *Scutellaria barbata* D. Don.	● Atherosclerosis; ● Diabetic retinopathy; ● Non-alcoholic fatty liver disease; ● Type 2 diabetes mellitus.	● Suppressing oxidative stress-induced vascular endothelial dysfunction and endothelial cell damage; ● Suppressing VEGF/ERK/FAK/Src pathway Signaling; ● Suppressing oxidative stress.	Long et al., 2015; Mo et al., 2018; Zhang X. et al., 2018; Long et al., 2019
Salvianolic acid B	*Salvia miltiorrhiza* Bge.	● Diabetic cardiomyopathy; ● Myocardial ischemic injury; ● Endothelial dysfunction; ● Obesity; ● Atherosclerosis; ● Non-alcoholic fatty liver disease; ● Type 2 diabetes mellitus.	● Suppressing insulin-like growth factor-binding protein 3 expression; ● Suppressing NLRP3 inflammasome; ● Suppressing apoptosis; ● Regulating gut microbiota abundances and LPS/TLR4 signaling pathway; ● Suppressing YAP/TAZ/JNK signaling pathway; ● Enhancing SIRT1-mediated inhibition of HMGB1; ● Enhancing insulin sensitivity.	Huang et al., 2015; Zeng et al., 2015; Hu et al., 2020; Ko et al., 2020; Li C.-L. et al., 2020; Li L. et al., 2020; Yang et al., 2020
Resveratrol	*Polygonum cuspidatum* Sieb.et Zucc.; *Belamcanda chinensis*(L.)Redouté; *Smilax davidiana* A. DC.; *Reynoutria cillinerve* C. F. Fang transl. nov.; *Ampelopsis japonica* (Thunb.) Makino; *Scirpus yagara* Ohwi.	● Metabolic syndrome; ● Type 2 diabetes mellitus; ● Atherosclerosis; ● Non-alcoholic fatty liver disease; ● Obesity; ● Diabetic cardiomyopathy; ● Myocardial ischemia.	● Suppressing inflammation response and oxidative stress; ● Enhancing insulin sensitivity; ● Enhancing mitochondrial function; ● Remodeling gut microbiota; ● Suppressing STIM1-mediated intracellular calcium accumulation.	Chen et al., 2016; Ma et al., 2017; de Ligt et al., 2018; Seyyedebrahimi et al., 2018; Tabrizi et al., 2018; Huang et al., 2019; Szkudelska et al., 2019; Xu et al., 2019; Huang et al., 2020
Curcumin	*Curcuma phaeocaulis* Valeton; *Curcuma longa* L.; *Radix Curcumae*.	● Metabolic syndrome; ● Type 2 diabetes mellitus; ● Atherosclerosis; ● Non-alcoholic fatty liver disease; ● Obesity; ● Diabetic cardiomyopathy; ● Myocardial ischemia.	● Suppressing hyperlipidemia; ● Suppressing oxidative stress; ● Enhancing insulin sensitivity; ● Regulating intestinal barrier function; ● Suppressing TLR4-related inflammation response; ● Enhancing autophagy; ● Suppressing cell apoptosis.	Bradford, 2013; Ghosh et al., 2018; Mokhtari-Zaer et al., 2018; Yao et al., 2018; Zhang S. et al., 2018; Ahmed et al., 2019; Azhdari et al., 2019; Pivari et al., 2019; Ren et al., 2020; Wu et al., 2020

Astragalus membranaceus (Fisch.) Bge., alleviates non-alcoholic fatty liver disease by enhancing PINK1/Parkin-dependent mitophagy in oleate/palmitate-induced HepG2 cells and high-fat diet-fed mice (Liu et al., 2018). Consistent with the above results, Li et al. also observe that cyanidin-3-O-glucoside inhibits hepatic oxidative stress, NLRP3 inflammasomes, hepatic lipid accumulation and improves insulin sensitivity in mice with NAFLD. In palmitic acid-induced alpha mouse liver 12 (AML-12) cells, cyanidin-3-O-glucoside also suppresses lipid accumulation, IL-1β and IL-18 levels and ROS content, and up-regulates the expressions of autophagosome formation genes including phosphatidylinositol 3-kinase catalytic subunit type 3 (PIK3C3), Beclin1, ATG5, ATG12, ATG7, transcription factor EB (TFEB) and LC3-II. Moreover, in palmitic acid-induced AML-12 cells and HepG2 cells, cyanidin-3-O-glucoside also increases the expressions of PINK1, Parkin and TOM20. In hepatocytes from NAFLD patients, cyanidin-3-O-glucoside significantly decreases triglyceride, NLRP3, Caspase-1, IL-1β, IL-18 and ROS levels, and increases the expressions of PINK1, Parkin and TOM20 proteins. Li et al. speculated that cyanidin-3-O-glucoside activated PINK1-mediated mitophagy to alleviate NAFLD. Corilagin, water-soluble tannin, is found in many herbs such as *Dimocarpus* longana, *Phyllanthus urinaria* and *Phyllanthus emblica* Linn. Corilagin markedly attenuates hepatic steatosis, which is manifested by decreased serum lipids, hepatic cholesterol and triglyceride contents, down-regulated expressions of fatty acid synthesis genes including ACC1 and SREBP-1c, decreased pro-inflammatory cytokine genes including TNF-a and IL-6, and up-regulated expressions of fatty acid oxidation genes including PPARα and ACOX1. Moreover, Corilagin can restore high-fat diet-mediated mitophagy blockage via activating the expressions of Parkin and LC3-II proteins. In line with these results, Corilagin can improve mitochondrial dysfunction, evidenced by reduced ROS and MDA levels, enhanced expressions of antioxidative enzymes including SOD, GSH-PX and CAT, increased mitochondrial membrane potential and reduced mitochondrial oxidative DNA damage. In conclusion, mitophagy plays an important role in the treatment of Corilagin in NAFLD (Zhang R. et al., 2019). Melatonin is a hormone found in bacteria, eukaryotic unicells, macroalgae, plants and fungi (Hardeland and Poeggeler, 2003). In high-fat diet-fed rats, melatonin administration can significantly alleviate mitochondrial dysfunction and NAFLD. In the setting of NAFLD, NR4A1/DNA-PKcs/p53 signal pathway can promote DRP1-dependent mitochondrial fission and suppress BNIP3-mediated mitophagy. However, melatonin can suppress NR4A1/DNA-PKcs/p53 signal pathway to restore mitophagy, thereby improving mitochondrial dysfunction in NAFLD, which is manifested by enhanced ATP production, restored mitochondrial membrane potential and improved mitochondrial respiratory function (Zhou et al., 2018). Choi et al. observe that fermented Korean red ginseng extract (RG) administration remarkably improves the high-fat diet-induced hepatic steatosis, liver injury and inflammation in the setting of NAFLD. And RG also inhibits lipid accumulation in the palmitate-induced primary hepatocytes. Mechanistically, RG inhibits the activation of mTORC1 to activate mitophagy and

PPARα signaling pathway to improve NAFLD (**Table 2** and **Figure 3**; Choi et al., 2019).

Obesity

In 2020, the last report of World Health Organization (WHO) categorizes 1.9 billion adults as overweight and more than 650 million as obese worldwide. Accumulating evidence confirms that mitophagy plays an important role in the regulation of mitochondrial content and function in the setting of obesity. In Parkin$^{-/-}$ mice, Gouspillou et al. show that Parkin ablation causes decreased mitochondrial respiration and increased ROS production in skeletal muscles (Gouspillou et al., 2018; Pileggi et al., 2021). In liver-specific Parkin knockout mice, hepatic steatosis increased by 45% compared with wild-type mice (Edmunds et al., 2020). Although there were no differences in the number of mitochondria in liver between wild-type mice and liver-specific Parkin knockout mice, mitochondrial respiratory were obviously decreased in liver-specific Parkin knockout mice. And whole-body insulin resistance and hepatic insulin resistance were observed in high-fat diet-fed liver-specific Parkin knockout mice (Edmunds et al., 2020). In high-fat diet-fed mice, cyanidin-3-O-glucoside, a kind of anthocyanins mainly found in black rice, black beans and purple potatoes, significantly reduces body weight by activating PINK1-mediated mitophagy (Li X. et al., 2020). Quercetin is proved to inhibit the body weight gain in high-fat diet-fed mice, simultaneously suppress the level of hepatic or serum cholesterol and triglyceride, and inhibit the expression of lipogenic gene fatty acid synthase (FAS) (Liu et al., 2018). Quercetin also prevents oleate/palmitate-induced lipid accumulation in HepG2 cells (Liu et al., 2018). Mechanistically, Quercetin activates PINK1/Parkin-dependent mitophagy to improve lipid metabolism in the setting of obesity. Since obesity is considered to be a concomitant symptom of various diseases such as metabolic syndrome and NAFLD, only a few studies have focused on it. Therefore, it will be very meaningful to clarify the role of mitophagy-mediated mitochondrial quality control in the prevention and treatment of obesity in future studies (**Table 2** and **Figure 3**).

Type 2 Diabetes

Growing evidence has proved that mitochondrial dysfunction is a risk factor of type 2 diabetes and its complications such as hyperglycemia, diabetic nephropathy and diabetic retinopathy (Rovira-Llopis et al., 2017). Therefore, targeting mitophagy is a promising pharmaceutical strategy for type 2 diabetes and its complications. The *Astragalus mongholicus* Bunge and *Panax* notoginseng (Burk.) F.H. Chen formula (APF) consists of *Astragalus mongholicus* Bunge, *Panax* notoginseng (Burkill) F.H. Chen, *Angelica sinensis* (Oliv.) Diels, *Achyranthes bidentata* Blume, and *Ecklonia kurome* Okamura. APF significantly improves the blood urea nitrogen, serum creatinine and 24-h albuminuria of mice with diabetic nephropathy, and prevents inflammatory response in high glucose-induced renal mesangial cells and the kidney tissue of mice with diabetic nephropathy. Furthermore, increased expressions of PINK1, Parkin, Beclin1 and LC3-II are recorded in renal mesangial cells and the kidney tissue of

TABLE 2 | Phytochemical enhances mitophagy to treat metabolic disorders.

Phytochemical	Disease	Type of mitophagy	Molecular mechanism	References
Akebia saponin D	Non-alcoholic fatty liver disease	BNIP3-mediated mitophagy	• Enhancing autophagy: p-AMPK ↑, p-mTOR ↓ and LC3-II ↑; • Enhancing mitophagy: BNIP3 ↑.	Gong et al., 2018
Quercetin	Non-alcoholic fatty liver disease	PINK1/Parkin-mediated mitophagy	• Suppressing hyperlipidemia: triglyceride↓ and cholesterol ↓; • Suppressing lipogenic gene expression: fatty acid synthase (FAS) ↓; • Enhancing β-oxidation enzyme: carnitine palmitoyltransferase I (CPT1) ↑; • Enhancing mitochondrial function: respiratory control ratio ↑ and mitochondrial membrane potential ↑; • Enhancing mitophagy: Frataxin ↑, Parkin ↑;PINK1 ↑, Beclin1 ↑, LC3-II ↑, p62 ↓, CISD1 ↓, VDAC1 ↑, TOM20 ↓ and HIF-1α ↓.	Liu et al., 2018
Cyanidin-3-O-glucoside	Non-alcoholic fatty liver disease	PINK1-mediated mitophagy	• Suppressing hyperlipidemia: cholesterol synthesis-related genes (HMGCR) ↓, fatty acid uptake related genes (FABP1 ↓, FATB1 ↓ and CD36 ↓), fatty acid synthesis related genes (FAS ↓, ACCα ↓, SREBF1 ↓ and PPAR-γ ↓), cholesterol efflux-related genes (CYP7A1 ↑) and fatty acid β-oxidation-related genes (PPARA ↑, CPT1A ↑, ACOX1 ↑ and MCAD ↑); • Suppressing inflammation: IL-1β ↓, IL-18 ↓, NLRP3 ↓, Caspase-1 ↓, Pro-Caspase-1 ↓ and IL-1β ↓; • Suppressing oxidative stress: H_2O_2 ↓, MDA ↓, SOD ↑, CAT ↑, GSH-PX ↑ and ROS ↓; • Enhancing mitochondrial function: peroxisome proliferative activated receptor- γ (NR1C3) ↑, nuclear respiratory factor 1 (NRF1) ↑, nuclear factor erythroid derived 2 like 2 (NRF2) ↑ and mitochondrial transcription factor A (TFAM) ↑; • Enhancing mitophagy: PINK1 ↑, Parkin ↑;LC3-II ↑, p62 ↓, TOM20 ↓, PIK3C3 ↑, Beclin1 ↑, ATG5 ↑, ATG12 ↑, ATG7 ↑ and TFEB ↑.	Li X. et al., 2020
Corilagin	Non-alcoholic fatty liver disease	Parkin-mediated mitophagy	• Suppressing hyperlipidemia: triglyceride ↓, cholesterol ↓, low-density lipoprotein cholesterol ↓, high-density lipoprotein cholesterol ↑; fatty acid synthesis genes (FASN ↓, ACC1 ↓, and SREBP-1c ↓) and fatty acid oxidation genes (PPARA ↑, CPT1A ↑, and ACOX1 ↑); • Suppressing inflammation: MCP1 ↓, F4/80 ↓, TNF-α ↓ and IL-6 ↓; • Enhancing mitophagy: LC3-II ↑, p62 ↓, Parkin ↑ and VDAC1 ↑; • Suppressing oxidative stress: ROS ↓, SOD ↑, GSH-PX ↑, CAT ↑, and MDA ↓; • Enhancing mitochondrial function: mitochondrial membrane potential ↑ and mitochondrial biogenesis related gene (NRF1 ↑, NRF2 ↑, and TFAM ↑).	Zhang R. et al., 2019
Melatonin	Non-alcoholic fatty liver disease	BNIP3-mediated mitophagy	• Suppressing hyperlipidemia: triglycerides ↓ and cholesterol ↓; • Suppressing inflammation: IL-6 ↓, TNF-α ↓ and TGF-β ↓; • Suppressing oxidative stress: ROS ↓, SOD ↑, GSH-PX ↑ and MDA ↓; • Enhancing mitochondrial function: ATP generation ↑ and mitochondrial respiratory function ↑; • Enhancing mitophagy: DRP ↓, BNIP3 ↑, LC3-II ↑, Beclin1 ↑, Atg5 ↑, DNA-PKcs ↓, p53 ↓ and NR4A1 ↑.	Zhou et al., 2018
Cyanidin-3-O-glucoside	Obesity	PINK1-mediated mitophagy	• Suppressing cholesterol synthesis-related genes (HMGCR ↓), fatty acid uptake related genes (FABP1 ↓, FATB1 ↓ and CD36 ↓) and fatty acid synthesis related genes (FAS ↓, ACCα ↓, SREBF1 ↓ and PPAR-γ ↓); • Enhancing cholesterol efflux-related genes (CYP7A1 ↑) and fatty acid β-oxidation-related genes (PPARA ↑, CPT1A ↑, ACOX1 ↑ and MCAD ↑); • Suppressing inflammation response: IL-1β ↓, IL-18 ↓, NLRP3 ↓, Caspase-1 ↓, Pro-Caspase-1 ↓ and IL-1β ↓; • Suppressing oxidative stress: H_2O_2 ↓, MDA ↓, SOD ↑, l-cysteine:2-oxoglutarate aminotransferase (CAT) ↑ and glutathione peroxidase (GSH-PX) ↑ and ROS ↓; • Enhancing mitochondrial function: peroxisome proliferative activated receptor- γ (NR1C3) ↑, nuclear respiratory factor 1 (NRF1) ↑, nuclear factor erythroid derived 2 like 2 (NRF2) ↑ and mitochondrial transcription factor A (TFAM) ↑; • Enhancing mitophagy: PINK1 ↑, Parkin ↑;LC3-II ↑, p62 ↓, TOM20 ↓, PIK3C3 ↑, Beclin 1 ↑, ATG5 ↑, ATG12 ↑, ATG7 ↑ and TFEB ↑.	Li X. et al., 2020
Quercetin	Obesity	PINK1/Parkin-mediated mitophagy	• Suppressing hyperlipidemia: triglyceride ↓ and cholesterol ↓; • Suppressing lipogenic gene expression: fatty acid synthase (FAS) ↓; • Enhancing β-oxidation enzyme: carnitine palmitoyltransferase I (CPT1) ↑; • Enhancing mitochondrial function: respiratory control ratio and mitochondrial membrane potential ↑; • Enhancing mitophagy: Frataxin ↑, Parkin ↑, PINK1 ↑, Beclin1 ↑, LC3-II ↑, p62 ↓, CISD1 ↓, VDAC1 ↑, TOM20 ↓ and HIF-1α ↓.	Liu et al., 2018
Notoginsenoside R1	Diabetic retinopathy	PINK1-mediated mitophagy	• Suppressing oxidative stress: ROS ↓, 4-HNE ↓, protein carbonyl ↓ and 8-OHdG ↓; • Suppressing inflammation: MCP-1 ↓, TNF-α ↓, IL-6 ↓ and ICAM-1 ↓; • Enhancing mitophagy: Parkin ↑, PINK1 ↑, LC3 ↑ and p62 ↓.	Zhou et al., 2019a

(Continued)

TABLE 2 | Continued

Phytochemical	Disease	Type of mitophagy	Molecular mechanism	References
Scutellarin	Diabetes-related vascular disease	PINK1/Parkin-mediated mitophagy	• Suppressing oxidative stress: ROS ↓, SOD ↑ and SOD2 ↑; • Enhancing mitophagy: LC3-II ↑, p62 ↓, Beclin1 ↑, Atg5 ↑, Parkin ↑, PINK1 ↑ and MFN2 ↑; • Suppressing vascular endothelial cell apoptosis: Bcl-2 ↑, Bax ↓, Cytochrome C ↓ and cleaved caspase-3 ↓.	Xi et al., 2021
Delphinidin-3-O-β-glucoside	Atherosclerosis	AMPK/SIRT1-dependent mitophagy	• Enhancing mitophagy: SIRT1 ↑, Phospho-AMPKα ↑, LC3-II ↑ and p62 ↓.	Jin et al., 2014
Salvianolic acid B	Atherosclerosis	SIRT1-mediated mitophagy	• Suppressing inflammation: NLRP3 ↓, IL-1β ↓, apoptosis-associated speck-like protein (ASC) ↓ and caspase-1 ↓; • Enhancing mitophagy: SIRT1 ↑, Parkin ↑, Beclin1 ↑, PINK1 ↓, LC3-II ↑ and p62 ↓; • Enhancing mitochondrial function: ROS ↓ and mitochondrial membrane potential ↑.	Hu et al., 2020
Melatonin	Atherosclerosis	Sirt3/FOXO3/Parkin-mediated mitophagy	• Suppressing inflammation: NLRP3 ↓, caspase-1 ↓ and IL-1β ↓; • Enhancing mitophagy: Sirt3 ↑, FOXO3a ↓, LC3-II ↑, TOM20 ↓, Parkin ↑ and Beclin1 ↑; • Enhancing mitochondrial function: ROS ↓ and mitochondrial membrane potential ↑.	Ma et al., 2018
Resveratrol	Atherosclerosis	BNIP3-related mitophagy	• Suppressing oxidative stress: SOD ↑, GSH ↑ and GSH-PX ↑; • Enhancing mitochondrial function: Mitochondrial respiration complex I and III ↑; • Enhancing mitophagy: BNIP3 ↑, Beclin1 ↑, Atg5 ↑, HIF1 ↑ and AMPK ↑.	Li C. et al., 2020

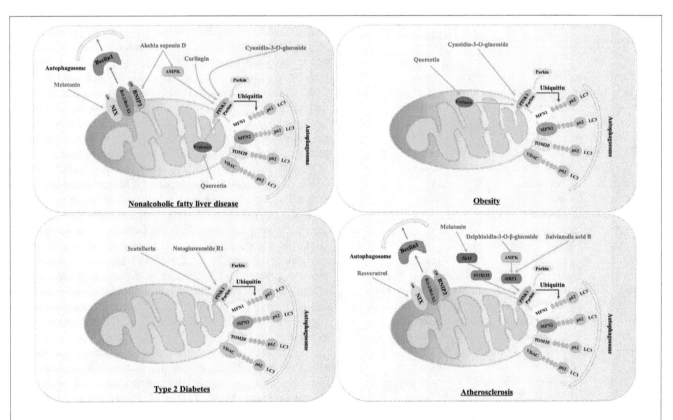

FIGURE 3 | Phytochemical activates mitophagy to treat metabolic disorders. Phytochemical activates PINK1-Parkin-dependent mitophagy and BNIP3/NIX-dependent mitophagy to treat metabolic disorders. In PINK1-Parkin-dependent mitophagy, PINK1 phosphorylates Ser65 in the ubiquitin and ubiquitin-like domain of Parkin and further facilitates its localization from the cytosol to the outer mitochondrial membrane of dysfunctional mitochondria. Moreover, Parkin can further promote the ubiquitination of MFN1, MFN2, TOM20 and VDAC, which can be identified by autophagy receptors p62 and then bind to LC3 positive autophagosomes to promote dysfunctional mitochondria to be captured by autophagosomes. Additionally, BNIP3 and NIX are easier to bind to Bcl-2 and Bcl-XL than Beclin1, which causes the release of Beclin-1 from Beclin1-Bcl-2-Bcl-XL complexes and subsequently induces mitophagy.

mice with diabetic nephropathy. These results remind that APF activates PINK1/Parkin-mediated mitophagy to protect the kidney from inflammatory injury in the setting of diabetes mellitus (Wen et al., 2020). Diabetic retinopathy is a serious complication of diabetes and remains the leading cause of blindness worldwide (Zhou et al., 2019a). Notoginsenoside

R1, a saponin from *Panax notoginseng*, is proved to prevent oxidative stress and inflammatory response in high glucose-treated rat retinal Müller cells and the retinas of diabetic *db/db* mice. Mechanistically, Notoginsenoside R1 improves diabetic retinopathy through activating PINK1-mediated mitophagy (Zhou et al., 2019a). There is a consensus that endothelial cell injury is a critical pathophysiological basis of diabetes-related vascular disease. Scutellarin, a main composition of *Scutellaria baicalensis* Georgi, inhibits mitochondrial-mediated apoptosis to increase cell viability of high glucose-induced human umbilical vein endothelial cells (HUVECs). Moreover, scutellarin can activate PINK1/Parkin-mediated mitophagy to improve mitochondrial function characterized by reduced ROS production, enhanced mitochondrial membrane potential and increased SOD activity. Many mechanisms involved in this effect include LC3-II, Atg5, P62, PINK1, Parkin, and MFN2. However, the effect is weakened by PINK1 gene knockdown. These results remind that scutellarin suppresses vascular endothelial cell damage caused by hyperglycemia through activating PINK1/Parkin-dependent mitophagy (**Table 2** and **Figure 3**; Xi et al., 2021).

Cardiovascular Disease

Cardiovascular disease is the leading cause of death in the world, including cardiac failure, coronary heart disease, myocardial infarction and atherosclerosis (Mir et al., 2021). Atherosclerosis is one of the most common causes of cardiovascular disease (Poznyak et al., 2021). It is known that mitochondrial dysfunction is an important cause of inflammatory response, lipid accumulation and oxidative stress, which are the pathogenic factors of atherosclerosis (Poznyak et al., 2021). Given the critical role of mitophagy in maintaining mitochondrial function in cardiovascular disease, the regulatory mechanism of mitophagy has captured the attention of researchers around the world. Among various pathogenic factors, vascular endothelial injury is the driving force for the development of atherosclerosis, and oxidized low-density lipoprotein (ox-LDL) plays a key role in this process (Fang et al., 2014). Delphinidin-3-O-β-glucoside, a natural anthocyanin, is abundant in black soybean, bilberries and cereals (Park et al., 2019). Jin et al. have demonstrated that delphinidin-3-O-β-glucoside suppresses ox-LDL-induced cell death in human umbilical vein endothelial cells. Further studies have suggested that activated AMPK/SIRT1-dependent mitophagy is the pivotal molecular mechanism for the protective effect of delphinidin-3-O-β-glucoside on human umbilical vein endothelial cells (Jin et al., 2014). Myocardial ischemic injury, a common kind of cardiovascular disease, can cause irreversible damage to heart. It is known that NLRP3 inflammasome-mediated inflammatory response is the pivotal mechanism of the development of myocardial ischemic injury (Zhu et al., 2015; Yao et al., 2020). Salvianolic acid B, an active constituent of *Salvia miltiorrhiza* Bge, significantly prevents acute myocardial ischemic injury in rats with isoproterenol-induced acute myocardial ischemia. In lipopolysaccharide + adenosine triphosphate-administrated H9C2 cells, salvianolic acid B markedly prevents ROS production, NLRP3 inflammasome-mediated inflammatory response and cell apoptosis, and

enhances mitochondrial membrane potential. Further evidence has confirmed that salvianolic acid B promotes SIRT1-mediated mitophagy to restore mitochondrial function, thereby preventing myocardial ischemic injury (Hu et al., 2020). Accumulating evidence has demonstrated that NLRP3 inflammasome-regulated inflammatory responses are responsible for the development of atherosclerosis. Recent evidence reminds that mitochondrion is a critical regulator for inflammatory responses because mitochondrial ROS is considered as a potent activator of NLRP3 inflammasome (Gurung et al., 2015; Jin et al., 2017). It is known that mitophagy plays a pivotal role in maintaining mitochondrial function though selectively eliminating dysfunctional mitochondria. Therefore, mitophagy is primarily considered as a regulator for NLRP3 inflammasome-mediated inflammatory response through scavenging mitochondrial ROS (Zhou et al., 2011; Kim et al., 2016). Ma et al. verify that melatonin activates Sirt3/FOXO3/Parkin-mediated mitophagy to scavenge excessive mitochondrial ROS, thereby suppressing NLRP3 inflammasome activation and then ameliorating atherosclerosis (Ma et al., 2018). Chen et al. also confirm that melatonin protects vascular smooth muscle cells against calcification by promoting AMPK/OPA1-dependent mitophagy. In ox-LDL-administrated human umbilical vein endothelial cells, cell apoptosis, cell proliferation arrest, impaired mitochondrial respiration, excessive mitochondrial ROS and mitochondrial dysfunction are observed. However, resveratrol, a potent natural antioxidant from *Vitis vinifera* L., enhances the expressions of hypoxia-inducible factor-1 (HIF-1) and AMPK protein to activate BNIP3-related mitophagy, thereby promoting mitochondrial respiration, scavenging excessive mitochondrial ROS and favoring endothelial cell survival (Li C. et al., 2020). The increased senescence of vascular endothelial cells evoked by high glucose and palmitate will cause endothelial dysfunction, leading to diabetic cardiovascular complications. The traditional Chinese medicine Ginseng-Sanqi-Chuanxiong (GSC) is composed of *Panax ginseng* C. A. Mey., *Panax notoginseng* (Burk.) F. H. Chen, and *Ligusticum chuanxiong* Hort. at a ratio of 2:3:4. Wang et al. find that GSC extract inhibits high glucose and palmitate-induced vascular endothelial cell senescence via activating AMPK-dependent mitophagy to suppress mitochondrial ROS production (**Table 2** and **Figure 3**; Wang et al., 2020).

At present, more and more clinical trials have confirmed the efficacies and mechanisms of phytochemicals for metabolic diseases, such as quercetin, melatonin and resveratrol (**Supplementary Table 1**). However, as more and more phytochemicals have been used to prevent or treat metabolic disorders, their side effects should also be taken seriously. For example, high-dose of quercetin can cause liver damage in an animal model of hyperhomocysteinemia (Meng, 2013). High concentration of resveratrol (50 μM) suppresses the cell viability of transformed macrophages and carcinoma cells. However, low concentration of resveratrol (5 μM) promotes the cell viability of these cells (Shaito et al., 2020). Moreover, low concentration of resveratrol (0.5–5μM) has no significant effect on the viability or function of rat pancreatic cells, while high concentration of resveratrol (50 μM) increases pancreatic

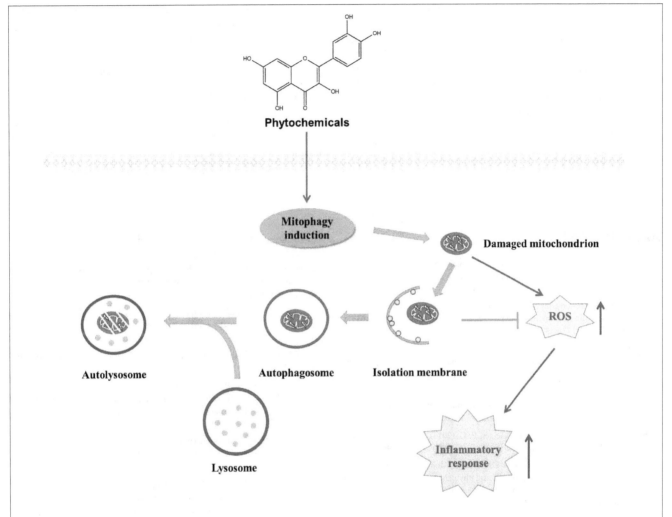

FIGURE 4 | Mechanisms of phytochemical-mediated mitophagy in the treatment of metabolic disorders. Phytochemical activates mitophagy to degrade damaged mitochondria to prevent the production of mitochondrial ROS which can trigger oxidative stress and inflammatory response, and eventually preventing and treating metabolic diseases.

cell apoptosis (Shaito et al., 2020). Surprisingly, resveratrol can stimulate oxidative stress to induce mitochondrial-mediated cancer cell apoptosis (Ashrafizadeh et al., 2020). In conclusion, exploring the optimal phytochemical dosage and the different molecular mechanisms shown in different disease models can maximize its health benefits without causing toxicity problems, which will be an area worthy of in-depth research.

SUMMARY AND FUTURE PERSPECTIVES

Mitochondrion is an important organelle responsible for various cellular processes including ATP generation, energy metabolism, ROS production and Ca^{2+} homeostasis, cell survival and death. Accumulating evidence proves that mitochondrial dysfunction is involved in various metabolic disorders such as NAFLD, obesity,

type 2 diabetes and cardiovascular disease. Mitophagy, a major mechanism of mitochondrial quality control, can selectively degrade dysfunctional mitochondria to maintain mitochondrial integrity and function. Generally speaking, mitophagy selectively degrades damaged mitochondria to suppress damaged mitochondria-derived ROS which will significantly damage healthy mitochondria and ultimately resulting in mitochondrial dysfunction. Despite increasing evidence has greatly improved our understanding of the underlying mechanisms involved in the regulation of mitophagy in metabolic disorders, some adverse results are also reported. Montgomery et al. consider that mitophagy-mediated elimination of damaged mitochondria inevitably decreases mitochondrial number, leading to decreased substrate oxidation, and finally impairing mitochondrial function (Montgomery and Turner, 2015). Now the association between mitophagy and mitochondrial homeostasis is still not fully understood, in part due to various methods for detecting mitochondrial function, different cell models and disease states (Chow et al., 2010; Montgomery and Turner, 2015). Fortunately, current studies have demonstrated that activated mitophagy will prevent damaged mitochondria-derived ROS triggering oxidative stress and inflammatory response, which are the leading causes of metabolic diseases. However, the research focused on the role of phytochemical-mediated mitophagy in the prevention and treatment of metabolic diseases is limited, and the definite relationship between phytochemical-regulated

mitophagy and the treatment of metabolic diseases still needs further experimental confirmation. One thing is for sure, looking for natural compounds with mitophagic activities will provide new insights into the therapeutic intervention for mitochondrial dysfunction-related metabolic diseases (**Figure 4**).

AUTHOR CONTRIBUTIONS

ZS, YG, XH, GZ, and YZ conceived of the topic for the review. All authors listed have made a substantial direct and intellectual contribution to the work, and approved it for publication.

REFERENCES

Ahmed, S., Khan, H., and Mirzaei, H. (2019). Mechanics insights of curcumin in myocardial ischemia: Where are we standing? *Eur. J. Med. Chem.* 183:111658.

Anderson, E. J., Lustig, M. E., Boyle, K. E., Woodlief, T. L., Kane, D. A., Lin, C.-T., et al. (2009). Mitochondrial H2O2 emission and cellular redox state link excess fat intake to insulin resistance in both rodents and humans. *J. Clin. Investig.* 119, 573–581. doi: 10.1172/jci37048

Angajala, A., Lim, S., Phillips, J. B., Kim, J.-H., Yates, C., You, Z., et al. (2018). Diverse Roles of Mitochondria in Immune Responses: Novel Insights Into Immuno-Metabolism. *Front. Immunol.* 9:1605. doi: 10.3389/fimmu.2018.01605

Anzell, A. R., Maizy, R., Przyklenk, K., and Sanderson, T. H. (2018). Mitochondrial Quality Control and Disease: Insights into Ischemia-Reperfusion Injury. *Mol. Neurobiol.* 55, 2547–2564. doi: 10.1007/s12035-017-0503-9

Archer, A. E., Von Schulze, A. T., and Geiger, P. C. (2018). Exercise, heat shock proteins and insulin resistance. *Philosoph. Transacti. Royal Soc. B* 19:373.

Ashrafizadeh, M., Javanmardi, S., Moradi-Ozarlou, M., Mohammadinejad, R., and Farkhondeh, T. (2020). Natural products and phytochemical nanoformulations targeting mitochondria in oncotherapy: an updated review on resveratrol. *Biosci. Rep.* 40: BSR20200257.

Azhdari, M., Karandish, M., and Mansoori, A. (2019). Metabolic benefits of curcumin supplementation in patients with metabolic syndrome: A systematic review and meta-analysis of randomized controlled trials. *Phytother. Res.* 33, 1289–1301. doi: 10.1002/ptr.6323

Ba Razzoni, R., Zanetti, M., Cappellari, G. G., Semolic, A., Boschelle, M., and Codarin, E. (2012). Fatty acids acutely enhance insulin-induced oxidative stress and cause insulin resistance by increasing mitochondrial reactive oxygen species (ROS) generation and nuclear factor-κB inhibitor (IκB)–nuclear factor-κB (NFκB) activation in rat muscle, in the absence of mitochondrial dysfunction. *Diabetologia* 55, 773–782. doi: 10.1007/s00125-011-2396-x

Bacanli, M., Dilsiz, S. A., Başaran, N., and Başaran, A. A. (2019). Effects of phytochemicals against diabetes. *Adv. Food Nutr. Res.* 89, 209–238. doi: 10. 1016/bs.afnr.2019.02.006

Bahrami, M., Cheraghpour, M., Jafarirad, S., Alavinejad, P., Asadi, F., and Hekmatdoost, A. (2020). The effect of melatonin on treatment of patients with non-alcoholic fatty liver disease: a randomized double blind clinical trial. *Compl. Ther. Med.* 52:102452. doi: 10.1016/j.ctim.2020.102452

Baker, M. J., Tatsuta, T., and Langer, T. (2011). Quality control of mitochondrial proteostasis. *Cold Spring Harbor Perspect. Biol.* 3:a007559. doi: 10.1101/cshperspect.a007559

Bhaswant, M., Fanning, K., Netzel, M., Mathai, M. L., Panchal, S. K., and Brown, L. (2015). Cyanidin 3-glucoside improves diet-induced metabolic syndrome in rats. *Pharmacol. Res.* 102, 208–217. doi: 10.1016/j.phrs.2015.10.006

Bhatti, J. S., Bhatti, G. K., and Reddy, P. H. (2017). Mitochondrial dysfunction and oxidative stress in metabolic disorders — A step towards mitochondria

based therapeutic strategies. *Biochim. Biophys. Acta* 1863, 1066–1077. doi: 10.1016/j.bbadis.2016.11.010

Bloch-Damti, A., and Bashan, N. (2005). Proposed mechanisms for the induction of insulin resistance by oxidative stress. *Antiox. Redox Signal.* 7, 1553–1567. doi: 10.1089/ars.2005.7.1553

Boland, M. L., He, H., Shah, R., Ali, A., and Macleod, K. F. (2014). BNip3 connects energy sensing to hepatic lipid metabolism and mitophagy. *Cancer Res.* 74, 4324–4324.

Bradford, P. G. (2013). Curcumin and obesity. *BioFactors* 39, 78–87. doi: 10.1002/biof.1074

Bradshaw, A., Campbell, P., Schapira, A., Morris, H., and Taanman, J.-W. (2020). The PINK1 – Parkin mitophagy signalling pathway is not functional in peripheral blood mononuclear cells. *bioRxiv* [preprint] doi: 10.1101/2020.02. 12.945469

Chan, D. C. (2020). Mitochondrial Dynamics and Its Involvement in Disease. *Annu. Rev. Pathol.* 15, 235–259. doi: 10.1146/annurev-pathmechdis-012419-032711

Chen, M.-L., Yi, L., Zhang, Y., Zhou, X., Ran, L., Yang, J., et al. (2016). Resveratrol Attenuates Trimethylamine-N-Oxide (TMAO)-Induced Atherosclerosis by Regulating TMAO Synthesis and Bile Acid Metabolism via Remodeling of the Gut Microbiota. *mBio* 7, e02210–e02215.

Chen, X. J., and Butow, R. A. (2005). The organization and inheritance of the mitochondrial genome. *Nat. Rev. Genet.* 6, 815–825.

Chen, X., Wei, R., Jin, T., and Du, H. (2019). Notoginsenoside R1 alleviates TNF-α-induced pancreatic β-cell Min6 apoptosis and dysfunction through up-regulation of miR-29a. *Artif. Cells Nanomed. Biotechnol.* 47, 2379–2388. doi: 10.1080/21691401.2019.1624368

Chen, Z., Siraj, S., Liu, L., and Chen, Q. (2017). MARCH5-FUNDC1 axis fine-tunes hypoxia-induced mitophagy. *Autophagy* 13, 1244–1245. doi: 10.1080/15548627.2017.1310789

Chiang, W. C., Wei, Y., Kuo, Y. C., Wei, S., Zhou, A., Zou, Z., et al. (2018). High Throughput Screens to Identify Autophagy Inducers that Function by Disrupting Beclin 1/Bcl-2 Binding. *Acs Chem. Biol.* 13, 2247–2260. doi: 10. 1021/acschembio.8b00421

Chiara, M., Gaetane, L. T., Alfredo, C., Jean-Christophe, R., Fabien, G., Philippe, J., et al. (2014). Functional and physical interaction between Bcl-X(L) and a BH3-like domain in Beclin-1. *EMBO J.* 26, 2527–2539. doi: 10.1038/sj.emboj. 7601689

Choi, S. Y., Park, J. S., Shon, C. H., Lee, C. Y., Ryu, J. M., Son, D. J., et al. (2019). Fermented Korean Red Ginseng Extract Enriched in Rd and Rg3 Protects against Non-Alcoholic Fatty Liver Disease through Regulation of mTORC1. *Nutrients* 11:2963. doi: 10.3390/nu11122963

Chow, L., From, A., and Seaquist, E. (2010). Skeletal muscle insulin resistance: the interplay of local lipid excess and mitochondrial dysfunction. *Metabolism* 59, 70–85. doi: 10.1016/j.metabol.2009.07.009

Cicero, A. F., and Colletti, A. (2016). Role of phytochemicals in the management of metabolic syndrome. *Phytomedicine* 23, 1134–1144. doi: 10.1016/j.phymed. 2015.11.009

Czech, M. P. (2020). Mechanisms of insulin resistance related to white, beige, and brown adipocytes. *Mol. Metabol.* 34, 27–42. doi: 10.1016/j.molmet.2019.12.014

de Ligt, M., Bruls, Y. M. H., Hansen, J., Habets, M.-F., Havekes, B., Nascimento, E. B. M., et al. (2018). Resveratrol improves ex vivo mitochondrial function but does not affect insulin sensitivity or brown adipose tissue in first degree relatives of patients with type 2 diabetes. *Mol. Metabol.* 12, 39–47. doi: 10.1016/j.molmet. 2018.04.004

Dehghani, F., Sezavar Seyedi, Jandaghi, S. H., Janani, L., Sarebanhassanabadi, M., Emamat, H., et al. (2021). Effects of quercetin supplementation on inflammatory factors and quality of life in post-myocardial infarction patients: A double blind, placebo-controlled, randomized clinical trial. *Phytother. Res.* 35, 2085–2098. doi: 10.1002/ptr.6955

Dombi, E., Mortiboys, H., and Poulton, J. (2018). Modulating Mitophagy in Mitochondrial Disease. *Curr. Med. Chem.* 25, 5597–5612. doi: 10.2174/0929867324666170616101741

Edmunds, L. R., Xie, B., Mills, A. M., Huckestein, B. R., Undamatla, R., Murali, A., et al. (2020). Liver-specific Prkn knockout mice are more susceptible to diet-induced hepatic steatosis and insulin resistance. *Mole. Metabol.* 41:101051. doi: 10.1016/j.molmet.2020.101051

Edwards, R. L., Lyon, T., Litwin, S. E., Rabovsky, A., Symons, J. D., and Jalili, T. (2007). Quercetin reduces blood pressure in hypertensive subjects. *J. Nutr.* 137, 2405–2411. doi: 10.1093/jn/137.11.2405

Egert, S., Boesch-Saadatmandi, C., Wolffram, S., Rimbach, G., and Müller, M. J. (2010). Serum lipid and blood pressure responses to quercetin vary in overweight patients by apolipoprotein E genotype. *J. nutr.* 140, 278–284. doi: 10.3945/jn.109.117655

Egert, S., Bosy-Westphal, A., Seiberl, J., Kürbitz, C., Settler, U., and Plachta-Danielzik, S. (2009). Quercetin reduces systolic blood pressure and plasma oxidised low-density lipoprotein concentrations in overweight subjects with a high-cardiovascular disease risk phenotype: a double-blinded, placebo-controlled cross-over study. *Br. J. Nutr.* 102, 1065–1074. doi: 10.1017/s0007114509359127

Eid, H. M., and Haddad, P. S. (2017). The Antidiabetic Potential of Quercetin: Underlying Mechanisms. *Curr. Med. Chem.* 24, 355–364. doi: 10.2174/0929867323666160909153707

Eid, N., Ito, Y., and Otsuki, Y. (2016). Triggering of parkin mitochondrial translocation in mitophagy: implications for liver diseases. *Front. Pharmacol.* 7:100.

Fang, Y., Li, J., Ding, M., Xu, X., Zhang, J., Jiao, P., et al. (2014). Ethanol extract of propolis protects endothelial cells from oxidized low density lipoprotein-induced injury by inhibiting lectin-like oxidized low density lipoprotein receptor-1-mediated oxidative stress. *Exp. Biol. Med.* 239, 1678–1687. doi: 10.1177/1535370214541911

Fisher-Wellman, K. H., and Neufer, P. D. (2012). Linking mitochondrial bioenergetics to insulin resistance via redox biology. *Trends Endocrinol. Metabol.* 23, 142–153. doi: 10.1016/j.tem.2011.12.008

Fujii, H., Kawada, N., and Japan Study Group Of Nafld JSG-NAFLD. (2020). The Role of Insulin Resistance and Diabetes in Nonalcoholic Fatty Liver Disease. *Int. J. Mole. Sci.* 21:3863.

Geng, Y., Faber, K. N., De Meijer, V. E., Blokzijl, H., and Moshage, H. (2021). How does hepatic lipid accumulation lead to lipotoxicity in non-alcoholic fatty liver disease? *Hepatol. Int.* 15, 21–35. doi: 10.1007/s12072-020-10121-2

Ghosh, S. S., He, H., Wang, J., Gehr, T. W., and Ghosh, S. (2018). Curcumin-mediated regulation of intestinal barrier function: The mechanism underlying its beneficial effects. *Tissue Barriers* 6:e1425085. doi: 10.1080/21688370.2018. 1425085

Glick, D., Zhang, W., Beaton, M., Marsboom, G., Gruber, M., Simon, M. C., et al. (2012). BNip3 regulates mitochondrial function and lipid metabolism in the liver. *Mol. Cell. Biol.* 32, 2570–2584. doi: 10.1128/mcb.00167-12

Gluvic, Z., Zaric, B., Resanovic, I., Obradovic, M., Mitrovic, A., Radak, D., et al. (2017). Link between Metabolic Syndrome and Insulin Resistance. *Curr. Vasc. Pharmacol.* 15, 30–39.

Gong, L., Yang, S., Zhang, W., Han, F., Lv, Y., Wan, Z., et al. (2018). Akebia saponin D alleviates hepatic steatosis through BNip3 induced mitophagy. *J. Pharmacol. Sci.* 136, 189–195. doi: 10.1016/j.jphs.2017.11.007

Gouspillou, G., Godin, R., Piquereau, J., Picard, M., Mofarrahi, M., Mathew, J., et al. (2018). Protective role of Parkin in skeletal muscle contractile and mitochondrial function. *J. Physiol.* 596, 2565–2579. doi: 10.1113/jp275604

Gurung, P., Lukens, J. R., and Kanneganti, T. D. (2015). Mitochondria: diversity in the regulation of the NLRP3 inflammasome. *Trends Mole. Med.* 21, 193–201. doi: 10.1016/j.molmed.2014.11.008

Hardeland, R., and Poeggeler, B. (2003). Non-vertebrate melatonin. *J. Pineal Res.* 34, 233–241. doi: 10.1034/j.1600-079x.2003.00040.x

Heebøll, S., Kreuzfeldt, M., Hamilton-Dutoit, S., Kjær Poulsen, M., Stødkilde-Jørgensen, H., Møller, H. J., et al. (2016). Placebo-controlled, randomised clinical trial: high-dose resveratrol treatment for non-alcoholic fatty liver disease. *Scand. J. Gastroenter.* 51, 456–464.

Hernando-Rodríguez, B., and Artal-Sanz, M. (2018). Mitochondrial Quality Control Mechanisms and the PHB (Prohibitin) Complex. *Cells* 7:238. doi: 10. 3390/cells7120238

Hu, Y., Wang, X., Li, Q., Pan, Y., and Xu, L. (2020). Salvianolic acid B alleviates myocardial ischemic injury by promoting mitophagy and inhibiting activation of the NLRP3 inflammasome. *Mole. Med. Rep.* 22, 5199–5208. doi: 10.3892/mmr.2020.11589

Huang, M., Wang, P., Xu, S., Xu, W., Xu, W., Chu, K., et al. (2015). Biological activities of salvianolic acid B from Salvia miltiorrhiza on type 2 diabetes induced by high-fat diet and streptozotocin. *Pharmaceut. Biol.* 53, 1058–1065. doi: 10.3109/13880209.2014.959611

Huang, Y., Lang, H., Chen, K., Zhang, Y., Gao, Y., Ran, L., et al. (2020). Resveratrol protects against nonalcoholic fatty liver disease by improving lipid metabolism and redox homeostasis via the PPARα pathway. *Appl. Physiol. Nutr. Metabol.* 45, 227–239. doi: 10.1139/apnm-2019-0057

Huang, Y., Zhu, X., Chen, K., Lang, H., Zhang, Y., Hou, P., et al. (2019). Resveratrol prevents sarcopenic obesity by reversing mitochondrial dysfunction and oxidative stress via the PKA/LKB1/AMPK pathway. *Aging* 11, 2217–2240. doi: 10.18632/aging.101910

Iacobazzi, R. M., Lopalco, A., Cutrignelli, A., Laquintana, V., Lopedota, A., Franco, M., et al. (2017). Bridging Pharmaceutical Chemistry with Drug and Nanoparticle Targeting to Investigate the Role of the 18-kDa Translocator Protein TSPO. *ChemMedChem* 12, 1261–1274. doi: 10.1002/cmdc.201700322

Jin, H. S., Suh, H. W., Kim, S. J., and Jo, E. K. (2017). Mitochondrial Control of Innate Immunity and Inflammation. *Immune Network* 17, 77–88. doi: 10.4110/in.2017.17.2.77

Jin, X., Chen, M., Yi, L., Chang, H., Zhang, T., Wang, L., et al. (2014). Delphinidin-3-glucoside protects human umbilical vein endothelial cells against oxidized low-density lipoprotein-induced injury by autophagy upregulation via the AMPK/SIRT1 signaling pathway. *Mole. Nutri. Food Res.* 58, 1941–1951. doi: 10.1002/mnfr.201400161

Kalyanaraman, B., Cheng, G., Zielonka, J., and Bennett, B. (2018). Low-Temperature EPR Spectroscopy as a Probe-Free Technique for Monitoring Oxidants Formed in Tumor Cells and Tissues: Implications in Drug Resistance and OXPHOS-Targeted Therapies. *Cell Biochem. Biophys.* 77, 89–98. doi: 10. 1007/s12013-018-0858-1

Keenan, S., Watt, M., and Montgomery, M. (2020). Inter-organelle Communication in the Pathogenesis of Mitochondrial Dysfunction and Insulin Resistance. *Curr. Diabet. Rep.* 20:20.

Kim, J.-A., Wei, Y., and Sowers, J. R. (2008). Role of mitochondrial dysfunction in insulin resistance. *Circul. Res.* 102, 401–414. doi: 10.1161/circresaha.107. 165472

Kim, M. J., Yoon, J. H., and Ryu, J. H. (2016). Mitophagy: a balance regulator of NLRP3 inflammasome activation. *BMB Rep.* 49, 529–535. doi: 10.5483/bmbrep. 2016.49.10.115

Kirtonia, A., Gala, K., Fernandes, S. G., Pandya, G., Pandey, A. K., Sethi, G., et al. (2021). Repurposing of drugs: An attractive pharmacological strategy for cancer therapeutics. *Semin. Cancer Biol.* 68, 258–278. doi: 10.1016/j.semcancer.2020. 04.006

Kirtonia, A., Sethi, G., and Garg, M. (2020). The multifaceted role of reactive oxygen species in tumorigenesis. *Cell. Mole. Life Sci.* 77, 4459–4483. doi: 10. 1007/s00018-020-03536-5

Ko, Y. S., Jin, H., Park, S. W., and Kim, H. J. (2020). Salvianolic acid B protects against oxLDL-induced endothelial dysfunction under high-glucose conditions by downregulating ROCK1-mediated mitophagy and apoptosis. *Biochem. Pharmacol.* 174:113815. doi: 10.1016/j.bcp.2020.113815

Koziróg, M., Poliwczak, A. R., Duchnowicz, P., Koter-Michalak, M., Sikora, J., and Broncel, M. (2011). Melatonin treatment improves blood pressure, lipid profile, and parameters of oxidative stress in patients with metabolic syndrome. *J. Pineal Res.* 50, 261–266. doi: 10.1111/j.1600-079x.2010.00835.x

Kuang, Y., Ma, K., Zhou, C., Ding, P., Zhu, Y., Chen, Q., et al. (2016). Structural basis for the phosphorylation of FUNDC1 LIR as a molecular switch of mitophagy. *Autophagy* 12, 2363–2373. doi: 10.1080/15548627.2016.1238552

Lampert, M. A., Orogo, A. M., Najor, R. H., Hammerling, B. C., Leon, L. J., Wang, B. J., et al. (2019). BNIP3L/NIX and FUNDC1-mediated mitophagy is required for mitochondrial network remodeling during cardiac progenitor cell differentiation. *Autophagy* 15, 1182–1198. doi: 10.1080/15548627.2019.1580095

Lemasters, J. (2005). Selective mitochondrial autophagy, or mitophagy, as a targeted defense against oxidative stress, mitochondrial dysfunction, and aging. *Rejuvenat. Res.* 8, 3–5. doi: 10.1089/rej.2005.8.3

Lemasters, J. J., Nieminen, A. L., Qian, T., Trost, L. C., Elmore, S. P., Nishimura, Y., et al. (1998). The mitochondrial permeability transition in cell death: a common mechanism in necrosis, apoptosis and autophagy. *Biochim. Biophys. Acta* 1366, 177–196.

Li, C., Liu, Z., Tian, J., Li, G., Jiang, W., Zhang, G., et al. (2010). Protective roles of Asperosaponin VI, a triterpene saponin isolated from Dipsacus asper Wall on acute myocardial infarction in rats. *Eur. J. Pharmacol.* 627, 235–241. doi: 10.1016/j.ejphar.2009.11.004

Li, C., Tan, Y., Wu, J., Ma, Q., Bai, S., Xia, Z., et al. (2020). Resveratrol Improves Bnip3-Related Mitophagy and Attenuates High-Fat-Induced Endothelial Dysfunction. *Front. Cell Devel. Biol.* 8:796.

Li, C.-L., Liu, B., Wang, Z.-Y., Xie, F., Qiao, W., Cheng, J., et al. (2020). Salvianolic acid B improves myocardial function in diabetic cardiomyopathy by suppressing IGFBP3. *J. Mole. Cell. Cardiol.* 139, 98–112. doi: 10.1016/j.yjmcc.2020.01.009

Li, H., Qi, J., and Li, L. (2019). Phytochemicals as potential candidates to combat obesity via adipose non-shivering thermogenesis. *Pharmacol. Res.* 147:104393. doi: 10.1016/j.phrs.2019.104393

Li, L., Li, R., Zhu, R., Chen, B., Tian, Y., Zhang, H., et al. (2020). Salvianolic acid B prevents body weight gain and regulates gut microbiota and LPS/TLR4 signaling pathway in high-fat diet-induced obese mice. *Food Funct.* 11, 8743–8756. doi: 10.1039/d0fo01116a

Li, X., Shi, Z., Zhu, Y., Shen, T., Wang, H., Shui, G., et al. (2020). Cyanidin-3-O-glucoside improves non-alcoholic fatty liver disease by promoting PINK1-mediated mitophagy in mice. *Br. J. Pharmacol.* 177, 3591–3607. doi: 10.1111/bph.15083

Li, Y., Liu, Z., Zhang, Y., Zhao, Q., Wang, X., Lu, P., et al. (2018). PEDF protects cardiomyocytes by promoting FUNDC1-mediated mitophagy via PEDF-R under hypoxic condition. *Int. J. Mole. Med.* 41, 3394–3404.

Li, Y., Wang, Y., Chen, Y., Wang, Y., Zhang, S., Liu, P., et al. (2020). Corilagin Ameliorates Atherosclerosis in Peripheral Artery Disease via the Toll-Like Receptor-4 Signaling Pathway in vitro and in vivo. *Front. Immunol.* 6: 1611.

Liu, H., Yang, J., Yang, W., Hu, S., Wu, Y., Zhao, B., et al. (2020). Focus on Notoginsenoside R1 in Metabolism and Prevention Against Human Diseases. *Drug Design. Devel. Ther.* 14, 551–565. doi: 10.2147/dddt.s240511

Liu, L., Liao, X., Wu, H., Li, Y., and Chen, Q. (2020). Mitophagy and Its Contribution to Metabolic and Aging-Associated Disorders. *Antiox. Redox Signal.* 32, 906–927. doi: 10.1089/ars.2019.8013

Liu, P., Lin, H., Xu, Y., Zhou, F., Wang, J., Liu, J., et al. (2018). Frataxin-Mediated PINK1-Parkin-Dependent Mitophagy in Hepatic Steatosis: The Protective Effects of Quercetin. *Mole. Nutr. Food Res.* 62:e1800164.

Liu, Z., and Butow, R. A. (2006). Mitochondrial Retrograde Signaling. *Annu. Rev. Genet.* 40, 159–185. doi: 10.1146/annurev.genet.40.110405.090613

Long, L., Li, Y., Yu, S., Li, X., Hu, Y., Long, T., et al. (2019). Scutellarin Prevents Angiogenesis in Diabetic Retinopathy by Downregulating VEGF/ERK/FAK/Src Pathway Signaling. *J. Diabet. Res.* 2019:4875421.

Long, L., Wang, J., Lu, X., Xu, Y., Zheng, S., Luo, C., et al. (2015). Protective effects of scutellarin on type II diabetes mellitus-induced testicular damages related to reactive oxygen species/Bcl-2/Bax and reactive oxygen species/microcirculation/staving pathway in diabetic rat. *J. Diabet. Res.* 2015:252530.

Luo, C., Sun, Z., Li, Z., Zheng, L., and Zhu, X. (2019). Notoginsenoside R1 (NGR1) Attenuates Chronic Atrophic Gastritis in Rats. *Med. Sci. Monitor* 25, 1177–1186. doi: 10.12659/msm.911512

Lv, H., Hong, L., Tian, Y., Yin, C., Zhu, C., and Feng, H. (2019). Corilagin alleviates acetaminophen-induced hepatotoxicity via enhancing the AMPK/GSK3β-Nrf2 signaling pathway. *Cell Commun. Signal.* 17:2.

Ma, B., Cao, W., Li, W., Gao, C., Qi, Z., Zhao, Y., et al. (2014). Dapper1 promotes autophagy by enhancing the Beclin1-Vps34-Atg14L complex formation. *Cell Res.* 24, 912–924. doi: 10.1038/cr.2014.84

Ma, K., Zhang, Z., Chang, R., Cheng, H., Mu, C., Zhao, T., et al. (2020). Dynamic PGAM5 multimers dephosphorylate BCL-xL or FUNDC1 to regulate mitochondrial and cellular fate. *Cell Death Different.* 27, 1036–1051. doi: 10.1038/s41418-019-0396-4

Ma, S., Chen, J., Feng, J., Zhang, R., Fan, M., Han, D., et al. (2018). Melatonin Ameliorates the Progression of Atherosclerosis via Mitophagy Activation and NLRP3 Inflammasome Inhibition. *Oxidative Med. Cell. Long.* 2018:9286458.

Ma, S., Feng, J., Zhang, R., Chen, J., Han, D., Li, X., et al. (2017). SIRT1 Activation by Resveratrol Alleviates Cardiac Dysfunction via Mitochondrial Regulation in Diabetic Cardiomyopathy Mice. *Oxidat. Med. Cell. Long.* 2017:4602715.

Ma, X., Mckeen, T., Zhang, J., and Ding, W. X. (2020). Role and Mechanisms of Mitophagy in Liver Diseases. *Cells* 9:837. doi: 10.3390/cells9040837

Magyar, K., Halmosi, R., Palfi, A., Feher, G., Czopf, L., Fulop, A., et al. (2012). Cardioprotection by resveratrol: A human clinical trial in patients with stable coronary artery disease. *Clin. Hemorheol. Microcirculat.* 50, 179–187. doi: 10.3233/ch-2011-1424

Mahdavi, A., Bagheriya, M., Mirenayat, M. S., Atkin, S. L., and Sahebkar, A. (2021). Medicinal Plants and Phytochemicals Regulating Insulin Resistance and Glucose Homeostasis in Type 2 Diabetic Patients: A Clinical Review. *Adv. Exp. Med. Biol.* 1308, 161–183. doi: 10.1007/978-3-030-64872-5_13

Marí, M., and Colell, A. (2021). Mitochondrial Oxidative and Nitrosative Stress as a Therapeutic Target in Diseases. *Antioxidants* 10:314. doi: 10.3390/antiox10020314

Martin, S. D., and McGee, S. L. (2014). The role of mitochondria in the aetiology of insulin resistance and type 2 diabetes. *Biochim. Biophys. Acta* 1840, 1303–1312. doi: 10.1016/j.bbagen.2013.09.019

Melber, A., and Haynes, C. M. (2018). UPR regulation and output: a stress response mediated by mitochondrial-nuclear communication. *Cell Res.* 28, 281–295. doi: 10.1038/cr.2018.16

Meng, B. (2013). *Effect of Quercetin on Regulation of Homocysteine Metabolism and Its Mechanism.* New York: Academy of Military Medical Sciences.

Mills, E. L., Kelly, B., and O'neill, L. A. J. (2017). Mitochondria are the powerhouses of immunity. *Nat. Immunol.* 18, 488–498. doi: 10.1038/ni.3704

Mir, R., Elfaki, I., Khullar, N., Waza, A. A., Jha, C., Mir, M. M., et al. (2021). Role of Selected miRNAs as Diagnostic and Prognostic Biomarkers in Cardiovascular Diseases, Including Coronary Artery Disease, Myocardial Infarction and Atherosclerosis. *J. Cardiovas. Devel. Dis.* 8:22. doi: 10.3390/jcdd8020022

Mo, J., Yang, R., Li, F., Zhang, X., He, B., Zhang, Y., et al. (2018). Scutellarin protects against vascular endothelial dysfunction and prevents atherosclerosis via antioxidation. *Phytomedicine* 42, 66–74. doi: 10.1016/j.phymed.2018.03.021

Mokhtari-Zaer, A., Marefati, N., Atkin, S. L., Butler, A. E., and Sahebkar, A. (2018). The protective role of curcumin in myocardial ischemia-reperfusion injury. *J. Cell. Physiol.* 234, 214–222.

Montgomery, M. K., and Turner, N. (2015). Mitochondrial dysfunction and insulin resistance: an update. *Endocr. Connect.* 4, 1–15.

Montgomery, M. K., De Nardo, W., and Watt, M. J. (2019). Impact of Lipotoxicity on Tissue "Cross Talk" and Metabolic Regulation. *Physiology* 34, 134–149. doi: 10.1152/physiol.00037.2018

Moreira, O. C., Estebanez, B., Martinez-Florez, S., De Paz, J. A., Cuevas, M. J., and Gonzalez-Gallego, J. (2017). Mitochondrial Function and Mitophagy in the Elderly: Effects of Exercise. *Oxidat. Med. Cell. Long.* 2017:2012798.

Moreno-Valdespino, C. A., Luna-Vital, D., Camacho-Ruiz, R. M., and Mojica, L. (2020). Bioactive proteins and phytochemicals from legumes: Mechanisms of action preventing obesity and type-2 diabetes. *Food Res. Int.* 130:108905. doi: 10.1016/j.foodres.2019.108905

Naraki, K., Rezaee, R., and Karimi, G. (2021). *A review on the protective effects of naringenin against natural and chemical toxic agents.* America: Wiley.

Nardin, A., Schrepfer, E., and Ziviani, E. (2016). Counteracting PINK/Parkin Deficiency in the Activation of Mitophagy: A Potential Therapeutic

Intervention for Parkinson's Disease. *Curr. Neuropharmacol.* 14, 250–259. doi: 10.2174/1570159x13666151030104414

Narendra, D., Tanaka, A., Suen, D. F., and Youle, R. J. (2009). Parkin is recruited selectively to impaired mitochondria and promotes their autophagy. *J. Cell Biol.* 183, 795–803. doi: 10.1083/jcb.200809125

Ni, H.-M., Williams, J. A., and Ding, W.-X. (2015). Mitochondrial dynamics and mitochondrial quality control. *Redox Biol.* 4, 6–13. doi: 10.1016/j.redox.2014.11.006

Nishida, Y., Nishijima, K., Yamada, Y., Tanaka, H., Matsumoto, A., Fan, J., et al. (2021). Whole-body insulin resistance and energy expenditure indices, serum lipids, and skeletal muscle metabolome in a state of lipoprotein lipase overexpression. *Metabolomics* 17:26.

Nishikawa, T., and Araki, E. (2007). Impact of mitochondrial ROS production in the pathogenesis of diabetes mellitus and its complications. *Antioxid. Redox Signal.* 9, 343–353. doi: 10.1089/ars.2006.1458

Ostadmohammadi, V., Soleimani, A., Bahmani, F., Aghadavod, E., Ramezani, R., Reiter, R. J., et al. (2020). The Effects of Melatonin Supplementation on Parameters of Mental Health, Glycemic Control, Markers of Cardiometabolic Risk, and Oxidative Stress in Diabetic Hemodialysis Patients: A Randomized, Double-Blind, Placebo-Controlled Trial. *J. Renal Nutr.* 30, 242–250. doi: 10.1053/j.jrn.2019.08.003

Palikaras, K., Lionaki, E., and Tavernarakis, N. (2018). Mechanisms of mitophagy in cellular homeostasis, physiology and pathology. *Nat. Cell Biol.* 20, 1013–1022. doi: 10.1038/s41556-018-0176-2

Park, M., Sharma, A., and Lee, H. J. (2019). Anti-Adipogenic Effects of Delphinidin-3-O-β-Glucoside in 3T3-L1 Preadipocytes and Primary White Adipocytes. *Molecules* 24:1848. doi: 10.3390/molecules24101848

Patel, R. V., Mistry, B. M., Shinde, S. K., Syed, R., Singh, V., and Shin, H. S. (2018). Therapeutic potential of quercetin as a cardiovascular agent. *Eur. J. Med. Chem.* 155, 889–904. doi: 10.1016/j.ejmech.2018.06.053

Patel, T. P., Rawal, K., Bagchi, A. K., Akolkar, G., Bernardes, N., Dias, D. D. S., et al. (2016). Insulin resistance: an additional risk factor in the pathogenesis of cardiovascular disease in type 2 diabetes. *Heart Failure Rev.* 21, 11–23. doi: 10.1007/s10741-015-9515-6

Pei, L., Wan, T., Wang, S., Ye, M., Qiu, Y., Jiang, R., et al. (2018). Cyanidin-3-O-β-glucoside regulates the activation and the secretion of adipokines from brown adipose tissue and alleviates diet induced fatty liver. *Biomed. Pharmacother.* 105, 625–632. doi: 10.1016/j.biopha.2018.06.018

Petersen, M. C., and Shulman, G. I. (2017). Roles of Diacylglycerols and Ceramides in Hepatic Insulin Resistance. *Trends Pharmacol. Sci.* 38, 649–665. doi: 10.1016/j.tips.2017.04.004

Petersen, M. C., Madiraju, A. K., Gassaway, B. M., Marcel, M., Nasiri, A. R., Butrico, G., et al. (2016). Insulin receptor Thr1160 phosphorylation mediates lipid-induced hepatic insulin resistance. *J. Clin. Investigat.* 126, 4361–4371. doi: 10.1172/jci86013

Pickles, S., Vigié, P., and Youle, R. J. (2018). Mitophagy and Quality Control Mechanisms in Mitochondrial Maintenance. *Curr. Biol.* 28, R170–R185.

Pileggi, C. A., Parmar, G., and Harper, M. E. (2021). The lifecycle of skeletal muscle mitochondria in obesity. *Obesity Rev.* 22:9793.

Pivari, F., Mingione, A., Brasacchio, C., and Soldati, L. (2019). Curcumin and Type 2 Diabetes Mellitus: Prevention and Treatment. *Nutrients* 11:1837. doi: 10.3390/nu11081837

Pop, R. M., Popolo, A., Trifa, A. P., and Stanciu, L. A. (2018). Phytochemicals in Cardiovascular and Respiratory Diseases: Evidence in Oxidative Stress and Inflammation. *Oxidat. Med. Cell. Long.* 2018:1603872.

Poulsen, M. M., Vestergaard, P. F., Clasen, B. F., Radko, Y., Christensen, L. P., Stødkilde-Jørgensen, H., et al. (2013). High-dose resveratrol supplementation in obese men: an investigator-initiated, randomized, placebo-controlled clinical trial of substrate metabolism, insulin sensitivity, and body composition. *Diabetes* 62, 1186–1195. doi: 10.2337/db12-0975

Poznyak, A. V., Nikiforov, N. G., Wu, W. K., Kirichenko, T. V., and Orekhov, A. N. (2021). Autophagy and Mitophagy as Essential Components of Atherosclerosis. *Cells* 10:443. doi: 10.3390/cells10020443

Qin, Y., Zhai, Q., Li, Y., Cao, M., Xu, Y., Zhao, K., et al. (2018). Cyanidin-3-O-glucoside ameliorates diabetic nephropathy through regulation of glutathione pool. *Biomed. Pharmacother.* 103, 1223–1230. doi: 10.1016/j.biopha.2018.04.137

Ren, B.-C., Zhang, Y.-F., Liu, S.-S., Cheng, X.-J., Yang, X., Cui, X.-G., et al. (2020). Curcumin alleviates oxidative stress and inhibits apoptosis in diabetic cardiomyopathy via Sirt1-Foxo1 and PI3K-Akt signalling pathways. *J. Cell. Mole. Med.* 24, 12355–12367. doi: 10.1111/jcmm.15725

Roque, W., Cuevas-Mora, K., and Romero, F. (2020). Mitochondrial Quality Control in Age-Related Pulmonary Fibrosis. *Int. J. Mole. Sci.* 21:643. doi: 10.3390/ijms21020643

Rovira-Llopis, S., Bañuls, C., Diaz-Morales, N., Hernandez-Mijares, A., Rocha, M., and Victor, V. M. (2017). Mitochondrial dynamics in type 2 diabetes: Pathophysiological implications. *Redox Biol.* 11, 637–645. doi: 10.1016/j.redox.2017.01.013

Rubio-Sastre, P., Scheer, F. A. J. L., Gómez-Abellán, P., Madrid, J. A., and Garaulet, M. (2014). Acute melatonin administration in humans impairs glucose tolerance in both the morning and evening. *Sleep* 37, 1715–1719. doi: 10.5665/sleep.4088

Sajadi Hezaveh, Z., Azarkeivan, A., Janani, L., and Shidfar, F. (2019). Effect of quercetin on oxidative stress and liver function in beta-thalassemia major patients receiving desferrioxamine: A double-blind randomized clinical trial. *J. Res. Med. Sci.* 24:91. doi: 10.4103/jrms.jrms_911_18

Sarparanta, J., García-Macia, M., and Singh, R. (2017). Autophagy and Mitochondria in Obesity and Type 2 Diabetes. *Curr. Diabet. Rev.* 13, 352–369.

Sattarinezhad, A., Roozbeh, J., Shirazi Yeganeh, B., Omrani, G. R., and Shams, M. (2019). Resveratrol reduces albuminuria in diabetic nephropathy: A randomized double-blind placebo-controlled clinical trial. *Diabet. Metabol.* 45, 53–59. doi: 10.1016/j.diabet.2018.05.010

Seyyedebrahimi, S., Khodabandehloo, H., Nasli Esfahani, E., and Meshkani, R. (2018). The effects of resveratrol on markers of oxidative stress in patients with type 2 diabetes: a randomized, double-blind, placebo-controlled clinical trial. *Acta Diabetol.* 55, 341–353. doi: 10.1007/s00592-017-1098-3

Shaito, A., Posadino, A. M., Younes, N., Hasan, H., Halabi, S., Alhababi, D., et al. (2020). Potential Adverse Effects of Resveratrol: A Literature Review. *Int. J. Mole. Sci.* 21:2084. doi: 10.3390/ijms21062084

Shamsi, M. B., Kumar, R., Bhatt, A., Bamezai, R. N. K., Kumar, R., Gupta, N. P., et al. (2008). Mitochondrial DNA Mutations in etiopathogenesis of male infertility. *Indian J. Urol.* 24, 150–154. doi: 10.4103/0970-1591.40606

Shi, Y., and Williamson, G. (2016). Quercetin lowers plasma uric acid in pre-hyperuricaemic males: a randomised, double-blinded, placebo-controlled, cross-over trial. *Br. J. Nutr.* 115, 800–806. doi: 10.1017/s0007114515005310

Simona, Mrakic, S., Alessandra, Vezzoli, Alex, Rizzato, et al. (2019). Oxidative stress assessment in breath-hold diving. *Eur. J. Appl. Physiol.* 119, 2449–2456.

St John, J. C., Jokhi, R. P., and Barratt, C. L. R. (2005). The impact of mitochondrial genetics on male infertility. *Int. J. Androl.* 28, 65–73. doi: 10.1111/j.1365-2605.2005.00515.x

Su, Z., Nie, Y., Huang, X., Zhu, Y., Feng, B., Tang, L., et al. (2019). Mitophagy in Hepatic Insulin Resistance: Therapeutic Potential and Concerns. *Front. Pharmacol.* 10:1193.

Sweetlove, L. J., Beard, K. F. M., Nunes-Nesi, A., Fernie, A. R., and Ratcliffe, R. G. (2010). Not just a circle: flux modes in the plant TCA cycle. *Trends Plant Sci.* 15, 462–470. doi: 10.1016/j.tplants.2010.05.006

Szkudelska, K., Deniziak, M., Hertig, I., Wojciechowicz, T., Tyczewska, M., Jaroszewska, M., et al. (2019). Effects of Resveratrol in Goto-Kakizaki Rat, a Model of Type 2 Diabetes. *Nutrients* 11:2480.

Tabrizi, R., Tamtaji, O. R., Lankarani, K. B., Mirhosseini, N., Akbari, M., Dadgostar, E., et al. (2018). The effects of resveratrol supplementation on biomarkers of inflammation and oxidative stress among patients with metabolic syndrome and related disorders: a systematic review and meta-analysis of randomized controlled trials. *Food Funct.* 9, 6116–6128. doi: 10.1039/c8fo01259h

Tahrir, F. G., Langford, D., Amini, S., Mohseni Ahooyi, T., and Khalili, K. (2019). Mitochondrial quality control in cardiac cells: Mechanisms and role in cardiac cell injury and disease. *J. Cell. Physiol.* 234, 8122–8133. doi: 10.1002/jcp.27597

Tan, Y. Q., Zhang, X., Zhang, S., Zhu, T., Garg, M., Lobie, P. E., et al. (2021). Mitochondria: The metabolic switch of cellular oncogenic transformation. *Biochim. Biophys. Acta.* 1876:188534. doi: 10.1016/j.bbcan.2021.188534

Theodotou, M., Fokianos, K., Mouzouridou, A., Konstantinou, C., Aristotelous, A., Prodromou, D., et al. (2017). The effect of resveratrol on hypertension: A clinical trial. *Exp. Therap. Med.* 13, 295–301. doi: 10.3892/etm.2016.3958

Timmers, S., Konings, E., Bilet, L., Houtkooper, R. H., Van De Weijer, T., Goossens, G. H., et al. (2011). Calorie restriction-like effects of 30 days of resveratrol supplementation on energy metabolism and metabolic profile in obese humans. *Cell Metab.* 14, 612–622. doi: 10.1016/j.cmet.2011.10.002

Turpin, S. M., Nicholls, H. T., Willmes, D. M., Mourier, A., Brodesser, S., Wunderlich, C. M., et al. (2014). Obesity-induced CerS6-dependent C16:0 ceramide production promotes weight gain and glucose intolerance. *Cell Metabol.* 20, 678–686. doi: 10.1016/j.cmet.2014.08.002

van der Bliek, A. M., Shen, Q., and Kawajiri, S. (2013). Mechanisms of mitochondrial fission and fusion. *Cold Spring Harbor Perspect. Biol.* 5:a011072.

Vargas, T. R., Cai, Z., Shen, Y., Dosset, M., Benoitlizon, I., Martin, T., et al. (2017). Selective degradation of PU.1 during autophagy represses the differentiation and antitumour activity of TH9 cells. *Nat. Commun.* 8:559.

Vásquez-Trincado, C., García-Carvajal, I., Pennanen, C., Parra, V., Hill, J. A., Rothermel, B. A., et al. (2016). Mitochondrial dynamics, mitophagy and cardiovascular disease. *J. Physiol.* 594, 509–525. doi: 10.1113/jp271301

Vazirani, R. P., Verma, A., Sadacca, L. A., Buckman, M. S., Picatoste, B., Beg, M., et al. (2016). Disruption of Adipose Rab10-Dependent Insulin Signaling Causes Hepatic Insulin Resistance. *Diabetes* 65, 1577–1589. doi: 10.2337/db15-1128

Wang, D., Xia, M., Gao, S., Li, D., Zhang, Y., Jin, T., et al. (2012). Cyanidin-3-O-β-glucoside upregulates hepatic cholesterol 7α-hydroxylase expression and reduces hypercholesterolemia in mice. *Mole. Nutr. Food Res.* 56, 610–621. doi: 10.1002/mnfr.201100659

Wang, H., Ni, H., Chao, X., Ma, X., Rodriguez, Y., Chavan, H., et al. (2019). Double deletion of PINK1 and Parkin impairs hepatic mitophagy and exacerbates acetaminophen-induced liver injury in mice. *Redox Biol.* 22:101148. doi: 10.1016/j.redox.2019.101148

Wang, R., Zhu, Y., Lin, X., Ren, C., Zhao, J., Wang, F., et al. (2019). Influenza M2 protein regulates MAVS-mediated signaling pathway through interacting with MAVS and increasing ROS production. *Autophagy* 15:1181.

Wang, S., Li, J., Du, Y., Xu, Y., Wang, Y., Zhang, Z., et al. (2017). The Class I PI3K Inhibitor S14161 induces autophagy in malignant blood cells by modulating the Beclin 1/Vps34 complex. *J. Pharmacol. Sci.* 134, 197–202. doi: 10.1016/j.jphs.2017.07.001

Wang, X., Zhang, J. Q., Xiu, C. K., Yang, J., Fang, J. Y., and Lei, Y. (2020). Ginseng-Sanqi-Chuanxiong (GSC) Extracts Ameliorate Diabetes-Induced Endothelial Cell Senescence through Regulating Mitophagy via the AMPK Pathway. *Oxidat. Med. Cell. Long.* 2020:7151946.

Wen, D., Tan, R. Z., Zhao, C. Y., Li, J. C., Zhong, X., Diao, H., et al. (2020). Astragalus mongholicus Bunge and Panax notoginseng (Burkill) F.H. Chen Formula for Renal Injury in Diabetic Nephropathy-In Vivo and In Vitro Evidence for Autophagy Regulation. *Front. Pharmacol.* 11:732.

Wrobel, L., Topf, U., Bragoszewski, P., Wiese, S., Sztolsztener, M. E., Oeljeklaus, S., et al. (2015). Mistargeted mitochondrial proteins activate a proteostatic response in the cytosol. *Nature* 524, 485–488. doi: 10.1038/nature14951

Wu, W., Xu, H., Wang, Z., Mao, Y., Yuan, L., Luo, W., et al. (2015). PINK1-Parkin-Mediated Mitophagy Protects Mitochondrial Integrity and Prevents Metabolic Stress-Induced Endothelial Injury. *PLoS One* 10:e0132499. doi: 10.1371/journal.pone.0132499

Wu, X., Huang, L., Zhou, X., and Liu, J. (2020). Curcumin protects cardiomyopathy damage through inhibiting the production of reactive oxygen species in type 2 diabetic mice. *Biochem. Biophys. Res. Commun.* 530, 15–21. doi: 10.1016/j.bbrc.2020.05.053

Xi, J., Rong, Y., Zhao, Z., Huang, Y., Wang, P., Luan, H., et al. (2021). Scutellarin ameliorates high glucose-induced vascular endothelial cells injury by activating PINK1/Parkin-mediated mitophagy. *J. Ethnopharmacol.* 271:113855. doi: 10.1016/j.jep.2021.113855

Xia, J. Y., Holland, W. L., Kusminski, C. M., Sun, K., Sharma, A. X., Pearson, M. J., et al. (2015). Targeted Induction of Ceramide Degradation Leads to Improved Systemic Metabolism and Reduced Hepatic Steatosis. *Cell Metabol.* 22, 266–278. doi: 10.1016/j.cmet.2015.06.001

Xu, H., Cheng, J., Wang, X., Liu, H., Wang, S., Wu, J., et al. (2019). Resveratrol pretreatment alleviates myocardial ischemia/reperfusion injury by inhibiting STIM1-mediated intracellular calcium accumulation. *J. Physiol. Biochem.* 75, 607–618. doi: 10.1007/s13105-019-00704-5

Xu, Y., Shen, J., and Ran, Z. (2020). Emerging views of mitophagy in immunity and autoimmune diseases. *Autophagy* 16, 3–17. doi: 10.1080/15548627.2019.1603547

Yang, H., Yang, T., Heng, C., Zhou, Y., Jiang, Z., Qian, X., et al. (2019). Quercetin improves nonalcoholic fatty liver by ameliorating inflammation, oxidative stress, and lipid metabolism in db/db mice. *Phytother. Res.* 33, 3140–3152. doi: 10.1002/ptr.6486

Yang, S., Hu, T., Liu, H., Lv, Y.-L., Zhang, W., Li, H., et al. (2021). Akebia saponin D ameliorates metabolic syndrome (MetS) via remodeling gut microbiota and attenuating intestinal barrier injury. *Biomed. Pharmacother.* 138, 111441. doi: 10.1016/j.biopha.2021.111441

Yang, S., Zhang, W., Xuan, L. L., Han, F. F., Lv, Y. L., Wan, Z. R., et al. (2019). Akebia Saponin D inhibits the formation of atherosclerosis in ApoE(-/-) mice by attenuating oxidative stress-induced apoptosis in endothelial cells. *Atherosclerosis* 285, 23–30. doi: 10.1016/j.atherosclerosis.2019.04.202

Yang, Y., Pei, K., Zhang, Q., Wang, D., Feng, H., Du, Z., et al. (2020). Salvianolic acid B ameliorates atherosclerosis via inhibiting YAP/TAZ/JNK signaling pathway in endothelial cells and pericytes. *Biochim. Biophys. Acta* 1865:158779. doi: 10.1016/j.bbalip.2020.158779

Yao, L., Song, J., Meng, X. W., Ge, J. Y., Du, B. X., Yu, J., et al. (2020). Periostin aggravates NLRP3 inflammasome-mediated pyroptosis in myocardial ischemia-reperfusion injury. *Mole. Cell. Probes* 53:101596. doi: 10.1016/j.mcp.2020.101596

Yao, Q., Ke, Z.-Q., Guo, S., Yang, X.-S., Zhang, F.-X., Liu, X.-F., et al. (2018). Curcumin protects against diabetic cardiomyopathy by promoting autophagy and alleviating apoptosis. *J. Mole. Cell. Cardiol.* 124, 26–34. doi: 10.1016/j.yjmcc.2018.10.004

Yaribeygi, H., Farrokhi, F. R., Butler, A. E., and Sahebkar, A. (2019). Insulin resistance: Review of the underlying molecular mechanisms. *J. Cellular Physiol.* 234, 8152–8161. doi: 10.1002/jcp.27603

Yazıcı, D., and Sezer, H. (2017). Insulin Resistance, Obesity and Lipotoxicity. *Adv. Exp. Med. Biol.* 960, 277–304. doi: 10.1007/978-3-319-48382-5_12

Younossi, Z. M., Koenig, A. B., Abdelatif, D., Fazel, Y., Henry, L., and Wymer, M. (2016). Global epidemiology of nonalcoholic fatty liver disease-Meta-analytic assessment of prevalence, incidence, and outcomes. *Hepatology* 64, 73–84. doi: 10.1002/hep.28431

Zahedi, M., Ghiasvand, R., Feizi, A., Asgari, G., and Darvish, L. (2013). Does Quercetin Improve Cardiovascular Risk factors and Inflammatory Biomarkers in Women with Type 2 Diabetes: A Double-blind Randomized Controlled Clinical Trial. *Int. J. Prev. Med.* 4, 777–785.

Zeng, W., Shan, W., Gao, L., Gao, D., Hu, Y., Wang, G., et al. (2015). Inhibition of HMGB1 release via salvianolic acid B-mediated SIRT1 up-regulation protects rats against non-alcoholic fatty liver disease. *Scientific Rep.* 5:16013.

Zhang, B., Zhang, X., Zhang, C., Shen, Q., Sun, G., and Sun, X. (2019). Notoginsenoside R1 Protects db/db Mice against Diabetic Nephropathy via Upregulation of Nrf2-Mediated HO-1 Expression. *Molecules* 24:247. doi: 10.3390/molecules24020247

Zhang, R., Chu, K., Zhao, N., Wu, J., Ma, L., Zhu, C., et al. (2019). Corilagin Alleviates Nonalcoholic Fatty Liver Disease in High-Fat Diet-Induced C57BL/6 Mice by Ameliorating Oxidative Stress and Restoring Autophagic Flux. *Front. Pharmacol.* 10:1693.

Zhang, S., Zou, J., Li, P., Zheng, X., and Feng, D. (2018). Curcumin Protects against Atherosclerosis in Apolipoprotein E-Knockout Mice by Inhibiting Toll-like Receptor 4 Expression. *J. Agricult. Food Chem.* 66, 449–456. doi: 10.1021/acs.jafc.7b04260

Zhang, W. (2020). *The mitophagy receptor FUN14 domain-containing 1 (FUNDC1): A promising biomarker and potential therapeutic target of human diseases.* Netherland: Elsevier.

Zhang, X., Ji, R., Sun, H., Peng, J., Ma, X., Wang, C., et al. (2018). Scutellarin ameliorates nonalcoholic fatty liver disease through the PPARγ/PGC-1α-Nrf2 pathway. *Free Radical Res.* 52, 198–211. doi: 10.1080/10715762.2017.1422602

Zhou, H., Du, W., Li, Y., Shi, C., Hu, N., Ma, S., et al. (2018). Effects of melatonin on fatty liver disease: The role of NR4A1/DNA-PKcs/p53 pathway, mitochondrial fission, and mitophagy. *J. Pineal Res.* 1:64.

Zhou, P., Xie, W., Meng, X., Zhai, Y., Dong, X., Zhang, X., et al. (2019a). Notoginsenoside R1 Ameliorates Diabetic Retinopathy through PINK1-Dependent Activation of Mitophagy. *Cells* 8:213. doi: 10.3390/cells8030213

Zhou, P., Yang, X., Yang, Z., Huang, W., Kou, J., and Li, F. (2019b). Akebia Saponin D Regulates the Metabolome and Intestinal Microbiota in High Fat Diet-Induced Hyperlipidemic Rats. *Molecules* 24:1268. doi: 10.3390/molecules24071268

Zhou, R., Yazdi, A. S., Menu, P., and Tschopp, J. (2011). A role for mitochondria in NLRP3 inflammasome activation. *Nature* 469, 221–225.

Zhou, X., Xiong, J., Lu, S., Luo, L., Chen, Z.-L., Yang, F., et al. (2019c). Inhibitory Effect of Corilagin on miR-21-Regulated Hepatic Fibrosis Signaling Pathway. *Am. J. Chin. Med.* 47, 1541–1569. doi: 10.1142/s0192415x1950 0794

Zhu, L., Wei, T., Gao, J., Chang, X., He, H., Luo, F., et al. (2015). The cardioprotective effect of salidroside against myocardial ischemia reperfusion injury in rats by inhibiting apoptosis and inflammation. *Apoptosis* 20, 1433–1443. doi: 10.1007/s10495-015-1174-5

Zhu, X., Xiong, T., Liu, P., Guo, X., Xiao, L., Zhou, F., et al. (2018). Quercetin ameliorates HFD-induced NAFLD by promoting hepatic VLDL assembly and lipophagy via the IRE1a/XBP1s pathway. *Food Chem. Toxicol.* 114, 52–60. doi: 10.1016/j.fct.2018.02.019

Zhu, Y., Massen, S., Terenzio, M., Lang, V., Chen-Lindner, S., Eils, R., et al. (2013). Modulation of serines 17 and 24 in the LC3-interacting region of Bnip3 determines pro-survival mitophagy versus apoptosis. *J. Biol. Chem.* 288, 1099–1113. doi: 10.1074/jbc.m112.399345

New Insights into the Role of Autophagy in Liver Surgery in the Setting of Metabolic Syndrome and Related Diseases

Ana Isabel Álvarez-Mercado[1,2,3†], Carlos Rojano-Alfonso[4†], Marc Micó-Carnero[4],
Albert Caballeria-Casals[4], Carmen Peralta[4*†] and Araní Casillas-Ramírez[5,6*†]

[1] Department of Biochemistry and Molecular Biology II, School of Pharmacy, Granada, Spain, [2] Institute of Nutrition and Food
Technology "José Mataix", Biomedical Research Center, Parque Tecnológico Ciencias de la Salud, Granada, Spain,
[3] Instituto de Investigación Biosanitaria ibs. GRANADA, Complejo Hospitalario Universitario de Granada, Granada, Spain,
[4] Institut d'Investigacions Biomèdiques August Pi i Sunyer (IDIBAPS), Barcelona, Spain, [5] Hospital Regional de Alta
Especialidad de Ciudad Victoria "Bicentenario 2010", Ciudad Victoria, Mexico, [6] Facultad de Medicina e Ingeniería en
Sistemas Computacionales de Matamoros, Universidad Autónoma de Tamaulipas, Matamoros, Mexico

*Correspondence:
Carmen Peralta
cperalta@clinic.cat
Araní Casillas-Ramírez
aranyc@yahoo.com

† These authors have contributed
equally to this work

Visceral obesity is an important component of metabolic syndrome, a cluster of diseases that also includes diabetes and insulin resistance. A combination of these metabolic disorders damages liver function, which manifests as non-alcoholic fatty liver disease (NAFLD). NAFLD is a common cause of abnormal liver function, and numerous studies have established the enormously deleterious role of hepatic steatosis in ischemia-reperfusion (I/R) injury that inevitably occurs in both liver resection and transplantation. Thus, steatotic livers exhibit a higher frequency of post-surgical complications after hepatectomy, and using liver grafts from donors with NAFLD is associated with an increased risk of post-surgical morbidity and mortality in the recipient. Diabetes, another MetS-related metabolic disorder, also worsens hepatic I/R injury, and similar to NAFLD, diabetes is associated with a poor prognosis after liver surgery. Due to the large increase in the prevalence of MetS, NAFLD, and diabetes, their association is frequent in the population and therefore, in patients requiring liver resection and in potential liver graft donors. This scenario requires advancement in therapies to improve postoperative results in patients suffering from metabolic diseases and undergoing liver surgery; and in this sense, the bases for designing therapeutic strategies are in-depth knowledge about the molecular signaling pathways underlying the effects of MetS-related diseases and I/R injury on liver tissue. A common denominator in all these diseases is autophagy. In fact, in the context of obesity, autophagy is profoundly diminished in hepatocytes and alters mitochondrial functions in the liver. In insulin resistance conditions, there is a suppression of autophagy in the liver, which is associated with the accumulation of lipids, being this is a risk factor for NAFLD. Also, oxidative stress occurring in hepatic I/R injury promotes autophagy. The present review aims to shed some light on the role of autophagy in livers undergoing surgery and also suffering from metabolic diseases, which may lead to the discovery of effective therapeutic targets that could be translated from laboratory to clinical practice, to improve postoperative results of liver surgeries when performed in the presence of one or more metabolic diseases.

Keywords: autophagy, metabolic syndrome, ischemia-reperfusion, liver surgery, transplantation

INTRODUCTION

Obesity is the major risk for the development of metabolic syndrome (MetS), a prevalent entity in Western societies that includes cardiovascular risk factors i.e., hypertension, diabetes mellitus, and, insulin resistance (Nakao et al., 2012). The combination of these metabolic disorders compromises liver function, manifested as non-alcoholic fatty liver disease (NAFLD), a risk marker in type 2 diabetes (T2D) and MetS. NAFLD compromises pre-existing hepatic disease and is progressively on the rise throughout the world (Gadiparthi et al., 2020). Albeit controversial, the use of fatty livers in liver transplantation is also increasing due to the paucity of available organs, but they tend to poorly tolerate the ischemia/reperfusion (I/R) process, leading to primary non-function, early graft dysfunction, and graft loss. Significant steatosis has also been more frequent in tumor-associated hepatic resections in which I/R is also sub-par, and carries high morbidity in the immediate postoperative period (Micó-Carnero et al., 2021).

Abbreviations: ADP, adenosine diphosphate; AGE, advanced glycation end product; Akt, serine-threonine protein kinase Akt; AMPK, adenosine 5′-monophosphate-activated protein kinase; ASNS, asparagine synthetase; Atg, autophagy gen; ATP, adenosine triphosphate; ATP6V1B2, vacuolar H + -ATPase, B2 subunit; BNIP3, BCL2 and adenovirus E1B 19-kDa-interacting protein 3; CRY1, cryptochrome 1; CXCR3, chemokine (C-X-C motif) receptor 3; DNA, desoxyribonucleic acid; ER, endoplasmic reticulum; ERK, extracellular signal-regulated kinase; FA, fatty acids; FGF21, fibroblast growth factor 21; FOXO, forkhead box O; GSK3b, glycogen synthase kinase 3 beta; HFD, high-fat diet; HOTAIR, homeobox (HOX) transcript antisense RNA; I/R, ischemia/reperfusion; IKK, inhibitor of NF-κB kinase; IL, interleukin; IRE1, inositol-requiring enzyme 1; IRF1, interferon regulatory factor 1; IRGM, immunity-related guanosine triphosphatase family M; IRS, insulin receptor substrate; JNK, c-Jun NH(2)-terminal kinase; LAMP, lysosome-associated membrane protein; LC3, microtubule-associated protein light-chain 3; LD, lipid droplets; lncRNAs, long-non-coding RNAs; MAPK, mitogen-activated protein kinase; MC3R, melanocortin 3 receptor; MCD, methionine/choline-deficient; MetS, metabolic sydrome; miR, microRNA; mTOR, mammalian target of rapamycin; mTORC1, mammalian target of rapamycin complex 1; NAD + , nicotinamide adenine dinucleotide; NAFLD, non-alcoholic fatty liver disease; NASH, non-alcoholic steatohepatitis; NF-kB, nuclear factor kappa B; NIX, BNIP3-like (BNIP3L), also known as NIX; NLRP3, nucleotide-binding oligomerization domain (NOD)-like receptor (NLR) family pyrin domain containing 3; NO, nitric oxide; NPC1, Niemann-Pick-type C1; PARP, poly (ADP-ribose) polymerase; PERK, protein kinase R (PKR)-like endoplasmic reticulum kinase; PGAM5, phosphoglycerate mutase family member 5; PI3K, phosphoinositide-3 kinase; PINK1, phosphatase and tensin homolog (PTEN)-induced putative kinase 1; PKC, protein kinase C; PLIN2, perilipin 2; PPAR-γ, peroxisome proliferator-activated receptor gamma; RAGE, receptor for AGE; RBP4, retinol binding protein 4; RNA, ribonucleic acid; ROS, reactive oxygen species; Rubicon, run domain beclin-1-interacting and cysteine-rich domain-containing protein; S6K1, ribosome S6 protein kinase 1; Sirt1, silencing information regulator 1; SOD, superoxide dismutase; SQSTM, p62/sequestosome; SRA, class A scavenger receptor; T2D, type 2 diabetes; TFEB, transcription factor EB; TNF-α, tumor necrosis factor alpha; UPR, unfolded protein response; Vps34, vacuolar protein sorting 34.

The complex molecular interrelation between obesity, MetS, insulin resistance, and diabetes does not allow us to clarify which is the precise concatenation of events driving NAFLD. However, a common denominator in all of such metabolic diseases is autophagy. Abnormal autophagy fails to restore homeostasis, promotes the development of obesity-associated diseases, and increases insulin resistance (Yang et al., 2010). The pathophysiology of diabetes mellitus types I and II, as well as β-cell dysfunction, has been associated with abnormal autophagy mechanisms (Gonzalez et al., 2011). Abnormal autophagy may also underlie I/R injury and NAFLD in partially resected or transplanted livers (Zhao et al., 2016). Moderate I/R injury causes cell dysfunction by autophagy and activates survival recovery systems, but prolonged I/R-mediated cell damage may lead to apoptosis and necrosis (Lopez-Neblina et al., 2005; Zhu J. et al., 2016; Ling et al., 2017). Furthermore, hyperglycemia exacerbates liver ischemic injury (Behrends et al., 2010). Patients with diabetes and requiring a liver resection are at great risk of hepatic injury during surgery (Han et al., 2014), and this also applies to potential liver transplant diabetic donors. Due to the great increase in the prevalence of NAFLD and diabetes, their association is frequently present in society and hence, in potential liver graft donors, and patients requiring a hepatic resection. This scenario requires the development of effective strategies to improve post-operative results in NAFLD and/or diabetic patients subjected to liver surgery; hence, a thorough understanding of the signaling pathways in NAFLD, MetS, diabetes, insulin resistance, and I/R injury are paramount.

Based on the previously presented challenges, we will specifically review the effects of obesity, MetS, insulin resistance, and/or diabetes in the postoperative outcomes from liver resection and transplantation, and the crucial role of autophagy in that setting. A better understanding of the molecular mechanisms related to autophagy underlying such conditions is extremely relevant to develop effective therapeutic targets to improve the post-operative outcomes of hepatic surgeries when associated with the mentioned comorbidities. In this sense, it is important the knowledge whether the autophagy process is different in livers affected by metabolic comorbidities with and without surgical intervention. Then, we will initially analyze the effects of MetS and related diseases as obesity, insulin resistance, NAFLD, and/or diabetes on livers without surgery, and the involvement of the autophagy process in such context. We will then focus on how metabolic diseases negatively affect hepatic I/R injury inherent to liver surgery. Finally, we will present the mechanisms underlying the role of autophagy in damage in surgically intervened livers, especially those suffering metabolic diseases.

INVOLVEMENT OF HEPATIC AUTOPHAGY IN THE EFFECTS OF METABOLIC DYSFUNCTIONS ON THE LIVER

Autophagy is a vacuolar self-digestion, whereby intracellular proteins, fatty acids (FA), organelles, and cellular detritus (cargo) are degraded by lysosomal enzymes and recycled into their basic units, to be reused in the cytoplasm for survival, differentiation, etc. (Mizushima et al., 2010; Miyamoto and Heller, 2016). Autophagy can be selective or non-selective since this cellular response can be directed to degrade a specific organelle (i.e., mitophagy or lipophagy) (Kim et al., 2016). Autophagy begins with the development and elongation of a membrane, the phagophore that in turn, is transformed into a vesicle surrounded by two membranes in which the cargo is isolated. Microtubule-associated protein light-chain 3 (LC3) participates in the formation of autophagosomes; its cleavage by autophagy gen (Atg)4B results in LC3-I, which conjugates with phosphatidylethanolamine via two consecutive reactions catalyzed by the E1-like enzyme Atg7, and the E2-like enzyme Atg3, thus forming lipidated LC3-II associated with the autophagosomal membrane. The autophagosome matures by fusing with lysosomes to create autophagolysosomes where its selected cargo is degraded (Kabeya et al., 2000; Kirisako et al., 2000). The p62/sequestosome (SQSTM) is a ubiquitin-binding protein that recognizes ubiquitinated cargo and links with autophagosomes through direct interaction with LC3-II (Lamark et al., 2003; Pankiv et al., 2007). Since LC3-II and p62 are both degraded in the autolysosome with autophagic cargo, accumulation of LC3-II and p62 is regarded as a robust marker of impaired autophagic flux (Lee et al., 2012). Lysosome-associated membrane proteins (LAMPs) are essential for autophagosome-lysosome fusion during autophagy and are responsible for lysosomal proteolytic activity. When LAMP1 and LAMP2 are inhibited, then autophagosome and lysosome fusion is inhibited, and this is associated with the accumulation of LC3-II and p62 suggesting a decrease in autophagy flux (Fortunato et al., 2009). Lysosomal proteases, such as cathepsin, also play a key role in autolysosome degradation (Uchiyama, 2001), and therefore, lysosome dysfunction may be involved with autophagic flux impairment. In line with this, defective cathepsin B, cathepsin D, and cathepsin L enzyme activity resulted in impaired lysosomal acidification and this occurred concomitantly with autophagic flux blockade, including autophagosome accumulation and decreased degradation of SQSTM1/p62 (Mareninova et al., 2009). Considering all autophagy stages, there exists an updated consensus that suggests that the real status of autophagy should be assessed not only by the number of autophagosomes and autolysosomes but also by evaluating the actual autophagic flux, such as monitoring the clearance of cell components in autolysosomes (du Toit et al., 2018).

The liver is rich in lysosomes and has a high level of stress-induced autophagy. In fact, reactive oxygen species (ROS) give rise to lysosomal dysfunction and autophagy flux impairment, avoiding the correct degradation of damaged cellular components (Jung et al., 2020). In addition, enhanced endoplasmic reticulum (ER) stress can deregulate lysosomal acidification and thus, blocking autophagy in hepatocytes (Chen et al., 2019a). This provokes hepatotoxicity, cell death, and alteration of hepatic function (Jung et al., 2020). A close association between autophagy functionality, obesity, and liver disease has been posited (He et al., 2016), and consequently, the understanding of the molecular mechanisms underlying this relationship occurring in the liver may be the basis for the design of new protective strategies for livers affected by metabolic diseases and undergoing a liver surgery process. The vast majority of reviews that address the role of autophagy in obesity, MetS, insulin resistance, NAFLD or diabetes, does not clearly distinguish which are the molecular signaling pathways related to autophagy that come about at the liver tissue. Therefore, the findings that have been reported about the effects of such metabolic diseases on the hepatic autophagy process are presented below.

Metabolic Syndrome and Associated Disorders

Although several studies have attempted to determine the origin of the MetS, due to its complexity, a clear etiology remains to be established. MetS refers to central obesity, insulin resistance, impaired glucose tolerance, dyslipidemia, and elevated blood pressure (Simmons et al., 2010). Excessive fat accumulation in obesity associated with the MetS and its macrovascular complications activates the immune system and chronic states of low-grade inflammation. Altered signaling at the molecular level in adipose tissue, negatively affects the liver as causes hepatic infiltration by macrophages and other immune cells (Esser et al., 2014). This event is not the only one that damages liver tissue. Once adipose tissue has reached its storage capacity, excess calories are redirected to other depots and lead to ectopic fat accumulation. Visceral fat drains into the portal vein, and then the liver is targeted by multiple metabolites and adipokines (Schleinitz et al., 2014). A connection between obesity, progressive lipid accumulation in the liver, and T2D in humans has been established (Goto et al., 2017). Diabetes is linked particularly to NAFLD, and indeed, up to 70% of diabetic patients develop NAFLD (Williamson et al., 2011). Hepatic lipids tend to further exacerbate insulin resistance by interfering with insulin signaling, thus perpetuating the vicious cycle. In fact, FA increases gluconeogenesis, lipogenesis, and chronic inflammation, which foster hepatic glucose production, resulting in hyperglycemia and hepatic insulin resistance (Pereira et al., 2015; Wang Z. et al., 2017).

Based on evidence obtained from *in vivo* and *in vitro* studies, autophagy has been suggested to underlie the pathophysiology of MetS, obesity, insulin resistance, and diabetes in the liver (Ogihara et al., 2002; Engeli et al., 2003; Yang et al., 2010; Putnam et al., 2012; Wang H.J. et al., 2015). Whether autophagy is a protective factor against obesity or a manifestation of impaired adipose tissue function, remains to be determined. Obesity is often associated with liver steatosis and insulin resistance. In obesity, autophagy decreases in hepatocytes, and metabolism is impaired. The release of lipids stored in droplets is mediated by autophagy; if inhibited, promotes fatty liver development. Mice with the hepatocyte-specific Atg7 deletion, develop fat droplets, whereas Atg7 reestablishment ameliorates hepatic function. Yang et al. described lower protein levels of Atg7, Beclin 1 (Atg6), LC3, Atg5, and elevated p62 in the livers of obese mice (Yang et al., 2010). Concerning other metabolic disorders, in rats with MetS increased hepatic autophagy activity manifested by elevated LC3-II/I, Beclin-1, mammalian target of rapamycin (mTOR), and p62 autophagy-related proteins, as well as phosphorylated adenosine 5′-monophosphate-activated protein kinase (AMPK) down-regulation, has been reported (Cui et al., 2020). These results appear to reflect an opposite role for autophagy in obesity and MetS, however, they must be carefully analyzed. Since an increase in autophagy-dependent protein expression can result from one of two mechanisms, it could reflect either an increase in autophagosome synthesis or an arrest in degradation.

Accumulation of autophagosomes in the liver in the setting of obesity has been demonstrated, and to explain this, a study carried out with a genetic obese experimental model found that a defect in lysosomal acidification and proteinase activity of cathepsin impaired hepatic autophagic degradation (Inami et al., 2011). On the other hand, an investigation performed with a diet-induced obese model indicated that impairment of autophagic flux was due to blockage of autophagosome-lysosome fusion, without alteration in lysosomal environment, including acidification and hydrolytic function; and this was associated with ER stress (Miyagawa et al., 2016). These results would indicate that possibly, different experimental models could induce variations in some autophagy signaling pathways. The autophagosome-lysosome degradation process plays a role in the pathogenesis of obesity-mediated diabetes. In mice, deficiencies in LAMP2, which is crucial in the fusion and degradation of autophagosomes with lysosomes, prevent the development of high-fat diet (HFD)-induced obese T2D and increases energy expenditure, in turn, associated with hepatic fibroblast growth factor 21 (FGF21) overproduction. The expression of ER stress-related proteins was increased in the liver of HFD-fed LAMP2-deficient mice and it was suggested that ER stress was involved in the hepatic induction of FGF21 (Yasuda-Yamahara et al., 2015). In line with these results, it has been also reported that insufficient autophagosome formation in the liver induced mitochondrial stress, increased ATF4-FGF21 pathway activity, and protected from diet-induced obesity and insulin resistance (Kim et al., 2013).

In the context of metabolic diseases, autophagy is a dynamic process in the liver that changes as a function of time. Experimental studies demonstrate an increased hepatic autophagy activity in HFD-induced obesity and hepatic steatosis. However, the raise of HFD-induced autophagy only lasts a few weeks and in fact, it decreases in chronic obesity due to cellular stress. In this sense, it has been observed that autophagy remains active for 7 weeks under HFD conditions, but disappears after the eighth week (Adkins et al., 2013). These results should be cautiously interpreted. Although in several investigations experimental results may indicate an increased expression of autophagy markers and autophagosome number, in such studies

the role and values of autophagic flux were not appropriately determined (the total process of autophagosome synthesis, substrate delivery, and lysosomal degradation) (Menikdiwela et al., 2020). Thus, it is not possible to ascertain whether such results are completely reliable as evidence of increased autophagic activity.

Several factors may regulate hepatic autophagy in MetS and related disorders. Hepatic ER stress suppresses autophagy in high-fat-fed mice and *ob/ob* mice, and disruption of autophagy function by genetic ablation of Atg proteins can lead to ER stress (Choi et al., 2018). Collectively, these data suggest that hepatic ER stress is directly related to the suppression of autophagy. In genetic and in diet-induced mouse models of obesity, lower levels of hepatic autophagy and increased ER stress with concomitant insulin resistance, appear to follow a pattern. Decreased autophagy led to greater ER stress and insulin resistance in murine hepatocytes (Menikdiwela et al., 2020). ER stress and increased lipogenesis are potential mechanisms accounting for insulin resistance mediated by high fructose feedings. Higher levels of calpain 2 in hepatocytes decrease autophagy in obese models, while its inhibition increases it; melanocortin 3 receptor (MC3R) also regulates hepatic autophagy by possibly acting on transcription factor EB (TFEB) signaling. Another mechanism that decreases hepatic autophagy is via the forkhead box O (FOXO) transcriptional factor. FOXO is a key regulator of vacuolar protein sorting 34 (Vps34) and Atg12, responsible for autophagy initiation. Its activity is suppressed by increased insulin levels and serine-threonine protein kinase Akt (Akt) activation, and hence, autophagy decreases in MetS (Liu et al., 2009). Nutrients and insulin also regulate the autophagy process in the liver, since they are two powerful suppressors of autophagy (Vanhorebeek et al., 2011). Regarding the effects of some nutrients, hepatic autophagy was suppressed in the presence of ER stress after mice were fed high fructose diets for 2–12 h, 2 weeks, as well as in liver explants incubated with fructose medium (Wang H. et al., 2015). Increased secretion of insulin by β-cells decreases hepatic autophagy and promotes insulin resistance in hepatocytes (Quan et al., 2012). In line with this, in MetS hyperinsulinemia up-regulates mammalian target of rapamycin complex 1 (mTORC1) activity and suppresses hepatic autophagy. Concurrently, activated hepatic mTORC1 further phosphorylates the insulin receptor through ribosome S6 protein kinase 1 (S6K1), and this leads to insulin resistance (Wang et al., 2012). As regards hyperglycemia and diabetes, hepatic autophagy comes to play an important role in glucose homeostasis (Wang H.J. et al., 2015). Cryptochrome 1 (CRY1) decreases hepatic glucose production, and its timely removal by autophagy promotes glucose production. Obesity increases CRY1 degradation by autophagy, thus increasing glucose production and circulating blood sugar levels (Toledo et al., 2018).

Whether defective autophagy is cause or consequence of hepatic insulin resistance remains to be determined. This distinction might be pivotal when managing diabetic patients undergoing liver surgery. For instance, if defective autophagy induces insulin resistance, a promising strategy for such patients may be to treat hyperglycemia with short-term intensive insulin therapy, since autophagy is already defective, and this treatment has proven effective in the control of glucose levels (Kramer et al., 2013). However, if an increase in insulin results in decreased hepatic autophagy, insulin therapy may render the liver vulnerable to other stressors. In diabetes conditions, research indicates that there is an upregulation of autophagy and therefore, a decrease in autophagy could be useful in hepatic glucose homeostasis regulation, and to a certain extent, prevent the development of diabetes and its complications. Although these findings contribute to a better understanding of the role of autophagy in the liver affected by diabetes, there is still very little literature on the molecular events underlying hepatic autophagy in diabetic conditions, indicating that more research is required in this regard.

NAFLD

Non-alcoholic fatty liver disease is the most common cause of abnormal liver function and it covers a broad spectrum of liver changes, ranging from simple steatosis to non-alcoholic steatohepatitis (NASH), liver cirrhosis, and hepatocellular carcinoma (Zhang et al., 2018). The prevalence of NAFLD is on the rise throughout the Western world since it is strongly associated with obesity, insulin resistance, MetS, and T2D. In fact, NAFLD is generally considered to be the hepatic manifestation of MetS, and research has confirmed that hepatic lipid accumulation is responsible for hepatic insulin resistance and whole-body insulin resistance. Lee et al. have reported that obese adolescents with fatty liver are at greater risk of developing systemic insulin resistance than those with a healthy liver (Lee et al., 2015). Thus, NAFLD has become a major public health issue, with potentially serious consequences (Parafati et al., 2015). In this sense, NAFLD is rapidly becoming the leading indication for liver transplantation (Zhang et al., 2018).

A consensus has been reached, suggesting that autophagy plays a crucial role in the pathogenesis of NAFLD, and in fact, several studies have indicated impaired autophagy (Samala et al., 2017). Autophagy is inhibited in the livers of NAFLD and NASH murine models. Furthermore, enhancing autophagy by overexpressing Atg7, improved hepatic steatosis in ob/ob mice and mice fed a HFD (Gong et al., 2016). Increased levels of LC3-II and p62 reflect a defect in the autophagic flux (a failure in the clearance of autophagosomes), and this has been observed in the liver of C57BL/6 mice when fed a HFD. Similar results have been reported in mice fed a methionine/choline-deficient (MCD) diet that is usually used to induce NASH (Wang et al., 2018). Also, autophagy markers, LC3-II and p62, were impaired in the liver of genetically leptin-deficient ob/ob mice that are obese and insulin resistant, and that develop NAFLD like that observed in humans (Yang et al., 2010). The presented body of evidence suggests that under these conditions, clearance of autophagosomes is impaired. In NAFLD and NASH patients, p62 and LC3-II levels are increased and reflect autophagic flux impairment in the diseased livers (González-Rodríguez et al., 2014). Regardless, normal p62 values have also been reported in NAFLD and NASH patient livers (Lee et al., 2017). This issue remains a controversial subject. In the context of these metabolic diseases, a deficient autophagic flux is related to lysosome dysfunction. Autolysosome acidification is critical to the degradation of

autophagosomal cargos for the maintenance of autophagic flux. In NASH, the precursor form of cathepsin D, an enzyme cleaved to its mature form upon acidification and involved in lysosome-dependent proteolysis, showed accumulation. In addition, the number of acidic lysosomes was reduced in steatotic hepatocytes. These events could be associated with the increased synthesis of asparagine by asparagine synthetase (ASNS). Expression of ASNS was elevated in steatohepatitis and knockdown of ASNS restored autophagic flux in MCD medium–cultured hepatocyte cell lines, as evidenced by the decreased accumulation of p62. As well, asparagine exposure in hepatocytes directly inhibited lysosome acidification, as evidenced by the failed cleavage of procathepsin D to its mature form, and the reduced number of acidic autolysosomes (Wang et al., 2018). In addition, to defects in acidification of lysosomes, other causes of lysosomal dysfunction related to worsened autophagic flux have been described in NAFLD-NASH. Chemokine (C-X-C motif) receptor 3 (CXCR3) inhibited autophagic flux in steatohepatitis since ablation of CXCR3 reduced p62 and LC3-II accumulation and ameliorated steatohepatitis. In this context, CXCR3 induced LAMP1 and LAMP2, which are membrane proteins crucial in autophagosome-lysosome fusion and proteolytic activity, indicating lysosome storage disorder (Zhang et al., 2016). According to what happens in other diseases, upregulation of LAMP might suggest an increase in the overall lysosomal mass that could be interpreted as an attempt to counteract lysosomal dysfunction (Houben et al., 2017). Last but not least, an increment in intracellular lipids, as occurs in NAFLD-NASH, altered the intracellular membrane lipid composition of both autophagosomes and lysosomes. This reduced the ability of autophagosomes to fuse with lysosomes and led to a decrease in autophagic flux (Koga et al., 2010).

Hepatic ER stress and autophagy dysfunction increase with the onset of NAFLD in patients and dietary-induced obese models, whereas suppressing ER stress and activating autophagy ameliorate high-fat-induced hepatocyte apoptosis (Wang H. et al., 2015). NAFLD development requires additional diverse signaling pathways and mediators. In steatotic livers, autophagy is mainly regulated by the AMPK-mTOR and silencing information regulator 1 (Sirt1)-FOXO pathways, which are activated by increased adenosine diphosphate (ADP)/adenosine triphosphate (ATP) ratios and nicotinamide adenine dinucleotide (NAD +), respectively (**Figure 1**). Several studies suggest that AMPK activation or Sirt1 induction restore impaired autophagy and ameliorate hepatic lipid accumulation (Huang et al., 2017). The TFEB is another autophagy regulator that positively modulates lipid catabolism, as a result of the direct induction of the "coordinated lysosomal expression and regulation" (CLEAR) network, which includes genes that control autophagy, lysosome biogenesis, and lipolysis (Wang Z. et al., 2017). Interestingly, TFEB overexpression in mice in which autophagy was genetically suppressed by deletion of hepatic Atg7, did not preclude the development of or decrease fatty infiltration in hepatic steatosis, suggesting that the effects of TFEB on lipid metabolism require a functional autophagic pathway (Settembre et al., 2013). The induction of autophagy is dependent upon nutrient conditions, whereby in nutrient-rich conditions,

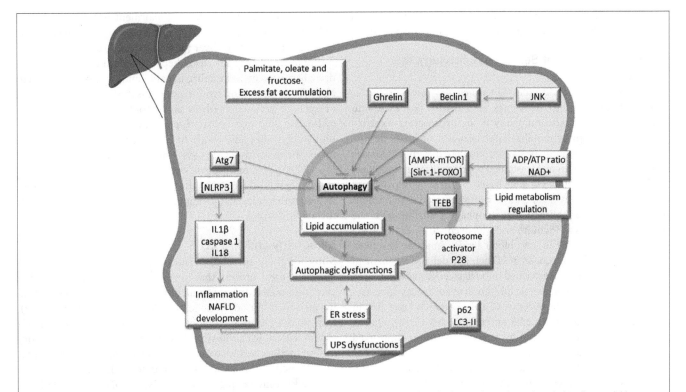

FIGURE 1 | Autophagy signaling pathway in steatotic liver. Atg7, Beclin1, LC3-II, and p62 has been described as markers of autophagy in fatty liver, and this process is regulated by AMPK-mTOR, Sirt1-FOXO, and TFEB. In this type of liver, autophagy is interrelated with UPS, ER stress, JNK, ghrelin, and NLRP3 inflammasome signaling pathways, among others. As a result of interaction between all these mediators, dysfunction in lipid accumulation and inflammation may occurs in steatotic liver. Some diet components such as excess fat, palmitate, oleate or fructose could alter hepatic autophagy in steatotic livers and therefore affect NAFLD progression.

mTOR inhibits the initiation of autophagy. Perhaps as a result of over-nutrition, mTOR signaling is frequently hyperactivated in the livers of obese mice and also suppresses TFEB activity (Singh et al., 2009). Hepatic steatosis improved in HFD-induced NAFLD, after mTOR inhibitor treatment, rapamycin (Gong et al., 2016). Autophagy is also dependent on c-Jun NH(2)-terminal kinase (JNK) whereby JNK activation contributes to Beclin-1 expression and modulates autophagy. Inhibition of JNK suppresses autophagy and decreases insulin resistance in NAFLD (Yan et al., 2017). Different ghrelin isoforms might upregulate autophagy and ameliorate liver disease, as proven in preclinical and clinical studies. It appears that acyl ghrelin up-regulation stimulates hepatic autophagy by suppressing tumor necrosis factor alpha (TNF-α) production via AMPK/mTOR. This protective mechanism leads to NAFLD improvement (Chorny et al., 2008). However, in experimental acute hepatitis and liver fibrosis, ghrelin administration decreases hepatic autophagy (Mao et al., 2015). These different ghrelin effects may result from differences in experimental conditions, drug doses, and cellular physiological states.

Dietary nutrients could affect autophagy in the liver and consequently regulate NAFLD progression. Under starvation, active autophagy leads to lipolysis and free FA production, providing additional energy sources. In conditions of excessive fat accumulation in the liver, autophagy is downregulated, leading to an additional increase in lipid accumulation in the liver, as it is observed in the liver of mice fed a HFD (Samala et al., 2017). Palmitate (one of the most abundant FA in the plasma of humans and rodents) is poorly converted into triglyceride-enriched lipid droplets (LD), and inhibits autophagy by inducing the caspase-dependent cleavage of Beclin1; its presence also induces a degree of lipid-induced apoptosis (lipoapoptosis) in hepatocytes (Ricchi et al., 2009). On the other hand, monounsaturated FA, such as oleate, stimulate the formation of triglyceride-enriched LD and induce autophagy but hardly affects lipoapoptosis. The formation of LD and the induction of autophagy are known to be protective mechanisms against saturated FA-induced lipotoxicity (Mei et al., 2011). These data indicate that not only excessive nutrition per se but also diet composition, are crucial factors fomenting NAFLD. Long-lasting intake of certain nutrients can also modulate hepatic autophagy. After 4 weeks of consuming a HFD, autophagy was activated to protect hepatocytes from lipotoxicity; further, apoptosis was activated after a HFD intake for 8 weeks, and autophagy initiation was suppressed. After 16 weeks on the HFD, an increase in the LC3II/LC3I ratio was demonstrated, suggesting that functional autophagy was disrupted after HFD consumption lasting more than 8 weeks (Hsu et al., 2016). A high fructose diet also suppresses liver autophagy and appears to be mediated by the activation of mTOR. High fructose-induced suppression of autophagy may cause ER stress, and the resulting changes in JNK/inhibitor of NF-κB kinase (IKK) and insulin signaling cascades. When autophagy is restored with pharmacological agents, ER stress is improved and all associated injurious events caused by a high fructose diet are corrected (Wang H. et al., 2015).

Lipophagy, a Form of Selective Autophagy, Is Significant in NAFLD

Lipophagy selectively degrades LD which are incorporated in vesicles, transported to lysosomes, and finally degraded into FA. This lipid degradation pathway in hepatocytes explains their ability to rapidly mobilize large amounts of lipids despite low levels of cytosolic lipases when compared with adipocytes (Zhang et al., 2018). In fact, sustained abnormalities in lipophagy in hepatocytes might be the basis of liver steatosis and steatohepatitis (Schott et al., 2019). Continuing studies in humans or animals have established that lipophagy contributes to the NAFLD development (Schulze and McNiven, 2014; Xiong et al., 2016; Chen et al., 2017b). As blood lipids infiltrate the liver, upregulation of the biogenesis of LD acts as a defense mechanism against toxic FA that are esterified into triglycerides and stored in LD. Pharmacological or genetic inhibition of autophagy increases triglyceride and cholesterol contents, and LD number and size, in hepatocytes treated with free FA and in mice fed a HFD. On the opposite, enhancing autophagy by Atg7 overexpression improved hepatic steatosis and insulin resistance in ob/ob mice and mice fed a HFD (Jeong Kim et al., 2017). Thus, this emerging evidence points that lipophagy could be a therapeutic target in NAFLD.

In the liver, lipophagy is mediated by complex transcriptional regulators of autophagy genes and is inhibited by the insulin and amino acid-mTOR signaling pathway via short- and long-term regulation mechanisms. Short-term inhibition is dependent on the mTOR complex, while long-term regulation is mediated by the transcription factors FOXO and TFEB (Stayrook et al., 2005; Oberkofler et al., 2010). Insulin receptor activation induces *de novo* lipogenesis and prevents autophagy-mediated LD degradation (Bechmann et al., 2012). Other regulators of lipophagy in the liver have been described. Oxidative stress appears to affect lipophagy, in fact, LD accumulated more readily in the liver in SOD1-knockout mice compared with the wild-type mouse, under fasting conditions. Lipophagy was abolished by oxidative stress, and lipoprotein secretion was suppressed in superoxide dismutase (SOD)1 deficiency, ultimately leading to LD accumulation (Kurahashi et al., 2015). Further, ROS increases perilipin 2 (PLIN2), which induces LD accumulation by blocking autophagy and negatively affecting droplet breakdown (Jin et al., 2018). Therefore, hepatic autophagy induction might modulate LD accumulation and ROS generation. Immunity-related guanosine triphosphatase family M (IRGM) is another key gene involved in lipophagy regulation, as IRGM knockdown inhibited autophagy and increased LD content in HepG2 and PLC/PRF/5 cells, and this process could be reversed by rapamycin (Lin et al., 2016). FGF21 can ameliorate NAFLD, partly re-establish insulin sensitivity, and correct several metabolic parameters through lipophagy in HepG2 cells overloaded with lipids (Zhu S. et al., 2016). The run domain beclin-1-interacting and cysteine-rich domain-containing protein (Rubicon) inhibit late-stage autophagy during the autophagosome-lysosome fusion. In livers with impaired Rubicon expression, ER stress and the accumulation of LD

decreased, and also autophagy impairment is attenuated, thus indicating that Rubicon could abolish lipophagy, and hence cause the deposit of LD in the liver (Tanaka et al., 2016).

Enhancing lipophagy clears hepatocellular LD and this could drive to a strategy to mobilize hepatic lipids and prevent human NAFLD. An important issue to ponder is the possible cooperation or synergy between lipolysis and lipophagy in the regulation of hepatic lipid metabolism. Lipophagy may degrade larger LD into smaller droplets, which in turn increases LD surface area upon which cytosolic lipases can exert their action (Zhang et al., 2018). Recognizing lipophagy as an elementary process regulating lipid clearance in the liver enlightens new possibilities to design therapies that promote hepatic lipophagy and improve metabolic diseases.

Mitophagy and NAFLD

Mitochondrial autophagy (mitophagy) is a mitochondrial quality control process that degrades damaged mitochondrion and suppresses their production of ROS that might lead to mitochondrial dysfunction (Adeva-Andany et al., 2019). Hepatic FA accumulation can cause damaged mitochondria accumulation, which in turn, hinders mitochondrial respiratory chain function, and FA oxidative degradation. The accumulation of dysfunctional mitochondria leads to BCL2 and adenovirus E1B 19-kDa-interacting protein 3 (BNIP3)/BNIP3-like (BNIP3L, also known as NIX) (NIX)-mediated mitophagy, clearance of mitochondrial debris, and the reestablishment of mitochondrial function. Phosphatase and tensin homolog (PTEN)-induced putative kinase 1 (PINK1)/Parkin is another molecular mechanism that could be involved in hepatic mitophagy (Sato and Furuya, 2017).

Studies on mitophagy in NAFLD and related metabolic comorbidities are still scarce, however, they show that this molecular pathway could have broad therapeutic possibilities. Impaired mitophagy promotes macrophage infiltration that activates mitogen-activated protein kinase (MAPK) pathway, and causes inflammation, impairing mitochondrial quality control, and fostering the development of insulin resistance and hepatic steatosis. It has been demonstrated that stimulating mitophagy can inhibit hepatic lipid accumulation and temper insulin resistance (Su et al., 2019). In an experimental model of NAFLD, abnormal PINK1/Parkin-dependent mitophagy might be responsible for hepatic FA accumulation and treatments aimed at increasing PINK1/Parkin-mediated mitophagy (as quercetin), accelerated mitochondrial FA oxidation, and suppressed FA accumulation. Quercetin also activated PINK1/Parkin-dependent mitophagy and prevented oleic acid/palmitic acid-induced lipid accumulation in HepG2 cells (Liu et al., 2018). Linseed oil, exenatide, melatonin, akebia saponin D, and sirtuin 3 have also evidenced to reduce hepatic lipid accumulation by enhancing mitophagy (Gong et al., 2018; Li R. et al., 2018; Shao et al., 2018; Zhou et al., 2018; Yu et al., 2019). On the other hand, it also has been described that in advanced NAFLD, mitophagy increases, and mitochondrial mass, mtDNA, and PGC-1α expression are reduced; this combines with compromised ATP production, resulting in a vicious cycle of mitochondrial depletion and liver dysfunction.

This later finding could mean that pharmacological interference with mitophagy molecular mechanisms may lead to therapeutic approaches (Lee et al., 2018). As can be seen, there are still serious controversies about the role of mitophagy in NAFLD that must be resolved in order to design efficient strategies in the treatment of metabolic liver diseases.

Future Directions From the Role of Hepatic Autophagy in Metabolic Liver Diseases

Currently, existing knowledge about the autophagic response in the liver when obesity, MetS, insulin resistance, NAFLD, or diabetes are present, does not allow one to establish if a defect in the capacity of the liver to induce autophagy is the underlying cause for the appearance of such metabolic diseases. Regulation of hepatic autophagy seems to change throughout a metabolic disease, since while in the first weeks of obesity there is an increase in autophagy markers, after a few months autophagy decreases considerably (Adkins et al., 2013). In addition, although most studies suggest that a defect in liver autophagy invariably accompanies obesity, MetS, insulin resistance, and NAFLD, some reports indicate that autophagy could be overactive in diabetes (Yasuda-Yamahara et al., 2015; Choi et al., 2018; Menikdiwela et al., 2020). The need to investigate in more detail the role of autophagy in livers affected by obesity, MetS, insulin resistance, NAFLD, and/or diabetes is evident since this step is crucial for the design of new therapies that can improve the postoperative results of this type of livers when they undergo surgery and are susceptible to being damaged by I/R injury. To achieve this, first, it is important to characterize whether one or more metabolic comorbidities are present in experimental models used at present, seeing that many studies use HFD models to induce and study obesity but do not include results that allow knowing if animal model also exhibits MetS or insulin resistance (Gracia-Sancho et al., 2013; Zaouali et al., 2017; Panisello-Roselló et al., 2018). On the other hand, although there have been multiple versions of consensus within the autophagy community on the use and interpretation of assays for monitoring autophagy (Klionsky et al., 2021), it is notorious that incompliance of investigations to the established guidelines led to a discrepancy in experimental results in hepatic autophagy in the setting of metabolic diseases. For example, while various publications indicate hepatic autophagy enhancement based on results showing high levels of LC3II or Beclin-1, other investigations interpret that the reduction in levels of these parameters means an increase in autophagic activity (Parafati et al., 2015; Gong et al., 2016; Shao et al., 2018; Cui et al., 2020). Therefore, to explain controversies of existing results on hepatic autophagy in obesity, MetS, insulin resistance, NAFLD, or diabetes, it is necessary to adhere to the existing consensus on autophagy parameters, which would permit to have the most appropriate autophagy mediators in the liver to indicate with greater certainty an increase in the formation of autophagosomes and if lysosomal degradation is being carried out properly. Once the role of hepatic autophagy in these pathological conditions is more precisely understood, it will be possible to design therapeutic strategies for livers affected by metabolic diseases and undergoing surgery.

There are many studies regarding the role of autophagy in NAFLD without surgery. In them decreased liver autophagy seems to be a common finding in various experimental models of NAFLD. However, it remains to be clarified whether the reduction in autophagy is the cellular event that results in hepatic steatosis or occurs after the liver has accumulated a significant amount of lipids. It is also unknown whether autophagy changes in the function of different degrees of steatosis. Additionally, although several molecular mechanisms related to autophagy have been described in the steatotic liver, there are controversies about which ones precede autophagy failure and which ones are a consequence of such dysfunction.

Regarding the selective forms of autophagy (lipophagy and mitophagy) in livers affected by metabolic diseases, more research is mandatory. In the case of NAFLD, very few underlying molecular mechanisms for lipophagy and mitophagy have been described, whereby more research is needed in this regard, being of special interest those mediators that could be directly or indirectly related to inflammation, damage, or cell death in the liver. Moreover, given the central role of mitochondrial quality control on lipid degradation and suppression of hepatic lipid accumulation, the active search, and understanding of the signaling pathways involved in lipophagy and mitophagy in metabolic liver diseases, could yield new therapeutic options in the prevention and treatment of insulin resistance, MetS, NAFLD or diabetes in patients requiring liver surgery.

EFFECTS OF METABOLIC SYNDROME AND RELATED DISEASES ON LIVER SURGERY

Non-alcoholic fatty liver disease is the MetS-associated disease whose effects in liver surgery have been studied the most. Numerous studies have established the enormously damaging role of hepatic steatosis in I/R injury in both liver resection and transplantation. Surgical removal remains the only therapy for liver tumors with an elevated risk of failure in steatotic livers. To avoid blood loss during liver resection, portal inflow is temporarily occluded, leading to a warm ischemic period that may provoke relevant liver damage upon reperfusion. Steatosis not only accentuates the liver's susceptibility toward ischemic insults but also hinders its regenerative capacity in terms of both repairing ischemic injury and counteracting for lost volume following resection. Together, these characteristics lead to an increased frequency of postoperative complications that restrain surgical possibilities in patients with fatty liver (Linecker et al., 2017). In addition, NAFLD makes liver grafts too sensitive to cold I/R inherent with transplantation, and thus, steatosis is correlated with a greater risk of graft malfunctioning, and consequently higher postoperative morbidity and mortality in the recipient. Because of so high a percentage of people with NAFLD, many potential donors are not eligible for donations (Forbes and Newsome, 2016). Due to the present epidemic of obesity, the repercussion of hepatic steatosis in the setting of liver surgery is expected to continue to rise (Tashiro et al., 2014).

Considering that steatotic livers tolerate I/R poorly, there is growing comprehension of molecular and cellular mechanisms underpinning the development of I/R injury in patients with fatty livers. These molecular mechanisms of damage are very different from those occurring in healthy livers (not affected by NAFLD) subjected to I/R. In this way, hepatocyte damage is markedly higher in steatotic livers than in non-steatotic ones and contributes to their poor tolerance to I/R (Selzner et al., 2000). Hepatocyte de-regulation has several causes, such as elevated susceptibility to ROS that affects mitochondrial processes and subsequently, ATP synthesis (Caraceni et al., 2005). Moreover, hepatocytes with fatty infiltration develop massive necrosis after I/R injury, rather than apoptosis observed in non-steatotic livers (Fernández et al., 2004). This fact might explicate why caspase inhibition, a protective strategy in non-steatotic livers, has no effects on hepatocyte injury in steatotic livers (Selzner et al., 2000). In experimental models of liver transplantation, exogenous nitric oxide (NO) administration reduce damage in non-steatotic grafts but is useless, or even harmful, in steatotic livers. The deleterious effects of exogenous NO are explained by exaggerated peroxynitrite generation caused by ROS overproduction (Carrasco-Chaumel et al., 2005). Steatotic livers also diverge from non-steatotic grafts in their response to the unfolded protein response (UPR) and ER stress, indeed the expression of inositol-requiring enzyme 1 (IRE1) and protein kinase R (PKR)-like endoplasmic reticulum kinase (PERK) is lower in the presence of steatosis (Ben Mosbah et al., 2010).

A very important aspect that must be contemplated, is that although in both, resection and transplantation, steatosis worsens postoperative outcomes, the signaling pathways underlying hepatic injury are substantially different in each surgical setting, this means, depending on warm or cold I/R occurs. Indeed, in each type of surgery there exist distinct therapeutic targets and therefore, treatments that work in one surgical situation might not function in the other. In accordance, increased adiponectin levels were observed in steatotic livers as a consequence of warm I/R associated with hepatic resection, and then, the treatment with adiponectin small interfering ribonucleic acid (RNA) protected steatotic livers against oxidative stress and hepatic injury (Massip-Salcedo et al., 2008). On the opposite, when subjected to transplantation, steatotic liver grafts exhibited downregulation of adiponectin. Adiponectin pre-treatment protected steatotic grafts activating the phosphoinositide-3 kinase (PI3K)/Akt pathway and unraveling AMPK as an upstream mediator of adiponectin's actions in steatotic grafts (Jiménez-Castro et al., 2013). Similarly, a therapy based on modulating retinol binding protein 4 (RBP4) has proven to impair damage and liver regeneration in steatotic livers in the setting of hepatectomy under warm I/R; whereas the same therapeutical strategy was beneficial in steatotic livers undergoing transplantation (Casillas-Ramírez et al., 2011; Elias-Miró et al., 2012). In addition, warm I/R produced an increase in angiotensin II which injured steatotic livers, and pharmacologic blockers of angiotensin II action, such as angiotensin II receptor antagonists, protected steatotic livers against I/R injury through

enhancement of peroxisome proliferator-activated receptor gamma (PPAR-γ) (Casillas-Ramírez et al., 2008). Interestingly, in liver transplantation, angiotensin II did not play a role in cold I/R in steatotic grafts, and therefore, treatment with angiotensin II receptor antagonists was useless in this type of grafts (Alfany-Fernandez et al., 2009). ER stress has shown to be a useful therapeutic target to reduce ischemic damage in steatotic livers submitted to resection under vascular occlusion (Ben Mosbah et al., 2010) but this did not happen in steatotic liver transplantation (Jiménez-Castro et al., 2012). Cortisol levels in the liver were elevated in steatotic livers undergoing resections (hepatectomy and warm I/R) and such elevations were attributed to a raise in cortisol production, and a decrease in cortisol clearance. Cortisol administration exacerbated tissue damage and regenerative failure, and such injurious effects were linked to high hepatic acetylcholine levels (Cornide-Petronio et al., 2017). Interestingly, although steatotic liver grafts also exhibited increased cortisol after transplantation due to the same causes that in hepatic resection (augment in cortisol generation and diminishment in cortisol clearance), in liver transplantation exogenous administration of cortisol treatment up-regulated the PI3K-protein kinase C (PKC) pathway, resulting in protection against the deleterious effects of brain death on damage and inflammatory response in steatotic liver transplantation (Jiménez-Castro et al., 2017). All these experimental results highlight a different role for several mediators in the regulation of damage in steatotic livers, depending on the type of surgery. This indicates that finding feasible and highly protective therapeutical strategies to reduce the adverse effects of NAFLD on liver surgery entails exhaustive evaluation of potential therapeutic targets and strategies based on its modulation in appropriated experimental models for each surgical setting.

The effects of obesity, insulin resistance, and MetS in liver surgery have not been separately investigated. There are some studies that, considering the experimental model used, one could assume that various metabolic diseases are present, such as NAFLD in combination with MetS, obesity, or insulin resistance; but unfortunately, they report confusing information about the precise diagnosis of such comorbidities. A great milestone for future research on I/R in the liver with metabolic comorbidities in appropriated experimental models would be to include parameters that facilitate the establishment of the presence of concurrent metabolic diseases and the effects of the tested treatments on them.

There are a few studies about the effects of hyperglycemia or diabetes in liver surgery. Hyperglycemia has been shown to worsen hepatic warm I/R injury by inducing hyperinflammatory immune responses through activation of advanced glycation end product (AGE)-receptor for AGE (RAGE) pathway in Kupffer cells (Wang Q. et al., 2020). Several factors may explain the mechanisms underlying the pathological and functional changes in liver injury-induced hyperglycemia, including insulin resistance, inflammation, and oxidative stress. Diabetic animals show the decreased hepatic activity of antioxidant enzymes such as catalase and SOD, thus increasing ROS, which can damage lipids, proteins, desoxyribonucleic acid (DNA), compromise mitochondria or ER function, thus leading to cell homeostasis failure and cell death. Considering that T2D is associated with hepatic lipid accumulation and that lipids are highly susceptible to being damaged by ROS, oxidative stress represents a major issue in liver function in these patients (Gjorgjieva et al., 2019). Pro-inflammatory mediators involved in hyperglycemic liver injury include interleukin (IL)-1 and IL-6, nuclear factor kappa B (NF-kB), MAPK, transforming growth factor (TGF), poly (ADP-ribose) polymerase (PARP), and TNF-α. Indeed, diabetic rat models have confirmed that in the liver, the induction of TNF-α results in increased NF-kB and JNK signaling, nitric oxide production, and apoptosis (Manna et al., 2010; Ingaramo et al., 2011). All these mediators and events occurring during oxidative stress and inflammation are part of the underlying signaling mechanisms in I/R, so when surgery occurs in the presence of hyperglycemia, the production of these mediators would be exacerbated and result in major liver injury. Inflammation and oxidative stress can negatively affect insulin sensitivity. In fact, ROS can inhibit insulin signaling by inducing Insulin Receptor Substrate (IRS) degradation in peripheral tissues, a cause of insulin desensitization (Archuleta et al., 2009). TNF-α has also been shown to induce insulin resistance (Alipourfard et al., 2019).

The negative effects of metabolic diseases in liver surgery have been described at the clinical level, and it has been shown that they can also affect a patient's condition in the medium or long term after surgery. Transoperative stress hyperglycemia is a common clinical finding due to a transient decrease in insulin responsiveness that may persist from days to weeks after major surgery. Patients without established diabetes mellitus and who develop stress hyperglycemia, are at higher risk of poor outcomes, depending on the severity and duration of stress hyperglycemia (Chae et al., 2020). For example, hemi-hepatectomy results in moderate disturbances in glucose homeostasis that are of no clinical relevance. However, early exacerbation of insulin resistance results in a greater risk of developing overt diabetes in the long term (Durczynski et al., 2013). Along the same lines, diabetes negatively impacts the surgical outcome of patients with cirrhosis after liver resection and transplantation, and the stress associated with the post-reperfusion syndrome further increases hyperglycemia and insulin resistance during surgery in recipients with reduced-size liver grafts (Chae et al., 2020). Although the exact mechanisms responsible for these adverse outcomes are not completely elucidated, a probable cause seems to be the increase in I/R injury resulting from the acute hyperglycemic disturbances. As a result, the early post-reperfusion period is critical since significant hepatic insults are inflicted, and graft regeneration is concurrently initiated with metabolic and detoxifying associated phenomena (Kang et al., 2018). Moreover, liver transplantation recipients have been shown to progressively develop MetS in a high proportion despite current efforts to mitigate their evolution (i.e., lifestyle modifications and aggressive management of hypertension, diabetes, and hyperlipidemia). Associated risk factors include age, increased body mass index, and pre- and post-transplantation serum glucose (Vida Perez et al., 2016). Importantly, increased recurrence of NASH and cryptogenic cirrhosis was associated with the presence of concomitant MetS, hypertension, and the

use of insulin. Recurrence should be further evaluated in larger studies, with special emphasis on the management of MetS and prevention strategies (El Atrache et al., 2012). Curtailing the development of postoperative MetS after orthotopic liver transplantation, may decrease readmissions and improve patient and graft outcomes (Chang et al., 2016).

AUTOPHAGY IN LIVER SURGERY IN THE SETTING OF METABOLIC SYNDROME

The majority of research about autophagy in liver surgery has been focused on healthy livers more than on livers affected by MetS or related metabolic diseases. Such investigations have allowed us to distinguish the relevance of autophagy in liver surgery outcomes and a better mechanistic understanding of the autophagy process in resection and transplantation, which makes it possible to conceive new therapeutic options that could be evaluated in livers suffering metabolic diseases and submitted to surgery. In some cases, findings on autophagy in I/R injury in healthy livers have been reflected in the clinical setting. This supports that results in autophagy in liver surgery in the setting of metabolic diseases might be translated from the laboratory toward a possible new clinical therapy. Therefore, this section first discusses the existing knowledge on the role of autophagy in liver surgery without the effect of MetS or related diseases; subsequently, published results regarding the role of autophagy in I/R in livers with MetS and associated diseases are analyzed; and finally, new lines of research that could be approached in the future to improve the results of liver surgery in the setting of metabolic diseases are discussed.

Autophagy in Hepatic I/R Injury

The pathogenic signaling pathways in hepatic I/R have been documented to be different in normothermic vs. cold ischemia, and even in livers in optimal conditions and those with underlying pathological conditions such as steatosis. Then, it is foreseeable that the autophagy process also works differently in I/R injury in livers depending on whether they undergo resection or transplantation. The design of therapeutic strategies based on autophagy modulation to protect livers suffering metabolic disorders and subjected to surgery, largely depends on a clear understanding of the molecular mechanisms of autophagy in liver I/R injury, distinguishing between liver resection and transplantation models.

Autophagy in Warm I/R Injury Associated With Hepatic Resection

Many reports in the literature strongly support a relevant role of autophagy in I/R injury in liver resection. Recent research on this topic has focused on the discovery of novel molecular signaling mechanisms that, in the first instance, are being studied in experimental models with optimal livers (without steatosis or other metabolic comorbidities). **Table 1** summarizes the studies in the literature on autophagy in warm I/R that have been conducted in the last 5 years. As shown, results have been contradictory, since some indicate that increased autophagy protects livers subjected to I/R, while others report that it is the inhibition of autophagic activity that leads to beneficial effects. These findings are most likely due to the different experimental models used, including the different durations of ischemia and/or reperfusion. It is widely known that experimental conditions influence the mechanisms underlying liver I/R, and hence, the results.

Some findings in signaling molecular pathways lately described in warm ischemia are included following. Long-non-coding RNAs (lncRNAs) homeobox (HOX) transcript antisense RNA (HOTAIR), regulated autophagy via the microRNA (miR)-20b-5p/ATG7 axis in I/R injury in mice subjected to partial hepatic ischemia (Tang et al., 2019). HOTAIR and ATG7 expression levels increased as did autophagy during I/R injury, while the knockdown of HOTAIR expression attenuated autophagy in isolated hepatocytes (Tang et al., 2019). During experimental hepatic I/R injury, the master transcription factor Interferon Regulatory Factor (IRF1) was upregulated and associated with activation of autophagic signaling (Yu et al., 2017). IRF1 also inhibited β-catenin expression in livers subjected to I/R injury, it activated autophagy and worsened hepatic injury (Yan et al., 2020). MicroRNA refers to a highly conserved, small, non-coded RNA, associated with basic cellular processes, such as apoptosis, proliferation, and stress responses. MicroRNAs have been shown to also play a role in autophagy regulation. *In vivo* and *in vitro* miR-30b levels are down-regulated after hepatic I/R injury, and simultaneously, activate autophagy. High levels of miR-17 upregulate autophagy and worsen hepatic I/R injury by suppressing Stat3 expression *in vitro* (Li et al., 2016). Interestingly, mitophagy is involved in warm hepatic ischemia, and some molecular mediators related to this process are the following: (a) Parkin expression and mitochondrial autophagy are up-regulated after I/R injury (Ning et al., 2018); (b) PINK1 (a mediator of mitophagy) protected against hepatic I/R injury by preventing nucleotide-binding oligomerization domain (NOD)-like receptor (NLR) family pyrin domain containing 3 (NLRP3) inflammasome activation in mice subjected to partial warm I/R (Xu et al., 2020), and (c) miR-330-3p suppresses phosphoglycerate mutase family member 5 (PGAM5)-induced mitophagy to dampen hepatic I/R injury (Sun et al., 2019).

Autophagy in Cold I/R Injury Inherent to Liver Transplantation

Table 2 summarizes the studies evaluating the role of autophagy in liver transplantation. In optimal liver transplantation models subjected to various cold storage times, a slight increase or no change in autophagy parameters are usually observed as a result of ischemic insult. The various strategies that have been used to increase autophagy activity have proven to be beneficial in decreasing liver injury and cell death (Pantazi et al., 2015; Nakamura et al., 2018, 2019; Wang J. et al., 2020). Only one study revealed that pharmacological inhibition of autophagy protected optimal grafts undergoing transplantation (Gotoh et al., 2009). However, it should be noted that in this study, the autophagy and liver injury parameters were evaluated after very short reperfusion periods (15 or 120 min) in comparison with the rest of the studies (6 to 24 h). In

studies using allogeneic optimal liver grafts (Lewis rat donor and Norway rat recipient), there are disagreements. In a study based on transplantation with a small-size liver graft, a discrete increase in some autophagy parameters was detected, and the grafts were protected by increasing autophagic activity through cell therapy combined with gene overexpression; this led to a decrease in the rejection rate. In another study, benefits for graft viability (reduction of injury and graft rejection) were obtained by administering drugs to inhibit autophagy (Wang R. R. et al., 2017; Chen et al., 2019b). In these cases, the main difference that could explain the contradictory results was the decrease in the liver graft size in one of the models. Small grafts are known to exhibit a much greater hepatic regeneration response than whole-size grafts (González et al., 2010). Perhaps, mechanisms underlying regeneration may influence other signaling pathways including autophagy; therefore, autophagy modulation in small-size transplants might induce different effects on liver injury than in whole-size transplants.

Investigations about the role of autophagy in clinical liver transplantation are very limited. Research conducted to date, indicates that in optimal and steatotic transplantation, there is usually a slight expression of autophagy markers (Degli Esposti et al., 2011; Ricca et al., 2015; Nakamura et al., 2018, 2019; Chen et al., 2019b). It is important to note that in steatotic grafts, published reports do not specify whether the donors presented any metabolic comorbidity such as insulin resistance or the MetS. Although no strategy to directly regulate autophagy has been applied yet in clinical practice, results suggest that steatotic and non-steatotic transplanted liver grafts may benefit from strategies promoting autophagy, such as ischemic postconditioning, ischemic preconditioning, and recipient treatment with antibiotics to modulate gut microbiota (Degli Esposti et al., 2011; Ricca et al., 2015). This indicates that the mechanisms underlying I/R injury and associated with autophagy that have been described at the experimental level, also seem to occur at the clinical level. It encourages the study of new experimental strategies that are capable of modulating autophagy to improve postsurgical outcomes in steatotic liver grafts that are also compromised by metabolic comorbidities, and that later can be translated to clinical practice.

Autophagy in Livers Affected by Metabolic Diseases and Undergoing Surgery

To date, there are only studies on autophagy involvement in liver surgery in the setting of NAFLD or hyperglycemia. However, findings described in the present review make it highly feasible that autophagy is also playing a crucial role in the damage of livers affected by the other metabolic diseases and that are submitted to surgery. As will be seen below, reports remain very limited and denote a huge area of opportunity in the field of liver surgery with underlying pathological conditions.

Experimentally, modulation of autophagy through various strategies protects livers affected by NAFLD and subjected to I/R intrinsic to resections. Lithium chloride-induced autophagy via modulating both glycogen synthase kinase 3 beta (GSK3b)

TABLE 1 | Outcomes about the role of autophagy in normothermic hepatic I/R injury, in the last 5 years.

Study	Animal species	Type of liver	Ischemia time	Reperfusion time	Parameters of autophagy in normothermic ischemia without modulation	Modulation of autophagy	Results from autophagy modulation vs. untreated groups
Lee et al., 2016	Hepatocytes from AML12 cell line	Optimal	1 h	0, 1, 3, 5, and 24 h	Autophagy parameters vs. Control group: ↓LC3 I to LC3II conversion, ↓Atg5. ↑mTOR phosphorylated.	Yes. Everolimus.	Autophagy enhancement: ↑LC3 I to LC3 II conversion, ↓p62. Cell injury: ↓Apoptosis.
Biel et al., 2016	C57BL/6 mice primary hepatocytes	Optimal	4 h	1 and 2 h	Autophagic parameters vs. Control group: Mild ↑LC3 I to LC3 II conversion. No expression of SIRT1	Yes. SIRT1 overexpression	Autophagy enhancement: ↑LC3 I to LC3 II conversion, ↑Autophagosomes number. ↑Mitophagy: Improved mitochondria structure and function. Cell injury: ↓Cell death percentage.
Xu D. et al., 2017	C57BL/6 mice primary hepatocytes	Optimal	4 h	2 h	Autophagy parameters vs. Control group: Mild ↑LC3 I to LC3 II conversion, mild ↑SQSTM1. ↑Autophagosomes number.	Yes. CDDO imidazole, a Nrf2 activator.	Autophagy enhancement: ↑LC3 I to LC3 II conversion, ↑Autophagosomes number, ↓SQSTM1. ↓Mitochondrial dysfunction. Cell injury: ↓Cytotoxicity percentage, ↓Apoptosis.
Khader et al., 2017	H4IIE hepatoma cells and Sprague-Dawley rat primary hepatocytes	Optimal	4 and 6 h	2, 4, and 24 h	Autophagy parameters vs. Control group: ↓LC3 I to LC3 II conversion.	Yes. SRT1720, a SIRT1 activator.	Autophagy enhancement: ↑LC3 I to LC3 II conversion, ↓SQSTM1. ↓Mitochondrial dysfunction. Cell injury: ↑Cell survival.
Cui et al., 2018	Hepatocytes from AML12 cell line	Optimal	90 min	12 h	Autophagy parameters: Notable LC3 and Beclin-1 expression.	Yes. Interferon regulatory factor-1 siRNA or Glycyrrhizin Acid, an HMGB1 inhibitor.	Autophagy inhibition: ↓LC3 and ↓Beclin-1 expression.
Kong et al., 2019	C57BL/6 mice primary hepatocytes	Optimal	4 h	2 h	Autophagy parameters: Mild LC3 I to LC3 II conversion and ATG5 expression. Notable expression of mTOR phosphorylated.	Yes. SB216763, inhibitor of GSK3β.	Autophagy enhancement: ↑LC3 I to LC3 II conversion, ↑ATG5. ↓mTOR phosphorylated. Cell injury: ↓Cytotoxicity percentage.
Li J. et al., 2020	C57BL/6 mice primary hepatocytes	Optimal	Not specified.	Not specified.	Autophagy parameters vs. Sham group: ↓ LC3 I to LC3 II conversion, ↓ATG7.	Yes. CD5-like (CD5L) protein, an apoptosis inhibitor of macrophage.	Autophagy enhancement: ↑LC3 I to LC3 II conversion, ↑ATG7. Cell injury: ↓Apoptosis, ↓Oxidative stress.
Bi et al., 2020	Sprague-Dawley rat primary hepatocytes	Aged hepatocytes	1 h	8 h	Autophagy parameters vs. Control old group: Mild ↑LC3 I to LC3 II conversion and mild ↓p62.	Yes. Irisin.	Autophagy enhancement: ↑LC3 I to LC3 II conversion, ↓p62.

(Continued)

TABLE 1 | Continued

Study	Animal species	Type of liver	Ischemia time	Reperfusion time	Parameters of autophagy in normothermic ischemia without modulation	Modulation of autophagy	Results from autophagy modulation vs. untreated groups
Lee et al., 2016	BALB/c mice.	Optimal	Partial normothermic ischemia (right lateral lobe). 45 min	24 h	Autophagy parameters vs. Sham group: ↓LC3B, mild ↑p62.	Yes. Everolimus.	Autophagy enhancement: ↑ LC3B, ↓p62. Liver damage: ↓ALT and AST, ↓Necrosis, ↓Apoptosis, ↓Inflammation.
Li M. et al., 2018	C57BL/6 mice	Optimal	Partial normothermic ischemia (right lateral lobe). 90 min	6 and 12 h	Autophagy parameters vs. Sham group: No changes in LC3 I to LC3II conversion or autophagosomes number, mild ↑p62.	Yes. Alda-1, an activator of ALDH2.	Autophagy enhancement: ↑LC3 I to LC3 II conversion, ↑Autophagosomes number, ↓p62. Liver damage: ↓ALT and AST, ↓Necrosis, ↓Apoptosis, ↓Inflammation, ↓Oxidative stress.
Xiang et al., 2020	Balb/c mice	Optimal	Partial normothermic ischemia of 70% (left and middle Lobes). 1 h	2, 8, and 24 h	Autophagy parameters vs. Sham group: ↑Beclin-1, ↑LC3-II, ↓p62.	Yes. Bergenin.	Autophagy inhibition: ↓Beclin-1, ↓LC3-II, ↑p62. Liver damage: ↓ALT and AST, ↓Necrosis, ↓Apoptosis, ↓Inflammation, ↓Oxidative stress.
Ji et al., 2020	BALB/c mice	Optimal	Partial normothermic ischemia of 70% (left and middle lobes). 45 min	2, 8, and 24 h	Autophagy parameters vs. Sham group: ↑Beclin-1, ↑LC3, ↓p62.	Yes. Cafestol, a natural diterpene extract from coffee beans.	Autophagy inhibition: ↓Beclin-1, ↓LC3, ↑p62. Liver damage: ↓ALT and AST, ↓Necrosis, ↓Apoptosis, ↓Inflammation.
Tan et al., 2018	C57BL/6 mice	Optimal	Partial normothermic ischemia of 70% (left and middle lobes). 1 h	6 h	Autophagy parameters: Mild LC3 I to LC3 II conversion and Beclin-1 expression. Low number of autophagosomes. Notable expression of phosphorylated mTOR.	Yes. Helix B surface peptide, an erythropoietin-derived peptide.	Autophagy enhancement: ↑LC3 I to LC3 II conversion, ↑Beclin-1, ↑Autophagosomes number. Liver damage: ↓ALT and AST, ↓Necrosis, ↓Apoptosis.
Li H. et al., 2020	Sprague-Dawley rats	Optimal	Partial normothermic ischemia of 70% (left and middle lobes). 45 min	6 h	Autophagy parameters vs. Sham group: ↑LC3, ↑Beclin-1, ↑ATG-7, ↓p62. Affected mitochondrial structure.	Yes. N-acetyl-L-tryptophan, a ROS scavenger.	Autophagy inhibition: ↓LC3, ↓Beclin-1, ↓ATG-7, ↑p62. ↓Mitophagy: Improved mitochondria morphology.
Kong et al., 2019	C57BL/6 mice	Optimal	Partial normothermic ischemia (cephalad lobes). 90 min	6 h	Autophagy parameters vs. Sham group: ↑LC3 I to LC3 II conversion, ↑ATG5, ↑Autophagosomes number. ↑mTOR phosphorylation.	Yes. SB216763, an inhibitor of GSK3β.	Autophagy enhancement: ↑LC3 I to LC3 II conversion, ↑ATG5, ↑Autophagosomes number. ↓ mTOR phosphorylated. Liver damage: ↓ALT and AST, ↓Necrosis, ↓Apoptosis.

(Continued)

TABLE 1 | Continued

Study	Animal species	Type of liver	Ischemia time	Reperfusion time	Parameters of autophagy in normothermic ischemia without modulation	Modulation of autophagy	Results from autophagy modulation vs. untreated groups
Wu et al., 2017	Balb/c mice	Optimal	Partial normothermic ischemia of 70% (left and middle lobes). 45 min	2, 8, and 24 h	Autophagy parameters vs. Sham group: ↑Beclin-1, ↑LC3, ↓p62.	Yes. Quercetin.	Autophagy inhibition: ↓Beclin-1, ↓LC3, ↑p62. Liver damage: ↓ALT and AST, ↓Necrosis, ↓Apoptosis, ↓Inflammation.
Biel et al., 2016	C57BL/6 mice	Optimal	Total hepatic ischemia. 45 min	20 min	Autophagy parameters vs. Control group: ↓LC3 I to LC3 II conversion. ↓SIRT1	Yes. SIRT1 overexpression	Autophagy enhancement: ↑LC3 I to LC3 II conversion. ↑Mitophagy: Improved mitochondria function.
Liu et al., 2020	Sprague-Dawley rats	Optimal	Partial normothermic ischemia of 70% (left and middle lobes). 1 h	6 and 24 h	Autophagy parameters vs. Sham group: ↓LC3 I to LC3 II conversion, ↓ATG7, ↑p62. ↑mTOR phosphorylated.	Yes. Alda-1, an activator of ALDH2.	Autophagy enhancement: ↑LC3 I to LC3 II conversion, ↑ATG7, ↓p62. ↓mTOR phosphorylated Liver damage: ↓ALT and AST, ↓Necrosis, ↓Apoptosis, ↓Inflammation, ↓Oxidative stress.
Yang et al., 2015	C57BL/6 mice	Optimal	Partial normothermic ischemia of 70% (left and middle lobes). 1 h	6 h	Autophagy parameters vs. Sham group: Mild ↑LC3I to LC3II conversion, mild ↑Beclin-1, mild ↑ATG7 and mild ↑Autophagic vacuoles.	Yes. Vitamin D	Autophagy enhancement: ↑LC3 I to LC3 II conversion, ↑Beclin-1, ↑ATG7, ↑autophagic vacuoles. Liver damage: ↓ALT and AST, ↓Necrosis, ↓Apoptosis, ↓Inflammation, ↓Oxidative stress.
Chen et al., 2017a	Balb/c mice	Optimal	Partial normothermic ischemia of 70% (left and middle lobes). 1 h	6, 12, and 24 h	Autophagy parameters vs. Sham group: ↑LC3I to LC3II conversion, ↑Beclin-1.	Yes. 15-Deoxy-Δ12,14-prostaglandin J2, a dehydration product of prostaglandin D2.	Autophagy inhibition: ↓LC3 I to LC3 II conversion, ↓Beclin-1. Liver damage: ↓ALT and AST, ↓Necrosis, ↓Apoptosis, ↓Inflammation, ↓Oxidative stress.
Feng et al., 2017	Balb/c mice	Optimal	Type of normothermic ischemia not specified. 45 min	2, 8, and 24 h	Autophagy parameters vs. Sham group: ↑LC3 I to LC3 II conversion, ↑Beclin-1, ↓p62, ↑Autophagosomes formation. ↓mTOR phosphorylated	Yes. Salidroside, main active component of *Rhodiola rosea*.	Autophagy inhibition: ↓LC3 I to LC3 II conversion, ↓Beclin-1, ↑p62, ↓Autophagosomes formation. ↑mTOR phosphorylated Liver damage: ↓ALT and AST, ↓Necrosis, ↓Apoptosis, ↓Inflammation.
Deng et al., 2018	Balb/c mice	Optimal	Partial normothermic ischemia of 70% (ischemic lobes not specified). 45 min	2, 8, and 24 h	Autophagy parameters vs. Sham group: ↑LC3 I to LC3 II conversion, ↑Beclin-1, ↓p62.	Yes. Beraprost sodium, an analog of prostacyclin.	Autophagy inhibition: ↓LC3 I to LC3 II conversion, ↓Beclin-1, ↑p62. Liver damage: ↓ALT and AST, ↓Necrosis, ↓Apoptosis, ↓Inflammation.

(Continued)

TABLE 1 | Continued

Study	Animal species	Type of liver	Ischemia time	Reperfusion time	Parameters of autophagy in normothermic ischemia without modulation	Modulation of autophagy	Results from autophagy modulation vs. untreated groups
Cui et al., 2018	C57BL/6 mice	Optimal	Partial normothermic ischemia of 70% (left and middle lobes). 90 min	2, 6, 12, and 24 h	Autophagy parameters vs. Sham group: ↑LC3 I to LC3 II conversion, ↑Autophagosomes number.	Yes. Knockout of Interferon regulatory factor-1.	Autophagy inhibition: ↓LC3 I to LC3 II conversion, ↓Autophagosomes number. Liver damage: ↓ALT and AST, ↓Necrosis.
Kou et al., 2020	Sprague Dawley rats	Optimal	Partial normothermic ischemia of 70% (left and middle lobes). 90 min	6 h	Autophagy parameters vs. Sham group: ↑LC3 I to LC3 II conversion, ↑Beclin-1.	Yes. Glycyrrhizin, an HMGB1 inhibitor.	Autophagy inhibition: ↓LC3 I to LC3 II conversion, ↓Beclin-1. Liver damage: ↓ALT and AST, ↓Necrosis, ↓Apoptosis, ↑NO, ↓Endothelin-1, ↓Inflammation, ↓Oxidative stress.
Yu et al., 2019	BALB/c mice	Optimal	Partial normothermic ischemia of 70% (ischemic lobes not specified). 45 min	2, 8, and 24 h	Autophagy parameters vs. Sham group: ↑LC3 and ↑Beclin-1.	Yes. Levo-tetrahydropalmatine (L-THP), an active component of *Corydalis yanhusuo*.	Autophagy inhibition: ↓LC3, ↓Beclin-1. Liver damage: ↓ALT and AST, ↓Necrosis, ↓Apoptosis, ↓Inflammation.
Dusabimana et al., 2019)	C57BL/6 mice	Optimal	Partial normothermic ischemia of 70% (left and middle lobes). 1 h	5 h	Autophagy parameters vs. Sham group: No changes in LC3 I to LC3 II conversion or ATG5. ↓ATG12, ↑p62. ↓SIRT1/FOXO3a	Yes. Nobiletin, a natural flavonoid.	Autophagy enhancement: ↑LC3 I to LC3 II conversion, ↑ATG5, ↑ATG12, ↓p62. ↑SIRT1/FOXO3a Liver damage: ↓ALT and AST, ↓Necrosis, ↓Apoptosis, ↓Inflammation, ↓Oxidative stress.
Xu D. et al., 2017	C57BL/6 mice	Optimal	Partial normothermic ischemia of 70% (cephalad lobes). 90 min	6 and 12 h	Autophagy parameters vs. Sham group: Mild ↑LC3 I to LC3 II conversion, ↑Autophagosomes number, ↑SQSTM1.	Yes. CDDO imidazole, a Nrf2 activator.	Autophagy enhancement: ↑LC3 I to LC3 II conversion, ↑Autophagosomes number, ↓SQSTM1. Liver damage: ↓ALT and AST, ↓Necrosis, ↓Apoptosis, ↓Inflammation, ↓Oxidative stress.
Wang et al., 2019	BALB/c mice	Optimal	Partial normothermic ischemia of 70% (left and middle lobes). 1 h	2, 8, and 24 h	Autophagy parameters vs. Sham group: ↑LC3 I to LC3 II conversion, ↑Beclin-1.	Yes. Oleanolic Acid.	Autophagy inhibition: ↓LC3 I to LC3 II conversion, ↓Beclin-1. Liver damage: ↓ALT and AST, ↓Necrosis, ↓Apoptosis.
Xu S. et al., 2017	Balb/c mice	Optimal	Partial normothermic ischemia of 70% (ischemic lobes not specified). 45 min	2, 8, and 24 h	Autophagy parameters vs. Sham group: ↑LC3 II, ↑Beclin-1, ↓p62.	Yes. Propylene glycol alginate sodium sulfate, a polysaccharide isolated from brown algae.	Autophagy inhibition: ↓LC3 II, ↓Beclin-1, ↑p62. Liver damage: ↓ALT and AST, ↓Necrosis, ↓Apoptosis, ↓Inflammation.

(Continued)

TABLE 1 | Continued

Study	Animal species	Type of liver	Ischemia time	Reperfusion time	Parameters of autophagy in normothermic ischemia without modulation	Modulation of autophagy	Results from autophagy modulation vs. untreated groups
Liu H. et al., 2019	C57BL/6 mice	Optimal	Partial normothermic ischemia of 70% (left and middle lobes). 1 h	8, 12, and 24 h	Autophagy parameters vs. Sham group: Mild ↑LC3 I to LC3 II conversion, mild ↑Beclin-1 and mild ↑Autophagic vacuoles number. Mild ↑AMPK phosphorylated, Mild ↑ULK-1 phosphorylated. ↑mTOR phosphorylated.	Yes. Spermidine	Autophagy enhancement: ↑LC3 I to LC3 II conversion, ↑Beclin-1, ↑Autophagic vacuoles number. ↑ULK-1 phosphorylated, ↓mTOR phosphorylated. Liver damage: ↓ALT and AST, ↓Necrosis, ↓Apoptosis, ↓Inflammation.
Li J. et al., 2017	BALB/C mice	Optimal	Partial normothermic ischemia of 70% (left and middle lobes). 1 h	2, 8, and 24 h	Autophagy parameters vs. Sham group: ↑LC3 I to LC3 II conversion, ↑Beclin-1, ↓p62, ↑Autophagosomes and Autolysosomes number.	Yes. Fucoidan.	Autophagy inhibition: ↓LC3 I to LC3 II conversion, ↓Beclin-1, ↑p62, ↓Autophagosomes and Autolysosomes number. Liver damage: ↓ALT and AST, ↓Necrosis, ↓Apoptosis, ↓Inflammation.
Miyauchi et al., 2019	C57BL/6 mice	Optimal	Partial normothermic ischemia of 70% (left and middle lobes). 1 h	1, 3, and 6 h	Autophagy parameters: Mild LC3B expression. Mild FOXO1/3 expression.	Yes. 12-h fasting β-hydroxybutyric acid	Autophagy enhancement: ↑LC3B ↑FOXO1/3 Liver damage: ↓ALT, ↓Necrosis, ↓Apoptosis, ↓Inflammation, ↓Oxidative stress.
Bai et al., 2018	Bama miniature pigs.	Optimal	Partial normothermic ischemia combined with partial resection. Ischemia time: 1 h	3 h, 1 and 3 days	Autophagy parameters vs. Sham group: ↑LC3B, ↑Beclin-1 ↓p62. ↓mTOR	Yes. Hydrogen-rich saline.	Autophagy inhibition: ↓LC3B, ↓Beclin-1, ↑p62. ↑mTOR Liver damage: ↓ALT and AST, ↓Oxidative stress.
Khader et al., 2017	C57BL/6 mice	Optimal	Partial normothermic ischemia of 70% (left and middle lobes). 1 h	24 h	Autophagy parameters vs. Control group: No changes in LC3 I to LC3 II conversion or SQSTM1.	Yes. SRT1720, a SIRT1 activator.	Autophagy enhancement: ↑LC3 I to LC3 II conversion, ↓SQSTM1. Liver damage: ↓ALT and AST, ↓Necrosis, ↓Apoptosis, ↓Inflammation, ↓Oxidative stress.
Jiang et al., 2019	C57BL/6 mice	Aged livers	Partial normothermic ischemia of 70% (cephalad lobes). 90 min	6 h	Autophagy parameters vs. Sham group: ↓ LC3 I to LC3 II conversion and ↑p62.	Yes. Ischemic preconditioning combined with Rapamycin.	Autophagy enhancement: ↑LC3 I to LC3 II conversion, ↓p62. Liver damage: ↓ALT, ↓Necrosis, ↓Apoptosis

(Continued)

TABLE 1 | Continued

Study	Animal species	Type of liver	Ischemia time	Reperfusion time	Parameters of autophagy in normothermic ischemia without modulation	Modulation of autophagy	Results from autophagy modulation vs. untreated groups
Bi et al., 2020	Sprague-Dawley rats	Aged liver	Partial normothermic ischemia of 70% (ischemic lobes not specified). 60 min	24 h	Autophagy parameters vs. Sham old group: ↑LC3 I to LC3 II conversion and ↓p62.	Yes. Irisin.	Autophagy enhancement: ↑LC3 I to LC3 II conversion, ↓p62. Liver damage: ↓ALT, ↓Necrosis, ↓Apoptosis, ↓Inflammation, ↓Oxidative stress.
Cho et al., 2017	C57BL/6 mice	Alcoholic fatty liver	Partial normothermic ischemia of 70% (left and middle lobes). 1 h	5 h	Autophagy parameters vs. Sham group: ↓LC3 I to LC3 II conversion, ↓ATG3, ↓ATG7, ↓ATG12-5, ↑p62, ↓LAMP-2, ↓Autophagic vacuoles number. ↓Mitophagy: ↑PINK1 and ↓Parkin. ↓SIRT1	Yes. 2-Methoxyestradiol	Autophagy enhancement: ↑LC3 I to LC3 II conversion, ↑ATG3, ↑ATG7, ↑ATG12-5, ↓p62, ↑LAMP-2 ↑Autophagic vacuoles number. ↑Mitophagy: ↓PINK1 and ↑Parkin ↑SIRT1 Liver damage: ↓ALT and AST, ↓Necrosis, ↓Inflammation,

and extracellular signal-regulated kinase (ERK) 1/2 pathways was beneficial for steatotic livers undergoing I/R (Kan et al., 2017). A therapeutic effect was also achieved by treatment with exogenous hydrogen sulfide, which reduced ER stress and the class A scavenger receptor (SRA) pathway, and promoted autophagy. This led to the amelioration of hepatic damage by reducing oxidative stress and inflammation (Ruan et al., 2019). Ischemic preconditioning, a surgical therapeutical strategy consisting of a short period of ischemia followed by a brief period of reperfusion before a sustained ischemic insult, proved beneficial in a mouse model of I/R injury in steatotic livers, by increasing autophagic flux. This surgical technique restored mitochondrial function via heme oxygenase-1 (HO-1)-mediated autophagy and protected against damage (Liu et al., 2016). Such outcomes mean that pharmacological treatments that stimulate autophagy could be potentially useful in livers affected by metabolic diseases and that are subjected to surgery. Accordingly, another study revealed that calpain 2 inhibition enhanced autophagy, decreased mitochondrial dysfunction, suppressed cell death, and improved injury in livers affected by NAFLD and obesity and undergoing I/R (Zhao et al., 2016). However, it should be mentioned that opposite results have also been described in HFD-fed mice exposed to I/R, since treatment with Exendin 4, a glucagon-like peptide 1 analog, mitigated autophagy thus ameliorating hepatocellular injury, and preserving mitochondrial integrity (Gupta et al., 2014). These controversies could be caused by the great diversity of experimental conditions described in the literature in warm I/R models, such as different times of ischemia or reperfusion, induction of ischemia in different liver regions, or various ways of inducing steatosis. To reach a consensus on the most convenient way to modulate autophagy in liver surgery in the presence of NAFLD, the effects of I/R on autophagy

occurring in each of these different experimental conditions must be characterized.

Very few experimental studies have evaluated the role of autophagy in transplantation of NAFLD grafts (Gracia-Sancho et al., 2013; Zaouali et al., 2013a,b, 2017; Panisello-Roselló et al., 2017, 2018; Zhang et al., 2019). To date, reported results differ depending on the experimental model used. Most of the studies on steatotic liver grafts have used an *ex vivo* reperfusion model. In these conditions, when autophagy parameters were analyzed after short reperfusion periods (1 to 2 h), results agreed with those reported in optimal liver grafts: (a) cold ischemia induces a mild increase or no change in autophagy parameters; and (b) grafts benefited from pharmacological strategies that increased autophagy activity (Gracia-Sancho et al., 2013; Zaouali et al., 2013b, 2017). However, results were altogether different in the only study conducted in an *in vivo* model, since autophagy parameters after a prolonged reperfusion period (6 h), increased as a result of I/R injury. Furthermore, under these conditions, the pharmacological inhibition of autophagy protected steatotic liver grafts. This study also generated another important result in the setting of transplantation: in steatotic grafts, berberine inhibited autophagy and protected the graft, but the same drug activated autophagy in optimal grafts and decreased liver injury (Lin et al., 2017; Zhang et al., 2019). This observation underscores the very different signaling mechanisms that act in optimal *vs.* steatotic grafts, despite being subjected to the same surgical maneuvers.

As to the role of autophagy among the mechanisms responsible for liver injury-induced hyperglycemia, reports in the literature are scarce. In a streptozotocin-induced hyperglycemic mouse model, hyperglycemia aggravated thioacetamide-induced acute liver injury. In this model, the inflammatory response was stimulated by promoting liver resident macrophage

TABLE 2 | Findings about the involvement of autophagy in liver transplantation.

Study	Animal species	Type of liver graft	Cold preservation time	Reperfusion time	Parameters of autophagy in transplantation without modulation	Modulation of autophagy	Results from autophagy modulation vs. untreated groups
Pantazi et al., 2015	Male SD rats	Optimal grafts	8 h	24 h	Autophagy parameters vs. Sham group: No changes in LC3B or Beclin-1. Mild ↑SIRT1/FOXO1 pathway activity. No changes in mTOR activity.	YES. Trimetazidine added to IGL-1 preservation solution.	Autophagy enhancement: ↑ LC3B and ↑Beclin-1. ↑SIRT1/FOXO1 pathway activity, ↓mTOR activity. Liver damage: ↓ALT, ↓Oxidative stress.
Nakamura et al., 2019	C57BL/6 mice	Optimal grafts in mice	18 h in mice	6 h	Autophagy parameters: Mild LC3 I to LC3II conversion. ↑ p-S6K (mTORC1 activity) and ↑CHOP (ER stress marker).	YES. Antibiotic pretreatment in recipient to modulate gut microbiome.	Autophagy enhancement: ↑LC3 I to LC3 II conversion. ↓ p-S6K (mTORC1 activity) and ↓ER stress (CHOP). Liver damage: ↓AST, ↓Necrosis, ↓Apoptosis, ↓Inflammation.
Xue et al., 2020	C57BL/6 mice	Optimal graft	20 h	6 h	Autophagy parameters vs. Sham group: ↓LC3 I to LC3II conversion, ↑ATG5 ↑Beclin-1, no changes in p62.	YES. Pituitary adenylate cyclase-activating polypeptide (PACAP).	Autophagy enhancement: ↑LC3 I to LC3 II conversion, ↑ATG5, ↑Beclin-1, ↓p62. Liver damage: ↑ Survival rate, ↓ALT, ↓Necrosis.
Nakamura et al., 2018	C57BL/6 mice	Optimal grafts in mice	20 h	6 h	Autophagy markers: Mild expression of LC3B and SIRT1.	YES. Heme oxygenase-1 overexpression.	Autophagy enhancement: ↑LC3B. ↑SIRT1. Liver damage: ↓ALT, ↓Necrosis, ↓Apoptosis, ↓Inflammatory mediators.
Gotoh et al., 2009	Wistar rats	Optimal grafts	24 h	15 and 120 min	Autophagy markers: Detected LC3 and nascent autophagosomes and autolysosomes, at 15 min of reperfusion.	YES. Wortmannin, a PI3K inhibitor.	Autophagy inhibition: ↓LC3, ↓Number of nascent autophagosomes and autolysosomes volume density, at 15 min of reperfusion. Liver damage: ↓ALT and AST at 120 min of reperfusion, ↑ Survival rate.
Wang J. et al., 2020	SD rats	Optimal graft	Not specified.	24 h	Autophagy parameters vs. Sham group: No changes in LC3 I to LC3II conversion, ATG5 or ATG16L1. ↑p62. ↑AKT/mTOR	YES. Suberoylanilide hydroxamic acid (SAHA), a pan-histone deacetylase inhibitor.	Autophagy enhancement: ↑LC3 I to LC3 II conversion, ↑ATG5, ↑ATG16L1, ↓p62. ↓AKT/mTOR Liver damage: ↓ALT and AST, ↓Apoptosis, ↓Inflammatory cytokines.
Lin et al., 2017	Wistar rats	Optimal grafts	Not specified	6 h	Autophagy parameters vs. Sham group: Mild ↑LC3 I to LC3 II conversion, ↑Beclin-1, mild ↓p62. Mild ↑SIRT1/FoxO3α pathway activity.	YES. Berberine.	Autophagy enhancement: ↑LC3 I to LC3 II conversion, ↑Beclin-1, ↓p62. ↑SIRT1/FoxO3α pathway activity. Liver damage: ↓ALT and AST, ↓Apoptosis, ↓Oxidative stress.

(Continued)

TABLE 2 | Continued

Study	Animal species	Type of liver graft	Cold preservation time	Reperfusion time	Parameters of autophagy in transplantation without modulation	Modulation of autophagy	Results from autophagy modulation vs. untreated groups
Chen et al., 2019b	Lewis rats as donors and Brown Norway rats as recipients.	Optimal grafts	35 min	14 days	Autophagy parameters vs. syngeneic control: ↑LC3 I to LC3 II conversion in CD8 + T cells.	YES. 3-Methyladenine, an autophagy inhibitor.	Autophagy inhibition: ↓LC3 I to LC3 II conversion in CD8 + T cells. Liver damage: ↓ALT and AST, ↓Rejection index, ↑ Survival rate.
Wang R. R. et al., 2017	Lewis rats as donors and Brown Norway rats as recipients.	Reduced-size liver grafts.	Not specified	0, 1, 3, 5, 7, and 14 days	Autophagy parameters: Mild LC3 I to LC3 II conversion and Beclin-1 expression. Notable expression of phosphorylated mTOR.	YES. HO-1 transduced Bone-marrow derived Mesenchymal Stem Cells.	Autophagy enhancement: ↑LC3 I to LC3 II conversion, ↑Beclin-1. ↓mTOR phosphorylated. Liver damage: ↓Rejection index, ↓Apoptosis.
Zeng et al., 2019	C57BL/6 mice	Grafts from donation after circulatory death (DCD).	4 h	2 h	Autophagy parameters vs. control: Mild ↑LC3B-II ULK1, mild ↑Atg5 and mild ↓p62. ↓mTOR. Not statistical significance.	YES. HOPE (Hypothermic oxygenated machine perfusion) treatment during 1 h	Autophagy enhancement: ↑LC3B-II,↑ULK1, ↑Atg5 and ↓p62. ↓mTOR. Liver damage: ↓ALT and AST, ↓ Necrosis and Apoptosis, ↓Oxidative stress. N/A.
Liu T. et al., 2019	Sprague Dawley rats.	Grafts from DCD.	Not specified	6, 12, and 24 h	Autophagy parameters at 6, 12, and 24 h of reperfusion in rats: Notable increased expression of LC3 and AMPK. Notable decreased expression of p62.	NO.	N/A
Zhang et al., 2019	Wistar rats fed with high-fat diet for 12 weeks.	Steatotic grafts. Not additional data about presence of metabolic comorbidities.	Not specified	6 h	Autophagy parameters vs. steatotic sham: ↑LC3 I to LC3 II conversion, ↑Beclin-1, ↑p62, ↑Autophagosomes number. ↑ER stress (p-PERK, CHOP, Bip).	YES. Berberine.	Autophagy inhibition: ↓LC3 I to LC3 II conversion, ↓Beclin-1, ↓p62, ↓Autophagosomes number. ↓ER stress (p-PERK, CHOP, Bip). Liver damage: ↓ALT and AST, ↓Necrosis, ↓Oxidative stress, ↓Inflammatory cytokines.
Panisello-Roselló et al., 2018	Zucker rats	Steatotic grafts. Obesity.	24 h	Not reperfusion. Liver samples collected at the end of cold storage.	Autophagy parameters vs. steatotic sham: No changes in, LC3B, Beclin-1 or ATG7. ↓mTOR activity	YES. IGL-1 preservation solution.	Autophagy enhancement: ↑ LC3B,↑Beclin-1, ↑ATG7. ↓mTOR activity. Liver damage: ↓ALT and AST, ↓Necrosis, ↓Apoptosis.
Gracia-Sancho et al., 2013	Wistar rats fed with high-fat diet for 3 days.	Steatotic grafts. Not additional data about presence of metabolic comorbidities.	16 h	1 h (ex vivo reperfusion)	Autophagy parameters vs. steatotic control: Mild ↓LC3 I to LC3 II conversion.	YES. Simvastatin.	Autophagy enhancement: ↑LC3 I to LC3 II conversion. Liver damage: ↓ALT and AST.

(Continued)

TABLE 2 | Continued

Study	Animal species	Type of liver graft	Cold preservation time	Reperfusion time	Parameters of autophagy in transplantation without modulation	Modulation of autophagy	Results from autophagy modulation vs. untreated groups
Zaouali et al., 2017	Zucker rats	Steatotic grafts. Obesity.	24 h	2 h (ex vivo reperfusion)	Autophagy parameters vs. steatotic control: No changes in LC3 I to LC3 II conversion, Beclin-1 No changes in SIRT1.	YES. Trimetazidene added to IGL-1 preservation solution.	Autophagy enhancement: ↑LC3 I to LC3 II conversion, ↑Beclin-1. ↑SIRT1. Liver damage: ↓ALT and AST ↓TNFα.
Zaouali et al., 2013b	Zucker rats	Steatotic grafts. Obesity.	24 h	2 h (ex vivo reperfusion)	Autophagy parameters vs. steatotic control: Mild ↑LC3 I to LC3 II conversion, ↑Beclin-1, ↑p62. ↑ER stress (GRP78, CHOP, p-PERK).	YES. Trimetazidene + Melatonin added to IGL-1 preservation solution.	Autophagy enhancement: ↑LC3 I to LC3 II conversion, ↑Beclin-1, ↑ATG7, ↓p62. ↓ER stress (GRP78, CHOP, p-PERK). Liver damage: ↓ALT and AST, ↓Oxidative stress.
Minor et al., 2011	German landrace pigs	Optimal grafts.	10 h	1 h, 7 days	Autophagy parameters: Mild LC3 II and Beclin-1 expression, at 1 h of reperfusion.	YES. Hypothermic reconditioning by gaseous oxygen persufflation treatment during 2 h.	Autophagy enhancement: ↑LC3-II, ↑Beclin-1, at 1 h of reperfusion. Liver damage: ↓ALT ↑ Survival rate, at 7 days after transplantation.
Liu T. et al., 2019	Bama miniature pigs	Grafts from DCD.	Not specified	6, 12, and 24 h	Autophagy parameters at 24 h of reperfusion in pigs: Notable increased expression of LC3 and AMPK. Notable decreased expression of p62.	NO.	N/A
Nakamura et al., 2019	Humans	Grafts from donors after brain or cardiac death.	7–8 h on average	2 h	Autophagy parameters: Mild LC3B expression. Notable CHOP expression.	YES. Pre-transplantation Antibiotics treatment ≥ 10 days in recipients.	Autophagy enhancement: ↑LC3B. ↓ER stress (CHOP). Liver damage: ↓ALT and AST.
Chen et al., 2019b	Humans	Liver transplant recipients with acute rejection.	Not specified	Not specified	Autophagy parameters vs. recipients without acute rejection: ↑LC3 expression in CD8 + T cells.	NO	N/A
Nakamura et al., 2018	Humans	Not specified	Not specified	2 h after portal reperfusion	Autophagy markers: Expression of LC3B and SIRT1.	NO	N/A
Ricca et al., 2015	Humans	Grafts from donors after brain death, including steatotic and non-steatotic liver grafts.	5 to 10 h	≤2 h after reperfusion	Autophagy markers: Expression of LC3.	YES. Ischemic postconditioning.	Autophagy enhancement: ↑LC3. Liver damage: ↓I/R injury at reperfusion biopsy, defined by the presence of both inflammatory infiltration and hepatocellular necrosis.
Degli Esposti et al., 2011	Humans	Grafts from donors after brain death, including steatotic and non-steatotic liver grafts.	5 to 10 h	Not specified (liver samples collected before abdomen closure).	*Steatotic grafts* Autophagy markers: Expression of LC3 and Beclin-1. *Non-steatotic grafts* Autophagy markers: Rarely observed LC3 o Beclin-1 expression.	YES. Ischemic preconditioning.	*Steatotic grafts* Autophagy enhancement: ↑LC3, ↑Beclin-1. Liver damage: No changes in transaminases, ↓Acute rejection. *Non-steatotic grafts* No changes in autophagy parameters. Liver damage: ↓ALT and AST in non-steatotic grafts.

NLRP3 inflammasome activation and inhibiting AMPK/mTOR autophagy signaling pathways. Autophagy restoration by AMPK activation or mTOR knockdown inhibited NLRP3 inflammasome activation in Kupffer cells and decreased thioacetamide-induced acute liver injury in hyperglycemic mice (Wang Q. et al., 2020). Considering that the autophagy-NLRP3 inflammasome pathway is also involved in NAFLD (Wan et al., 2016), perhaps the regulation of this signaling pathway could be useful to protect against damage in liver surgery with other metabolic comorbidities in addition to hyperglycemia.

Liver dysfunctions in the immediate postoperative period of liver resection or transplantation, especially in livers affected by underlying metabolic conditions, are still an unsolved problem. As the prevalence of metabolic diseases such as NAFLD, MetS, insulin resistance, obesity, or diabetes is increasing worldwide, the development of therapeutic options in patients affected by these diseases and also undergo liver surgery are required. There is no doubt that regulation of autophagy improves warm I/R injury in optimal livers, but is uncertain whether these benefits are maintained when livers affected by metabolic diseases face I/R injury. The relevance of autophagy steatotic liver transplantation associated with other related metabolic comorbidities has not been investigated. To date, in studied models of steatotic liver transplantation, only some mention specifically that the experimental animals were obese aside from harboring fatty liver disease; and in all published studies, information on the parameters that would reflect the associated presence of insulin resistance or MetS in the animals is omitted. To the best of our knowledge, the role of autophagy in experimental conditions in which the donor has steatosis and diabetes has not been evaluated. Thus, in the coming years, research should be carried out on autophagy and its associated molecular mediators in livers undergoing surgery with one or more metabolic diseases, as it is what happens in the clinical practice. So, concerning laboratory approaches, to use experimental models the closest to clinical practice is the best to design new therapeutic strategies to be developed and successfully applied in patients.

The lack of studies describing how metabolic diseases affect post-operative results of liver surgery in the medium and long term is evident, and even less is known to what extent autophagy is relevant in this setting. Intensive research is also necessary to establish whether autophagy is involved in post-surgical events such as transient hyperglycemia and the development of MetS in liver transplantation recipients. This information will allow us to elucidate whether autophagy regulation could lead to the generation of effective therapeutic strategies that could improve the current results of transplantation and resection, not only in the immediate postoperative period but also in the long term.

Future Perspectives on Research in Autophagy and I/R Injury, in Livers Affected by Metabolic Comorbidities

To date, no experimental or clinical investigations have been carried out, in which the fatty liver undergoing surgery is combined with the presence of obesity, insulin resistance, MetS, and/or hyperglycemia, nor on the effects of autophagy under these conditions. The combination of several of these conditions is commonplace in clinical practice, due to their high prevalence. In those multiple disease scenarios, autophagy most likely plays a predominant role since it contributes to the development of each of these pathological entities when manifested separately. There are even some mediators of autophagy that are common to hepatic ischemia, steatosis, obesity, MetS, and diabetes, such as ER stress, AMPK, MAPK, or oxidative stress. Importantly, it should be taken into account that the effectiveness of treatments could be different depending on the combination of metabolic comorbidities that occurs in each situation, given that a beneficial therapy for steatotic livers in presence of obesity or MetS, may not be effective in the case of steatotic livers also suffering diabetes. This hypothesis is originated based on existing reports showing that some therapies that have been described to reduce hepatic I/R injury exhibit different effectiveness depending on the underlying pathological condition in the liver. By way of example, therapies that have been found to reduce injury in steatotic livers do not offer any benefit in non-steatotic grafts (Álvarez-Mercado et al., 2019). Therefore, in order to consider the autophagy pathway as a possible therapeutic target in patients with several metabolic comorbidities and that are subjected to transplantation or resection, autophagic molecular signaling must first be exquisitely characterized in experimental or clinical models of fatty livers with obesity, diabetes, and/or MetS (separately or in different combinations of these pathologies).

Much work is required before experimental results can be translated into clinical practice, and the first important step is to make use of experimental models that best mimic clinical conditions. In several experimental models of hepatic steatosis used nowadays, insulin resistance does not always develop, and then insufficiently would reflect the pathogenesis of NAFLD in patients. There are several NAFLD animal models available, among which the most common are mice fed the MCD or HFD. The MCD diet causes hepatic steatosis, and body weight loss but no insulin resistance. The HFD causes obesity, hepatic steatosis with mild injury, and insulin resistance. Genetically deficient ob/ob or db/db mice or Zucker rats, develop obesity and steatosis, but in some cases, this does not occur automatically, and they often need to be fed either the MCD or the HFD (Adkins et al., 2013). Combinations of fat- and carbohydrate-rich dietary components have been used in rodents to mimic MetS. Among such diets, the "cafeteria" diet has been used to induce severe obesity with glucose intolerance and liver steatosis classifiable as NAFLD. After following the cafeteria diet for 8 and 15 weeks, insulin resistance and high plasma triglyceride levels are greater than in animals fed a traditional lard-based HFD (Parafati et al., 2015). It is important to characterize which metabolic comorbidities (obesity, MetS, diabetes, insulin resistance, fatty liver) are present or predominant in each experimental model, in order to determine with greater accuracy which combination of pathological entities to study when submitting a fatty liver obtained from these models to liver surgery. Another highly relevant consideration when selecting an experimental model is to evaluate whether if it mimics clinical liver surgery. Regarding liver resection, there is a paucity of research using experimental models that best mimic the ischemic times commonly used or including partial hepatectomy in combination with vascular occlusion. Post-operative outcomes after liver resection are influenced by the magnitude of I/R injury, but also by the regenerative response. Hepatic ischemia causes liver injury and impairs regeneration, and these phenomena are further compromised if livers with underlying diseases (steatosis, cirrhosis, diabetes, etc.) are resected and undergo I/R injury (McCormack et al., 2007). In terms of modeling liver transplantation, experimental studies have been carried out in the absence of brain death or cardiac death, which means in surgical conditions very different to those occurring in clinical practice. Brain death and cardiac death cause important hemodynamic changes, hypoperfusion in the mesenteric microcirculation and warm hepatic ischemia, which might result in significant modifications in the mediators generated in the liver, and the concomitant inflammation. This could alter the autophagy pathways, and have deleterious effects on liver grafts used for transplantation. It is necessary to include pathological liver grafts in experimental studies, since the success, dysfunction or loss of liver grafts may be affected by the presence of steatosis, diabetes, MetS, etc. in potential donors. These conditions should be considered in future research to establish how they influence autophagy and post-operative outcomes. Since the effectiveness of a therapeutic modality aimed at improving post-surgical outcomes in patients undergoing liver surgery could differ depending on the surgical conditions, the type and characteristics of the liver and other factors, the use of experimental models that reproduce as closely as possible real clinical conditions is key to the effective translation of laboratory results into the clinical realm.

Several molecular mediators of autophagy in the steatotic liver are key in hepatic I/R injury, which represents an area of opportunity to explore treatments for protecting livers affected by metabolic diseases such as NAFLD, and those undergoing surgery. AMPK and ER stress are closely related at the level of molecular signaling mechanisms associated with autophagy in NAFLD models (Homma and Fujii, 2020), as also occurs in I/R. In fact, activation of AMPK, as well as inhibition of ER stress through drugs, are beneficial to regulate autophagy and protect steatotic livers that undergo surgery (Carrasco-Chaumel et al., 2005; Zaouali et al., 2013b), but its usefulness at the clinical level has not yet been evaluated. These findings indicate that regulation of AMPK and ER stress could be promising therapies. On the other hand, although JNK and ghrelin are also mediators involved in autophagy in fatty liver and I/R, their pharmacological modulation in livers with NAFLD and undergoing surgery could lead to serious difficulties. In non-surgical NAFLD models, activation of JNK, or ghrelin is associated with activation of autophagy, which is beneficial (Singh et al., 2009; Mao et al., 2015). However, it has been widely demonstrated that JNK activation is implicated with steatotic liver damage in transplantation, and warm ischemia alone or combined with resection (Lehmann et al., 2003; Massip-Salcedo et al., 2006; Ben Mosbah et al., 2010; Shaker et al., 2016; Li S. et al., 2017); and, although pharmacological regulation of ghrelin has been scarcely explored in liver surgery, first published reports in this regard indicate that treatments increasing hepatic ghrelin

levels are harmful in non-steatotic liver grafts from brain dead donor, which represents an experimental model very close to clinical practice (Álvarez-Mercado et al., 2019). Therefore, to design effective strategies for protecting livers with metabolic diseases and undergoing surgery, it is required to perform meticulous research on the regulation of molecular mediators involved in both hepatic autophagy and I/R, using experimental models that include NAFLD and even other metabolic diseases, and that should be studied in diverse variants of liver surgery.

When attempting to develop new therapeutic strategies, one should consider mediators that have been recently described to modulate autophagy in obesity, NAFLD, or diabetes, but not yet been studied in conditions in which one or more of these comorbidities are combined with hepatic surgery. **Table 3** shows some examples of this type of mediator. However, we must consider that the regulation of autophagy could also cause serious side effects that would be a serious inconvenience in hepatic surgery. Recent studies have demonstrated that pharmacological upregulation of autophagy decreases hepatotoxicity and steatosis in NAFLD. However, further studies are needed before autophagy activation can be considered a viable treatment against I/R injury in steatotic livers affected by other metabolic comorbidities, because upregulation of autophagy in hepatic stellate cells has been shown to foment their activation, and consequently, initiate liver fibrosis. Inhibition of mTOR activity can induce autophagy, but also inhibits cell proliferation. Thus, in liver resection with vascular occlusion, cell proliferation is detrimental, since it precludes or impairs liver regeneration (Matter et al., 2014). The liver responds to some stressors through global activation of autophagy, causing lipid, protein, and organelle degradation; but in some instances, upregulation of autophagy as a protective mechanism against liver injury could only involve a specific form of autophagy, such as lipophagy. For instance, autophagy upregulated as the first line of defense against alcohol-induced toxicity in the liver, selectively targets mitochondria, and LD, while excluding cytosolic proteins and other organelles. Future efforts should focus on establishing how selective forms of autophagy can be individually modulated for therapeutic purposes (Singh and Cuervo, 2012).

Recent findings on autophagy signaling pathways in NAFLD could also be useful in the development of markers for hepatic injury progression. In NAFLD, lipolysosomes appear to reflect the progressive impairment of lysosomal function, and particularly, the capability of lysosomal hydrolases to catabolize fat. This is supported by the correlation between an increase in the number of lipolysosomes and disease activity, in terms of necroinflammation. Upregulation of lysosomal genes such as cathepsin D, LAMP1, LAMP2, Niemann-Pick-type C1 (NPC1), vacuolar H + -ATPase, B2 subunit (ATP6V1B2), TFEB, suggests an increase in the overall lysosomal mass and could be interpreted as an attempt to counteract lysosomal dysfunction (Houben et al., 2017). Cathepsin D expression is greater in NAFLD patients compared with controls, and a direct correlation has been observed between cathepsin D expression and both NASH and fibrosis. Thus, molecular markers of lipophagy impairment could help to identify hepatic injury in patients on time (Carotti et al., 2020). Further studies are required

TABLE 3 | New promising autophagy regulators to be evaluated as therapeutical strategies in livers affected by metabolic diseases and submitted to surgery.

Study	Modulation of autophagy	Type of liver pathology	Animal species or cell culture	Experimental model used to induce hepatic metabolic diseases	Results from administration of exogenous regulator of autophagy vs. untreated groups
Lee et al., 2020	Iridoids of *Valeriana fauriei*	Steatotic cells	Huh7 cells	Treatment with oleic acid.	Autophagy enhancement: ↑LC3 I to LC3 II conversion, ↑Autophagic vacuoles. ↑Lipophagy: ↓Lipid droplets. ↓mTORC1, ↓ULK1 phosphorylated. Other cellular effects: ↓Lipid accumulation.
	Valeriana fauriei 70% ethanol extract	Fatty liver, obesity.	C57BL/6 J mice	High fat diet for 13 weeks.	Autophagy enhancement: ↑LC3 I to LC3 II conversion, ↑Autophagic vacuoles. ↓mTOR phosphorylated, ↓ULK1 phosphorylated. Other liver effects: ↓Lipid accumulation, ↓Lipogenesis-related genes.
Sinha et al., 2014	Caffeine	Steatotic cells	HepG2 cells	Treatment with oleic acid and palmitic acid.	Autophagy enhancement: ↑LC3 I to LC3 II conversion, ↑ATG7, ↑ATG5, ↑Beclin, ↓p62 ↑Autophagosome formation. ↓mTOR phosphorylated. Other cellular effects: ↑Lipid clearance.
	Caffeine	Fatty liver	C57BL6 mice	High fat diet for 8 weeks.	Autophagy enhancement: ↑LC3 I to LC3 II conversion, ↓p62. ↓mTOR phosphorylated. Other liver effects: ↓Lipid accumulation, ↑Lipid uptake in lysosomes, ↑Fatty acid β-oxidation
Kuo et al., 2020	Magnolol	Steatotic cells	HepG2 cells and C57BL/6 mice primary hepatocytes	Treatment with palmitic acid.	Autophagy enhancement: ↑LC3 I to LC3 II conversion, ↑ATG7, ↓p62. ↓mTOR phosphorylated. Other cellular effects: ↓Cellular triglycerides, ↓Lipogenesis, ↑Lipolysis, ↓Inflammation.
	Magnolol	Hypertriglyceri-demia	Male Wistar Rats	Tyloxapol	Autophagy enhancement: ↑LC3 I to LC3 II conversion, ↑ATG5-12, ↑ATG7, ↑Beclin-1, ↓p62. ↓mTOR phosphorylated. Other liver effects: ↓Oxidative stress, ↓Lipogenesis, ↑Lipolysis, ↓Inflammation.
Baldini et al., 2020	Silybin	Steatotic cells	Rat hepatoma FaO cells	Treatment with oleic acid and palmitic acid.	Autophagy inhibition: ↓LC3 I to LC3 II conversion. Other cellular effects: ↓Lipid droplet diameter.
Wang C. et al., 2017	TFEB agonists: Digoxin, Ikarugamycin or Aloxidine dihydrochloride.	Fatty liver, hyperglycemia, hyperinsulinemia.	C57BL/6J mice	High fat diet for 1 month.	Autophagy enhancement: ↓p62. Other metabolic and hepatic effects: ↓Circulating glucose, ↓Circulating insulin, ↓Liver steatosis.
Li X. et al., 2017	Pectic bee pollen polysaccharide	Steatotic cells with insulin resistance	HepG2 cells	Treatment with high glucose and oleic acid and palmitic acid.	Autophagy enhancement: ↑LC3 I to LC3 II conversion, ↓p62. Other cellular effects: ↓Insulin resistance.
	Pectic bee pollen polysaccharide	Fatty liver, type 2 diabetes.	C57BL/6J mice	High fat diet for 8 weeks.	Autophagy enhancement: ↑LC3 I to LC3 II conversion, ↓p62. ↓mTOR phosphorylated Other metabolic and hepatic effects: ↓Glucose intolerance, ↓Insulin resistance, ↓Liver steatosis, ↓AST, ↑Lipolysis.
Gong et al., 2016	Akebia saponin D	Steatotic cells	Buffalo rat liver (BRL) cells	Treatment with oleic acid.	Autophagy enhancement: ↓LC3 I to LC3 II conversion, ↓Beclin, ↓p62, ↑Autolysosomes. ↓mTOR phosphorylated. Other cellular effects: ↓Lipid droplets.
	Akebia saponin D	Fatty liver, insulin resistance.	Ob/ob mice	High fat diet.	Autophagy enhancement: ↓LC3 I to LC3 II conversion, ↓Beclin, ↓p62, ↑Autophagosomes. Other metabolic and hepatic effects: ↓Circulating Glucose, ↓Circulating Insulin, ↓Insulin resistance, ↓Liver steatosis, ↓ALT and AST, ↓Apoptosis, ↓Oxidative stress.

(Continued)

TABLE 3 | Continued

Study	Modulation of autophagy	Type of liver pathology	Animal species or cell culture	Experimental model used to induce hepatic metabolic diseases	Results from administration of exogenous regulator of autophagy vs. untreated groups
Parafati et al., 2015	Bergamot polyphenol fraction.	Metabolic syndrome: Fatty liver, Obesity, Hyperglycemia, Hypertriglyceridemia.	Rcc:Han WIST rats	Cafeteria diet (15% protein, 70% carbohydrates, 15% fat) for 13 weeks.	Autophagy enhancement: ↑LC3 I to LC3 II conversion, ↑Beclin-1, ↓p62. ↑Lipophagy: ↓Lipid droplets. Other metabolic and hepatic effects: ↓Circulating Glucose, ↓Circulating Triglycerides, ↓Liver steatosis.
Huang et al., 2017	Ginsenoside Rb2	Steatotic cells	HepG2 cells and C57BL mice primary hepatocytes.	Treatment with high glucose and oleic acid.	Autophagy enhancement: ↑LC3 I to LC3 II conversion, ↓p62. ↑Lipophagy: ↓Lipid droplets. ↑SIRT1
	Ginsenoside Rb2	Fatty liver, obesity, diabetes.	C57BL/KsJ-Lepdb (db/db) mice	N/A	Autophagy enhancement: ↑LC3 I to LC3 II conversion, ↓p62. ↑SIRT1, ↓mTOR phosphorylated. Other metabolic and hepatic effects: ↓Circulating Glucose, ↓Insulin resistance, ↓Liver steatosis, ↓ALT and AST.
Shao et al., 2018	Exenatide	Fatty liver, diabetes.	C57BL/6 mice	High fat diet for 10 weeks and treatment with streptozocin.	Autophagy enhancement: ↑LC3 I to LC3 II conversion, ↑Beclin, ↑Autophagosomes. ↑Mitophagy: ↑Parkin, ↑BNIP3L. Other metabolic and hepatic effects: ↓Circulating Glucose, ↓Liver steatosis, ↓ALT, ↓Oxidative stress.
Cui et al., 2020	Chronic intermittent hypobaric hypoxia	Metabolic syndrome: Fatty liver, Obesity, Hypertension, Hyperglycemia, Hypertriglyceridemia, Insulin resistance.	Sprague Dawley rats	High fat diet and water supplemented with fructose for 16 weeks.	Autophagy enhancement: ↓LC3 I to LC3 II conversion, ↓Beclin-1, ↓p62. ↓mTOR phosphorylated, ↓ER stress (GRP78, CHOP). Other metabolic and hepatic effects: ↓Circulating Glucose, ↓Circulating Triglycerides, ↓Insulin resistance, ↓Liver steatosis, ↓ALT and AST.

to verify whether quantification of lipolysosomes could be a feasible and reproducible tool to assess the severity of NAFLD and its propensity to progress. The p62/SQSTM1 is essential for LC3B recruitment in LD in ethanol-induced lipophagy, while p62/SQSTM1 knockdown triggers the accumulation of triglycerides and cholesterol. Recent reports suggest that serum p62/SQSTM1 levels could also become a potential biomarker in the diagnosis of patients with steatosis and lobular inflammation (Kuo et al., 2020). These may all become very valuable non-invasive tools to evaluate liver injury in the immediate postoperative period in patients subjected to liver resection or transplantation.

CONCLUSION

Due to the high prevalence of obesity, MetS, NAFLD, and diabetes, in the coming years, there may be a need to use liver grafts from donors with these metabolic diseases to reduce the waiting list for liver transplantation. In the same way, the prevalence of such diseases causes an increasing presence of such diseases in liver resections. Livers with underlying pathological conditions possess higher sensitivity to I/R injury inherent to transplantation and resection and are at high risk of morbidity or mortality in the immediate postoperative period. Therefore, there is a growing need to

develop therapies to improve the postoperative results of livers affected by obesity, MetS, NAFLD, or diabetes that are subjected to surgery.

As described in this review, autophagy is closely involved in signaling pathways underlying effects of obesity, MetS, and obesity on the liver; and also is implicated as molecular mechanisms to NAFLD and the extent of the damage caused by I/R as well as in surgical outcomes. These characteristics make autophagy regulation the basis of promising treatments in patients suffering from the conditions aforementioned and submitted to liver surgery. Unfortunately, whether hepatic autophagy following warm or cold I/R protects or contributes to the damage is still unsolved since results are controversial. There are even controversies as to how the regulation of hepatic autophagia occurs in conditions of obesity, MetS, NAFLD, or diabetes. This lack of understanding hampers their translation from bench to bedside.

Therefore, it is mandatory to increase the knowledge about autophagic molecular signaling in experimental or clinical models of obesity, MetS, NAFLD, or diabetes subjected to resection or transplantation. In this last surgical situation, it is

important to clarify the mechanisms taking place in the recipient and donor. It should be bearing in mind that in clinical practice the most common scenario is patients combining NAFLD, obesity, MetS, or diabetes, and for this reason, preclinical studies must use adequate experimental ischemia when evaluating the important to clarify the mechanisms taking place in the recipient and donor. It should be bearing in mind that in clinical practice the most common scenario is patients combining NAFLD, obesity, MetS, or diabetes, and for this reason, preclinical studies must use adequate experimental ischemia when evaluating the relevance of autophagy in the setting of I/R. This knowledge is the premise for finding not only therapeutic strategies to prevent damage in patients with these metabolic diseases who undergo surgery but also to find useful and non-invasive biomarkers to monitor the progression of liver damage in these conditions. These advances would undoubtedly improve the clinical prognosis of liver surgery in the coming years.

AUTHOR CONTRIBUTIONS

AÁ-M, CR-A, MM-C, and AC-C gathered the related literature, prepared the figures, and drafted the manuscript. CP and AC-R participated in the design of the review and drafted the manuscript. All authors read and approved the final manuscript.

REFERENCES

Adeva-Andany, M. M., Carneiro-Freire, N., Seco-Filgueira, M., Fernandez-Fernandez, C., and Mourino-Bayolo, D. (2019). Mitochondrial beta-oxidation of saturated fatty acids in humans. *Mitochondrion* 46, 73–90. doi: 10.1016/j.mito.2018.02.009

Adkins, Y., Schie, I. W., Fedor, D., Reddy, A., Nguyen, S., Zhou, P., et al. (2013). A novel mouse model of nonalcoholic steatohepatitis with significant insulin resistance. *Lab. Investig.* 93, 1313–1322. doi: 10.1038/labinvest.2013.123

Alfany-Fernandez, I., Casillas-Ramirez, A., Bintanel-Morcillo, M., Brosnihan, K. B., Ferrario, C. M., Serafin, A., et al. (2009). Therapeutic targets in liver transplantation: angiotensin II in nonsteatotic grafts and angiotensin-(1-7) in steatotic grafts. *Am. J. Transplant.* 9, 439–451. doi: 10.1111/j.1600-6143.2008.02521.x

Alipourfard, I., Datukishvili, N., and Mikeladze, D. (2019). TNF-α downregulation modifies insulin receptor substrate 1 (IRS-1) in metabolic signaling of diabetic insulin-resistant hepatocytes. *Mediators Inflamm.* 2019:3560819. doi: 10.1155/2019/3560819

Álvarez-Mercado, A. I., Negrete-Sánchez, E., Gulfo, J., Ávalos De León, C. G., Casillas-Ramírez, A., Cornide-Petronio, M. E., et al. (2019). EGF-GH axis in rat steatotic and non-steatotic liver transplantation from brain-dead donors. *Transplantation* 103, 1349–1359. doi: 10.1097/TP.0000000000002636

Archuleta, T. L., Lemieux, A. M., Saengsirisuwan, V., Teachey, M. K., Lind-borg, K. A., Kim, J. S., et al. (2009). Oxidant stress-induced loss of IRS-1 and IRS-2 proteins in rat skeletal muscle: role of p38 MAPK. *Free. Radic. Biol. Med.* 47, 1486–1493. doi: 10.1016/j.freeradbiomed.2009.08.014

Bai, G., Li, H., Ge, Y., Zhang, Q., Zhang, J., Chen, M., et al. (2018). Influence of hydrogen-rich saline on hepatocyte autophagy during laparoscopic liver ischaemia-reperfusion combined resection injury in miniature pigs. *J. Vet. Res.* 62, 395–403. doi: 10.2478/jvetres-2018-0056

Baldini, F., Portincasa, P., Grasselli, E., Damonte, G., Salis, A., Bonomo, M., et al. (2020). Aquaporin-9 is involved in the lipid-lowering activity of the nutraceutical silybin on hepatocytes through modulation of autophagy and lipid droplets composition. *Biochim. Biophys. Acta - Mol. Cell Biol. Lipids* 1865:158586. doi: 10.1016/j.bbalip.2019.158586

Bechmann, L. P., Hannivoort, R. A., Gerken, G., Hotamisligil, G. S., Trauner, M., and Canbay, A. (2012). The interaction of hepatic lipid and glucose metabolism in liver diseases. *J. Hepatol.* 56, 952–964. doi: 10.1016/j.jhep.2011.08.025

Behrends, M., Martinez-Palli, G., Niemann, C. U., Cohen, S., Ramachandran, R., and Hirose, R. (2010). Acute hyperglycemia worsens hepatic ischemia/reperfusion injury in rats. *J. Gastrointest. Surg.* 14, 528–535. doi: 10.1007/s11605-009-1112-3

Ben Mosbah, I., Alfany-Fernández, I., Martel, C., Zaouali, M. A., Bintanel-Morcillo, M., Rimola, A., et al. (2010). Endoplasmic reticulum stress inhibition protects steatotic and non-steatotic livers in partial hepatectomy under ischemia-reperfusion. *Cell Death Dis.* 1, 1–12. doi: 10.1038/cddis.2010.29

Bi, J., Yang, L., Wang, T., Zhang, J., Li, T., Ren, Y., et al. (2020). Irisin improves autophagy of aged hepatocytes via increasing telomerase activity in liver injury. *Oxid. Med. Cell. Longev.* 2020:6946037. doi: 10.1155/2020/6946037

Biel, T. G., Lee, S., Flores-Toro, J. A., Dean, J. W., Go, K. L., Lee, M. H., et al. (2016). Sirtuin 1 suppresses mitochondrial dysfunction of ischemic mouse livers in a mitofusin 2-dependent manner. *Cell Death. Differ* 23, 279–290. doi: 10.1038/cdd.2015.96

Caraceni, P., Domenicali, M., Vendemiale, G., Grattagliano, I., Pertosa, A., Nardo, B., et al. (2005). The reduced tolerance of rat fatty liver to ischemia reperfusion is associated with mitochondrial oxidative injury. *J. Surg. Res.* 124, 160–168. doi: 10.1016/j.jss.2004.10.007

Carotti, S., Aquilano, K., Zalfa, F., Ruggiero, S., Valentini, F., Zingariello, M., et al. (2020). Lipophagy impairment is associated with disease progression in NAFLD. *Front. Physiol.* 11:850. doi: 10.3389/fphys.2020.00850

Carrasco-Chaumel, E., Rosselló-Catafau, J., Bartrons, R., Franco-Gou, R., Xaus, C., Casillas, A., et al. (2005). Adenosine monophosphate-activated protein kinase and nitric oxide in rat steatotic liver transplantation. *J. Hepatol.* 43, 997–1006. doi: 10.1016/j.jhep.2005.05.021

Casillas-Ramírez, A., Alfany-Fernández, I., Massip-Salcedo, M., Juan, M. E., Planas, J. M., Serafín, A., et al. (2011). Retinol-binding protein 4 and peroxisome proliferator-activated receptor-γ in steatotic liver transplantation. *J. Pharmacol. Exp. Ther.* 338, 143–153. doi: 10.1124/jpet.110.177691

Casillas-Ramírez, A., Amine-Zaouali, M., Massip-Salcedo, M., Padrissa-Altés, S., Bintanel-Morcillo, M., Ramalho, F., et al. (2008). Inhibition of angiotensin II action protects rat steatotic livers against ischemia-reperfusion injury. *Crit. Care Med.* 36, 1256–1266. doi: 10.1097/CCM.0b013e31816a023c

Chae, S., Choi, J., Lim, S., Choi, H. J., Park, J., Hong, S. H., et al. (2020). Stress burden related to postreperfusion syndrome may aggravate hyperglycemia with insulin resistance during living donor liver transplantation: a propensity score-matching analysis. *PLoS One* 15:e0243873. doi: 10.1371/journal.pone.0243873

Chang, A. L., Cortez, A. R., Bondoc, A., Schauer, D. P., Fitch, A., Shah, S. A., et al. (2016). Metabolic syndrome in liver transplantation: a preoperative and postoperative concern. *Surgery* 160, 1111–1117. doi: 10.1016/j.surg.2016.06.015

Chen, K., Li, J. J., Li, S. N., Feng, J., Liu, T., Wang, F., et al. (2017a). 15-Deoxy-Δ12,14-prostaglandin J2 alleviates hepatic ischemia-reperfusion injury in mice via inducing antioxidant response and inhibiting apoptosis and autophagy. *Acta Pharmacol. Sin.* 38, 672–687. doi: 10.1038/aps.2016.108

Chen, K., Yuan, R., Zhang, Y., Geng, S., and Li, L. (2017b). Tollip deficiency alters atherosclerosis and steatosis by disrupting lipophagy. *J. Am. Heart Assoc.* 6:e004078. doi: 10.1161/JAHA.116.004078

Chen, X., Chan, H., Zhangm, L., Liu, X., Hom, I. H. T., Zhang, X., et al. (2019a). The phytochemical polydatin ameliorates non-alcoholic steatohepatitis by restoring lysosomal function and autophagic flux. *J. Cell. Mol. Med.* 23, 4290–4300. doi: 10.1111/jcmm.14320

Chen, X., Wang, L., Deng, Y., Li, X., Li, G., Zhou, J., et al. (2019b). Inhibition of autophagy prolongs recipient survival through promoting CD8+ T cell apoptosis in a rat liver transplantation model. *Front. Immunol.* 10:1356. doi: 10.3389/fimmu.2019.01356

Cho, H. I., Seo, M. J., and Lee, S. M. (2017). 2-Methoxyestradiol protects against ischemia/reperfusion injury in alcoholic fatty liver by enhancing sirtuin 1-mediated autophagy. *Biochem. Pharmacol.* 131, 40–51. doi: 10.1016/j.bcp.2017. 02.008

Choi, J. W., Ohn, J. H., Jung, H. S., Park, Y. J., Jang, H. C., Chung, S. S., et al. (2018). Carnitine induces autophagy and restores high-fat diet-induced mitochondrial dysfunction. *Metabolism* 78, 43–51. doi: 10.1016/j.metabol.2017.09.005

Chorny, A., Anderson, P., Gonzalez-Rey, E., and Delgado, M. (2008). Ghrelin protects against experimental sepsis by inhibiting high-mobility group box 1 release and by killing bacteria. *J. Immunol.* 180, 8369–8377. doi: 10.4049/jimmunol.180 12.8369

Cornide-Petronio, M. E., Bujaldon, E., Mendes-Braz, M., Avalos de León, C. G., Jiménez-Castro, M. B., Álvarez-Mercado, A. I., et al. (2017). The impact of cortisol in steatotic and non-steatotic liver surgery. *J. Cell. Mol. Med.* 21, 2344–2358. doi: 10.1111/jcmm.13156

Cui, F., Hu, H. F., Guo, J., Sun, J., and Shi, M. (2020). The effect of autophagy on chronic intermittent hypobaric hypoxia ameliorating liver damage in metabolic syndrome rats. *Front. Physiol.* 11:13. doi: 10.3389/fphys.2020.00013

Cui, Z., Li, S., Liu, Z., Zhang, Y., and Zhang, H. (2018). Interferon regulatory factor 1 activates autophagy to aggravate hepatic ischemia-reperfusion injury by increasing high mobility group box 1 release. *Cell. Physiol. Biochem.* 48, 328–338. doi: 10.1159/000491732

Degli Esposti, D., Sebagh, M., Pham, P., Reffas, M., Poüs, C., Brenner, C., et al. (2011). Ischemic preconditioning induces autophagy and limits necrosis in human recipients of fatty liver grafts, decreasing the incidence of rejection episodes. *Cell Death Dis.* 2:e111. doi: 10.1038/cddis.2010.89

Deng, J., Feng, J., Liu, T., Lu, X., Wang, W., Liu, N., et al. (2018). Beraprost sodium preconditioning prevents inflammation, apoptosis, and autophagy during hepatic ischemia-reperfusion injury in mice via the P38 and JNK pathways. *Drug Des. Devel. Ther.* 12, 4067–4082. doi: 10.2147/DDDT.S182292

du Toit, A., Hofmeyr, J. S., Gniadek, T. J., and Loos, B. (2018). Measuring autophagosome flux. *Autophagy* 14, 1060–1071. doi: 10.1080/15548627.2018. 1469590

Durczynski, A., Strzelczyk, J., Wojciechowska-Durczynska, K., Borkowska, A., Hogendorf, P., Szymanski, D., et al. (2013). Major liver resection results in early exacerbation of insulin resistance, and may be a risk factor of developing overt diabetes in the future. *Surg. Today* 43, 534–538. doi: 10.1007/s00595-012-0 268-8

Dusabimana, T., Kim, S. R., Kim, H. J., Kim, H., and Park, S. W. (2019). Nobiletin ameliorates hepatic ischemia and reperfusion injury through the activation of SIRT-1/FOXO3a-mediated autophagy and mitochondrial biogenesis. *Exp. Mol. Med.* 51, 1–16. doi: 10.1038/s12276-019-0245-z

El Atrache, M. M., Abouljoud, M. S., Divine, G., Yoshida, A., Kim, D. Y., Kazimi, M. M., et al. (2012). Recurrence of non-alcoholic steatohepatitis and cryptogenic cirrhosis following orthotopic liver transplantation in the context of the metabolic syndrome. *Clin. Transplant.* 26, 505–512. doi: 10.1111/ctr. 12014

Elias-Miró, M., Massip-Salcedo, M., Raila, J., Schweigert, F., Mendes-Braz, M., Ramalho, F., et al. (2012). Retinol binding protein 4 and retinol in steatotic and nonsteatotic rat livers in the setting of partial hepatectomy under ischemia/reperfusion. *Liver Transpl.* 18, 1198–1208. doi: 10.1002/lt. 23489

Engeli, S., Schling, P., Gorzelniak, K., Boschmann, M., Janke, J., Ailhaud, G., et al. (2003). The adipose-tissue renin-angiotensin-aldosterone system: role in the metabolic syndrome? *Int. J. Biochem. Cell Biol.* 35, 807–825. doi: 10.1016/s1357-2725(02)00311-4

Esser, N., Legrand-Poels, S., Piette, J., Scheen, A. J., and Paquot, N. (2014). Inflammation as a link between obesity, metabolic syndrome and type 2 diabetes. *Diabetes Res. Clin. Pract.* 105, 141–150. doi: 10.1016/j.diabres.2014. 04.006

Feng, J., Zhang, Q., Mo, W., Wu, L., Li, S., Li, J., et al. (2017). Salidroside pretreatment attenuates apoptosis and autophagy during hepatic ischemia-reperfusion injury by inhibiting the mitogen-activated protein kinase pathway in mice. *Drug Des. Devel. Ther.* 11, 1989–2006. doi: 10.2147/DDDT.S136792

Fernández, L., Carrasco-Chaumel, E., Serafín, A., Xaus, C., Grande, L., Rimola, A., et al. (2004). Is ischemic preconditioning a useful strategy in steatotic liver transplantation? *Am. J. Transplant.* 4, 888–899. doi: 10.1111/j.1600-6143.2004. 00447.x

Forbes, S. J., and Newsome, P. N. (2016). Liver regeneration - mechanisms and models to clinical application. *Nat. Rev. Gastroenterol. Hepatol.* 13, 473–485. doi: 10.1038/nrgastro.2016.97

Fortunato, F., Burgers, H., Bergmann, F., Rieger, P., Buchler, M. W., Kroemer, G., et al. (2009). Impaired autolysosome formation correlates with Lamp-2 depletion: role of apoptosis, autophagy, and necrosis in pancreatitis. *Gastroenterology* 137, 350–360. doi: 10.1053/j.gastro.2009.04.003

Gadiparthi, C., Spatz, M., Greenberg, S., Iqbal, U., Kanna, S., Satapathy, S. K., et al. (2020). NAFLD Epidemiology, Emerging Pharmacotherapy, Liver Transplantation Implications and the Trends in the United States. *J. Clin. Transl. Hepatol.* 8, 215–221. doi: 10.14218/JCTH.2020.00014

Gjorgjieva, M., Mithieux, G., and Rajas, F. (2019). Hepatic stress associated with pathologies characterized by disturbed glucose production. *Cell Stress* 3, 86–99. doi: 10.15698/cst2019.03.179

Gong, L. L., Li, G. R., Zhang, W., Liu, H., Lv, Y. L., Han, F. F., et al. (2016). Akebia saponin D decreases hepatic steatosis through autophagy modulation. *J. Pharmacol. Exp. Ther.* 359, 392–400. doi: 10.1124/jpet.116.236562

Gong, L. L., Yang, S., Zhang, W., Han, F. F., Lv, Y. L., Wan, Z. R., et al. (2018). Akebia saponin D alleviates hepatic steatosis through BNip3 induced mitophagy. *J. Pharmacol. Sci.* 136, 189–195. doi: 10.1016/j.jphs.2017.11.007

Gonzalez, C. D., Lee, M. S., Marchetti, P., Pietropaolo, M., Towns, R., Vaccaro, M. I., et al. (2011). The emerging role of autophagy in the pathophysiology of diabetes mellitus. *Autophagy* 7, 2–11. doi: 10.4161/auto.7.1.13044

González, H. D., Liu, Z. W., Cashman, S., and Fusai, G. K. (2010). Small for size syndrome following living donor and split liver transplantation. *World J. Gastrointest. Surg.* 2, 389–394. doi: 10.4240/wjgs.v2.i12.389

González-Rodríguez, A., Mayoral, R., Agra, N., Valdecantos, M. P., Pardo, V., Miquilena-Colina, M. E., et al. (2014). Impaired autophagic flux is associated with increased endoplasmic reticulum stress during the development of NAFLD. *Cell Death Dis.* 5:e1179. doi: 10.1038/cddis.2014.162

Goto, T., Elbahrawy, A., Furuyama, K., Horiguchi, M., Hosokawa, S., Aoyama, Y., et al. (2017). Liver-specific Prox1 inactivation causes hepatic injury and glucose intolerance in mice. *FEBS Lett.* 591, 624–635. doi: 10.1002/1873-3468.12570

Gotoh, K., Lu, Z., Morita, M., Shibata, M., Koike, M., Waguri, S., et al. (2009). Participation of autophagy in the initiation of graft dysfunction after rat liver transplantation. *Autophagy* 5, 351–360. doi: 10.4161/auto.5.3.7650

Gracia-Sancho, J., García-Calderó, H., Hide, D., Marrone, G., Guixé-Muntet, S., Peralta, C., et al. (2013). Simvastatin maintains function and viability of steatotic rat livers procured for transplantation. *J. Hepatol.* 58, 1140–1146. doi: 10.1016/j.jhep.2013.02.005

Gupta, N. A., Kolachala, V. L., Jiang, R., Abramowsky, C., Shenoi, A., Kosters, A., et al. (2014). Mitigation of autophagy ameliorates hepatocellular damage following ischemia-reperfusion injury in murine steatotic liver. *Am. J. Physiol. Gastrointest. Liver Physiol.* 307, G1088–G1099. doi: 10.1152/ajpgi.002 10.2014

Han, S., Ko, J. S., Jin, S. M., Park, H. W., Kim, J. M., Joh, J. W., et al. (2014). Intraoperative hyperglycemia during liver resection: predictors and association with the extent of hepatocytes injury. *PLoS One* 9:e0109120. doi: 10.1371/journal.pone.0109120

He, Q., Mei, D., Sha, S., Fan, S., Wang, L., and Dong, M. (2016). ERK-dependent mTOR pathway is involved in berberine-induced autophagy in hepatic steatosis. *J. Mol. Endocrinol.* 57, 251–260. doi: 10.1530/JME-16-0139

Homma, T., and Fujii, J. (2020). Emerging connections between oxidative stress, defective proteolysis, and metabolic diseases. *Free Radic. Res.* 0, 1–16. doi: 10.1080/10715762.2020.1734588

Houben, T., Oligschlaeger, Y., Hendrikx, T., Bitorina, A. V., Walenbergh, S. M. A., Van Gorp, P. J., et al. (2017). Cathepsin D regulates lipid metabolism in murine steatohepatitis. *Sci. Rep.* 7:3494. doi: 10.1038/s41598-017-03796-5

Hsu, H. C., Liu, C. H., Tsai, Y. C., Li, S. J., Chen, C. Y., Chu, C. H., et al. (2016). Time-dependent cellular response in the liver and heart in a dietary-induced obese mouse model: the potential role of ER stress and autophagy. *Eur. J. Nutr.* 55, 2031–2043. doi: 10.1007/s00394-015-1017-8

Huang, Q., Wang, T., Yang, L., and Wang, H. Y. (2017). Ginsenoside Rb2 alleviates hepatic lipid accumulation by restoring autophagy via induction of sirt1 and activation of AMPK. *Int. J. Mol. Sci.* 18, 1–15. doi: 10.3390/ijms18 051063

Inami, Y., Yamashina, S., Izumi, K., Ueno, T., Tanida, I., Ikejima, K., et al. (2011). Hepatic steatosis inhibits autophagic proteolysis via impairment of autophagosomal acidification and cathepsin expression. *Biochem. Biophys. Res. Commun.* 412, 618–625. doi: 10.1016/j.bbrc.2011.08.012

Ingaramo, P. I., Ronco, M. T., Francés, D. E. A., Monti, J. A., Pisani, G. B., Ceballos, M. P., et al. (2011). Tumor necrosis factor alpha pathways develops liver apoptosis in type 1 diabetes mellitus. *Mol. Immunol.* 48, 1397–1407. doi: 10.1016/j.molimm.2011.03.015

Jeong Kim, H., Joe, Y., Kim, S. K., Park, S. U., Park, J., Chen, Y., et al. (2017). Carbon monoxide protects against hepatic steatosis in mice by inducing sestrin-2 via the PERK-eIF2α-ATF4 pathway. *Free Radic. Biol. Med.* 110, 81–91. doi: 10.1016/j.freeradbiomed.2017.05.026

Ji, J., Wu, L., Feng, J., Mo, W., Wu, J., Yu, Q., et al. (2020). Cafestol preconditioning attenuates apoptosis and autophagy during hepatic ischemia-reperfusion injury by inhibiting ERK/PPARγ pathway. *Int. Immunopharmacol.* 84:106529. doi: 10.1016/j.intimp.2020.106529

Jiang, T., Zhan, F., Rao, Z., Pan, X., Zhong, W., Sun, Y., et al. (2019). Combined ischemic and rapamycin preconditioning alleviated liver ischemia and reperfusion injury by restoring autophagy in aged mice. *Int. Immunopharmacol.* 74:105711. doi: 10.1016/j.intimp.2019.105711

Jiménez-Castro, M. B., Casillas-Ramírez, A., Mendes-Braz, M., Massip-Salcedo, M., Gracia-Sancho, J., Elias-Miró, M., et al. (2013). Adiponectin and resistin protect steatotic livers undergoing transplantation. *J. Hepatol.* 59, 1208–1214. doi: 10.1016/j.jhep.2013.07.015

Jiménez-Castro, M. B., Elias-Miro, M., Mendes-Braz, M., Lemoine, A., Rimola, A., Rodés, J., et al. (2012). Tauroursodeoxycholic acid affects PPARγ and TLR4 in Steatotic liver transplantation. *Am. J. Transplant.* 12, 3257–3271. doi: 10.1111/j.1600-6143.2012.04261.x

Jiménez-Castro, M. B., Negrete-Sánchez, E., Casillas-Ramírez, A., Gulfo, J., Álvarez-Mercado, A. I., Cornide-Petronio, M. E., et al. (2017). The effect of cortisol in rat steatotic and non-steatotic liver transplantation from brain-dead donors. *Clin. Sci.* 131, 733–746. doi: 10.1042/CS20160676

Jin, Y., Tan, Y., Chen, L., Liu, Y., and Ren, Z. (2018). Reactive oxygen species induces lipid droplet accumulation in HepG2 cells by increasing perilipin 2 expression. *Int. J. Mol. Sci.* 19:3445. doi: 10.3390/ijms19113445

Jung, S. H., Lee, W., Park, S. H., Lee, K. Y., Choi, Y. J., Choi, S., et al. (2020). Diclofenac impairs autophagic flux via oxidative stress and lysosomal dysfunction: implications for hepatotoxicity. *Redox. Biol.* 37:101751. doi: 10.1016/j.redox.2020.101751

Kabeya, Y., Mizushima, N., Ueno, T., Yamamoto, A., Kirisako, T., Noda, T., et al. (2000). LC3, a mammalian homologue of yeast Apg8p, is localized in autophagosome membranes after processing. *EMBO J.* 19, 5720–5728. doi: 10.1093/emboj/19.21.5720

Kan, C., Liu, A., Fang, H., Dirsch, O., Dahmen, U., and Boettcher, M. (2017). Induction of autophagy reduces ischemia/reperfusion injury in steatotic rat livers. *J. Surg. Res.* 216, 207–218. doi: 10.1016/j.jss.2017.04.012

Kang, R. A., Han, S., Lee, K. W., Kim, G. S., Choi, S. J., Ko, J. S., et al. (2018). Portland intensive insulin therapy during living donor liver transplantation: association with postreperfusion hyperglycemia and clinical outcomes. *Sci. Rep.* 8:16306. doi: 10.1038/s41598-018-34655-6

Khader, A., Yang, W.-L., Godwin, A., Prince, J. M., Nicastro, J. M., Coppa, G. F., et al. (2017). Sirtuin 1 stimulation attenuates ischemic liver injury and enhances mitochondrial recovery and autophagy. *Crit. Care Med.* 44, 651–663. doi: 10.1097/CCM.0000000000001637

Kim, B. W., Kwon, D. H., and Song, H. K. (2016). Structure biology of selective autophagy receptors. *BMB Rep.* 49, 73–80. doi: 10.5483/BMBRep.2016.49.2.265

Kim, K. H., Jeong, Y. T., Oh, H., Kim, S. H., Cho, J. M., Kim, Y. N., et al. (2013). Autophagy deficiency leads to protection from obesity and insulin resistance by inducing Fgf21 as a mitokine. *Nat. Med.* 19, 83–92. doi: 10.1038/nm.3014

Kirisako, T., Ichimura, Y., Okada, H., Kabeya, Y., Mizushima, N., Yoshimori, T., et al. (2000). The reversible modification regulates the membrane-binding state of Apg8/Aut7 essential for autophagy and the cytoplasm to vacuole targeting pathway. *J. Cell Biol.* 151, 263–276. doi: 10.1083/jcb.151.2.263

Klionsky, D. J., Abdel-Aziz, A. K., Abdelfatah, S., Abdellatif, M., Abdoli, A., Abel, S., et al. (2021). Guidelines for the use and interpretation of assays for monitoring autophagy (4th edition). *Autophagy* 17, 1–382. doi: 10.1080/15548627.2020.1797280

Koga, H., Kaushik, S., and Cuervo, A. M. (2010). Altered lipid content inhibits autophagic vesicular fusion. *FASEB J.* 24, 3052–3065. doi: 10.1096/fj.09-144519

Kong, D., Hua, X., Qin, T., Zhang, J., He, K., and Xia, Q. (2019). Inhibition of glycogen synthase kinase 3ß protects liver against ischemia/reperfusion injury by activating 5′ adenosine monophosphate-activated protein kinase-mediated autophagy. *Hepatol. Res.* 49, 462–472. doi: 10.1111/hepr.13287

Kou, X., Zhu, J., Xie, X., Hao, M., and Zhao, Y. (2020). The protective effect of glycyrrhizin on hepatic ischemia-reperfusion injury in rats and possible related signal pathway. *Iran. J. Basic Med. Sci.* 23, 1232–1238. doi: 10.22038/ijbms.2020.44101.10334

Kramer, C. K., Zinman, B., and Retnakaran, R. (2013). Short-term intensive insulin therapy in type 2 diabetesmellitus: a systematic review and meta-analysis. *Lancet Diabetes Endocrinol.* 1, 28–34. doi: 10.1016/S2213-8587(13)70006-8

Kuo, N. C., Huang, S. Y., Yang, C. Y., Shen, H. H., and Lee, Y. M. (2020). Involvement of HO-1 and autophagy in the protective effect of magnolol in hepatic steatosis-induced NLRP3 inflammasome activation in vivo and in vitro. *Antioxidants* 9, 1–19. doi: 10.3390/antiox9100924

Kurahashi, T., Hamashima, S., Shirato, T., Lee, J., Homma, T., Kang, E. S., et al. (2015). An SOD1 deficiency enhances lipid droplet accumulation in the fasted mouse liver by aborting lipophagy. *Biochem. Biophys. Res. Commun.* 467, 866–871. doi: 10.1016/j.bbrc.2015.10.052

Lamark, T., Perander, M., Outzen, H., Kristiansen, K., Overvatn, A., Michaelsen, E., et al. (2003). Interaction codes within the family of mammalian Phox and Bem1p domain-containing proteins. *J. Biol. Chem.* 278, 34568–34581. doi: 10.1074/jbc.M303221200

Lee, D. H., Park, S. H., Huh, Y. H., Jung Kim, M., Seo, H. D., Ha, T. Y., et al. (2020). Iridoids of Valeriana fauriei contribute to alleviating hepatic steatosis in obese mice by lipophagy. *Biomed. Pharmacother.* 125:109950. doi: 10.1016/j.biopha.2020.109950

Lee, H. S., Daniels, B. H., Salas, E., Bollen, A. W., Debnath, J., and Margeta, M. (2012). Clinical utility of LC3 and p62 immunohistochemistry in diagnosis of drug-induced autophagic vacuolar myopathies: a case-control study. *PLoS One* 7:e36221. doi: 10.1371/journal.pone.0036221

Lee, K., Haddad, A., Osme, A., Kim, C., Borzou, A., Ilchenko, S., et al. (2018). Hepatic mitochondrial defects in a nonalcoholic fatty liver disease mouse model are associated with increased degradation of oxidative phosphorylation subunits. *Mol. Cell Proteomics* 17, 2371–2386. doi: 10.1074/mcp.RA118.000961

Lee, S., Kim, S., Hwang, S., Cherrington, N. J., and Ryu, D. Y. (2017). Dysregulated expression of proteins associated with ER stress, autophagy and apoptosis in tissues from nonalcoholic fatty liver disease. *Oncotarget* 8, 63370–63381. doi: 10.18632/oncotarget.18812

Lee, S., Rivera-Vega, M., Alsayed, H. M., Boesch, C., and Libman, I. (2015). Metabolic inflexibility and insulin resistance in obese adolescents with non-alcoholic fatty liver disease. *Pediatr. Diabetes.* 16, 211–218. doi: 10.1111/pedi.12141

Lee, S. C., Kim, K. H., Kim, O. H., Lee, S. K., and Kim, S. J. (2016). Activation of autophagy by everolimus confers hepatoprotection against ischemia-reperfusion injury. *Am. J. Transplant.* 16, 2042–2054. doi: 10.1111/ajt.13729

Lehmann, T. G., Wheeler, M. D., Froh, M., Schwabe, R. F., Bunzendahl, H., Samulski, R. J., et al. (2003). Effects of three superoxide dismutase genes delivered with an adenovirus on graft function after transplantation of fatty livers in the rat. *Transplantation* 76, 28–37. doi: 10.1097/01.TP.0000065299.29900.17

Li, H., Pan, Y., Wu, H., Yu, S., Wang, J., Zheng, J., et al. (2020). Inhibition of excessive mitophagy by N-acetyl-L-tryptophan confers hepatoprotection against Ischemia-Reperfusion injury in rats. *PeerJ* 2020, 1–18. doi: 10.7717/peerj.8665

Li, J., Lin, W., and Zhuang, L. (2020). CD5L-induced activation of autophagy is associated with hepatoprotection in ischemic reperfusion injury via the CD36/ATG7 axis. *Exp. Ther. Med.* 19, 2588–2596. doi: 10.3892/etm.2020.8497

Li, J., Zhang, Q. H., Li, S., Dai, W., Feng, J., Wu, L., et al. (2017). The natural product fucoidan ameliorates hepatic ischemia–reperfusion injury in mice. *Biomed. Pharmacother.* 94, 687–696. doi: 10.1016/j.biopha.2017.07.109

Li, M., Xu, M., Li, J., Chen, L., Xu, D., Tong, Y., et al. (2018). Alda-1 ameliorates liver ischemia-reperfusion injury by activating aldehyde dehydrogenase 2 and enhancing autophagy in mice. *J. Immunol. Res.* 2018:9807139. doi: 10.1155/2018/9807139

Li, R., Xin, T., Li, D., Wang, C., Zhu, H., and Zhou, H. (2018). Therapeutic effect of sirtuin 3 on ameliorating nonalcoholic fatty liver disease: the role of the ERK–CREB pathway and Bnip3-mediated mitophagy. *Redox. Biol.* 18, 229–243. doi: 10.1016/j.redox.2018.07.011

Li, S., Takahara, T., Fujino, M., Fukuhara, Y., Sugiyama, T., Li, X. K., et al. (2017). Astaxanthin prevents ischemia-reperfusion injury of the steatotic liver in mice. *PLoS One* 12:e0187810. doi: 10.1371/journal.pone.0187810

Li, S., Zhang, J., Wang, Z., Wang, T., Yu, Y., He, J., et al. (2016). MicroRNA-17 regulates autophagy to promote hepatic ischemia/reperfusion injury via suppression of signal transductions and activation of transcription-3 expression. *Liver Transplant.* 22, 1697–1709. doi: 10.1002/lt.24606

Li, X., Gong, H., Yang, S., Yang, L., Fan, Y., and Zhou, Y. (2017). Pectic bee pollen polysaccharide from *Rosa rugosa* alleviates diet-induced hepatic steatosis and insulin resistance via induction of AMPK/mTOR-mediated autophagy. *Molecules* 22:699. doi: 10.3390/molecules22050699

Lin, Y., Sheng, M., Weng, Y., Xu, R., Lu, N., Du, H., et al. (2017). Berberine protects against ischemia/reperfusion injury after orthotopic liver transplantation via activating Sirt1/FoxO3α induced autophagy. *Biochem. Biophys. Res. Commun.* 483, 885–891. doi: 10.1016/j.bbrc.2017.01.028

Lin, Y. C., Chang, P. F., Lin, H. F., Liu, K., Chang, M. H., and Ni, Y. H. (2016). Variants in the autophagy-related gene IRGM confer susceptibility to non-alcoholic fatty liver disease by modulating lipophagy. *J. Hepatol.* 65, 1209–1216. doi: 10.1016/j.jhep.2016.06.029

Linecker, M., Limani, P., Kambakamba, P., Kron, P., Tschuor, C., Calo, N., et al. (2017). Omega-3 fatty acids protect fatty and lean mouse livers after major hepatectomy. *Ann. Surg.* 266, 324–332. doi: 10.1097/SLA.0000000000001968

Ling, Q., Yu, X., Wang, T., Wang, S. G., Ye, Z. Q., and Liu, J. H. (2017). Roles of the exogenous H2S-mediated SR a signaling pathway in renal ischemia/reperfusion injury in regulating endoplasmic reticulum stress-induced autophagy in a rat model. *Cell Physiol. Biochem.* 41, 2461–2474. doi: 10.1159/000475915

Liu, A., Guo, E., Yang, J., Li, R., Yang, Y., Liu, S., et al. (2016). Ischemic preconditioning attenuates ischemia/reperfusion injury in rat steatotic liver: role of heme oxygenase-1-mediated autophagy. *Oncotarget* 7, 78372–78386. doi: 10.18632/oncotarget.13281

Liu, H., Dong, J., Song, S., Zhao, Y., Wang, J., Fu, Z., et al. (2019). Spermidine ameliorates liver ischaemia-reperfusion injury through the regulation of autophagy by the AMPK-mTOR-ULK1 signalling pathway. *Biochem. Biophys. Res. Commun.* 519, 227–233. doi: 10.1016/j.bbrc.2019.08.162

Liu, H. Y., Han, J., Cao, S. Y., Hong, T., Zhuo, D., Shi, J., et al. (2009). Hepatic autophagy is suppressed in the presence of insulin resistance and hyperinsulinemia: inhibition of FoxO1-dependent expression of key autophagy genes by insulin. *J. Biol. Chem.* 284, 31484–31492. doi: 10.1074/jbc.M109.033936

Liu, P., Lin, H., Xu, Y., Zhou, F., Wang, J., Liu, J., et al. (2018). Frataxin-mediated PINK1-parkin-dependent mitophagy in hepatic steatosis: the protective effects of quercetin. *Mol. Nutr. Food. Res.* 62:e1800164. doi: 10.1002/mnfr.201800164

Liu, T., Han, Y., Lv, W., Qi, P., Liu, W., Cheng, Y., et al. (2019). GSK-3β mediates ischemia-reperfusion injury by regulating autophagy in DCD liver allografts. *Int. J. Clin. Exp. Pathol.* 12, 640–656.

Liu, Z., Ye, S., Zhong, X., Wang, W., Lai, C. H., Yang, W., et al. (2020). Pretreatment with the ALDH2 activator Alda-1 protects rat livers from ischemia/reperfusion injury by inducing autophagy. *Mol. Med. Rep.* 22, 2373–2385. doi: 10.3892/mmr.2020.11312

Lopez-Neblina, F., Toledo, A. H., and Toledo-Pereyra, L. H. (2005). Molecular biology of apoptosis in ischemia and reperfusion. *J. Invest. Surg.* 18, 335–350. doi: 10.1080/08941930500328862

Manna, P., Das, J., Ghosh, J., and Sil, P. C. (2010). Contribution of type 1 diabetes to rat liver dysfunction and cellular damage via activation of NOS, PARP, IkappaBalpha/NF-kappaB, MAPKs, and mitochondria-dependent pathways: prophylactic role of arjunolic acid. *Free Radic. Biol. Med.* 48, 1465–1484. doi: 10.1016/j.freeradbiomed.2010.02.025

Mao, Y., Zhang, S., Yu, F., Li, H., Guo, C., and Fan, X. (2015). Ghrelin attenuates liver fibrosis through regulation of TGF-β1 expression and autophagy. *Int. J. Mol. Sci.* 16, 21911–21930. doi: 10.3390/ijms160921911

Mareninova, O. A., Hermann, K., French, S. W., O'Konski, M. S., Pandol, S. J., Webster, P., et al. (2009). Impaired autophagic flux mediates acinar cell vacuole

formation and trypsinogen activation in rodent models of acute pancreatitis. *J. Clin. Invest.* 119, 3340–3355. doi: 10.1172/JCI38674

Massip-Salcedo, M., Casillas-Ramirez, A., Franco-Gou, R., Bartrons, R., Mosbah, I. B., Serafin, A., et al. (2006). Heat shock proteins and mitogen-activated protein kinases in steatotic livers undergoing ischemia-reperfusion: some answers. *Am. J. Pathol.* 168, 1474–1485. doi: 10.2353/ajpath.2006.050645

Massip-Salcedo, M., Zaouali, M. A., Padrissa-Altés, S., Casillas-Ramirez, A., Rodés, J., Rosselló-Catafau, J., et al. (2008). Activation of peroxisome proliferator-activated receptor-alpha inhibits the injurious effects of adiponectin in rat steatotic liver undergoing ischemia-reperfusion. *Hepatology* 47, 461–472. doi: 10.1002/hep.21935

Matter, M. S., Decaens, T., Andersen, J. B., and Thorgeirsson, S. S. (2014). Targeting the mTOR pathway in hepatocellular carcinoma: current state and future trends. *J. Hepatol.* 60, 855–865. doi: 10.1016/j.jhep.2013.11.031

McCormack, L., Petrowsky, H., Jochum, W., Furrer, K., and Clavien, P. A. (2007). Hepatic steatosis is a risk factor for postoperative complications after major hepatectomy: a matched case-control study. *Ann. Surg.* 245, 923–930. doi: 10.1097/01.sla.0000251747.80025.b7

Mei, S., Ni, H. M., Manley, S., Bockkus, A., Kassel, K. M., Luyendyk, J. P., et al. (2011). Differential roles of unsaturated and saturated fatty acids on autophagy and apoptosis in hepatocytes. *J. Pharmacol. Exp. Ther.* 339, 487–498. doi: 10.1124/jpet.111.184341

Menikdiwela, K. R., Ramalingam, L., Rasha, F., Wang, S., Dufour, J. M., Kalupahana, N. S., et al. (2020). Autophagy in metabolic syndrome: breaking the wheel by targeting the renin–angiotensin system. *Cell Death Dis.* 11:87. doi: 10.1038/s41419-020-2275-9

Micó-Carnero, M., Rojano-Alfonso, C., Álvarez-Mercado, A. I., Gracia-Sancho, J., Casillas-Ramírez, A., and Peralta, C. (2021). Effects of gut metabolites and microbiota in healthy and marginal livers submitted to surgery. *Int. J. Mol. Sci.* 22, 1–28. doi: 10.3390/ijms22010044

Minor, T., Koetting, M., Koetting, M., Kaiser, G., Efferz, P., Lüer, B., et al. (2011). Hypothermic reconditioning by gaseous oxygen improves survival after liver transplantation in the pig. *Am. J. Transplant.* 11, 2627–2634. doi: 10.1111/j.1600-6143.2011.03731.x

Miyagawa, K., Oe, S., Honma, Y., Izumi, H., Baba, R., and Harada, M. (2016). Lipid-induced endoplasmic reticulum stress impairs selective autophagy at the step of autophagosome-lysosome fusion in hepatocytes. *Am. J. Pathol.* 186, 1861–1873. doi: 10.1016/j.ajpath.2016.03.003

Miyamoto, S., and Heller, B. J. (2016). Drp1 and mitochondrial autophagy lend a helping hand in adaptation to pressure overload. *Circulation* 133:1225. doi: 10.1161/CIRCULATIONAHA.116.021796

Miyauchi, T., Uchida, Y., Kadono, K., Hirao, H., Kawasoe, J., Watanabe, T., et al. (2019). Up-regulation of FOXO1 and reduced inflammation by β-hydroxybutyric acid are essential diet restriction benefits against liver injury. *Proc. Natl. Acad. Sci. U.S.A.* 116, 13533–13542. doi: 10.1073/pnas.1820282116

Mizushima, N., Yoshimori, T., and Levine, B. (2010). Methods in mammalian autophagy research. *Cell* 140, 313–326. doi: 10.1016/j.cell.2010.01.028

Nakamura, K., Kageyama, S., Ito, T., Hirao, H., Kadono, K., Aziz, A., et al. (2019). Antibiotic pretreatment alleviates liver transplant damage in mice and humans. *J. Clin. Invest.* 129, 3420–3434. doi: 10.1172/JCI127550

Nakamura, K., Kageyama, S., Yue, S., Huang, J., Fujii, T., Sosa, R. A., et al. (2018). Heme oxygenase-1 regulates sirtuin-1 – autophagy pathway in liver transplantation: from mouse-to-human. *Am. J. Transplant.* 18, 1110–1121. doi: 10.1111/ajt.14586.Heme

Nakao, Y. M., Miyawaki, T., Yasuno, S., Nakao, K., Tanaka, S., Ida, M., et al. (2012). Intra-abdominal fat area is a predictor for new onset of individual components of metabolic syndrome: MEtabolic syndRome and abdominaL ObesiTy (MERLOT study). *Proc. Jpn. Acad. Ser. B. Phys. Biol. Sci.* 88, 454–461. doi: 10.2183/pjab.88.454

Ning, X. J., Yan, X., Wang, Y. F., Wang, R., Fan, X. L., Zhong, Z. B., et al. (2018). Parkin deficiency elevates hepatic ischemia/reperfusion injury accompanying decreased mitochondrial autophagy, increased apoptosis, impaired DNA damage repair and altered cell cycle distribution. *Mol. Med. Rep.* 18, 5663–5668. doi: 10.3892/mmr.2018.9606

Oberkofler, H., Pfeifenberger, A., Soyal, S., Felder, T., Hahne, P., Miller, K., et al. (2010). Aberrant hepatic TRIB3 gene expression in insulin-resistant obese humans. *Diabetologia* 53, 1971–1975. doi: 10.1007/s00125-010-1772-2

Ogihara, T., Asano, T., Ando, K., Chiba, Y., Sakoda, H., Anai, M., et al. (2002). Angiotensin II-induced insulin resistance is associated with enhanced insulin signaling. *Hypertension* 40, 872–879. doi: 10.1161/01.hyp.0000040262.48405.a8

Panisello-Roselló, A., Verde, E., Lopez, A., Flores, M., Folch-Puy, E., Rolo, A., et al. (2018). Cytoprotective mechanisms in fatty liver preservation against cold ischemia injury: a comparison between IGL-1 and HTK. *Int. J. Mol. Sci.* 19:348. doi: 10.3390/ijms19020348

Panisello-Roselló, A., Verde, E., Zaouali, M. A., Flores, M., Alva, N., Lopez, A., et al. (2017). The relevance of the UPS in fatty liver graft preservation: a new approach for IGL-1 and HTK solutions. *Int. J. Mol. Sci.* 18, 1–10. doi: 10.3390/ijms18112287

Pankiv, S., Clausen, T. H., Lamark, T., Brech, A., Bruun, J. A., Outzen, H., et al. (2007). p62/SQSTM1 binds directly to Atg8/LC3 to facilitate degradation of ubiquitinated protein aggregates by autophagy. *J. Biol. Chem.* 282, 24131–24145. doi: 10.1074/jbc.M702824200

Pantazi, E., Zaouali, M. A., Bejaoui, M., Folch-Puy, E., Abdennebi, H. B., Varela, A. T., et al. (2015). Sirtuin 1 in rat orthotopic liver transplantation: an IGL-1 preservation solution approach. *World J. Gastroenterol.* 21, 1765–1774. doi: 10.3748/wjg.v21.i6.1765

Parafati, M., Lascala, A., Morittu, V. M., Trimboli, F., Rizzuto, A., Brunelli, E., et al. (2015). Bergamot polyphenol fraction prevents nonalcoholic fatty liver disease via stimulation of lipophagy in cafeteria diet-induced rat model of metabolic syndrome. *J. Nutr. Biochem.* 26, 938–948. doi: 10.1016/j.jnutbio.2015.03.008

Pereira, S., Shah, A., George Fantus, I., Joseph, J. W., and Giacca, A. (2015). Effect of N-acetyl-l-cysteine on insulin resistance caused by prolonged free fatty acid elevation. *J. Endocrinol.* 225, 1–7. doi: 10.1530/JOE-14-0676

Putnam, K., Shoemaker, R., Yiannikouris, F., and Cassis, L. A. (2012). The renin-angiotensin system: a target of and contributor to dyslipidemias, altered glucose homeostasis, and hypertension of the metabolic syndrome. *Am. J. Physiol. Heart Circ. Physiol.* 302, H1219–H1230. doi: 10.1152/ajpheart.00796.2011

Quan, W., Hur, K. Y., Lim, Y., Oh, S. H., Lee, J. C., Kim, K. H., et al. (2012). Autophagy deficiency in beta cells leads to compromised unfolded protein response and progression from obesity to diabetes in mice. *Diabetologia* 55, 392–403. doi: 10.1007/s00125-011-2350-y

Ricca, L., Lemoine, A., Cauchy, F., Hamelin, J., Sebagh, M., Esposti, D. D., et al. (2015). Ischemic postconditioning of the liver graft in adult liver transplantation. *Transplantation* 99, 1633–1643. doi: 10.1097/TP.0000000000000685

Ricchi, M., Odoardi, M. R., Carulli, L., Anzivino, C., Ballestri, S., Pinetti, A., et al. (2009). Differential effect of oleic and palmitic acid on lipid accumulation and apoptosis in cultured hepatocytes. *J. Gastroenterol. Hepatol.* 24, 830–840. doi: 10.1111/j.1440-1746.2008.05733.x

Ruan, Z., Liang, M., Deng, X., Lai, M., Shang, L., and Su, X. (2019). Exogenous hydrogen sulfide protects fatty liver against ischemia-reperfusion injury by regulating endoplasmic reticulum stress-induced autophagy in macrophage through mediating the class A scavenger receptor pathway in rats. *Cell Biol. Int.* 44, 306–316. doi: 10.1002/cbin.11234

Samala, N., Tersey, S. A., Chalasani, N., Anderson, R. M., and Mirmira, R. G. (2017). Molecular mechanisms of nonalcoholic fatty liver disease: potential role for 12-lipoxygenase. *J. Diabetes Complications* 31, 1630–1637. doi: 10.1016/j.jdiacomp.2017.07.014

Sato, S., and Furuya, N. (2017). Induction of PINK1/Parkin-mediated mitophagy. *Methods Mol. Biol.* 1759, 9–17. doi: 10.1007/7651_2017_7

Schleinitz, D., Böttcher, Y., Blüher, M., and Kovacs, P. (2014). The genetics of fat distribution. *Diabetologia* 57, 1276–1286. doi: 10.1007/s00125-014-3214-z

Schott, M. B., Weller, S. G., Schulze, R. J., Krueger, E. W., Drizyte-Miller, K., Casey, C. A., et al. (2019). Lipid droplet size directs lipolysis and lipophagy catabolism in hepatocytes. *J. Cell Biol.* 218, 3320–3335. doi: 10.1083/jcb.201803153

Schulze, R. J., and McNiven, M. A. (2014). A well-oiled machine: DNM2/dynamin 2 helps keep hepatocyte lipophagy running smoothly. *Autophagy* 10, 388–389. doi: 10.4161/auto.27486

Selzner, M., Rüdiger, H. A., Sindram, D., Madden, J., and Clavien, P. A. (2000). Mechanisms of ischemic injury are different in the steatotic and normal rat liver. *Hepatology.* 32, 1280–1288. doi: 10.1053/jhep.2000.20528

Settembre, C., De Cegli, R., Mansueto, G., Saha, P. K., Vetrini, F., Visvikis, O., et al. (2013). TFEB controls cellular lipid metabolism through a starvation-induced autoregulatory loop. *Nat. Cell Biol.* 15, 647–658. doi: 10.1038/ncb2718

Shaker, M. E., Trawick, B. N., and Mehal, W. Z. (2016). The novel TLR9 antagonist COV08-0064 protects from ischemia/reperfusion injury in non-steatotic and steatotic mice livers. *Biochem. Pharmacol.* 112, 90–101. doi: 10.1016/j.bcp.2016.05.003

Shao, N., Yu, X. Y., Ma, X. F., Lin, W. J., Hao, M., and Kuang, H. Y. (2018). Exenatide delays the progression of nonalcoholic fatty liver disease in C57BL/6 Mice, which may involve inhibition of the NLRP3 inflammasome through the mitophagy pathway. *Gastroenterol. Res. Pract.* 2018:1864307. doi: 10.1155/2018/1864307

Simmons, R. K., Alberti, K. G., Gale, E. A., Colagiuri, S., Tuomilehto, J., Qiao, Q., et al. (2010). The metabolic syndrome: useful concept or clinical tool? Report of a WHO expert consultation. *Diabetologia* 53, 600–605. doi: 10.1007/s00125-009-1620-4

Singh, R., and Cuervo, A. M. (2012). Lipophagy: connecting autophagy and lipid metabolism. *Int. J. Cell Biol.* 2012:282041. doi: 10.1155/2012/282041

Singh, R., Kaushik, S., Wang, Y., Xiang, Y., Novak, I., Komatsu, M., et al. (2009). Autophagy regulates lipid metabolism. *Nature* 458, 1131–1135. doi: 10.1038/nature07976

Sinha, R. A., Farah, B. L., Singh, B. K., Siddique, M. M., Li, Y., Wu, Y., et al. (2014). Caffeine stimulates hepatic lipid metabolism by the autophagy-lysosomal pathway in mice. *Hepatology* 59, 1366–1380. doi: 10.1002/hep.26667

Stayrook, K. R., Bramlett, K. S., Savkur, R. S., Ficorilli, J., Cook, T., Christe, M. E., et al. (2005). Regulation of carbohydrate metabolism by the farnesoid X receptor. *Endocrinology* 146, 984–991.

Su, Z., Nie, Y., Huang, X., Zhu, Y., Feng, B., Tang, L., et al. (2019). Mitophagy in hepatic insulin resistance: therapeutic potential and concerns. *Front. Pharmacol.* 10:1193. doi: 10.3389/fphar.2019.01193

Sun, X.-L., Zhang, Y.-L., Xi, S.-M., Ma, L.-J., and Li, S.-P. (2019). MiR-330-3p suppresses phosphoglycerate mutase family member 5 -inducted mitophagy to alleviate hepatic ischemia-reperfusion injury. *J. Cell. Biochem.* 120, 4255–4267. doi: 10.1002/jcb.27711

Tan, R., Tian, H., Yang, B., Zhang, B., Dai, C., Han, Z., et al. (2018). Autophagy and Akt in the protective effect of erythropoietin helix B surface peptide against hepatic ischaemia/reperfusion injury in mice. *Sci. Rep.* 8, 1–9. doi: 10.1038/s41598-018-33028-3

Tanaka, S., Hikita, H., Tatsumi, T., Sakamori, R., Nozaki, Y., Sakane, S., et al. (2016). Rubicon inhibits autophagy and accelerates hepatocyte apoptosis and lipid accumulation in nonalcoholic fatty liver disease in mice. *Hepatology* 64, 1994–2014. doi: 10.1002/hep.28820

Tang, B., Bao, N., He, G., and Wang, J. (2019). Long noncoding RNA HOTAIR regulates autophagy via the miR-20b-5p/ATG7 axis in hepatic ischemia/reperfusion injury. *Gene* 686, 56–62. doi: 10.1016/j.gene.2018.10.059

Tashiro, H., Kuroda, S., Mikuriya, Y., and Ohdan, H. (2014). Ischemia–reperfusion injury in patients with fatty liver and the clinical impact of steatotic liver on hepatic surgery. *Surg. Today* 44, 1611–1625. doi: 10.1007/s00595-013-0736-9

Toledo, M., Batista-Gonzalez, A., Merheb, E., Aoun, M. L., Tarabra, E., Feng, D., et al. (2018). Autophagy regulates the liver clock and glucose metabolism by degrading CRY1. *Cell Metab.* 28, 268.e4–281.e4. doi: 10.1016/j.cmet.2018.05.023

Uchiyama, Y. (2001). Autophagic cell death and its execution by lysosomal cathepsins. *Arch. Histol. Cytol.* 64, 233–246. doi: 10.1679/aohc.64.233

Vanhorebeek, I., Gunst, J., Derde, S., Derese, I., Boussemaere, M., Güiza, F., et al. (2011). Insufficient activation of autophagy allows cellular damage to accumulate in critically ill patients. *J. Clin. Endocrinol. Metab.* 96, 633–645. doi: 10.1210/jc.2010-2563

Vida Perez, L., Montero Alvarez, J. L., Poyato Gonzalez, A., Briceño Delgado, J., Costan Rodero, G., Fraga Rivas, E., et al. (2016). Prevalence and predictors of metabolic syndrome after liver transplantation. *Transplant. Proc.* 48, 2519–2524. doi: 10.1016/j.transproceed.2016.08.029

Wan, X., Xu, C., Yu, C., and Li, Y. (2016). Role of NLRP3 Inflammasome in the Progression of NAFLD to NASH. *Can. J. Gastroenterol. Hepatol.* 2016:6489012. doi: 10.1155/2016/6489012

Wang, C., Niederstrasser, H., Douglas, P. M., Lin, R., Jaramillo, J., Li, Y., et al. (2017). Small-molecule TFEB pathway agonists that ameliorate metabolic syndrome in mice and extend *C. elegans* lifespan. *Nat. Commun.* 8:2270. doi: 10.1038/s41467-017-02332-3

Wang, H., Sun, R. Q., Zeng, X. Y., Zhou, X., Li, S., Jo, E., et al. (2015). Restoration of autophagy alleviates hepatic ER stress and impaired insulin signalling transduction in high fructose-fed male mice. *Endocrinology* 156, 169–181. doi: 10.1210/en.2014-1454

Wang, H. J., Park, J. Y., Kwon, O., Choe, E. Y., Kim, C. H., Hur, K. Y., et al. (2015). Chronic HMGCR/HMG-CoA reductase inhibitor treatment contributes to dysglycemia by upregulating hepatic gluconeogenesis through autophagy induction. *Autophagy* 11, 2089–2101. doi: 10.1080/15548627.2015. 1091139

Wang, H., Zhang, Q., Wen, Q., Zheng, Y., Lazarovici, P., Jiang, H., et al. (2012). Proline-rich Akt substrate of 40kDa (PRAS40): a novel downstream target of PI3k/Akt signaling pathway. *Cell. Signal.* 24, 17–24. doi: 10.1016/j.cellsig.2011. 08.010

Wang, J., Deng, M., Wu, H., Wang, M., Gong, J., Bai, H., et al. (2020). Suberoylanilide hydroxamic acid alleviates orthotopic liver transplantation-induced hepatic ischemia-reperfusion injury by regulating the AKT/GSK3ß/NF-?B and AKT/mTOR pathways in rat Kupffer cells. *Int. J. Mol. Med.* 45, 1875–1887. doi: 10.3892/ijmm.2020.4551

Wang, Q., Wei, S., Zhou, S., Qiu, J., Shi, C., Liu, R., et al. (2020). Hyperglycemia aggravates acute liver injury by promoting liver-resident macrophage NLRP3 inflammasome activation via the inhibition of AMPK/mTOR-mediated autophagy induction. *Immunol. Cell Biol.* 98, 54–66. doi: 10.1111/imcb.12297

Wang, R. R., Shen, Z. Y., Yang, L., Yin, M. L., Zheng, W. P., Wu, B., et al. (2017). Protective effects of heme oxygenase-1-transduced bone marrow-derived mesenchymal stem cells on reduced-size liver transplantation: role of autophagy regulated by the ERK/mTOR signaling pathway. *Int. J. Mol. Med.* 40, 1537–1548. doi: 10.3892/ijmm.2017.3121

Wang, W., Wu, L., Li, J., Ji, J., Chen, K., Yu, Q., et al. (2019). Alleviation of hepatic ischemia reperfusion injury by oleanolic acid pretreating via reducing HMGB1 release and inhibiting apoptosis and autophagy. *Mediators Inflamm.* 2019:3240713. doi: 10.1155/2019/3240713

Wang, X., Zhang, X., Chu, E. S. H., Chen, X., Kang, W., Wu, F., et al. (2018). Defective lysosomal clearance of autophagosomes and its clinical implications in nonalcoholic steatohepatitis. *FASEB J.* 32, 37–51. doi: 10.1096/fj.201601393R

Wang, Z., Hou, L., Huang, L., Guo, J., and Zhou, X. (2017). Exenatide improves liver mitochondrial dysfunction and insulin resistance by reducing oxidative stress in high fat diet-induced obese mice. *Biochem. Biophys. Res. Commun.* 486, 116–123. doi: 10.1016/j.bbrc.2017.03.010

Williamson, R. M., Price, J. F., Glancy, S., Perry, E., Nee, L. D., Hayes, P. C., et al. (2011). Prevalence of and risk factors for hepatic steatosis and nonalcoholic fatty liver disease in people with type 2 diabetes: the edinburgh type 2 diabetes study. *Diabetes Care* 34, 1139–1144. doi: 10.2337/dc10-2229

Wu, L., Zhang, Q., Dai, W., Li, S., Feng, J., Li, J., et al. (2017). Quercetin Pretreatment Attenuates Hepatic Ischemia Reperfusion-Induced Apoptosis and Autophagy by Inhibiting ERK/NF-κ B pathway. *Gastroenterol. Res. Pract.* 2017:9724217. doi: 10.1155/2017/9724217

Xiang, S., Chen, K., Xu, L., Wang, T., and Guo, C. (2020). Bergenin exerts hepatoprotective effects by inhibiting the release of inflammatory factors, apoptosis and autophagy via the PPAR-γ pathway. *Drug Des. Devel. Ther.* 14, 129–143. doi: 10.2147/DDDT.S229063

Xiong, J., Wang, K., He, J., Zhang, G., Zhang, D., and Chen, F. (2016). TFE3 alleviates hepatic steatosis through autophagy-induced lipophagy and PGC1α-mediated fatty acid β-oxidation. *Int. J. Mol. Sci.* 17:387. doi: 10.3390/ ijms17030387

Xu, D., Chen, L., Chen, X., Wen, Y., Yu, C., Yao, J., et al. (2017). The triterpenoid CDDO-imidazolide ameliorates mouse liver ischemia-reperfusion injury through activating the Nrf2/HO-1 pathway enhanced autophagy. *Cell Death Dis.* 8:e2983. doi: 10.1038/cddis.2017.386

Xu, S., Niu, P., Chen, K., Xia, Y., Yu, Q., Liu, N., et al. (2017). The liver protection of propylene glycol alginate sodium sulfate preconditioning against ischemia reperfusion injury: focusing MAPK pathway activity. *Sci. Rep.* 7, 1–12. doi: 10.1038/s41598-017-15521-3

Xu, Y., Tang, Y., Lu, J., Zhang, W., Zhu, Y., Zhang, S., et al. (2020). PINK1-mediated mitophagy protects against hepatic ischemia/reperfusion injury by restraining NLRP3 inflammasome activation. *Free Radic. Biol. Med.* 160, 871–886. doi: 10.1016/j.freeradbiomed.2020.09.015

Xue, Z., Zhang, Y., Liu, Y., Zhang, C., Shen, X., Gao, F., et al. (2020). PACAP neuropeptide promotes hepatocellular protection via CREB-KLF4 dependent autophagy in mouse liver ischemia reperfusion injury. *Theranostics* 10, 4453–4465. doi: 10.7150/thno.42354

Yan, B., Luo, J., Kaltenmeier, C., Du, Q., Stolz, D. B., Loughran, P., et al. (2020). Interferon Regulatory Factor-1 (IRF1) activates autophagy to promote liver ischemia/reperfusion injury by inhibiting β-catenin in mice. *PLoS One* 15:e0239119. doi: 10.1371/journal.pone.0239119

Yan, H., Gao, Y., and Zhang, Y. (2017). Inhibition of JNK suppresses autophagy and attenuates insulin resistance in a rat model of nonalcoholic fatty liver disease. *Mol. Med. Rep.* 15, 180–186. doi: 10.3892/mmr.201 6.5966

Yang, J. H., Chen, Q., Tian, S. Y., Song, S. H., Liu, F., Wang, Q. X., et al. (2015). The role of 1,25-dyhydroxyvitamin D3 in mouse liver ischemia reperfusion injury: regulation of autophagy through activation of mek/erk signaling and pten/pi3k/akt/mtorc1 signaling. *Am. J. Transl. Res.* 7, 2630–2645.

Yang, L., Li, P., Fu, S., Calay, E. S., and Hotamisligil, G. S. (2010). Defective hepatic autophagy in obesity promotes ER stress and causes insulin resistance. *Cell Metab.* 11, 467–478. doi: 10.1016/j.cmet.2010.04.005

Yasuda-Yamahara, M., Kume, S., Yamahara, K., Nakazawa, J., Chin-Kanasaki, M., Araki, H., et al. (2015). Lamp-2 deficiency prevents high-fat diet-induced obese diabetes via enhancing energy expenditure. *Biochem. Biophys. Res. Commun.* 465, 249–255. doi: 10.1016/j.bbrc.2015.08.010

Yu, Q., Wu, L., Liu, T., Li, S., Feng, J., Mao, Y., et al. (2019). Protective effects of levo-tetrahydropalmatine on hepatic ischemia/reperfusion injury are mediated by inhibition of the ERK/NF-κB pathway. *Int. Immunopharmacol.* 70, 435–445. doi: 10.1016/j.intimp.2019.02.024

Yu, X., Huang, S., Deng, Q., Tang, Y., Yao, P., Tang, H., et al. (2019). Linseed oil improves hepatic insulin resistance in obese mice through modulating mitochondrial quality control. *J. Funct. Foods* 53, 166–175. doi: 10.1016/j.jff. 2018.12.016

Yu, Y., Li, S., Wang, Z., He, J., Ding, Y., Zhang, H., et al. (2017). Interferon regulatory factor-1 activates autophagy to aggravate hepatic ischemia-reperfusion injury via the P38/P62 pathway in mice. *Sci. Rep.* 7:43684. doi: 10.1038/srep43684

Zaouali, M. A., Bardag-Gorce, F., Carbonell, T., Oliva, J., Pantazi, E., Bejaoui, M., et al. (2013a). Proteasome inhibitors protect the steatotic and non-steatotic liver graft against cold ischemia reperfusion injury. *Exp. Mol. Pathol.* 94, 352–359. doi: 10.1016/j.yexmp.2012.12.005

Zaouali, M. A., Boncompagni, E., Reiter, R. J., Bejaoui, M., Freitas, I., Pantazi, E., et al. (2013b). AMPK involvement in endoplasmic reticulum stress and autophagy modulation after fatty liver graft preservation: a role for melatonin and trimetazidine cocktail. *J. Pineal Res.* 55, 65–78. doi: 10.1111/jpi. 12051

Zaouali, M. A., Panisello, A., Lopez, A., Folch, E., Castro-Benítez, C., Adam, R., et al. (2017). Cross-talk between sirtuin 1 and high-mobility box 1 in steatotic liver graft preservation. *Transplant. Proc.* 49, 765–769. doi: 10.1016/ j.transproceed.2017.01.071

Zeng, X., Wang, S., Li, S., Yang, Y., Fang, Z., Huang, H., et al. (2019). Hypothermic oxygenated machine perfusion alleviates liver injury in donation after circulatory death through activating autophagy in mice. *Artif. Organs* 43, E320–E332. doi: 10.1111/aor.13525

Zhang, N., Sheng, M., Wu, M., Zhang, X., Ding, Y., Lin, Y., et al. (2019). Berberine protects steatotic donor undergoing liver transplantation via inhibiting endoplasmic reticulum stress-mediated reticulophagy. *Exp. Biol. Med.* 244, 1695–1704. doi: 10.1177/1535370219878651

Zhang, X., Han, J., Man, K., Li, X., Du, J., Chu, E. S., et al. (2016). CXC chemokine receptor 3 promotes steatohepatitis in mice through mediating inflammatory cytokines, macrophages and autophagy. *J. Hepatol.* 64, 160–170. doi: 10.1016/j. jhep.2015.09.005

Zhang, Z., Yao, Z., Chen, Y., Qian, L., Jiang, S., Zhou, J., et al. (2018). Lipophagy and liver disease: new perspectives to better understanding and therapy. *Biomed. Pharmacother.* 97, 339–348. doi: 10.1016/j.biopha.2017.07.168

Zhao, Q., Guo, Z., Deng, W., Fu, S., Zhang, C., Chen, M., et al. (2016). Calpain 2-mediated autophagy defect increases susceptibility of fatty livers to ischemia-reperfusion injury. *Cell Death Dis.* 7:e2186. doi: 10.1038/cddis.2016.66

Zhou, H., Du, W., Li, Y., Shi, C., Hu, N., Ma, S., et al. (2018). Effects of melatonin on fatty liver disease: the role of NR4A1/DNA-PKcs/p53 pathway, mitochondrial fission, and mitophagy. *J. Pineal. Res.* 64:1. doi: 10.1111/jpi. 12450

Zhu, J., Yao, K., Wang, Q., Guo, J., Shi, H., Mam, L., et al. (2016). Ischemic postconditioning-regulated miR-499 protects the rat heart against ischemia/reperfusion injury by inhibiting apoptosis through

PDCD4. *Cell Physiol. Biochem.* 39, 2364–2380. doi: 10.1159/000 452506

Zhu, S., Wu, Y., Ye, X., Ma, L., Qi, J., Yu, D., et al. (2016). FGF21 ameliorates nonalcoholic fatty liver disease by inducing autophagy. *Mol. Cell. Biochem.* 420, 107–119. doi: 10.1007/s11010-016-2774-2

From Metabolic Syndrome to Neurological Diseases: Role of Autophagy

Jessica Maiuolo[1]*, Micaela Gliozzi[1], Vincenzo Musolino[1], Cristina Carresi[1],
Federica Scarano[1], Saverio Nucera[1], Miriam Scicchitano[1], Francesca Bosco[1],
Stefano Ruga[1], Maria Caterina Zito[1], Roberta Macri[1], Rosamaria Bulotta[1],
Carolina Muscoli[1,2] and Vincenzo Mollace[1,2]

[1] IRC-FSH Department of Health Sciences, University "Magna Graecia" of Catanzaro, Catanzaro, Italy, [2] IRCCS San Raffaele, Rome, Italy

*Correspondence:
Jessica Maiuolo
jessicamaiuolo@virgilio.it

Metabolic syndrome is not a single pathology, but a constellation of cardiovascular disease risk factors including: central and abdominal obesity, systemic hypertension, insulin resistance (or type 2 diabetes mellitus), and atherogenic dyslipidemia. The global incidence of Metabolic syndrome is estimated to be about one quarter of the world population; for this reason, it would be desirable to better understand the underlying mechanisms involved in order to develop treatments that can reduce or eliminate the damage caused. The effects of Metabolic syndrome are multiple and wide ranging; some of which have an impact on the central nervous system and cause neurological and neurodegenerative diseases. Autophagy is a catabolic intracellular process, essential for the recycling of cytoplasmic materials and for the degradation of damaged cellular organelle. Therefore, autophagy is primarily a cytoprotective mechanism; even if excessive cellular degradation can be detrimental. To date, it is known that systemic autophagic insufficiency is able to cause metabolic balance deterioration and facilitate the onset of metabolic syndrome. This review aims to highlight the current state of knowledge regarding the connection between metabolic syndrome and the onset of several neurological diseases related to it. Furthermore, since autophagy has been found to be of particular importance in metabolic disorders, the probable involvement of this degradative process is assumed to be responsible for the attenuation of neurological disorders resulting from metabolic syndrome.

Keywords: metabolic syndrome, vascular endothelium, neurological disorders, autophagy, brain-derived neurotrophic factor

INTRODUCTION

Metabolic syndrome (MetS), also known as syndrome X, insulin resistance syndrome, or Reaven syndrome; is not a single pathology, but a constellation of cardiovascular disease risk factors. These clinical conditions comprise: (a) central and abdominal obesity, (b) systemic hypertension, (c) insulin resistance (or 2 diabetes mellitus), and (d) atherogenic dyslipidemia, the so-defined "deadly quartet" (McCracken et al., 2018). There are several definitions to indicate the characteristics of MetS; among these, we point out the one provided by the International Federation of Diabetes (IDF) of 2006 (Saklayen, 2018), which states that metabolic syndrome is represented by glucose in the blood above 5.6 mmol/L (100 mg/dl) (or diabetes already diagnosed) along with the presence of two or more of the following conditions:

- HDL cholesterol (HDL-C) < 1.0 mmol/L (40 mg/dl) in men; < 1.3 mmol/L (50 mg/dl) in women or drug treatment for low HDL-C;
- blood triglycerides > 1.7 mmol/L (150 mg/dl) or drug treatment for elevated triglycerides;
- blood pressure > 130/85 mmHg or drug treatment for hypertension;
- waist > 94 cm (men) or > 80 cm (women). Obesity is diagnosed using waist circumference, which correlates better with visceral adiposity than Body Mass Index (BMI) (Alberti et al., 2005).

The presence of three of the five main risk factors is sufficient to confirm a MetS diagnosis (Altieri et al., 2015). All other MetS definitions are very similar; however, parameters indicated may vary by a few units. The global incidence of MetS is very high, afflicting one third of adults 18 years or older in the United States alone (Aguilar et al., 2015). To date, we can estimate the global prevalence to be about one quarter of the world population (Li et al., 2008). In general, the prevalence of MetS has been found to increase with age, involving about 20% of males and 16% of females under 40 years of age; 41% of males and 37% of females between the ages of 40–59; and 52% of males and 54% of females over 60 years of age (Ervin, 2009; Aoki et al., 2014). During the last 15 years, the prevalence of MetS has increased (Pucci et al., 2017) and the main motivation is related to significant changes in lifestyle; the western lifestyle consists of numerous risk factors such as: high-fat diet, cigarette smoking, alcohol consumption, obesity, and physical inactivity (O'Doherty et al., 2016; Sarmiento Quintero et al., 2016; Finicelli et al., 2019). In particular, the western diet is based on high consumption of salt, refined sugars, and saturated fats that determine significant effects on body composition and metabolism such as: increased BMI, generalized and abdominal obesity, dyslipidemia, and type 2 diabetes (Misra and Khurana, 2008). In addition to lifestyle changes, we should include other concomitant factors such as: chronic inflammation, endothelial dysfunction, genetic susceptibility, hypercoagulability, and chronic stress (Srikanthan et al., 2016; Motamedi et al., 2017; Woo et al., 2019). The main features of MetS are summarized in **Figure 1**.

The first part of this review, after describing the main features of MetS, deepens the involvement of the vascular endothelium in this metabolic disorder based on current scientific literature. Subsequently, the development of neurological disorders resulting from metabolic syndrome is considered. Lastly, the importance of autophagic function has discussed with the aim of proposing this element as molecular target to reduce and/or eliminate the dangerous symptoms of MetS and the consequent neurological symptoms.

THE ROLE OF THE ENDOTHELIUM IN METABOLIC SYNDROME

MetS can, as already stated, increase the risk of developing type 2 diabetes mellitus, obesity, and cardiovascular diseases; contributing, therefore, to high rates of mortality and morbidity (Alberti et al., 2009). The common denominators between MetS and its metabolic disorders are chronic low-grade inflammation and activation of the immune system (Chawla et al., 2011; Ouchi et al., 2011; El-Benna et al., 2016). MetS demonstrates a central role in promoting tissue inflammation in the adipose tissue of the liver, muscles, and pancreas; with concomitant infiltration of macrophages, and production of pro-inflammatory cytokines including Tumor Necrosis Factor alpha (TNFα), Interleukin 6 (IL-6), IL1β, activation of the c-JUN N-terminal kinase (JNK), and nuclear factor-kappa B (NF-κB) pathways (Chawla et al., 2011; Elmarakby and Sullivan, 2012; Grandl and Wolfrum, 2018). Macrophages are classically classified into two distinct subtypes: the activated phenotype secreting pro-inflammatory cytokines (M1), and the alternatively activated phenotype which produces anti-inflammatory cytokines such as IL-10 (M2) (Chawla et al., 2011). Under normal conditions, macrophages have been described as being a mix between M1 and M2 phenotypes, while in MetS, a phenotypic shift from M2 to M1 has been noted, both in mice and in humans (Wentworth et al., 2010) which shows a marked proinflammatory response. The inflammatory process includes increased vascular permeability to immune cells with the endothelium playing a fundamental role in this process (Bañuls et al., 2017; Bruno et al., 2017; Friesen and Cowan, 2019). The endothelium is composed of a layer of cells and constitutes the internal lining of the blood vessels; playing the role of a selectively permeable barrier. Endothelial cells do not play a passive role; instead, they regulate very important physiological functions such as: maintaining homeostatic balance, controlling vasomotor tone, ensuring proper permeability, and managing innate immunity reactions (Godo and Shimokawa, 2017). Precisely for this reason, the endothelium can be considered as an organ. The permeability of the endothelium allows the transport of only a few necessary molecules; this selectivity is ensured by a fine regulation carried out by junction proteins that have the function of keeping endothelial cells closely adjacent; thereby preventing the passage of unwanted molecules or cells (Babushkina et al., 2015). Junction proteins can be classified into two categories: tight junctions, also known as zonula occludens, and adherens junctions. Ensuring the cell adhesions and junctions, cytoskeleton proteins play a particularly key role (Maiuolo et al., 2018). When the expression of these proteins is nullified or reduced, endothelial disassembly and dysfunction occurs (Kiseleva et al., 2018).

Vascular endothelium cells (VEC) play a fundamental role in the human body; ensuring the regulation of vasomotor functions, the maintenance of vessel walls, anti-platelet aggregation, and endocrine functions. Numerous harmful stimuli can lead to endothelial cell dysfunction (ECD) with consequential increases in the risk of many diseases including cardiovascular diseases (Vykoukal and Davies, 2011; Khaddaj Mallat et al., 2017;

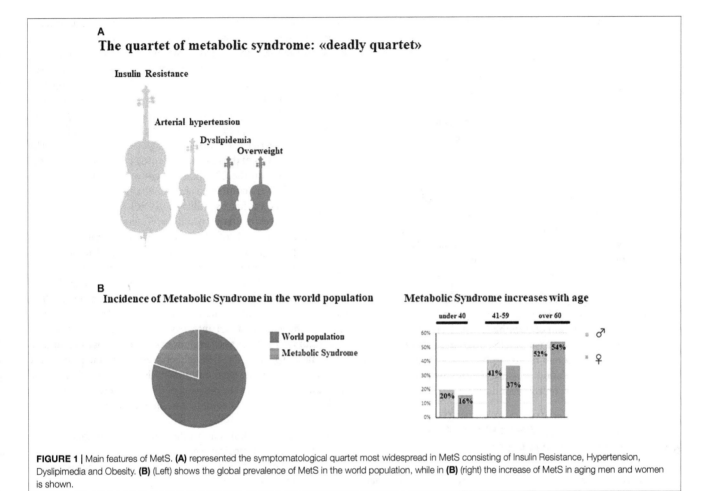

FIGURE 1 | Main features of MetS. **(A)** represented the symptomatological quartet most widespread in MetS consisting of Insulin Resistance, Hypertension, Dyslipimedia and Obesity. **(B)** (Left) shows the global prevalence of MetS in the world population, while in **(B)** (right) the increase of MetS in aging men and women is shown.

Kaplan et al., 2018; Maiuolo et al., 2020a). In MetS patients, the ECD is a specific early pathophysiological indicator of cardiovascular disorders; its recognition and early intervention are of extreme importance in the prevention, treatment, and prognosis of cardiovascular diseases (Wei et al., 2014; Dalal et al., 2020). In particular, many substances secreted by VEC are considered important indicators of the function of endothelial cells, these include: Plasminogen Activator Inhibitor-1 (PAI-1), von Willebrand factor (vWF), vascular endothelial cadherin (VE-cad), Thrombomodulin (TM), and Vascular endothelial growth factor (VEGF). PAI-1 is mainly produced by the endothelium but is also secreted by other types of tissue, such as adipose tissue. PAI-1 is a fibrinolysis inhibitor; preventing the physiological process that degrades blood clots and contributing to the formation of atherosclerotic plaques (Deng et al., 2012; Yarmolinsky et al., 2016). vWF is a macromolecular plasma glycoprotein involved in hemostasis with important implications in blood viscosity; an increase can predict the risk of thrombosis (Shahidi, 2017). VE-cad is a classic cadherin, belonging to the cadherin superfamily; it is expressed specifically on the endothelial surface and concentrated in existing cell-cell junctions. VE-cad is known to be necessary to maintain a restrictive endothelial barrier; early studies, using blocking antibodies against VE-caderin, resulted in increased endothelial

permeability *in vitro* (Hakanpaa et al., 2018) and in hemorrhage *in vivo* (Corada et al., 2002). TM is an integral membrane protein expressed on the surface of endothelial cells and serves as a cofactor for thrombin. TM reduces blood clotting by converting thrombin from a pro-clotting factor to an anti-coagulant factor (Loghmani and Conway, 2018). In normal conditions, plasma TM levels are low; but when vascular endothelial cells are damaged, TM increases significantly; highlighting that its level can be used as a marker of endothelial injury (Stadtmann et al., 2011; Kishi et al., 2020). VEGF is a selective signaling protein that promotes the growth of new blood vessels and restores the supply of oxygenated blood to cells and tissues that have been deprived due to impaired blood circulation. VEGF also improves vascular permeability by increasing exudation of blood components and inflammatory cytokines (Sack et al., 2016). Scientific studies have shown that serum levels of PAI-1, vWF, VE-cad, TM, and VEGF were increased in patients with MetS compared to healthy individuals (Georgieva et al., 2004; Hajiluian et al., 2017; Mazidi et al., 2017; Wang et al., 2018). Moreover, an increase has also been found in children and adolescents with MetS, evidencing that these parameters can be considered predictors of early vascular changes (Wei et al., 2014). MetS negatively affects the function of the vascular endothelium; increasing vasoconstriction and prothrombotic state through different mechanisms (Aggoun, 2007; O'Shea et al., 2015; Pomero et al., 2015; Domingueti et al., 2016):

- Hyperglycemia, hyperlipemia, and hypertension increase the release of numerous cytokines, such as: IL-1β, IL-6, and growth factor PDGF; triggering the process of endothelial dysfunction (Varghese et al., 2018).
- Carbohydrate metabolism (hyperinsulinemia/insulin resistance or hyperglycemia/diabetes), dyslipidemia, obesity, and hypertension can all determine vascular contractility (Cuspidi et al., 2018).
- Altered carbohydrate metabolism, dyslipidemia, hypertension, and obesity lead to increased PAI-1, vWF, VE-cad, TM, and VEGF production; a condition responsible for impaired anticoagulant and fibrinolytic activity which can cause hypercoagulability: a low fibrinolytic and high viscosity state, and promote the formation of microthrombi (Wei et al., 2014).

The main stages of endothelial inflammation, involved in Mets are represented in **Figure 2**. In the light of what has been stated, a clinical evaluation of endothelial involvement should be carried out both in patients with MetS and in people not affected who show clear risk factors related to body weight, metabolism of carbohydrates, and blood pressure. In this way, it could be possible to prevent and control secondary disorders of MetS.

FROM METABOLIC SYNDROME TO NEUROLOGICAL DISEASES

The effects of MetS are multiple and wide ranging; some of which have an impact on the central nervous system (CNS); causing neurodegenerative and neurological diseases (Kathy et al., 2012; Błaszczyk and Gawlik, 2016; Van Dyken and Lacoste, 2018). The CNS is the most complex and organized system in the human body and proper neuron functioning requires a correct biochemical balance (which includes suitable chemical and electrical signaling) in order to support and maintain adequate intracellular and intercellular communication. In addition, the correct concentration of ionic and signaling molecules must be guaranteed to remove catabolites and maintain a low concentration of neurotoxic mediators (Corasaniti et al., 2007; Maiuolo et al., 2018). A key role is played by the Blood Brain Barrier (BBB), which provides all these functions and represents a physical, selective, and highly lipophilic barrier; protecting brain tissue and separating it from systemic circulation (Daneman and Prat, 2015). The basic structure of the BBB consists of endothelial cells, tightly joined by junction proteins; while other constituents, including the basal membrane (BM), pericytes, and astrocytes, perform support and regulation functions (Andreone et al., 2015; O'Brown et al., 2018). The BBB endothelium is rich in specific proteins that act as carriers and receptors; responsible for the passage of metabolites, macronutrients, micronutrients, and junction proteins; which significantly limit their intercellular exchange. Endothelial cells consist of five or six times more mitochondria than other tissues in the human body as these organelles provide the energy required

for endothelial cells to maintain cerebral homeostasis (Gentil et al., 2005). Endothelial dysfunction leads to "frailty" of the BBB; characterized by increased vascular permeability, impaired ability to preserve brain tissue homeostasis, infiltration of toxic blood-derived molecules, cells, microbial agents; which together trigger inflammatory and immune neurodegeneration (Maiuolo et al., 2018, 2019). Basement membrane (BM) is composed of collagen, laminin, heparin, and other glycoproteins; it determines an additional barrier in the BBB, although it can be interrupted by metalloproteinases of the matrix (Thomsen et al., 2017). Pericytes are in contact with the BM, juxtaposed to the endothelial cells, with which they are connected and are involved in the regulation of angiogenesis, vascular stability, and BBB control (ElAli et al., 2014). Astrocytes regulate vasomotor responses and the brain blood flow as a result of changes in neural activity; they also release regulating factors for the maturation and maintenance of the BBB (Lacoste and Gu, 2015). Integrity of the BBB is essential to ensure the proper functioning of the CNS and many neurological disorders are caused by its rupture (Zhao et al., 2015; Chakraborty et al., 2017; Maiuolo et al., 2020b). The fundamental cause of the loss of barrier integrity is the inflammatory process that occurs in the CNS as a result of neuronal damage (Varatharaj and Galea, 2017). Under normal conditions, the integrity of the BBB prevents the passage of immune cells into the CNS; however, inflammation induces the opening of the BBB thereby altering the various components. The main consequences are:

- release of cytokines and inflammation mediators (Incalza et al., 2018; Oppedisano et al., 2020);
- leukocyte extravasation (diapedesis) across the endothelium (Rudziak et al., 2019);
- destruction of BBB cells (Chen et al., 2019).

The first important step for the diapedesis is the interaction between the leukocytes and adhesion molecules on endothelial cells, including P-selectin (a cell adhesion molecule on the surfaces of activated endothelial cells); E-selectin (endothelial-leukocyte adhesion molecule 1 expressed only on endothelial cells and activated by cytokines) (Laird et al., 2018); ICAM-1 (intercellular adhesion molecule-1 typically expressed on endothelial cells and cells of the immune system) (Schaefer et al., 2017); and VCAM-1 (vascular cell adhesion molecule-1 that mediates the adhesion of lymphocytes, monocytes, eosinophils, and basophils to vascular endothelium) (Fan et al., 2019). The next step involves the rolling of leukocytes along the wall of the vessel; the release of chemokines that strengthen contact with the endothelium; and the extension of pseudopods, from leukocytes, that allow the attack of endothelial cells (Lutz et al., 2017). The leukocyte crossing of the endothelium is defined as "transendothelial cell migration" and the correct direction to follow is provided by chemotactic and haptotactic stimuli outside of the vascular lumen and beyond. This movement occurs at the same time as the morphological variations of the leukocytes, which guide the cell nucleus through tight endothelial junctions and pores. Transendothelial leukocyte migration can take place through junctions between adjacent endothelial cells (paracellular migration) or through the

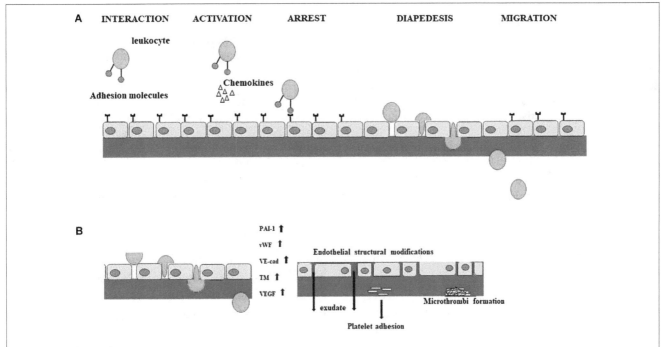

FIGURE 2 | Inflammation of the endothelium is involved in MetS and subsequent neurological manifestations. A portion of the inflammatory process, occurring both in MetS and in neurological disorders related to MetS, is schematized in Figure. In particular, **(A)** shows the sequence of leukocyte extravasation across the endothelium. **(B)** Important indicators of the dysfunction of endothelial cells are shown. The increases in PAI-1, vWF, VE-cad, TM and VEGF determine endothelial structural modifications, exudate production, platelet adhesion, and microthrombi formation.

body of the endothelium (transcellular migration) (Nourshargh and Alon, 2014). Although paracellular migration occurs in 70–80% of cases, the cerebral vascular endothelial cells appear to be an exception to this rule and prefer transcellular migration. This phenomenon is motivated by the particularly narrow specialized junction structures expressed by the brain endothelial cells (Engelhardt and Ransohoff, 2012). It has been widely demonstrated that increased inflammation facilitates BBB breakage (Varatharaj and Galea, 2017); with several mechanisms that include: downregulation of many junction proteins and important amino acid transporters (Yoo et al., 2016), alteration of transcytosis (Ransohoff et al., 2015), up-regulation of transporters for TNF-α, lysosomal degradation enzymes, VCAM-1 P/E-selectin (Varatharaj and Galea, 2017), and the accumulation of insoluble fibrin; responsible for the alteration of the immune response and blood clotting (Davalos and Akassoglou, 2012). Ultimately, these activated inflammatory processes are responsible for the destruction of cellular components of the BBB. In particular, the integrity of astrocytes is compromised, the leukocyte infiltration is increased, and the input of pathogens and toxins in the central nervous system is allowed (Van Dyken and Lacoste, 2018). Astrocytes are very susceptible to oxidative stress and inflammation; becoming unable to perform their role of maintaining ions and neurotransmitters in physiological conditions for BBB integrity (Bhat et al., 2012).

A positive feedback cycle has recently been described where activated microglia produce ROS; leading to cell death and increased levels of local glutamate. This condition results in increased secretion of proinflammatory cytokines, a further activation of microglia, and destruction of endothelial BBB cells (Mittal et al., 2014; Cai et al., 2017). Increased systemic inflammation impacts many of the systems in the body including the brain, in fact, inflammation is closely associated with neuropathology (Fan et al., 2014). To date, a series of epidemiological studies have shown that MetS increases the risk of developing neurodegenerative diseases, CNS dysfunction (Islam, 2017; Motamedi et al., 2017; Ricci et al., 2017; Arshad et al., 2018; Karaca and Karaca, 2018; Palta et al., 2021), and reduced cognitive performance including deficits in memory, visuospatial abilities, executive functioning, processing speed, and overall intellectual functioning. MetS was found to be a factor of risk for: ischemic stroke, intracranial arteriosclerosis, periventricular white matter hyperintensities, and subcortical white matter lesions (Yates et al., 2012). In this regard, changes in brain metabolism have been shown to be responsible for the onset of neuroinflammation; these brain changes may represent an early associated brain impairment with peripheral metabolic disorders.

MetS: Obesity, Diabetes, and Cognitive Functions

Obesity is the excess accumulation of body fat caused by an imbalance between energy intake and consumption. The effects of obesity are largely mediated through inflammation and, in these mouse models, neural inflammation can be detected even earlier than weight gain (Van Dyken and Lacoste, 2018). Obesity is directly related to impairment of cognitive function and an increased risk of different forms of dementia. Clinical and experimental evidence indicates that obesity and/or a high-fat diet is associated with impairment of learning, memory, and executive functioning (Anstey et al., 2011; Bremer and Jialal, 2013; Miller and Spencer, 2014; Saltiel and Olefsky, 2017; Costello and Petzold, 2020). Many studies have been carried out on the correlation of BMI-cognitive function and waist circumference-cognitive function. In general, it has been found that BMI is inversely related to cognitive function, including memory and executive functioning. In addition to cognitive performance, obesity can affect brain structure; leading to atrophy (Climie et al., 2015; Gogniat et al., 2018). Moreover, a relationship has also been described regarding particular areas of the brain; the temporal and frontal lobes appear to be particularly vulnerable to the effects of obesity and gray matter volumes of these brain regions are reduced in obese patients; resulting in the reduction of neuronal viability (Gómez-Apo et al., 2018; Lee et al., 2020). The first area of the brain to be affected is the hypothalamus; the subsequent damage reduces the number of synapses on hypothalamic neurons and increases neural apoptosis (Sohn, 2015). The obese mice showed a lower yield than the control group, thus confirming involvement of the hippocampus and cognitive impairment (Pendlebury and Rothwell, 2009; Hargrave et al., 2016; Van Dyken and Lacoste, 2018).

The activation of the inflammatory process, present in obesity, seems to be the fundamental cause of the alteration of the health of the brain (function and structure). In particular, a chain reaction occurs in which the activation of transcription factor NF-kB can be appreciated (Jais and Brüning, 2017), followed by upregulation of pro-inflammatory cytokines, such as: IL-1β, TNF-α, and IL-6 (Lawrence, 2009). It is also important to note that the observed cognitive decline was preceded by the reduction of protein TJ expression and loss of BBB integrity (Gustafson et al., 2007; Davidson et al., 2013; Dorfman and Thaler, 2015).

Scientific evidence has shown, both in animal models and in humans, a close correlation between diabetes mellitus [type 1 (T1DM) and type 2 (T2DM)] and cognitive decline leading to dementia; although T2DM has shown a stronger association with brain disorders (Monette et al., 2014; Zilliox et al., 2016; Black et al., 2018). Among the components of MetS, hyperglycemia has the strongest association with the risk of developing cognitive deterioration (Šmahelová, 2017). Numerous studies have shown reduced performance in cognitive activities in diabetic compared to non-diabetic controls which include memory, mental speed, mental flexibility, and executive function. These dysfunctions have been correlated with a reduced density of gray matter of the prefrontal and temporal cortex (van den Berg et al., 2010). It is not perfectly clear when cognitive impairment occurs in the course of diabetes; in some cases these events can be very early, while in other cases they are later events (Hassing et al., 2004). It is known that insulin signaling improves synaptic plasticity in the hippocampus; playing an important role in memory and learning. In fact, insulin facilitates long-term enhancement of the hippocampus (LTP) and, in the healthy mammalian brain, is associated with learning and memory; increasing the expression of N-methyl-D-aspartate receptors. In addition, insulin regulates

the concentration of several important neurotransmitters in memory maintenance such as: acetylcholine, norepinephrine, and epinephrine (Boyd et al., 1985; Figlewicz et al., 1993; Patterson et al., 2016). Insulin dysregulation in patients with diabetes could facilitate cognitive disorders (Kullmann et al., 2016; Denver et al., 2018; Tumminia et al., 2018). Insulin in the brain also has the function of regulating mitochondria (Heras-Sandoval et al., 2012). It has been shown that, in a condition of overt diabetes, highly altered insulin acts on the pre-synaptic terminals causing the mitochondrial DNA mutations responsible for functional and structural changes of the organelles (Lu et al., 2004). Dysfunction of the mitochondria causes the depletion of energy reserves; the enzymatic complexes of the electronic transport chain (complexes I and III) are altered, leading to neuronal synaptic loss and cognitive deficits (Kim et al., 2009; Choi et al., 2014).

MetS: Cognitive Dysfunction and the Possible Role of Brain-Derived Neurotrophic Factor

In the early 1950s, the neurotrophic theory was developed. This theory is based on the functional mechanisms adopted by effecter cells to control growth, survival, differentiation, and neural function through the production of biomolecules, identified as neurotrophins (Lewin and Barde, 1996; Dechant and Neumann, 2002). To date, it is known that the family of these molecules includes: Nerve Growth Factor (NGF), Brain-Derived Neurotrophic Factor (BDNF), Neurotrophin3 (NT3), NT4, NT5, NT6, and NT7 (Emanueli et al., 2014; West et al., 2014; Skup, 2018). BDNF is the most abundant neurotrophin in the mammalian CNS and is synthesized and expressed in different cerebral regions. BDNF is a protein encoded by the *BDNF* gene found in humans on chromosome 11; it is initially synthesized as a precursor, pro-BDNF, consisting of 129 amino acids in the endoplasmic reticulum. Subsequently, pro-BDNF is split through the action of proconvertase; in a mature form of 118 amino acids in the trans-Golgi. The mature shape dimerizes; forming the BDNF active factor (Hempstead, 2015). BDNF is synthesized in the cytoplasm of neurons and glia; although it is also found in the skeletal and smooth muscles, liver, lymphocytes, endocrine system, pancreas, endothelial cells, and adipose tissue (Ansari et al., 2016). BDNF is involved in many neurological processes such as: neural growth, differentiation, synaptic conductivity, plasticity, neurogenesis, neuroregeneration, cognition, memory, learning, and dendrite growth (Smith et al., 2015; Morales-Marín et al., 2016). For this reason, structural and functional alteration of BDNF, determined by several factors, has been implicated in a number of neurodegenerative diseases and psychiatric disorders such as Alzheimer's disease, Huntington's disease, Parkinson's disease, schizophrenia, intellectual disability, autism, depression, and the development of mood disorders (Björkholm and Monteggia, 2016). It has been shown that neurotrophins exert a metabotropic effect with respect to glucose, lipid, and energy; therefore, they have an important role in MetS (Chaldakov et al., 2014; Kim et al., 2020). Recent studies have shown a correlation between BDNF and MetS. In fact, there is a reduction of BDNF levels, especially in the stages of advancement of MetS (Morales-Marín et al., 2016). BDNF, which is reduced in MetS, performs critical functions within the CNS and alterations determine neurological diseases. Therefore, we can indirectly conclude that cognitive dysfunctions in MetS are correlated with BDNF. However, in order to better understand this topic, further studies should be carried out.

CAN AUTOPHAGY INTERFERE WITH METS AND ASSOCIATED NEURONAL DISORDERS?

Autophagy is a catabolic intracellular process evolutionarily preserved and finely regulated; essential for the recycling of cytoplasmic materials (proteins, lipids, carbohydrates) and for the degradation of damaged organelles (mitochondria, endoplasmic reticulum and peroxisomes), whose accumulation can be toxic to cells (Lapaquette et al., 2015). In this way, the renewal and proper functioning of intracellular organelles is also guaranteed. In lysosomes, autophagy determines: the recycling of cell portions that can still be used, the reduction of cell waste, the protection and maintenance of cellular energy and cellular adaptation to environmental challenges; all processes that contribute to cell survival (Madrigal-Matute and Cuervo, 2016). Therefore, autophagy is primarily a cytoprotective mechanism; even if excessive self-degradation can be detrimental. To date, it is known that autophagic activity is also connected to other important roles such as: the maintenance of cellular metabolism, control of cell cycle, immune response, development, and differentiation or cell death (Hu et al., 2019). In addition, when cells are subjected to a wide range of stressful conditions (physical, chemical, or metabolic), the autophagic process is activated in order to maintain cellular homeostasis. Since autophagy is critical for the maintenance of cellular metabolic homeostasis of whole body, its dysregulation may be the cause of the onset of pathologies which can affect liver, heart, brain, myopathies, diabetes, obesity, and cancer (Lim et al., 2018). Four main forms of autophagy have been described in mammalians:

- Macroautophagy (herein autophagy) is a catabolic process in which old cytoplasmic proteins, lipids, or damaged organelles are incorporated in double-membrane vesicular structures called autophagosomes. Autophagosomal membranes may derive from a number of sources such as: endoplasmic reticulum, Golgi apparatus, mitochondria, endosomes, and the plasma membrane. The movement of the autophagosomes takes place along the microtubules until reaching the lysosomes where the degradation process occurs (Feng et al., 2015).
- Microautophagy, a non-selective lysosomal process, refers to the direct engulfment of small amounts of cytosolic material (Li and Hochstrasser, 2020).
- Chaperone-mediated autophagy refers to the process in which some protein complexes are recognized by the cytosolic chaperones that deliver them to the surface of the lysosomes (Tekirdag and Cuervo, 2018).

- Selective autophagy that requires the respect of three criteria to ensure an efficient process (Zaffagnini and Martens, 2016): (i) the specific recognition of the cargo to be phagocytized; (ii) an efficient bonding of the cargo to a nascent autophagosome; (iii) the exclusion of components not part of the cargo.

The autophagy mechanism requires the expression of a set of evolutionarily conserved autophagy related genes (ATGs) whose protein products combine to form several useful complexes in the various stages of this process. All ATG genes, originally discovered in yeast, are needed for the efficient formation of autophagosomes that blend with the lysosomes, orchestrating and mediating the intra-cytoplasmic cargo degradation (Mizushima, 2018). The whole autophagic process is divided into six main steps which need to be tightly regulated both spatially and temporally: initiation, nucleation of vesicles, membrane elongation, closure, maturation, and degradation (Grumati and Dikic, 2018). In particular, the induction of autophagy occurs with the recruitment of Atg proteins and other proteic complexes in a specific subcellular position, called Phagophore Assembly Site, and with the nucleation of an insulating membrane forming a structure called phagophore (Yu et al., 2018). The very first autophagy-specific complex is termed Unc-51-Like Kinase 1 (ULK1) and is composed by ULK1 itself, Atg13, Focal adhesion kinase family Interacting Protein (FIP200) and Atg101 (Zachari and Ganley, 2017). When activated, ULK1 phosphorylates other autophagy pathway components, including Beclin1 and Atg9 and the onset of phagophore formation occurs when ULK1 complex is moved to a specific place in the endoplasmic reticulum membrane marked by the activated Atg9 protein (Levine and Kroemer, 2019). Elongation of the autophagosome membrane determines the expansion of the autophagosome in a sphere, around to the portion of the cytosol that must be degraded (Yoshii and Mizushima, 2017). This step involves Atg7 and Atg10 complexes that combine Atg12 and Atg5 proteins. The Atg12-Atg5 conjugate, along with Atg16L1, adds phosphatidylethanolamine monomers, determining the elongation of the autophagosome (Kauffman et al., 2018). The protein Atg9 is partly regulated by the Atg1 complex and other Atg proteins such as Atg17, Atg2, Atg18, Atg14L, Atg8, Atg21, Atg16, Atg12, and Atg5 (Nishimura and Tooze, 2020). The next step is the clearance of most Atgs proteins and the fusion of the autophagosome with the lysosomal membrane to form an autolysosome. Finally, the authophagic load is degraded by the hydrolytic environment into the autolysosome (Yu et al., 2018).

To date it is known that a dysfunction of autophagy is related to the onset of some diseases including cancer (White et al., 2015; Li Y. J. et al., 2017; Li et al., 2020), aging (Wong et al., 2020), neurodegenerative diseases (Menzies et al., 2015; Boland et al., 2018; Kumar et al., 2018; Suresh et al., 2020) and metabolic diseases (Ren and Anversa, 2015; van Niekerk et al., 2018; Wu N. N. et al., 2019; Almeida et al., 2020).

From the structural point of view, the neuron can be divided into three compartments: the soma, the axon and the dendrites. Axons can grow from a few micrometers up to many feet to reach their targets while dendrites are much shorter but can form highly branched nets. Since neurons are post-mitotic and long-lived cells, they must handle external stress removing aggregated and/or damaged proteins and organelles. For this reason, autophagy can perform this function in each neuronal compartment (Stavoe and Holzbaur, 2019). The interruption of homeostasis and physiological functions in the CNS, due to numerous pathophysiological events, can generate a wide range of diseases or pathological consequences. In particular, alteration of the redox state, inflammation, metabolic disorders, and failure in quality control of cellular proteins and organelles have been implicated in neurological and neurodegenerative disorders. In fact, a similar concept is also valid for psychiatric disorders (Menzies et al., 2015; Guo et al., 2018; Tomoda et al., 2020).

Numerous scientific studies have shown that the basal activity of autophagy is fundamental for the maintenance of homeostasis and neuronal vitality: in fact, it is known that neurons are particularly vulnerable in case of altered and/or switched off autophagy (Yamamoto and Yue, 2014; Kulkarni et al., 2018). It is important to stress that autophagy in CNS is important not only to maintain neuronal homeostasis, but also to ensure neurodevelopment (Stavoe and Holzbaur, 2019). Studies conducted in cultured embryonic peripheral neurons showed a retrogradely transport of large acidified vesicles from axons toward the soma along microtubules, suggesting that autophagosomes formed in the distal axon and were subsequently transported to the neuronal soma. The neuronal soma is rich in lysosomes and late endosomes with which autophagosomes fuse to lead autolysosomes (Maday and Holzbaur, 2014). Maintaining the integrity of proteins, neurotransmitters, receptors (localized at the synaptic level), and organelles (synaptic vesicles, mitochondria) is essential to support neuronal functionality (Lu et al., 2017; Conway et al., 2020).

Recent studies have revealed that autophagosomes are not only present in axons but also in the site of synaptic activation and these data suggest the possibility that neuronal autophagy regulates synaptic functions and neuroplasticity of the nervous system (Wang et al., 2015; Vanhauwaert et al., 2017; Tomoda et al., 2020). Synaptic plasticity requires intense biochemical activity that includes the synthesis of presynaptic neurotransmitters, postsynaptic receptor, signal transduction activity, gene expression, proper regulation of synapse, synaptic vesicle formation, and proper control of mitochondria (Binotti et al., 2015; Alvarez-Castelao and Schuman, 2015; Cohen and Ziv, 2017; Wang et al., 2017). All of these synaptic components are susceptible to wear and damage due to the frequencies of neuronal activation. Consequently, synapses are a site of great demand for cellular catabolic activities, for which an efficient degradation to support synaptic functions is indispensable (Vijayan and Verstreken, 2017). BDNF is also an inductor of long-term potentiation (LTP), considered one of the major cellular mechanisms that underlies learning and memory. Scientific evidence has shown that a receptor for BDNF is localized on the autophagosomic membrane, supporting the role of autophagy in transduction of BDNF signals (Nikoletopoulou et al., 2017; Nikoletopoulou and Tavernarakis, 2018). To date, it is known that failure of autophagy functions

causes neuronal death, while impaired autophagy functions are associated with neurodegenerative disorders such as: Alzheimer's disease, Huntington's disease, and Parkinson's disease (Menzies et al., 2017; Conway et al., 2020). Studies in mice with ablation of autophagy genes *ATG5* and *ATG7* showed degeneration of axonic terminals, progressive axonal swelling, and no signs of the autophagosome formation (Komatsu et al., 2006; Komatsu et al., 2007).

In addition, a recent study conducted on an *in vivo* model of knockout mice conditionally lacking the essential autophagy protein Atg5, showed that the loss of this neuronal mechanism led to a selective accumulation of the endoplasmic reticulum in axons. Increased endoplasmic reticulum leads to increased excitatory neurotransmission due to high release of calcium from the organelle and compromises neuronal viability. These results have suggested, therefore, that neuronal autophagy could control the axonal calcium reserves of endoplasmic reticulum to regulate neurotransmission in healthy neurons and in the brain (Kuijpers et al., 2021).

Autophagy and Neurodegenerative Diseases

To date, it is known that failure of autophagy causes neuronal death, while impaired autophagy is associated with neurodegenerative disorders such as: Alzheimer's Disease (AD), Huntington's Disease (HD), Parkinson's Disease (PD), and Amyotrophic Lateral Sclerosis (ALS) (Menzies et al., 2017; Conway et al., 2020). These pathologies are characterized by the formation of intracellular aggregates that result from misfolding and oligomerization of proteins. AD, the most common neurodegenerative disease, is characterized by extracellular β-amyloid plaques and intracellular neurofibrillary tangles composed of aggregated hyperphosphorylated tau protein (Hanzel et al., 2014; Cheignon et al., 2018). A dysfunctional autophagy is present in AD suffering patients, characterized by the loss of lysosome acidification, lysosomal alteration, failure to fusion between autophagosome and lysosomes and accumulation of autophagosomes (Yoon and Kim, 2016). Beclin1 is a key factor in the formation of autophagosomes and has been shown to be transcriptionally suppressed in the brain of AD (Salminen et al., 2013); in addition, caspase-3, an executive enzyme in the apoptosis pathway, can split the beclin1 protein and lead to the destruction of autophagy (Guo et al., 2018). Based on these observations, it is reasonable to assume that restoring lysosome function can increase the removal of protein aggregations. Finally, *in vitro* treatment with rapamycin, an enhancer of autophagy, has been shown to significantly increase the fusion of the autophagosomes with the lysosomes, improving the autophagic result (Li Q. et al., 2017).

PD, the second most common neurodegenerative disease, is characterized by selective loss of dopamine neurons in substantia nigra and accumulation of Lewy bodies, composed in misfolded and aggregated α-synuclein protein (Dauer and Przedborski, 2003; Lashuel et al., 2013). A close connection between this neurodegenerative disease and autophagy was indicated by the finding of dysfunctional lysosomes and accumulation of autophagosomes in the post-mortem brain samples of PD patients (Dehay et al., 2010; Xilouri et al., 2016). Additionally, if lysosomes are inhibited the levels of α-synuclein are increased, suggesting a link between α-synuclein degradation and autophagy (Guo et al., 2018). Lysosomal hydrolases, the enzymes responsible for degradation in lysosome, can be altered by autosomal recessive mutations: the consequence is the induction of defects in autophagosome-lysosome pathway and the aggregation of α-synuclein. Finally depletion of ATP6AP2, a transmembrane protein essential for lysosomal acidification, has been associated with PD (Abeliovich and Gitler, 2016).

HD is an autosomal dominant neurodegenerative disease, characterized by the repetition of trinucleotide CAG in the gene related to the protein huntingtin which leads to the expansion and pathogenic aggregation of the protein (Saudou and Humbert, 2016; Jimenez-sanchez et al., 2017). Huntingtin protein plays a key role in the autophagic process: in fact, its reduction results in an abnormal accumulation of autophagosomes (Wong and Holzbaur, 2014) and non-mutant huntingtin binds P62 to interact with ULK1 and activate it (Ravikumar et al., 2005).

ALS is a fatal disease characterized by the selective loss of motor neurons in the brain and spinal cord that causes weakness and muscle atrophy (Guo et al., 2018). The main cause of ALS is a mutation in *superoxide dismutase 1* and other genes that produce dysfunctional proteins, toxic cellular effects and oxidative stress (Medinas et al., 2018). To date, it is known that autophagy is closely associated with ALS (Morimoto et al., 2007); in fact, autophagic processes are also activated in degenerated motor neurons, although a reduced digestion of lysosomal load has been suggested (Sasaki, 2011). Finally, it has been highlighted that mutated and autophagy-related proteins are involved in the onset of ALS (Filimonenko et al., 2007). Scientific evidences

indicate that dysregulated autophagy plays a key role in the neurodegenerative diseases; for this reason, the regulation of autophagy is a potential therapeutic strategy to improve the course of neurodegenerative diseases.

Autophagy is also involved in higher brain functions, such as learning, memory, mood, social interaction, and cognition. In fact, it has been pointed out that deregulated autophagy is responsible for the predisposition to neurological disorders such as schizophrenia, bipolar disorder, psychosis, attention deficit disorder, hyperactivity, autism, cognitive decline, and depression (Tomoda et al., 2020). In addition, autophagic activity is known to gradually decrease during aging, in conjunction with the reduction of these brain functions (Vilchez et al., 2014). This apparent correlation has been demonstrated by studies that have shown that the intake of substances that enhance autophagy, are responsible for an increase in life span. The same substances may reduce memory deterioration associated with aging (Eisenberg et al., 2009). Since autophagic regulation has been shown to alleviate the deficit in synaptic plasticity and improve cognition, its regulation can be therapeutic and diagnostic in neurological and neuropsychiatric disorders.

In summary, we can say that the strategies used by neuronal autophagy to ensure the proper functioning of the CNS are basically five (Tomoda et al., 2020):

- degradation of dysfunctional cytosolic proteins;
- degradation of damaged organelles;
- selective surface presentation of neurotransmitter receptors;
- degradation of neurotransmitter activity and their receptors;
- morphological and functional regulation of synapses.

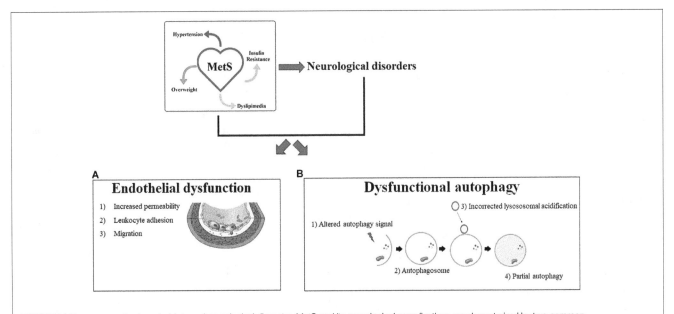

FIGURE 3 | Common mechanisms in Mets and neurological diseases. MetS and its neurological complications are characterized by two common pathophysiological mechanisms described in panels a and b. In particular, **(A)** endothelial dysfunction is shown with the main characteristics: (1) Increased permeability (2) Leukocyte adhesion (3) Cellular Migration. **(B)** Shows a dysfunctional autophagy due to an altered signal. An incorrect lysosomal acidification is responsible for the changed formation of the autofagosoma-lisosome complex and a consequent partial autophagy.

Autophagy and Metabolic Syndrome

Inflammatory diseases can trigger autophagy dysfunction (Deretic and Klionsky, 2018). It has been highlighted that autophagy is fundamental for the maintenance of cellular metabolic homeostasis and that it plays a crucial role in the control of body metabolism, whose dysregulation could participate in the onset of Mets (Lim et al., 2018). The role of autophagy in MetS was widely studied using animal models in which genetic alterations were induced (Lim et al., 2018). An example of this can be observed in a scientific study that highlighted how knockout mice of *ATG7*, an essential autophagy gene in pancreatic β-cells, showed structural and functional defects of these cells; with subsequent glucose intolerance and increased predisposition to develop diabetes (Ebato et al., 2008; Jung et al., 2008; Quan et al., 2012). Additionally, in another study, overexpression of *ATG5* another essential autophagic gene, improved the metabolic profile of older mice (Pyo et al., 2013). A further example of the effects of autophagy is confirmed by important results showing how systemic autophagic insufficiency is able to cause deterioration of adaptation to metabolic stress and facilitate progression from obesity to diabetes (Lim et al., 2014). Recently it has been shown that Mets is characterized by a dysfunctional mitophagy (Wu H. et al., 2019) and present alterations which manifest as inadequate acidification in lysosomes (Yamamoto et al., 2017; Park et al., 2020; Yamamoto et al., 2020).

CONCLUSION

MetS is a clustering of several disorders including dyslipidemia, obesity and hyperglycemia/insulin resistance and every component is close connected with a high risk of developing atherosclerotic cardiovascular disease and type 2 diabetes. In addition, Mets has been shown to develop secondary disorders that affect the nervous system; the altered physiological state, due to Mets, can generate neurological deficits and a cognitive metabolic syndrome (Gasparova et al., 2018).

A physiopathological mechanism that links Mets and the neurological disorders is the endothelial dysfunction. In fact, in both cases, we can find an alteration of the endothelium of the cardiocirculatory system and of the BBB, respectively. In this review we wanted to better characterize the important correlation MetS-Neuronal disorders associated with another key process of cellular homeostasis: the autophagy. It has been highlighted that autophagy is fundamental for the maintenance of cellular metabolic homeostasis and that its dysregulation could participate in the onset of Mets (Lim et al., 2018). Moreover, neuronal autophagy is important also for the maintenance of homeostasis and vitality of neurons and these cells are particularly vulnerable in case of altered and/or switched off autophagy (Yamamoto and Yue, 2014; Kulkarni et al.,

2018). It is important to stress that neuronal autophagy regulates also presynaptic excitatory neurotransmission by controlling the axonal cellular organelle ER. In particular, scientific experiments have shown that the deprivation of the Atg5, essential autophagic protein, leads to a selective accumulation of the tubular endoplasmic reticulum in axons, an increased release of the calcium ion, increased excitatory neurotransmission and impairment of postnatal viability *in vivo* Therefore, the main consequence is an altered control of neuronal neurotransmission that, to occur properly, needs physiological autophagy (Kuijpers et al., 2021). Dysregulated autophagy can occur for multiple reasons but current scientific literature highlighted a common link in both Mets and neurological or neurodegenerative disorders. In fact, dysfunctional lysososomal acidification may be involved, leading to consequent failure of the fusion between autophagosomes and lysosomes (Yamamoto et al., 2017; Park et al., 2020; Yamamoto et al., 2020). Although this hypothesis is very fascinating, further studies are needed to confirm this link. In this direction, autophagy may be considered a target to reduce MetS risk factors and related disorders.

In summary, the model we propose is as follows:

- MetS involves, in addition to the risks already mentioned, the predisposition to the onset of neurological disorders;
- The inflammatory process is constantly present in MetS and participates in the onset of the neurological component. In fact, the subsequent dysfunction of the vascular endothelium involves the suffering of the nerve cells and the loss of integrity of the BBB;
- The autophagic process, notoriously involved in MetS, is a fundamental actor also in neurological disorders;
- Dysfunctional lysososomal acidification occurs in both MetS and neurological pathologies;
- Maintaining proper autophagic regulation, could reduce the constellation of primary and secondary MetS risk factors.

A summary cartoon of this described model is shown in **Figure 3**.

AUTHOR CONTRIBUTIONS

JM and VMo conceptualized, designed, and wrote the manuscript. MG, CC, VMu, SN, FB, FS, RM, SR, MZ, and CM revised the manuscript critically. All authors contributed to the article and approved the submitted version.

REFERENCES

Abeliovich, A., and Gitler, A. D. (2016). Defects in trafficking bridge Parkinson's disease pathology and genetics. *Nature* 539, 207–216. doi: 10.1038/nature20414

Aggoun, Y. (2007). Obesity, metabolic syndrome, and cardiovascular disease. *Pediatr. Res.* 61, 653–656.

Aguilar, M., Bhuket, T., Torres, S., Liu, B., and Wong, R. J. (2015). Prevalence of the metabolic syndrome in the United States, 2003-2012. *JAMA* 313, 1973–1974. doi: 10.1001/jama.2015.4260

Alberti, K. G., Zimmet, P., and Shaw, J. (2005). The metabolic syndrome–a new worldwide definition. *Lancet*. 366, 1059–1062.

Alberti, K. G., Eckel, R. H., Grundy, S. M., Zimmet, P. Z., Cleeman, J., Donato, K. A., et al. (2009). Harmonizing the metabolic syndrome: a joint interim statement of the international diabetes federation task force on epidemiology and prevention; national heart, lung, and blood institute; american heart association; world heart federation; international atherosclerosis society; and international association for the study of obesity. *Circulation* 120, 1640–1645. doi: 10.1161/circulationaha.109.192644

Almeida, M. F., Bahr, B. A., and Kinsey, S. T. (2020). Endosomal-lysosomal dysfunction in metabolic diseases and Alzheimer's disease. *Int. Rev. Neurobiol.* 154, 303–324. doi: 10.1016/bs.irn.2020.02.012

Altieri, P. I., Marcial, J., Banchs, H. L., Escobales, N., and Crespo, Ml (2015). The metabolic syndrome in Hispanics–the role of inflammation. *Glob. J. Obes. Diabetes Metab. Syndr.* 2, 12–17.

Alvarez-Castelao, B., and Schuman, E. M. (2015). The regulation of synaptic protein turnover. *J. Biol. Chem.* 290, 28623–28630. doi: 10.1074/jbc.r115.657130

Andreone, B. J., Lacoste, B., and Gu, C. (2015). Neuronal and vascular interactions. *Annu. Rev. Neurosci.* 38, 25–46. doi: 10.1146/annurev-neuro-071714-033835

Ansari, S., Djalali, M., Mohammadzadeh, N., Mohammadzadeh Honarvar, N., Mazaherioun, M., Zarei, M., et al. (2016). Assessing the effect of omega-3 fatty acids supplementation on serum BDNF (brain derived neurotrophic factor) in patients with type 2 diabetes: a randomized, double-blind, placebo-controlled study. *Int. Res. J. Appl. Basic Sci.* 10, 380–383.

Anstey, K. J., Cherbuin, N., Budge, M., and Young, J. (2011). Body mass index in midlife and late-life as a risk factor for dementia: a meta-analysis of prospective studies. *Obes. Rev.* 12:e426-e437.

Aoki, Y., Yoon, S. S., Chong, Y., and Carroll, M. D. (2014). Hypertension, abnormal cholesterol, and high body mass index among non-Hispanic Asian adults: United States, 2011-2012. *NCHS Data Brief.* 140, 1–8.

Arshad, N., Lin, T. S., and Yahaya, M. F. (2018). Metabolic syndrome and its effect on the brain: possible mechanism. *CNS Neurol. Disord. Drug Targets* 17, 595–603. doi: 10.2174/1871527317666180724143258

Babushkina, I. V., Sergeeva, A. S., Pivovarov, I., Kuril'skaia, T. E., and Koriakina, L. B. (2015). Structural and functional properties of vascular endothelium. *Kardiologiia.* 55, 82–86.

Bañuls, C., Rovira-Llopis, S., Martinez de Marañon, A., Veses, S., Jover, A., Gomez, M., et al. (2017). Metabolic syndrome enhances endoplasmic reticulum, oxidative stress and leukocyte-endothelium interactions in PCOS. *Metabolism* 71, 153–162. doi: 10.1016/j.metabol.2017.02.012

Bhat, R., Crowe, E. P., Bitto, A., Moh, M., Katsetos, C. D., Garcia, F. U., et al. (2012). Astrocyte senescence as a component of Alzheimer's disease. *PLoS One* 7:e45069. doi: 10.1371/journal.pone.0045069

Binotti, B., Pavlos, N. J., Riedel, D., Wenzel, D., Vorbrüggen, G., Schalk, A. M., et al. (2015). The GTPase Rab26 links synaptic vesicles to the autophagy pathway. *Elife* 4:e05597.

Björkholm, C., and Monteggia, L. M. (2016). BDNF - a key transducer of antidepressant effects. *Neuropharmacology.* 102, 72–79. doi: 10.1016/j.neuropharm.2015.10.034

Black, S., Kraemer, K., Shah, A., Simpson, G., Scogin, F., and Smith, A. (2018). Diabetes, depression, and cognition: a recursive cycle of cognitive dysfunction and glycemic dysregulation. *Curr. Diab. Rep.* 18:118.

Błaszczyk, E., and Gawlik, A. (2016). Neurotrophins, VEGF and matrix metalloproteinases: new markers or causative factors of metabolic syndrome components? *Pediatr. Endocrinol. Diab. Metab.* 22. doi: 10.18544/PEDM-22.03.0060

Boland, B., Yu, W. H., Corti, O., Mollereau, B., Henriques, A., Bezard, E., et al. (2018). Promoting the clearance of neurotoxic proteins in neurodegenerative disorders of ageing. *Nat. Rev. Drug Discov.* 17, 660–688. doi: 10.1038/nrd.2018.109

Boyd, F. T. Jr., Clarke, D. W., Muther, T. F., and Raizada, M. K. (1985). Insulin receptors and insulin modulation of norepinephrine uptake in neuronal cultures from rat brain. *J. Biol. Chem.* 260, 15880–15884. doi: 10.1016/s0021-9258(17)36340-8

Bremer, A. A., and Jialal, I. (2013). Adipose tissue dysfunction in nascent metabolic syndrome. *J. Obes.* 2013:393192.

Bruno, R. M., Reesink, K. D., and Ghiadoni, L. (2017). Advances in the non-invasive assessment of vascular dysfunction in metabolic syndrome and diabetes: focus on endothelium, carotid mechanics and renal vessels. *Nutr. Metab. Cardiovasc. Dis.* 27, 121–128. doi: 10.1016/j.numecd.2016.09.004

Cai, W., Zhang, K., Li, P., Zhu, L., Xu, J., Yang, B., et al. (2017). Dysfunction of the neurovascular unit in ischemic stroke and neurodegenerative diseases: an aging effect. *Ageing Res. Rev.* 34, 77–87. doi: 10.1016/j.arr.2016.09.006

Chakraborty, A., de Wit, N. M., van der Flier, W. M., and de Vries, H. E. (2017). The blood brain barrier in Alzheimer's disease. *Vascul. Pharmacol.* 89, 12–18.

Chaldakov, G. N., Fiore, M., Rančić, G., Beltowski, J., Tunçel, N., and Aloe, L. (2014). An integrated view: neuroadipocrinology of diabesity. *Ser. J. Expclin. Res.* 15, 61–69. doi: 10.2478/sjecr-2014-0008

Chawla, A., Nguyen, K. D., and Goh, Y. P. (2011). Macrophage-mediated inflammation in metabolic disease. *Nat. Rev. Immunol.* 11, 738–749. doi: 10.1038/nri3071

Cheignon, C., Tomas, M., Bonnefont-Rousselot, D., Faller, P., Hureau, C., and Collin, F. (2018). Oxidative stress and the amyloid beta peptide in Alzheimer's disease. *Redox Biol.* 14, 450–464.

Chen, A. Q., Fang, Z., Chen, X. L., Yang, S., Zhou, Y. F., Mao, L., et al. (2019). Microglia-derived TNF-alpha mediates endothelial necroptosis aggravating blood brain-barrier disruption after ischemic stroke. *Cell Death Dis.* 10:487.

Choi, J., Chandrasekaran, K., Demarest, T. G., Kristian, T., Xu, S., Vijaykumar, K., et al. (2014). Brain diabetic neurodegeneration segregates with low intrinsic aerobic capacity. *Ann. Clin. Transl. Neurol.* 1, 589–604. doi: 10.1002/acn3.86

Climie, R. E., Moran, C., Callisaya, M., Blizzard, L., Sharman, J. E., Venn, A., et al. (2015). Abdominal obesity and brain atrophy in type 2 diabetes mellitus. *PLoS One* 10:e0142589. doi: 10.1371/journal.pone.0142589

Cohen, L. D., and Ziv, N. E. (2017). Recent insights on principles of synaptic protein degradation. *F1000Res* 6:675. doi: 10.12688/f1000research.10599.1

Conway, O., Akpinar, H. A., Rogov, V. V., and Kirkin, V. (2020). Selective autophagy receptors in neuronal health and disease. *J. Mol. Biol.* 432, 2483–2509. doi: 10.1016/j.jmb.2019.10.013

Corada, M., Zanetta, L., Orsenigo, F., Breviario, F., Lampugnani, M. G., Bernasconi, S., et al. (2002). A monoclonal antibody to vascular endothelial-cadherin inhibits tumor angiogenesis without side effects on endothelial permeability. *Blood* 100, 905–911. doi: 10.1182/blood.v100.3.905

Corasaniti, M. T., Maiuolo, J., Maida, S., Fratto, V., Navarra, M., Russo, R., et al. (2007). Cell signaling pathways in the mechanisms of neuroprotection afforded by bergamot essential oil against NMDA-induced cell death in vitro. *Br. J. Pharmacol.* 151, 518–529. doi: 10.1038/sj.bjp.0707237

Costello, F., and Petzold, A. (2020). Weighting evidence in MS: obesity and neurodegeneration. *Mult. Scler.* 26, 748–750. doi: 10.1177/1352458520912171

Cuspidi, C., Sala, C., Provenzano, F., Tadic, M., Gherbesi, E., Grassi, G., et al. (2018). Metabolic syndrome and subclinical carotid damage: a meta-analysis from population-based studies. *J. Hypertens.* 36, 23–30. doi: 10.1097/hjh.0000000000001575

Dalal, P. J., Muller, W. A., and Sullivan, D. P. (2020). Endothelial cell calcium signaling during barrier function and inflammation. *Am. J. Pathol.* 190, 535–542. doi: 10.1016/j.ajpath.2019.11.004

Daneman, R., and Prat, A. (2015). The blood-brain barrier. *Cold Spring Harb Perspect Biol.* 7:a020412.

Dauer, W., and Przedborski, S. (2003). Parkinson's disease: mechanisms and models. *Neuron.* 39, 889–909.

Davalos, D., and Akassoglou, K. (2012). Fibrinogen as a key regulator of inflammation in disease. *Semin. Immunopathol.* 34, 43–62. doi: 10.1007/s00281-011-0290-8

Davidson, T. L., Hargrave, S. L., Swithers, S. E., Sample, C. H., Fu, X., Kinzig, K. P., et al. (2013). Inter-relationships among diet, obesity and hippocampaldependent cognitive function. *Neuroscience* 253, 110–122. doi: 10.1016/j.neuroscience.2013.08.044

Dechant, G., and Neumann, H. (2002). Neurotrophins. *Adv. Exp. Med. Biol.* 513, 303–334.

Dehay, B., Bové, J., Rodríguez-Muela, N., Perier, C., Recasens, A., Boya, P., et al. (2010). Pathogenic lysosomal depletion in Parkinson's disease. *J. Neurosci.* 30, 12535–12544. doi: 10.1523/jneurosci.1920-10.2010

Deng, J., Liu, S., Zou, L., Xu, C., Geng, B., and Xu, G. (2012). Lipolysis response to endoplasmic reticulum stress in adipose cells. *J. Biol. Chem.* 2012, 6240–6249. doi: 10.1074/jbc.m111.299115

Denver, P., English, A., and McClean, P. L. (2018). Inflammation, insulin signaling and cognitive function in aged APP/PS1 mice. *Brain Behav. Immun.* 70, 423–434. doi: 10.1016/j.bbi.2018.03.032

Deretic, V., and Klionsky, D. J. (2018). Autophagy and inflammation: a special review issue. *Autophagy* 14, 179–180. doi: 10.1080/15548627.2017.1412229

Domingueti, C. P., Dusse, L. M., Carvalho, M., de Sousa, L. P., Gomes, K. B., and Fernandes, A. P. (2016). Diabetes mellitus: the linkage between oxidative stress, inflammation, hypercoagulability and vascular complications. *J. Diabetes Complications.* 30, 738–745. doi: 10.1016/j.jdiacomp.2015.12.018

Dorfman, M. D., and Thaler, J. P. (2015). Hypothalamic inflammation and gliosis in obesity. *Curr. Opin. Endocrinol. Diabetes Obes.* 22, 325–330. doi: 10.1097/med.0000000000000182

Ebato, C., Uchida, T., Arakawa, M., Komatsu, M., Ueno, T., Komiya, K., et al. (2008). Autophagy is important in islet homeostasis and compensatory increase of beta cell mass in response to high-fat diet. *Cell Metab.* 8:32.

Eisenberg, T., Knauer, H., Schauer, A., Büttner, S., Ruckenstuhl, C., Carmona-Gutierrez, D., et al. (2009). Induction of autophagy by spermidine promotes longevity. *Nat. Cell Biol.* 11, 1305–1314.

ElAli, A., Thériault, P., and Rivest, S. (2014). The role of pericytes in neurovascular unit remodeling in brain disorders. *Int. J. Mol. Sci.* 15, 6453–6474. doi: 10.3390/ijms15046453

El-Benna, J., Hurtado-Nedelec, M., Marzaioli, V., Marie, J. C., Gougerot-Pocidalo, M. A., and Dang, P. M. (2016). Priming of the neutrophil respiratory burst: role in host defense and inflammation. *Immunol. Rev.* 273, 180–193. doi: 10.1111/imr.12447

Elmarakby, A. A., and Sullivan, J. C. (2012). Relationship between oxidative stress and inflammatory cytokines in diabetic nephropathy. *Cardiovasc. Ther.* 30, 49–59. doi: 10.1111/j.1755-5922.2010.00218.x

Emanueli, C., Meloni, M., Hasan, W., and Habecker, B. A. (2014). The biology of neurotrophins: cardiovascular function. *Handb. Exp Pharmacol.* 220, 309–328. doi: 10.1007/978-3-642-45106-5_12

Engelhardt, B., and Ransohoff, R. M. (2012). Capture, crawl, cross: the T cell code to breach the blood-brain barriers. *Trends Immunol.* 33, 579–589. doi: 10.1016/j.it.2012.07.004

Ervin, R. B. (2009). Prevalence of metabolic syndrome among adults 20 years of age and over, by sex, age, race and ethnicity, and body mass index: United States, 2003-2006. *Natl. Health Stat. Report* 13, c1–c7.

Fan, L., Wang, T., Chang, L., Song, Y., Wu, Y., and Ma, D. (2014). Systemic inflammation induces a profound long term brain cell injury in rats. *Acta Neurobiol. Exp.* 74, 298–306.

Fan, X., Chen, X., Feng, Q., Peng, K., Wu, Q., Passerini, A. G., et al. (2019). Downregulation of GATA6 in mTOR-inhibited human aortic endothelial cells: effects on TNF-alpha-induced VCAM-1 expression and monocytic cell adhesion. *Am. J. Physiol. Heart Circ. Physiol.* 316, H408–H420.

Feng, Y., Yao, Z., and Klionsky, D. J. (2015). How to control self-digestion: transcriptional, post-transcriptional, and post-translational regulation of autophagy. *Trends Cell Biol.* 25, 354–363. doi: 10.1016/j.tcb.2015.02.002

Figlewicz, D. P., Bentson, K., and Ocrant, I. (1993). The effect of insulin on norepinephrine uptake by PC12 cells. *Brain Res. Bull.* 32, 425–431. doi: 10.1016/0361-9230(93)90210-3

Filimonenko, M., Stuffers, S., Raiborg, C., Yamamoto, A., Malerød, L., Fisher, E. M. C., et al. (2007). Functional multivesicular bodies are required for autophagic clearance of protein aggregates associated with neurodegenerative disease. *J. cell Biol.* 179, 485–500. doi: 10.1083/jcb.200702115

Finicelli, M., Squillaro, T., Di Cristo, F., Di Salle, A., Melone, M. A. B., Galderisi, U., et al. (2019). Metabolic syndrome, mediterranean diet, and polyphenols: evidence and perspectives. *J. Cell Physiol.* 234, 5807–5826.

Friesen, M., and Cowan, C. A. (2019). Adipocyte metabolism and insulin signaling perturbations: insights from genetics. *Trends Endocrinol. Metab.* 30, 396–406. doi: 10.1016/j.tem.2019.03.002

Gasparova, Z., Janega, P., Weismann, P., El Falougy, H., Tyukos Kaprinay, B., Liptak, B., et al. (2018). Effect of metabolic syndrome on neural plasticity and morphology of the hippocampus: correlations of neurological deficits with physiological status of the rat. *Gen. Physiol. Biophys.* 37, 619–632. doi: 10.4149/gpb_2018016

Gentil, B. J., Benaud, C., Delphin, C., Remy, C., Berezowski, V., Cecchelli, R., et al. (2005). Specific AHNAK expression in brain endothelial cells with barrier properties. *J. Cell Physiol.* 203, 362–371. doi: 10.1002/jcp.20232

Georgieva, A. M., Cate, H. T., Keulen, E. T., van Oerle, R., Govers-Riemslag, J. W., Hamulyák, K., et al. (2004). Prothrombotic markers in familial combined hyperlipidemia: evidence of endothelial cell activation and relation to metabolic syndrome. *Atherosclerosis* 175, 345–351. doi: 10.1016/j.atherosclerosis.2004.04.006

Godo, S., and Shimokawa, H. (2017). Endothelial functions. *Arterioscler. Thromb. Vasc. Biol.* 37, e108–e114.

Gogniat, M. A., Robinson, T. L., Mewborn, C. M., Jean, K. R., and Miller, L. S. (2018). Body mass index and its relation to neuropsychological functioning and brain volume in healthy older adults. *Behav. Brain Res.* 348, 235–240. doi: 10.1016/j.bbr.2018.04.029

Gómez-Apo, E., García-Sierra, A., Silva-Pereyra, J., Soto-Abraham, V., Mondragón-Maya, A., Velasco-Vales, V., et al. (2018). A postmortem study of frontal and temporal gyri thickness and cell number in human obesity. *Obesity* 26, 94–102. doi: 10.1002/oby.22036

Grandl, G., and Wolfrum, C. (2018). Hemostasis, endothelial stress, inflammation, and the metabolic syndrome. *Semin. Immunopathol.* 40, 215–224. doi: 10.1007/s00281-017-0666-5

Grumati, P., and Dikic, I. (2018). Ubiquitin signaling and autophagy. *J. Biol. Chem.* 293, 5404–5413. doi: 10.1074/jbc.tm117.000117

Guo, F., Liu, X., Cai, H., and Le, W. (2018). Autophagy in neurodegenerative diseases: pathogenesis and therapy. *Brain Pathol.* 28, 3–13. doi: 10.1111/bpa.12545

Gustafson, D. R., Karlsson, C., Skoog, I., Rosengren, L., Lissner, L., and Blennow, K. (2007). Mid-life adiposity factors relate to blood-brain barrier integrity in late life. *J. Intern. Med.* 262, 643–650. doi: 10.1111/j.1365-2796.2007.01869.x

Hajiluian, G., Abbasalizad Farhangi, M., and Jahangiry, L. (2017). Mediterranean dietary pattern and VEGF +405 G/C gene polymorphisms in patients with metabolic syndrome: an aspect of gene-nutrient interaction. *PLoS One.* 12:e0171637. doi: 10.1371/journal.pone.0171637

Hakanpaa, L., Kiss, E. A., Jacquemet, G., Miinalainen, I., Lerche, M., Guzmán, C., et al. (2018). Targeting β1-integrin inhibits vascular leakage in endotoxemia. *Proc. Natl. Acad. Sci. U.S.A.* 115, E6467–E6476.

Hanzel, C. E., Pichet-Binette, A., Pimentel, L. S., Iulita, M. F., Allard, S., Ducatenzeiler, A., et al. (2014). Neuronal driven pre-plaque inflammation in a transgenic rat model of Alzheimer's disease. *Neurobiol. Aging* 35, 2249–2262. doi: 10.1016/j.neurobiolaging.2014.03.026

Hargrave, S. L., Davidson, T. L., Zheng, W., and Kinzig, K. P. (2016). Western diets induce blood-brain barrier leakage and alter spatial strategies in rats. *Behav. Neurosci.* 130, 123–135. doi: 10.1037/bne0000110

Hassing, L. B., Grant, M. D., Hofer, S. M., Pedersen, N. L., Nilsson, S. E., Berg, S., et al. (2004). Type 2 diabetes mellitus contributes to cognitive decline in old age: a longitudinal population-based study. *J. Int. Neuropsychol. Soc.* 10, 599–607. doi: 10.1017/s1355617704104165

Hempstead, B. L. (2015). Brain-Derived neurotrophic factor: three ligands, many actions. *Trans. Am. Clin. Climatol. Assoc.* 126, 9–19.

Heras-Sandoval, D., Ferrera, P., and Arias, C. (2012). Amyloid-beta protein modulates insulin signaling in presynaptic terminals. *Neurochem. Res.* 37, 1879–1885. doi: 10.1007/s11064-012-0800-7

Hu, Y. X., Han, X. S., and Jing, Q. (2019). Autophagy in development and differentiation. *Adv. Exp. Med. Biol.* 1206, 469–487. doi: 10.1007/978-981-15-0602-4_22

Incalza, M. A., D'Oria, R., Natalicchio, A., Perrini, S., Laviola, L., and Giorgino, F. (2018). Oxidative stress and reactive oxygen species in endothelial dysfunction associated with cardiovascular and metabolic diseases. *Vascul. Pharmacol.* 100, 1–19. doi: 10.1016/j.vph.2017.05.005

Islam, M. T. (2017). Oxidative stress and mitochondrial dysfunction linked neurodegenerative disorders. *Neurol. Res.* 39, 73–82. doi: 10.1080/01616412.2016.1251711

Jais, A., and Brüning, J. C. (2017). Hypothalamic inflammation in obesity and metabolic disease. *J. Clin. Invest.* 127, 24–32. doi: 10.1172/jci88878

Jimenez-sanchez, M., Licitra, F., Underwood, B. R., and Rubinsztein, D. C. (2017). Huntington's disease: mechanisms of pathogenesis and therapeutic strategies. *Cold Spring Harb Perspect Med.* 7:a024240.

Jung, H. S., Chung, K. W., Kim, J. W., Kim, J., Komatsu, M., Tanaka, K., et al. (2008). Loss of autophagy diminishes pancreatic b-cell mass and function with resultant hyperglycemia. *Cell. Metab.* 8, 318–324. doi: 10.1016/j.cmet.2008. 08.013

Kaplan, H. M., Kuyucu, Y., Polat, S., Pazarci, P., Yegani, A. A., Şingirik, E., et al. (2018). Molecular basis of vascular damage caused by cigarette smoke exposure and a new approach to the treatment: alpha-linolenic acid. *Biomed Pharmacother.* 102, 458–463. doi: 10.1016/j.biopha.2018.03.112

Karaca, C., and Karaca, Z. (2018). Beyond hyperglycemia, evidence for retinal neurodegeneration in metabolic syndrome. *Invest. Ophthalmol. Vis. Sci.* 59, 1360–1367. doi: 10.1167/iovs.17-23376

Kathy, F. Y., Ma, V. S., Po Lai, Y., Turchianoa, M. M., and Convit, A. (2012). Impact of metabolic syndrome on cognition and brain: a selected review of the literature. *Arterioscler. Thromb. Vasc. Biol.* 32, 2060–2067. doi: 10.1161/ atvbaha.112.252759

Kauffman, K. J., Yu, S., Jin, J., Mugo, B., Nguyen, N., O'Brien, A., et al. (2018). Delipidation of mammalian Atg8-family proteins by each of the four ATG4 proteases. *Autophagy* 14, 992–1010.

Khaddaj Mallat, R., Mathew John, C., Kendrick, D. J., and Braun, A. P. (2017). The vascular endothelium: a regulator of arterial tone and interface for the immune system. *Crit. Rev. Clin. Lab. Sci.* 54, 458–470. doi: 10.1080/10408363. 2017.1394267

Kim, B., Backus, C., Oh, S., Hayes, J. M., and Feldman, E. L. (2009). Increased tau phosphorylation and cleavage in mouse models of type 1 and type 2 diabetes. *Endocrinology* 150, 5294–5301. doi: 10.1210/en.2009-0695

Kim, H. W., Shi, H., Winkler, M. A., Lee, R., and Weintraub, N. L. (2020). Perivascular adipose tissue and vascular perturbation/atherosclerosis. *Arterioscler. Thromb. Vasc. Biol.* 40, 2569–2576. doi: 10.1161/atvbaha.120. 312470

Kiseleva, R. Y., Glassman, P. M., Greineder, C. F., Shuvaev, V. V., and Muzykantov, V. R. (2018). Targeting therapeutics to endothelium: are we there yet? *Drug Deliv. Transl. Res.* 8, 883–902. doi: 10.1007/s13346-017-0464-6

Kishi, T., Chipman, J., Evereklian, M., Nghiem, K., Stetler-Stevenson, M., Rick, M. E., et al. (2020). Endothelial activation markers as disease activity and damage measures in juvenile dermatomyositis. *J. Rheumatol.* 47, 1011–1018. doi: 10.3899/jrheum.181275

Komatsu, M., Waguri, S., Chiba, T., Murata, S., Iwata, J., Tanida, I., et al. (2006). Loss of autophagy in the central nervous system causes neurodegeneration in mice. *Nature* 441, 880–884. doi: 10.1038/nature04723

Komatsu, M., Wang, Q. J., Holstein, G. R., Friedrich, V. L. Jr., Iwata, J., Kominami, E., et al. (2007). Essential role for autophagy protein Atg7 in the maintenance of axonal homeostasis and the prevention of axonal degeneration. *Proc. Natl. Acad. Sci. U.S.A.* 104, 14489–14494. doi: 10.1073/pnas.0701311104

Kuijpers, M., Kochlamazashvili, G., Stumpf, A., Puchkov, D., Swaminathan, A., Lucht, M. T., et al. (2021). Neuronal autophagy regulates presynaptic neurotransmission by controlling the axonal endoplasmic reticulum. *Neuron* 109, 299–313.e9.

Kulkarni, A., Chen, J., and Maday, S. (2018). Neuronal autophagy and intercellular regulation of homeostasis in the brain. *Curr. Opin. Neurobiol.* 51, 29–36. doi: 10.1016/j.conb.2018.02.008

Kullmann, S., Heni, M., Hallschmid, M., Fritsche, A., Preissl, H., and Häring, H. U. (2016). Brain insulin resistance at the crossroads of metabolic and cognitive disorders in humans. *Physiol. Rev.* 96, 1169–1209. doi: 10.1152/physrev.00032. 2015

Kumar, A., Dhawan, A., Kadam, A., and Shinde, A. (2018). Autophagy and mitochondria: targets in neurodegenerative disorders. *CNS Neurol. Disord. Drug Targets* 17, 696–705. doi: 10.2174/1871527317666180816 100203

Lacoste, B., and Gu, C. (2015). Control of cerebrovascular patterning by neural activity during postnatal development. *Mech. Dev.* 138(Pt. 1), 43–49. doi: 10.1016/j.mod.2015.06.003

Laird, C. T., Hassanein, W., O'Neill, N. A., French, B. M., Cheng, X., Fogler, W. E., et al. (2018). P- and E-selectin receptor antagonism prevents human leukocyte adhesion to activated porcine endothelial monolayers and attenuates porcine endothelial damage. *Xenotransplantation* 25:e12381. doi: 10.1111/xen.12381

Lapaquette, P., Guzzo, J., Bretillon, L., and Bringer, M. A. (2015). Cellular and molecular connections between autophagy and inflammation. *Mediators Inflamm.* 2015:398483.

Lashuel, H. A., Overk, C. R., Oueslati, A., and Masliah, E. (2013). The many faces of alpha-synuclein: from structure and toxicity to therapeutic target. *Nat. Rev. Neurosci.* 14, 38–48. doi: 10.1038/nrn3406

Lawrence, T. (2009). The nuclear factor NF-kappaB pathway in inflammation. *Cold Spring Harb. Perspect. Biol.* 1:a001651.

Lee, S., Joo, Y. J., Kim, R. Y., Hwang, J., Lim, S. M., Yoon, S., et al. (2020). Obesity may connect insulin resistance to decreased neuronal viability in human diabetic brain. *Obesity* 28, 1626–1630. doi: 10.1002/oby.22869

Levine, B., and Kroemer, G. (2019). Biological functions of autophagy genes: a disease perspective. *Cell* 176, 11–42. doi: 10.1016/j.cell.2018.09.048

Lewin, G. R., and Barde, Y. A. (1996). Physiology of the neurotrophins. *Annu. Rev. Neurosci.* 19, 289–317. doi: 10.1146/annurev.ne.19.030196.001445

Li, J., and Hochstrasser, M. (2020). Microautophagy regulates proteasome homeostasis. *Curr. Genet.* 66, 683–687. doi: 10.1007/s00294-020-01059-x

Li, Q., Liu, Y., and Sun, M. (2017). Autophagy and Alzheimer's disease. *Cell Mol. Neurobiol.* 37, 377–388.

Li, W. J., Xue, H., Sun, K., Song, X. D., Wang, Y. B., Zhen, Y. S., et al. (2008). Cardiovascular risk and prevalence of metabolic syndrome by differing criteria. *Chin. Med. J.* 121, 1532–1536. doi: 10.1097/00029330-200808020-00006

Li, X., He, S., and Ma, B. (2020). Autophagy and autophagy-related proteins in cancer. *Mol. Cancer* 19:12.

Li, Y. J., Lei, Y. H., Yao, N., Wang, C. R., Hu, N., Ye, W. C., et al. (2017). Autophagy and multidrug resistance in cancer. *Chin. J. Cancer* 36:52.

Lim, H., Lim, Y. M., Kim, K. H., Jeon, Y. E., Park, K., Kim, J., et al. (2018). A novel autophagy enhancer as a therapeutic agent against metabolic syndrome and diabetes. *Nat. Commun.* 9:1438.

Lim, Y.-M., Lim, H., Hur, K. H., Quan, W., Lee, H. Y., and Cheon, H. (2014). Systemic autophagy insufficiency compromises adaptation to metabolic stress and facilitates progression from obesity to diabetes. *Nat. Commun.* 5:4934.

Loghmani, H., and Conway, E. M. (2018). Exploring traditional and nontraditional roles for thrombomodulin. *Blood.* 132, 148–158. doi: 10.1182/blood-2017-12- 768994

Lu, K., den Brave, F., and Jentsch, S. (2017). Receptor oligomerizationguides pathway choice between proteasomal and autophagic degradation. *Nat. Cell Biol.* 19, 732–739. doi: 10.1038/ncb3531

Lu, T., Pan, Y., Kao, S. Y., Li, C., Kohane, I., Chan, J., et al. (2004). Gene regulation and DNA damage in the ageing human brain. *Nature* 429, 883–891. doi: 10.1038/nature02661

Lutz, S. E., Smith, J. R., Kim, D. H., Olson, C. V. L., Ellefsen, K., Bates, J. M., et al. (2017). Caveolin1 is required for Th1 cell infiltration, but not tight junction remodeling, at the blood-brain barrier in autoimmune neuroinflammation. *Cell Rep.* 21, 2104–2117. doi: 10.1016/j.celrep.2017.10.094

Maday, S., and Holzbaur, E. L. (2014). Autophagosome biogenesis in primary neurons follows an ordered and spatially regulated pathway. *Dev. Cell* 30, 71–85. doi: 10.1016/j.devcel.2014.06.001

Madrigal-Matute, J., and Cuervo, A. M. (2016). Regulation of liver metabolism by autophagy. *Gastroenterology* 150, 328–339. doi: 10.1053/j.gastro.2015. 09.042

Maiuolo, J., Gliozzi, M., Musolino, V., Carresi, C., Nucera, S., Macrì, R., et al. (2019). The role of endothelial dysfunction in peripheral blood nerve barrier: molecular mechanisms and pathophysiological implications. *Int. J. Mol. Sci.* 20:3022. doi: 10.3390/ijms20123022

Maiuolo, J., Gliozzi, M., Musolino, V., Carresi, C., Nucera, S., Scicchitano, M., et al. (2020b). Environmental and nutritional "Stressors" and oligodendrocyte dysfunction: role of mitochondrial and endoplasmatic reticulum impairment. *Biomedicines* 8:553. doi: 10.3390/biomedicines8120553

Maiuolo, J., Gliozzi, M., Musolino, V., Scicchiatano, M., Carresi, C., Scarano, F., et al. (2018). The "Frail" brain blood barrier in neurodegenerative diseases: role of early disruption of endothelial Cell-to-Cell connections. *Int. J. Mol. Sci.* 19:2693. doi: 10.3390/ijms19092693

Maiuolo, J., Mollace, R., Gliozzi, M., Musolino, V., Carresi, C., Paone, S., et al. (2020a). The contribution of endothelial dysfunction in systemic injury subsequent to SARS-Cov-2 infection. *Int. J. Mol. Sci.* 21:9309. doi: 10.3390/ijms21239309

Mazidi, M., Rezaie, P., Kengne, A. P., Stathopoulou, M. G., Azimi-Nezhad, M., and Siest, S. (2017). VEGF, the underlying factor for metabolic syndrome; fact or fiction? *Diab. Metab. Syndr.* 11(Suppl. 1), S61–S64.

McCracken, E., Monaghan, M., and Sreenivasan, S. (2018). Pathophysiology of the metabolic syndrome. *Clin. Dermatol.* 36, 14–20.

Medinas, D. B., Rozas, P., Martinez Traub, F., Woehlbier, U., Brown, R. H., Bosco, D. A., et al. (2018). Endoplasmic reticulum stress leads to accumulation of wild-type SOD1 aggregates associated with sporadic amyotrophic lateral sclerosis. *Proc. Natl. Acad. Sci. U.S.A.* 115, 8209–8214. doi: 10.1073/pnas.1801109115

Menzies, F. M., Fleming, A., Caricasole, A., Bento, C. F., Andrews, S. P., Ashkenazi, A., et al. (2017). Autophagy and neurodegeneration: pathogenic mechanisms and therapeutic opportunities. *Neuron* 93, 1015–1034. doi: 10.1016/j.neuron.2017.01.022

Menzies, F. M., Fleming, A., and Rubinsztein, D. C. (2015). Compromised autophagy and neurodegenerative diseases. *Nat. Rev. Neurosci.* 16, 345–357. doi: 10.1038/nrn3961

Miller, A. A., and Spencer, S. J. (2014). Obesity and neuroinflammation: a pathway to cognitive impairment. *Brain Behav. Immun.* 42, 10–21. doi: 10.1016/j.bbi.2014.04.001

Misra, A., and Khurana, L. (2008). Obesity and the metabolic syndrome in developing countries. *J. Clin. Endocrinol. Metab.* 93, S9–S30.

Mittal, M., Siddiqui, M. R., Tran, K., Reddy, S. P., and Malik, A. B. (2014). Reactive oxygen species in inflammation and tissue injury. *Antioxid. Redox Signal.* 20, 1126–1167. doi: 10.1089/ars.2012.5149

Mizushima, N. (2018). A brief history of autophagy from cell biology to physiology and disease. *Nat. Cell Biol.* 20, 521–527. doi: 10.1038/s41556-018-0092-5

Monette, M. C., Baird, A., and Jackson, D. L. (2014). A meta-analysis of cognitive functioning in nondemented adults with type 2 diabetes mellitus. *Can. J. Diabetes* 38, 401–408. doi: 10.1016/j.jcjd.2014.01.014

Morales-Marín, M. E., Genis-Mendoza, A. D., Tovilla-Zarate, C. A., Lanzagorta, N., Escamilla, M., and Nicolini, H. (2016). Association between obesity and the brain-derived neurotrophic factor gene polymorphism Val66Met in individuals with bipolar disorder in Mexican population. *Neuropsychiatr. Dis. Treat.* 12, 1843–1848. doi: 10.2147/ndt.s104654

Morimoto, N., Nagai, M., Ohta, Y., Miyazaki, K., Kurata, T., Morimoto, M., et al. (2007). Increased autophagy in transgenic mice with a G93A mutant SOD1 gene. *Brain Res.* 1167, 112–117. doi: 10.1016/j.brainres.2007.06.045

Motamedi, S., Karimi, I., and Jafari, F. (2017). The interrelationship of metabolic syndrome and neurodegenerative diseases with focus on brain-derived neurotrophic factor (BDNF): kill two birds with one stone. *Metab. Brain Dis.* 32, 651–665. doi: 10.1007/s11011-017-9997-0

Nikoletopoulou, V., Sidiropoulou, K., Kallergi, E., Dalezios, Y., and Tavernarakis, N. (2017). Modulation of autophagy by BDNF underlies synaptic plasticity. *Cell Metab.* 26, 230–242.e5.

Nikoletopoulou, V., and Tavernarakis, N. (2018). Regulation and roles of autophagy at synapses. *Trends Cell Biol.* 28, 646–661. doi: 10.1016/j.tcb.2018.03.006

Nishimura, T., and Tooze, S. A. (2020). Emerging roles of ATG proteins and membrane lipids in autophagosome formation. *Cell Discov.* 6:32.

Nourshargh, S., and Alon, R. (2014). Leukocyte migration into inflamed tissues. *Immunity* 41, 694–707. doi: 10.1016/j.immuni.2014.10.008

O'Brown, N. M., Pfau, S. J., and Gu, C. (2018). Bridging barriers: a comparative look at the blood–brain barrier across organisms. *Genes Dev.* 32, 466–478. doi: 10.1101/gad.309823.117

O'Shea, J. J., Schwartz, D. M., Villarino, A. V., Gadina, M., McInnes, I. B., and Laurence, A. (2015). The JAK-STAT pathway: impact on human disease and therapeutic intervention. *Annu. Rev. Med.* 66, 311–328. doi: 10.1146/annurev-med-051113-024537

O'Doherty, M. G., Cairns, K., O'Neill, V., Lamrock, F., Jørgensen, T., Brenner, H., et al. (2016). Effect of major lifestyle risk factors, independent and jointly, on life expectancy with and without cardiovascular disease: results from the Consortium on Health and Ageing Network of Cohorts in Europe and the United States (CHANCES). *Eur. J. Epidemiol.* 31, 455–468. doi: 10.1007/s10654-015-0112-8

Oppedisano, F., Maiuolo, J., Gliozzi, M., Musolino, V., Carresi, C., Nucera, S., et al. (2020). The potential for natural antioxidant supplementation in the early

stages of neurodegenerative disorders. *Int. J. Mol. Sci.* 21:2618. doi: 10.3390/ijms21072618

Ouchi, N., Parker, J. L., Lugus, J. J., and Walsh, K. (2011). Adipokines in inflammation and metabolic disease. *Nat. Rev. Immunol.* 11, 85–97. doi: 10.1038/nri2921

Palta, P., Rippon, B., Tahmi, M., Sherwood, G., Soto, L., Ceballos, F., et al. (2021). Metbolic syndrome and its components in relation to in vivo brain amyloid and neurodegeneration in late middle age. *Neurobiol. Aging.* 97, 89–96. doi: 10.1016/j.neurobiolaging.2020.09.023

Park, H. S., Song, J. W., Park, J. H., Lim, B. K., Moon, O. S., Son, H. Y., et al. (2020). TXNIP/VDUP1 attenuates steatohepatitis via autophagy and fatty acid oxidation. *Autophagy* 16, 1–16. doi: 10.1080/15548627.2020.1834711

Patterson, S., Irwin, N., Guo-Parke, H., Moffett, R. C., Scullion, S. M., Flatt, P. R., et al. (2016). Evaluation of the role of N-methyl-D-aspartate (n.d.) receptors in insulin secreting beta-cells. *Eur. J. Pharmacol.* 771, 107–113. doi: 10.1016/j.ejphar.2015.12.015

Pendlebury, S. T., and Rothwell, P. M. (2009). Prevalence, incidence, and factors associated with pre-stroke and post-stroke dementia: a systematic review and meta-analysis. *Lancet Neurol.* 8, 1006–1018. doi: 10.1016/s1474-4422(09)70236-4

Pomero, F., Di Minno, M. N., Fenoglio, L., Gianni, M., Ageno, W., and Dentali, F. (2015). Is diabetes a hypercoagulable state? A critical appraisal. *Acta Diabetol.* 52, 1007–1016. doi: 10.1007/s00592-015-0746-8

Pucci, G., Alcidi, R., Tap, L., Battista, F., Mattace-Raso, F., and Schillaci, G. (2017). Sex- and gender-related prevalence, cardiovascular risk and therapeutic approach in metabolic syndrome: a review of the literature. *Pharmacol. Res.* 120, 34–42. doi: 10.1016/j.phrs.2017.03.008

Pyo, J. O., Yoo, S. M., Ahn, H. H., Nah, J., Hong, S. H., Kam, T. I., et al. (2013). Overexpression of Atg5 in mice activates autophagy and extends lifespan. *Nat. Commun.* 4:2300.

Quan, W., Hur, K. Y., Lim, Y., Oh, S. H., Lee, J.-C., Kim, K. H., et al. (2012). Autophagy deficiency in beta cells leads to compromised unfolded protein response and progression from obesity to diabetes in mice. *Diabetologia* 55, 392–403. doi: 10.1007/s00125-011-2350-y

Ransohoff, R. M., Schafer, D., Vincent, A., Blachère, N. E., and Bar-Or, A. (2015). Neuroinflammation: ways in which the immune system affects the brain. *Neurotherapeutics* 12, 896–909. doi: 10.1007/s13311-015-0385-3

Ravikumar, B., Acevedo-Arozena, A., Imarisio, S., Berger, Z., Vacher, C., O'Kane, C. J., et al. (2005). Dynein mutations impair autophagic clearance of aggregate-prone proteins. *Nat. Genet.* 37, 771–776. doi: 10.1038/ng1591

Ren, J., and Anversa, P. (2015). The insulin-like growth factor I system: physiological and pathophysiological implication in cardiovascular diseases associated with metabolic syndrome. *Biochem. Pharmacol.* 93, 409–417. doi: 10.1016/j.bcp.2014.12.006

Ricci, G., Pirillo, I., Tomassoni, D., Sirignano, A., and Grappasonni, I. (2017). Metabolic syndrome, hypertension, and nervous system injury: epidemiological correlates. *Clin. Exp. Hypertens.* 39, 8–16. doi: 10.1080/10641963.2016.1210629

Rudziak, P., Ellis, C. G., and Kowalewska, P. M. (2019). Role and molecular mechanisms of pericytes in regulation of leukocyte diapedesis in inflamed tissues. *Mediators Inflamm.* 2019:4123605.

Sack, K. D., Teran, M., and Nugent, M. A. (2016). Extracellular matrix stiffness controls VEGF signaling and processing in endothelial cells. *J. Cell Physiol.* 231, 2026–2039. doi: 10.1002/jcp.25312

Saklayen, M. G. (2018). The global epidemic of the metabolic syndrome. *Curr. Hypertens. Reports* 20:12.

Salminen, A., Kaarniranta, K., Kauppinen, A., Ojala, J., Haapasalo, A., Soininen, H., et al. (2013). Impaired autophagy and APP processing in Alzheimer's disease: the potential role of Beclin 1 interactome. *Prog. Neurobiol.* 10, 33–54. doi: 10.1016/j.pneurobio.2013.06.002

Saltiel, A. R., and Olefsky, J. M. (2017). Inflammatory mechanisms linking obesity and metabolic disease. *J. Clin. Invest.* 127, 1–4. doi: 10.1172/jci92035

Sarmiento Quintero, F., Ariza, A. J., Barboza García, F., Canal de Molano, N., Castro Benavidesm, M., Cruchet Muñoz, S., et al. (2016). Overweight and obesity: review and update. *Acta Gastroenterol. Latinoam.* 46, 131–159.

Sasaki, S. (2011). Autophagy in spinal cord motor neurons in sporadic amyotrophic lateral sclerosis. *J. Neuropathol. Exp. Neurol.* 70, 349–359. doi: 10.1097/nen.0b013e3182160690

Saudou, F., and Humbert, S. (2016). The biology of huntingtin. *Neuron* 89, 910–926. doi: 10.1016/j.neuron.2016.02.003

Schaefer, A., van Duijn, T. J., Majolee, J., Burridge, K., and Hordijk, P. L. (2017). Endothelial CD2AP binds the receptor ICAM-1 to control mechanosignaling, leukocyte adhesion, and the route of leukocyte diapedesis in vitro. *J. Immunol.* 198, 4823–4836. doi: 10.4049/jimmunol.1601987

Shahidi, M. (2017). Thrombosis and von willebrand factor. *Adv. Exp. Med. Biol.* 906, 285–306.

Skup, M. (2018). Neurotrophins: evolution of concepts on rational therapeutic approaches. *Postepy Biochem.* 64, 231–241.

Šmahelová, A. (2017). Diabetes mellitus and cognitive disorders from the diabetologists perspective. *Vnitr Lek.* 63, 717–720.

Smith, A. J., Malan, L., Uys, A. S., Malan, N. T., Harvey, B. H., and Ziemssen, T. (2015). Attenuated brain-derived neurotrophic factor and hypertrophic remodelling: the SABPA study. *J. Hum. Hypertens.* 29, 33–39. doi: 10.1038/jhh.2014.39

Sohn, J. W. (2015). Network of hypothalamic neurons that control appetite. *BMB Rep.* 48, 229–233. doi: 10.5483/bmbrep.2015.48.4.272

Srikanthan, K., Feyh, A., Visweshwar, H., Shapiro, J. I., and Sodhi, K. (2016). Systematic review of metabolic syndrome biomarkers: a panel for early detection, management, and risk stratification in the west virginian population. *Int. J. Med. Sci.* 13, 25–38. doi: 10.7150/ijms.13800

Stadtmann, A., Brinkhaus, L., Mueller, H., Rossaint, J., Bolomini-Vittori, M., Bergmeier, W., et al. (2011). Rap1a activation by CalDAG-GEFI and p38 MAPK is involved in E-selectin-dependent slow leukocyte rolling. *Eur. J. Immunol.* 41, 2074–2085. doi: 10.1002/eji.201041196

Stavoe, A. K. H., and Holzbaur, E. L. F. (2019). Autophagy in neurons. *Annu. Rev. Cell Dev. Biol.* 35, 477–500.

Suresh, S. N., Chakravorty, A., Giridharan, M., Garimella, L., and Manjithaya, R. (2020). Pharmacological tools to modulate autophagy in neurodegenerative diseases. *J. Mol. Biol.* 432, 2822–2842. doi: 10.1016/j.jmb.2020.02.023

Tekirdag, K., and Cuervo, A. M. (2018). Chaperone-mediated autophagy and endosomal microautophagy: joint by a chaperone. *J. Biol. Chem.* 293, 5414–5424. doi: 10.1074/jbc.r117.818237

Thomsen, M. S., Routhe, L. J., and Moos, T. (2017). The vascular basement membrane in the healthy and pathological brain. *J. Cereb. Blood Flow Metab.* 37, 3300–3317. doi: 10.1177/0271678x17722436

Tomoda, T., Yang, K., and Sawa, A. (2020). Neuronal autophagy in synaptic functions and psychiatric disorders. *Biol. Psychiat.* 87, 787–796. doi: 10.1016/j.biopsych.2019.07.018

Tumminia, A., Vinciguerra, F., Parisi, M., and Frittitta, L. (2018). Type 2 diabetes mellitus and Alzheimer's Disease: role of insulin signalling and therapeutic implications. *Int. J. Mol. Sci.* 19:3306. doi: 10.3390/ijms19113306

van den Berg, E., Reijmer, Y. D., de Bresser, J., Kessels, R. P., Kappelle, L. J., and Biessels, G. J. (2010). A 4 year followup study of cognitive functioning in patients with type 2 diabetes mellitus. *Diabetologia* 53, 58–65.

Van Dyken, P., and Lacoste, B. (2018). Impact of metabolic syndrome on neuroinflammation and the blood–brain barrier. *Front. Neurosci.* 12:930. doi: 10.3389/fnins.2018.00930

van Niekerk, G., du Toit, A., Loos, B., and Engelbrecht, A. M. (2018). Nutrient excess and autophagic deficiency: explaining metabolic diseases in obesity. *Metabolism.* 82, 14–21. doi: 10.1016/j.metabol.2017.12.007

Vanhauwaert, R., Kuenen, S., Masius, R., Bademosi, A., Manetsberger, J., Schoovaerts, N., et al. (2017). The SAC1 domain in synaptojanin is required for autophagosome maturation at presynaptic terminals. *EMBO J.* 36, 1392–1411. doi: 10.15252/embj.201695773

Varatharaj, A., and Galea, I. (2017). The blood-brain barrier in systemic inflammation. *Brain Behav. Immun.* 60, 1–12. doi: 10.1016/j.bbi.2016.03.010

Varghese, J. F., Patel, R., and Yadav, U. C. S. (2018). Novel insights in the metabolic syndrome-induced oxidative stress and inflammation-mediated atherosclerosis. *Curr. Cardiol. Rev.* 14, 4–14. doi: 10.2174/1573403x14666171009112250

Vijayan, V., and Verstreken, P. (2017). Autophagy in the presynaptic compartment in health and disease. *J. Cell Biol.* 216, 1895–1906. doi: 10.1083/jcb.201611113

Vilchez, D., Saez, I., and Dillin, A. (2014). The role of protein clearance mechanisms in organismal ageing and age-related diseases. *Nat. Commun.* 5:5659.

Vykoukal, D., and Davies, M. G. (2011). Vascular biology of metabolic syndrome. *J. Vasc. Surg.* 54, 819–831. doi: 10.1016/j.jvs.2011.01.003

Wang, L., Chen, L., Liu, Z., Liu, Y., Luo, M., Chen, N., et al. (2018). PAI-1 exacerbates white adipose tissue dysfunction and metabolic dysregulation in high fat diet-induced obesity. *Front. Pharmacol.* 9:1087. doi: 10.3389/fphar.2018.01087

Wang, S., Livingston, M. J., Su, Y., and Dong, Z. (2015). Reciprocal regulation of cilia and autophagy via the MTOR and proteasome pathways. *Autophagy* 11, 607–616. doi: 10.1080/15548627.2015.1023983

Wang, Y. C., Lauwers, E., and Verstreken, P. (2017). Presynaptic protein homeostasis and neuronal function. *Curr. Opin. Genet. Dev.* 44, 38–46. doi: 10.1016/j.gde.2017.01.015

Wei, Y., Liu, G. L., Yang, J. Y., Zheng, R. Z., Jiang, L. H., Li, Y. P., et al. (2014). Association between metabolic syndrome and vascular endothelium dysfunction in children and adolescent. *Genet. Mol. Res.* 13, 8671–8678. doi: 10.4238/2014.october.27.7

Wentworth, J. M., Naselli, G., Brown, W. A., Doyle, L., Phipson, B., Smyth, G. K., et al. (2010). Proinflammatory CD11c+CD206+ adipose tissue macrophages are associated with insulin resistance in human obesity. *Diabetes* 59, 1648–1656. doi: 10.2337/db09-0287

West, A. E., Pruunsild, P., and Timmusk, T. (2014). Neurotrophins: transcription and translation. *Handb. Exp. Pharmacol.* 220, 67–100. doi: 10.1007/978-3-642-45106-5_4

White, E., Mehnert, J. M., and Chan, C. S. (2015). Autophagy, metabolism, and cancer. *Clin. Cancer Res.* 21, 5037–5046. doi: 10.1158/1078-0432.ccr-15-0490

Wong, S. Q., Kumar, A. V., Mills, J., and Lapierre, L. R. (2020). Autophagy in aging and longevity. *Hum. Genet.* 139, 277–290.

Wong, Y. C., and Holzbaur, E. L. (2014). The regulation of autophagosome dynamics by huntingtin and HAP1 is disrupted by expression of mutant huntingtin, leading to defective cargo degradation. *J. Neurosci.* 34, 1293–1305. doi: 10.1523/jneurosci.1870-13.2014

Woo, C. Y., Jang, J. E., Lee, S. E., Koh, E. H., and Lee, K. U. (2019). Mitochondrial dysfunction in adipocytes as a primary cause of adipose tissue inflammation. *Diabetes Metab. J.* 43, 247–256. doi: 10.4093/dmj.2018.0221

Wu, H., Wang, Y., Li, W., Chen, H., Du, L., and Liu, D. (2019). Deficiency of mitophagy receptor FUNDC1 impairs mitochondrial quality and aggravates dietary-induced obesity and metabolic syndrome. *Autophagy* 15, 1882–1898. doi: 10.1080/15548627.2019.1596482

Wu, N. N., Zhang, Y., and Ren, J. (2019). Mitophagy, mitochondrial dynamics, and homeostasis in cardiovascular aging. *Oxid Med Cell Longev.* 2019:9825061.

Xilouri, M., Brekk, O. R., and Stefanis, L. (2016). Autophagy and alpha-synuclein: relevance to Parkinson's Disease and related synucleopathies. *Mov. Disord.* 31, 178–192. doi: 10.1002/mds.26477

Yamamoto, A., and Yue, Z. (2014). Autophagy and its normal and pathogenic states in the brain. *Annu. Rev. Neurosci.* 37, 55–78. doi: 10.1146/annurev-neuro-071013-014149

Yamamoto, T., Takabatake, Y., Takahashi, A., Kimura, T., Namba, T., Matsuda, J., et al. (2017). High-fat diet-induced lysosomal dysfunction and impaired autophagic flux contribute to lipotoxicity in the kidney. *J. Am. Soc. Nephrol.* 28, 1534–1551. doi: 10.1681/asn.2016070731

Yamamoto, T., Takabatake, Y., Minami, S., Sakai, S., Fujimura, R., Takahashi, A., et al. (2020). Eicosapentaenoic acid attenuates renal lipotoxicity by restoring autophagic flux. *Autophagy.* 28, 1–14. doi: 10.1080/15548627.2020.1782034

Yarmolinsky, J., Barbieri, N. B., Weinmann, T., Ziegelmann, P. K., Duncan, B. B., and Schmidt, M. I. (2016). Plasminogen activator inhibitor-1 and type 2 diabetes: a systematic review and meta-analysis of observational studies. *Sci. Rep.* 6:17714.

Yates, K. F., Sweat, V., Po Lai Yau, Turchiano, M. M., and Convit, A. (2012). Impact of metabolic syndrome on cognition and brain: a selected review of the literature. *Arterioscler. Thromb. Vasc. Biol.* 32, 2060–2067.

Yoo, D. Y., Yim, H. S., Jung, H. Y., Nam, S. M., Kim, J. W., Choi, J. H., et al. (2016). Chronic type 2 diabetes reduces the integrity of the blood-brain barrier by reducing tight junction proteins in the hippocampus. *J. Vet. Med. Sci.* 78, 957–962. doi: 10.1292/jvms.15-0589

Yoon, S. Y., and Kim, D. H. (2016). Alzheimer's disease genes and autophagy. *Brain Res.* 1649(Pt B), 201–209.

Yoshii, S. R., and Mizushima, N. (2017). Monitoring and measuring autophagy. *Int. J. Mol. Sci.* 18:1865. doi: 10.3390/ijms18091865

Yu, L., Chen, Y., and Tooze, S. A. (2018). Autophagy pathway: cellular and molecular mechanisms. *Autophagy.* 14, 207–215. doi: 10.1080/15548627.2017. 1378838

Zachari, M., and Ganley, I. G. (2017). The mammalian ULK1 complex and autophagy initiation. *Essays Biochem.* 61, 585–596. doi: 10.1042/ebc20170021

Zaffagnini, G., and Martens, S. (2016). Mechanisms of selective autophagy. *J. Mol. Biol.* 428 (9 Pt. A), 1714–1724. doi: 10.1016/j.jmb.2016.02.004

Zhao, Z., Nelson, A. R., Betsholtz, C., and Zlokovic, B. V. (2015). Establishment and dysfunction of the blood-brain barrier. *Cell* 163, 1064–1078. doi: 10.1016/j.cell.2015.10.067

Zilliox, L. A., Chadrasekaran, K., Kwan, J. Y., and Russell, J. W. (2016). Diabetes and cognitive impairment. *Curr. Diab. Rep.* 16:87.

4

Communication Between Autophagy and Insulin Action: At the Crux of Insulin Action-Insulin Resistance?

Scott Frendo-Cumbo[1,2], Victoria L. Tokarz[1,2], Philip J. Bilan[1], John H. Brumell[1,3,4,5] and Amira Klip[1,2,6]*

[1] Cell Biology Program, Hospital for Sick Children, Toronto, ON, Canada, [2] Department of Physiology, University of Toronto, Toronto, ON, Canada, [3] Department of Molecular Genetics, University of Toronto, Toronto, ON, Canada, [4] Institute of Medical Science, University of Toronto, Toronto, ON, Canada, [5] SickKids Inflammatory Bowel Disease (IBD) Centre, Hospital for Sick Children, Toronto, ON, Canada, [6] Department of Biochemistry, University of Toronto, Toronto, ON, Canada

*Correspondence:
Amira Klip
amira@sickkids.ca

Insulin is a paramount anabolic hormone that promotes energy-storage in adipose tissue, skeletal muscle and liver, and these responses are significantly attenuated in insulin resistance leading to type 2 diabetes. Contrasting with insulin's function, macroautophagy/autophagy is a physiological mechanism geared to the degradation of intracellular components for the purpose of energy production, building-block recycling or tissue remodeling. Given that both insulin action and autophagy are dynamic phenomena susceptible to the influence of nutrient availability, it is perhaps not surprising that there is significant interaction between these two major regulatory mechanisms. This review examines the crosstalk between autophagy and insulin action, with specific focus on dysregulated autophagy as a cause or consequence of insulin resistance.

Keywords: insulin resistance, autophagy, insulin action, obesity, type 2 diabetes, adipose tissue, skeletal muscle, liver

INTRODUCTION

Autophagy as a Metabolic Process

Macroautophagy (hereafter referred to as autophagy) is an evolutionary conserved, bulk degradation process that facilitates the deconstruction of cytosolic components, including organelles and proteins (Shibutani and Yoshimori, 2014; Yu et al., 2018). This process is initiated by the formation of a vesicular double membrane structure, termed the autophagosome, which engulfs cytosolic cargo and fuses with the lysosome, wherein internalized contents are digested (**Figure 1**). As such, autophagy is dependent on both the rate of flow through the vesicular pathway (autophagic flux), as well as the rate of substrate clearance by the lysosome (Loos et al., 2014). These steps are controlled by a series of autophagy-related (ATG) proteins and protein complexes such as LC3, p62, Beclin1, WIPI, ATG2, the ULK1 complex (ULK1, ATG13, FIP200, and ATG101), the PI3K complex (Vps34, Vps15, Beclin1/2, and ATG14L) and the ATG12 complex (ATG12, ATG5, and ATG16L1), illustrated in **Figure 1** (Shibutani and Yoshimori, 2014; Yu et al., 2018). Studies in the past decade have highlighted the physiological importance of autophagy, identifying associations between defects in autophagy and human diseases, including diabetes and insulin resistance. The challenge is to understand how autophagy contributes to, or is impacted by disease states.

Autophagy is a highly nutrient-sensitive, catabolic process important for cellular responses to nutrient stress and, thus, it is vital in maintaining metabolic homeostasis. During starvation and caloric restriction, low nutrient availability induces autophagy to provide substrates for energy provision (Wohlgemuth et al., 2007; Russell et al., 2014). Alternatively, nutrient availability activates anabolic pathways, such as insulin signaling, that directly attenuate autophagy (Codogno and Meijer, 2005; Mammucari et al., 2007; Meijer and Codogno, 2008; Russell et al., 2014). Regulation of autophagy by nutrient plenty occurs through two primary mechanisms: (1) phosphorylation events facilitated by the kinase mTORC1, and (2) induction of gene expression via the Forkhead box O (FOXO) family of transcription factors (Mammucari et al., 2007; Zhao et al., 2007; Liu et al., 2009; Xu et al., 2011; Sanchez et al., 2012; Xiong et al., 2012; Di Malta et al., 2019; **Figure 1**). Downstream of mTORC1 lies the ULK1 complex, required for initiation of autophagy. mTORC1 directly phosphorylates the kinase ULK1 and its associated ATG13. In states of nutrient availability mTORC1 is activated and ULK1 and ATG13 become phosphorylated, the complex is inactive, thereby attenuating autophagy (Kim et al., 2011). During starvation, mTORC1 is inhibited, promoting dephosphorylation of ULK1 and ATG13, activating the complex to promote autophagy. In addition, ATG gene expression is highly controlled by various transcription factors that contribute to the regulation of autophagy (reviewed by Füllgrabe et al., 2016). In parallel to ULK1 inhibition, the FOXO1/3-induced expression of genes in the autophagy machinery is reduced in conditions of nutrient availability, independently of mTORC1 (Mammucari et al., 2007; Liu et al., 2009). Instead, FOXO1/3 is regulated through other kinases including AKT. Together, these phosphorylation and transcriptional responses to nutrient availability regulate autophagy induction and, in turn, autophagic flux.

Insulin Signaling and Autophagy—A Balance of Anabolic and Catabolic Processes

Secreted postprandially in response to high nutrient availability (glucose, amino acids), insulin is critical to maintain blood glucose levels. Insulin acts by reducing hepatic glucose production in the liver and inducing disposal of dietary glucose in skeletal muscle and adipose tissue for the purpose of energy storage in the form of glycogen and triglycerides, respectively (Tokarz et al., 2018). Additionally, it is well-recognized that insulin can inhibit autophagy, through the aforementioned activation of mTORC1 leading to ULK1 phosphorylation (inhibition), and inactivation of FOXO transcription factors. In turn, ULK1 inhibits kinase activity of mTORC1 by inducing phosphorylation of raptor (Lee et al., 2007; Jung et al., 2009, 2011), creating a autoregulatory feedback loop. Recapping, the mTORC1-ULK1 nexus emerges as a key junction of insulin signaling and regulation of autophagy. Nutrient availability/insulin action activates mTORC1 leading to anabolic responses, and nutrient deprivation inhibits mTORC1 and thereby activates ULK1, leading to catabolic energy utilization. In parallel, FOXO1 integrates signaling from insulin (liberated

in response to nutrient availability) by regulating autophagy gene expression.

The PI3K-AKT signaling pathway is a major canonical component of insulin signaling, essential for insulin inhibition of autophagy (**Figure 2**). Upon binding to its receptor, insulin induces receptor autophosphorylation on tyrosine residues that provide a docking site for insulin receptor substrates 1 and 2 (IRS1 and IRS2). The insulin receptor then tyrosine phosphorylates IRS1 and IRS2, inducing recruitment of PI3K and subsequent conversion of PIP_2 to PIP_3 at the cellular membrane. In turn, the serine-threonine kinase AKT/PKB binds PIP_3 and is subsequently activated by mTORC2- and PDK1-mediated phosphorylation (Hemmings and Restuccia, 2012). Diverse signaling downstream of AKT induces tissue-specific outcomes of enhanced glucose disposal and diminished hepatic glucose production (Tokarz et al., 2018).

Importantly, AKT regulates both mTORC1 and FOXO1/3 activity through phosphorylation, and thereby represents a key nodule of intersection between insulin signaling and autophagy (**Figure 2**). AKT induces the activation of mTORC1 and inhibits FOXO1/3, consequently inhibiting autophagy (Codogno and Meijer, 2005; Mammucari et al., 2007; Meijer and Codogno, 2008). Interestingly, work in mice indicates that both deficient and enhanced autophagy lead to alterations in insulin sensitivity, as discussed in detail below. This bimodal influence suggests that the relationship between insulin signaling and autophagy is complex, and begs analysis of the contextual nature of their reciprocal cross regulation.

Autophagy in the Development of Insulin Resistance

A poor response to insulin commonly arises with obesity and predisposes to type 2 diabetes (T2D). Insulin resistance occurs when insulin is unable to sufficiently stimulate glucose uptake in muscle and inhibit hepatic glucose production. This condition develops as a result of diminished insulin action in skeletal muscle, liver and adipose tissue, often observed as decreased phosphorylation of AKT on serine and threonine residues regulating its activity. Although the decrease in AKT activity may not be solely responsible for the ample and diverse insulin-resistant outcomes, AKT phosphorylation remains a useful index of insulin resistance. Downstream, defects in insulin signaling result in reduced activation of mTORC1 and overactivation of FOXO proteins.

In the past decade, the relationship between autophagy and insulin resistance has gained momentum. In insulin-resistant humans and mouse models of diet-induced or genetic obesity, changes in ATG gene expression and protein content have been observed in insulin target tissues, although a causal role has not been established. Here, we briefly review the changes in autophagy in insulin resistant humans and rodents, and discuss the effects of deficient autophagy on insulin signaling and whole-body insulin action in *Atg* knockout rodent models, focusing on the fundamental insulin target tissues—adipose tissue, skeletal muscle and liver.

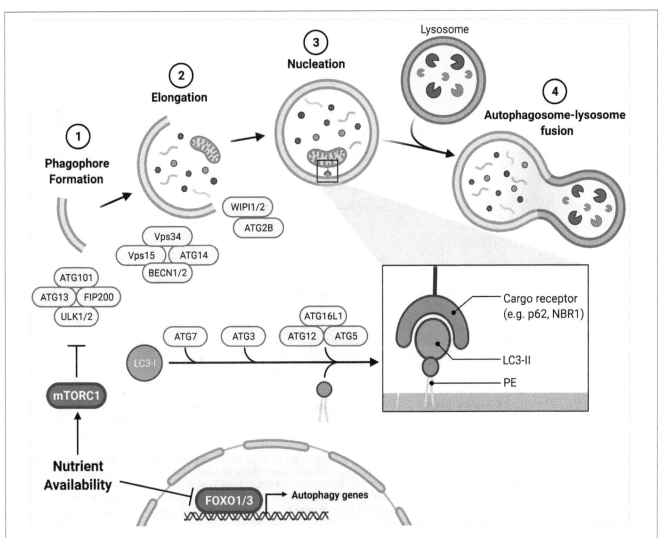

FIGURE 1 | Autophagy and its regulation by nutrient availability. The autophagic process is divided into defined segments: (1) phagophore formation, (2) elongation, (3) nucleation, and (4) autophagosome-lysosome fusion. In phagophore formation, the ULK1 complex, comprising ULK1, ATG13, FIP200, and ATG101, acts as a scaffold recruiting other ATG proteins to the phagophore. The PI3K complex, including Vps34, Vps15, Beclin1/2, and ATG14L, then produces PI3P on the phagophore, promoting membrane elongation via recruitment of WIPI/ATG2. Lastly, ATG7, ATG3, and ATG12-ATG5-ATG16L1 conjugate LC3-I to phosphatidylethanolamine (PE), forming LC3-II which is vital for autophagy target recognition and autophagosome nucleation. Nutrient availability attenuates autophagy via inhibition of FOXO1 and, crucially, mTORC1 inhibition of ULK1, with the mTORC1-ULK1 and FOXO1 nodes representing critical nexus between insulin action and autophagy regulation (Shibutani and Yoshimori, 2014; Yu et al., 2018).

ADIPOSE TISSUE: THE ENERGY RESERVE

Adipocytes are fat-storing cells that regulate energy balance and glucose homeostasis in the whole organism by regulating their fat content and secreting adipokines that act on distal tissues. White adipocytes store energy as triglycerides that can be mobilized through lipolysis to release fatty acids during times of nutrient depletion of the organism, to fuel other organs. In the fed state, insulin promotes energy storage in white adipocytes by increasing their capacity to take up and store fatty acids and glucose as triglycerides in a large lipid droplet. In contrast to white adipocytes that are "energy storing," brown adipocytes are "energy burning" (i.e., thermogenic), through their increased

mitochondrial content and expression of UCP1. As their lipid is constantly turned over, it segregates into smaller lipid droplets rather than in a single large lipid droplet, and at the whole body level brown adipocytes are associated with insulin sensitization (Saely et al., 2012). Changes in white adipose tissue (WAT) autophagy impinge on the levels of "browning" of the tissue by diverting metabolism from lipid storage to lipid utilization.

The insulin-dependent uptake of fatty acids and glucose in fat cells is mediated by translocation of their respective transporters, CD36 and GLUT4, from intracellular stores to the plasma membrane (**Figure 2**). While only responsible for 10–15% of post-prandial glucose uptake, perturbations in adipose tissue function impair whole-body insulin sensitivity and glycemic control (as reviewed by Guilherme et al., 2008).

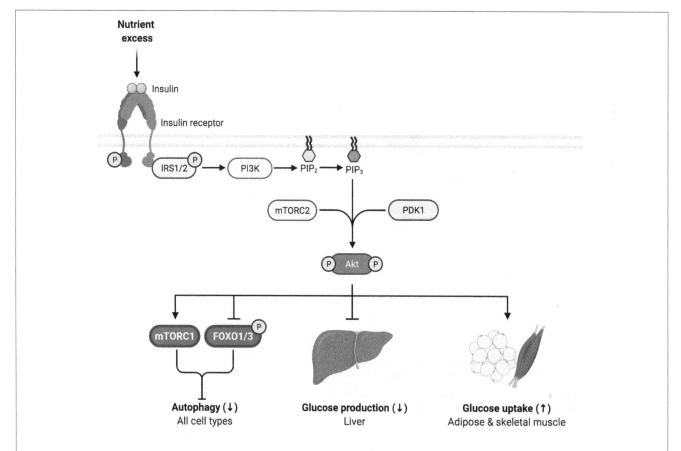

FIGURE 2 | Insulin signaling regulates glycemia and inhibits autophagy. Insulin binds to the insulin receptor, inducing receptor tyrosine autophosphorylation. Insulin receptor 1 (IRS1) and IRS2 then bind to the insulin receptor and are in turn tyrosine phosphorylated. PI3K is recruited to IRS1/IRS2 and produces PI(3,4,5)P$_3$ (PIP$_3$) at the cell membrane, onto which AKT binds, promoting its phosphorylation by PDK1 (T308) and mTORC2 (S473). Phosphorylated AKT is active and essential for insulin inhibition of autophagy, via inhibiting FOXO1 and activating mTORC1. Thus, as in **Figure 1**, mTORC1 and FOXO1 are critical nexus between insulin action and autophagy regulation. AKT is also vital for insulin regulation of glycemia, representing a key signaling node in attenuating glucose production in the liver and promoting glucose uptake in skeletal muscle and adipose tissue.

Autophagy and Metabolism in Human Adipose Tissue

The relative ease to sample subcutaneous WAT in humans, compared to liver and skeletal muscle, has enabled the study of autophagy in obesity and/or diabetes in this tissue. The majority of such studies have relied on measuring protein or mRNA levels of autophagy-related proteins in whole tissue explants. However, caution must be exercised when interpreting data on the expression levels of ATGs, as expression alone is not a *bona fide* measurement of autophagic flux (reviewed by Klionsky et al., 2021). Nonetheless, those values establish a baseline of defects that a functional analysis should build upon. Estimates of autophagic flux in general involve the detection of LC3-I and LC3-II levels and abundance of LC3-II-containing particles in the cytosol, denoting autophagosome formation (**Figure 1**). In addition, LC3-II abundance and autophagosome accumulation are impacted by both autophagic flux and the rate of lysosomal degradation (Loos et al., 2014). Lysosomal inhibitors that act by reducing lysosomal acidification are used to measure autophagic flux, as they eliminate the influence of cargo

degradation in this organelle (Shibutani and Yoshimori, 2014; Yoshii and Mizushima, 2017).

As recently reviewed by Clemente-Postigo et al. (2020), WAT from obese individuals presents elevated levels of the autophagic markers ATG5, ATG7, ATG12, LC3-II, p62, and Beclin-1, at either the mRNA and/or protein levels. This amplified expression of autophagy genes in obese WAT is likely mediated by increased activity of both FOXO and E2F family of transcription factors (Haim et al., 2015; Maixner et al., 2016). Examination of WAT explants in the presence of lysosomal inhibitors provides a more accurate measure of autophagic flux by blocking autophagosome degradation. Importantly, such studies have been performed and support that autophagic flux is in fact enhanced in WAT of obese individuals (Kovsan et al., 2011).

WAT explants contain not only adipocytes, but also fibroblasts, immune cells and vascular cells—collectively referred to as the stromal vascular fraction. Although these cells display a relative paucity of autophagy gene and protein expression compared to isolated adipocytes from WAT biopsies (Kovsan et al., 2011), measurements performed on whole explants include the joint contribution of all cells present in the tissue. Macrophages, are of particular interest given that they exhibit increased infiltration into WAT during obesity and impact insulin sensitivity and glucose homeostasis (Heilbronn and Campbell, 2008), and these cells display decreased autophagic flux in insulin-resistant mice (Liu et al., 2015a). Importantly, macrophage-specific knockout of *Atg5* or *Atg7* impairs glucose tolerance and insulin sensitivity (Liu et al., 2015a; Kang et al., 2016).

To directly assess the impact of obesity on adipocyte autophagy independent of the contributions of stromal vascular cells present in WAT biopsies, Soussi et al. (2015) isolated adipocytes from obese and control individuals. Obesity reduced LC3-II protein accumulation, indicating attenuated adipocyte autophagic flux, and that these changes were inversely correlated to fat cell size. Further, the obesity-induced reductions in adipocyte autophagy were reversible and improved after bariatric surgery (a strategy that diminishes energy intake and restores systemic insulin sensitivity). On the other hand, Öst et al. (2010) found that autophagic flux is elevated in adipocytes isolated from patients with T2D, measured by scoring phagosome content via electron microscopy and scoring LC3-II by immunofluorescence. This increased autophagic flux was associated with insulin resistance induced attenuation of mTORC1 activity (Öst et al., 2010). Of note, the latter study compared T2D subjects to a heterogenous population of control subjects consisting of lean, obese and insulin resistant subjects who did not have T2D, and were thus unable to discern differences induced by obesity from those of overt diabetes. A plausible reconciliation of the findings by Öst et al. (2010) and Soussi et al. (2015) is that adipocyte autophagy is attenuated in obesity, but as this condition progresses to T2D autophagy is conversely enhanced. In support of temporal changes in autophagy in the progression of obesity and T2D, Rodríguez et al. (2012) found that expression of *ATG7* and *BECN1* were unchanged in obese omental WAT compared to lean, while these genes exhibited increased expression in T2D WAT. However, autophagic flux, *per se*, was not assessed and therefore more work is required to confirm a functional contribution of autophagy in the diabetic phenotype. Therefore, whether adipocyte autophagic flux is increased or decreased in obesity, insulin resistance and diabetes remains controversial and may follow a biphasic pattern. Importantly, autophagic responses in various disease states are often biphasic, with measures of autophagic flux varying throughout disease progression (Schneider and Cuervo, 2014), although this has yet to be established with regard to insulin resistance and T2D. Overall, findings in whole WAT explants indicate that obesity and insulin resistance are accompanied by elevated autophagic flux and expression of autophagic markers (reviewed in Clemente-Postigo et al., 2020). Intriguingly, adipocytes isolated from tissue explants of obese individuals have lower autophagic flux than controls, unlike those from explants from type 2 diabetes (Öst et al., 2010; Soussi et al., 2015), suggesting that obesity, but not diabetes, impart adipose cell-autonomous changes in the autophagic process (**Table 1**).

Beyond their importance as an insulin responsive energy reserve, adipocytes contribute to whole body insulin sensitivity

TABLE 1 | Impact of obesity and insulin resistance on autophagy.

	Human subjects Obesity/T2D	Rodent models HFD/*ob/ob*
Adipose tissue	↑ PC/GE (Clemente-Postigo et al., 2020) ↑ AF (Öst et al., 2010; Kovsan et al., 2011) ↓ AF (Soussi et al., 2015)	↑ AF/PC (Nuñez et al., 2013; Mizunoe et al., 2017) ↓ AF (Yoshizaki et al., 2012)
Skeletal muscle	≈ PC/GE (Kruse et al., 2015) ↓ PC/GE (Møller et al., 2017)	↑ PC (Liu et al., 2015b) ≈ PC (Turpin et al., 2009; He et al., 2012)
Liver	≈/↑ PC/GE (Ezquerro et al., 2019)	↓ AF/PC/GE (Liu et al., 2009; Yang et al., 2010) ≈ PC/GE (Ezquerro et al., 2016)

Arrows indicate changes in autophagic flux (AF), ATG protein content (PC) and/or ATG gene expression (GE), where indicated.

through secretion of paracrine and autocrine acting cytokines, termed "adipokines." In addition to the influence of alterations of autophagy on metabolism, adipocyte endocrine function is also impacted. Genetic variants in *Atg7* correlate with circulating levels of the adipokine chemerin. Mechanistically, *Atg7* knockdown in adipocytes *in vitro* reduced secretion of the chemokine chemerin (Heinitz et al., 2019). This would suggest that there is a reduction in adipocyte-mediated macrophage recruitment in conditions of deficient autophagy. Illustrating a reciprocal cellular crosstalk between cytokines and autophagy, the adipokine leptin moderately enhanced autophagosome dynamics in cultured adipocytes (Goldstein et al., 2019). This finding is of particular interest, as leptin is considered and insulin sensitizing adipokine (Amitani et al., 2013) and therefore future work should examine whether leptin mediated changes in autophagy contribute to its whole-body insulin sensitizing actions.

Autophagy and Metabolism in Mouse Adipose Tissue

Animal models offer a degree of manipulability impossible to achieve in human studies and have been instrumental in our understanding of the relationship between autophagy and insulin resistance. Autophagy poses a critical influence on adipocyte differentiation, lipid droplet degradation (via lipophagy) and thermogenesis (Ferhat et al., 2019). Mice with adipocyte-specific congenital knockout of *Atg7*, a gene required for autophagy, display severely underdeveloped white adipocytes, with features characteristic of brown adipocytes (Singh et al., 2009b; Zhang et al., 2009). Metabolically, adipocytes from adipocyte-specific *Atg7* knockout mice display enhanced β-oxidation, leading systemic changes in free fatty acid homeostasis (Singh et al., 2009b; Zhang et al., 2009). These differentiation and metabolic changes induced by inhibition of autophagy have important implications in the context of insulin resistance.

High fat diet (HFD) feeding is a widely used strategy to drive weight gain and insulin resistance (Winzell and Ahren, 2004), and has been used to study the effects of high caloric intake on autophagy in insulin-responsive tissues. WAT from HFD-fed mice has augmented protein expression of LC3-II and p62, but not ATG5, while Beclin1 is either elevated or remains unchanged (Nuñez et al., 2013; Mizunoe et al., 2017). When autophagic flux was measured in the presence of a lysosomal inhibitors, HFD enhanced autophagic flux in WAT explants and caused accumulation of autophagosomes, presumably because clearance failed to match the rate of stimulated autophagy (Mizunoe et al., 2017). Opposite to these findings, Yoshizaki et al. (2012) reported that HFD impaired formation of LC3-II puncta in WAT. The discrepant results may be due to the length of HFD feeding, 16 weeks in Yoshizaki et al. (2012) and 30 weeks in Mizunoe et al. (2017), creating the possibility that shorter durations of HFD initially increase autophagic flux, but longer durations suppress it. Together, studies in mouse WAT mirror those of humans, as HFD increases expression of autophagic markers, but alterations in autophagic flux depend on the duration of HFD-feeding in animals or disease state (obesity *vs.* overt type 2 diabetes) in humans (**Table 1**).

While these studies indicate that overnutrition dysregulates autophagy in WAT, it is not clear whether dysregulated autophagy impairs insulin sensitivity or is a consequence of insulin resistance. To answer this question, Singh et al. (2009b) and Zhang et al. (2009) studied insulin sensitivity in mice with congenital, adipocyte-specific knockout of *Atg7*. Interestingly, loss of *Atg7* in adipocytes enhances WAT and whole-body insulin sensitivity compared to control mice, even when challenged with a HFD (Singh et al., 2009b; Zhang et al., 2009). However, in both studies, these independent groups attributed the insulin-sensitizing effects of adipocyte-specific *Atg7* knockout to "browning" of WAT brought on by the indispensable role of autophagy in adipocyte differentiation (Singh et al., 2009b; Zhang et al., 2009). Under conditions of overnutrition, these metabolically active "energy burning" brown adipocytes were protective against insulin resistance. Notably, insulin signaling to AKT was enhanced in WAT of HFD-fed adipocyte-specific *Atg7* knockout mice compared to WT controls (Singh et al., 2009b). Therefore, it appears that impaired adipocyte differentiation, not the inhibition of autophagy *per se*, is responsible for the insulin-sensitizing effects of congenital inhibition of autophagy in WAT (**Figure 3**).

To circumvent the detrimental effect of inhibiting autophagy on adipocyte development, and examine the effect on insulin action of a more acute reduction in autophagy Cai et al. (2018) generated mice with inducible, adipocyte-specific knockout of *Atg16l1* or *Atg3*. This system allowed them to examine the effect of inhibiting autophagy in mature adipocytes on insulin signaling. In stark contrast to the effects of congenital adipocyte autophagy inhibition, knockout of *Atg16l1* or *Atg3* in the adipose tissue of 8-week old mice with mature WAT depots caused insulin resistance (**Figure 3**). More specifically, autophagy inhibition in the adipocytes impaired insulin signaling to AKT not only in the WAT, but also in the liver and skeletal muscle (Cai et al., 2018). Further support for the development of insulin resistance from deficient autophagy comes from mice with adipocyte-specific depletion of p62. These mice experience

increased weight gain and fat mass and have impaired glucose and insulin tolerance compared to wild-type controls (Müller et al., 2013). Complementing these findings, Yamamoto et al. (2018) reported that constitutive activation of autophagy (by whole-body expression of Beclin1^{F121A}) preserved insulin signaling to AKT in WAT of HFD-fed mice by mitigating endoplasmic reticulum (ER) stress, a well described contributor to the development of insulin resistance. The mechanistic connections between autophagy and ER stress and the connection between ER stress and insulin resistance are beyond the scope of this review, but excellent reviews exist on these topics (Hotamisligil, 2010; Rashid et al., 2015; Salvadó et al., 2015). As a collective interpretation of these studies, congenital inhibition of autophagy obstructs adipogenesis and results in enhanced insulin sensitivity due to adipocyte browning, but selective inhibition of autophagy in mature adipocytes causes insulin resistance (**Table 2**).

SKELETAL MUSCLE: THE ENERGY USER

Skeletal muscle primarily functions to sustain position and movement, and therefore must extract from nutrients the mechanical energy required for these processes. Despite only accounting for 40% of total body weight in humans (Frontera and Ochala, 2015), skeletal muscle is responsible for ~80% of insulin-stimulated whole-body glucose uptake (**Figure 2**). Accordingly, skeletal muscle insulin sensitivity is paramount for whole body glucose homeostasis and skeletal muscle insulin resistance is a requisite precursor to the development of T2D (DeFronzo and Tripathy, 2009). Autophagy is critical for the maintenance of skeletal muscle integrity and mass (Masiero et al., 2009) and mounting evidence indicates that autophagy is also crucial for skeletal muscle energy metabolism (Neel et al., 2013).

Autophagy and Metabolism in Human Muscle

Given the complexity expected from analyzing an integrated function such as autophagy in humans, skeletal muscle biopsies have been examined to score indices of autophagy. Perhaps not surprisingly, this has met with contrasting results across studies (**Table 1**). Kruse et al. (2015) found no differences between lean, obese and T2D patients in the expression of various autophagy markers (mRNA of *ULK1*, *BECN1*, *ATG5*, *ATG7*, *ATG12*, *GABARAPL1*, *p62*; proteins ATG7, BNIP3, LC3B-I, and II, p62). However, a more recent study found lower expression of autophagy-related genes (*ATG14*, *RB1CC1/FIP200*, *GABARAPL1*, *p62*, and *WIPI1*) and proteins (LC3-II, p62, and ATG5) in skeletal muscle biopsies from individuals with T2D, suggesting suppression of autophagy (Møller et al., 2017). Insulin infusion during hyperinsulinemic-euglycemic clamp conditions (where glucose levels were maintained at 5.5 mmol/l) lowered the content of LC3-II protein in biopsies of lean and obese humans, but not of T2D patients (Kruse et al., 2015). These findings suggest that T2D, but not obesity, disrupts insulin action on autophagosome formation. Interestingly, insulin inhibition of autophagy was restored when

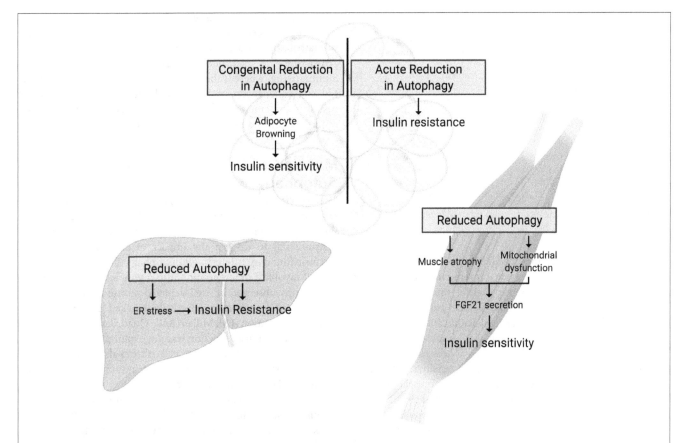

FIGURE 3 | Autophagy deficient rodent models present tissue specific alterations in insulin action. Tissue specific knockout of *Atg* genes in mice has provided a wealth of knowledge guiding our understanding of the potential for deficient autophagy to induce insulin resistance. In WAT, autophagy is essential for adipocyte differentiation, and thus congenital *Atg* knockout in these cells promotes a brown adipocyte phenotype that drives whole-body insulin sensitivity. In contrast, inducible adipocyte knockout of autophagy genes in mature white adipose tissue induces insulin resistance. Autophagy is also essential for skeletal muscle maintenance and development, and thus skeletal muscle-specific *Atg* gene knockout in mice induces muscle atrophy and mitochondrial dysfunction. These muscle impairments paradoxically promote FGF21 secretion and hence whole-body insulin sensitivity. Lastly, hepatocyte-specific *Atg* knockout induces insulin resistance associated with the induction of ER stress.

T2D patients were studied under isoglycemic clamp conditions (where glucose levels were maintained at the prevailing level of fasting hyperglycemia, i.e., isoglycemia) (Kruse et al., 2015). The distinct responses during euglycemia and isoglycemia in T2D patients led the authors to speculate that the failure of insulin to inhibit autophagy under euglycemic conditions represents a putative adaptation of autophagy to hyperglycemic conditions that ultimately preserves muscle mass (Kruse et al., 2015). In this context, the drop in autophagy markers in insulin resistant individuals is posited to reflect a chronic suppression of autophagy that occurs during hyperinsulinemic-hyperglycemic conditions.

Autophagy in Mouse Muscle

Numerous studies have aimed to characterize the relationship between overnutrition, insulin resistance and autophagy (**Table 1**). Six weeks of HFD-feeding elevated LC3-II expression and lowered p62 protein expression, indicating that HFD induced skeletal muscle autophagy (Liu et al., 2015b). On the other hand, after 12 weeks, LC3-II levels were similar in skeletal muscle biopsies from chow- and HFD-fed mice, indicating that

HFD-feeding did not alter basal autophagy (Turpin et al., 2009; He et al., 2012). A potential reconciliation of these observations would again be that varying durations of overnutrition have biphasic consequence on the regulation of autophagy, akin to that observed in adipose tissue. This scenario highlights the pressing need to resolve the temporal effects of overnutrition on skeletal muscle autophagy.

In order to directly assess whether HFD-induced insulin resistance impinges on insulin's ability to regulate skeletal muscle autophagy, Ehrlicher et al. (2018) performed hyperinsulinemic-euglycemic clamps on HFD-fed (12 weeks) mice (or chow-fed controls) and assessed insulin suppression of autophagy by measuring the LC3-II/LC3-I ratio in skeletal muscle. Despite demonstrating that HFD-mice developed whole-body insulin resistance (measured by increased glucose infusion rate during hyperinsulinemic-euglycemic clamps), insulin suppressed autophagy in both groups to the same extent. Thus autophagy remained insulin-responsive in the muscle of obese and otherwise insulin-resistant mice. Notably, while insulin suppressed autophagy to similar levels in chow and HFD-fed mice, potential differences may have been obscured by the

TABLE 2 | Impact of altered autophagy on insulin action.

	Congenital ATG knockout	Inducible ATG knockout	Enhanced autophagy
Adipose tissue	↑ WB/TS (Singh et al., 2009b; Zhang et al., 2009)	↓ WB/TS (Cai et al., 2018)	↑ WB/TS (Yamamoto et al., 2018)
Skeletal muscle	↑ WB (Kim et al., 2013)	NA	↑ WB/TS (Yamamoto et al., 2018)
Liver	↓ WB/TS (Yang et al., 2010) ↑ WB (Kim et al., 2013)	NA	↑ WB/TS (Yang et al., 2010; Yamamoto et al., 2018)

Arrows indicate changes in whole-body insulin action (WB) and/or tissue insulin signaling (TS), where indicated. NA, No available data.

higher insulin concentrations needed to maintain euglycemia in the latter mice. Moreover, the aforementioned studies of autophagy in human and mouse skeletal muscle are limited in their interpretation, as autophagy flux, *per se*, cannot be measured without the use of lysosomal acidification inhibitors.

Studies in skeletal muscle-specific *Atg7* knockout mice have been instrumental in our understanding of how skeletal muscle autophagy reciprocally impinges on insulin sensitivity (**Table 2**). However, *Atg7* knockout results in profound muscle atrophy, emphasizing the requirement of autophagy in skeletal muscle development and maintaining skeletal muscle mass (Masiero et al., 2009; Kim et al., 2013). Thus, the delicate balance between activation and suppression of autophagy is integral to skeletal muscle development and any perturbations in this equilibrium has aggravating consequences. Despite this perturbation in skeletal muscle mass, glucose tolerance is enhanced in chow-fed, skeletal muscle-specific *Atg7* knockout mice, and these mice were protected from diet-induced insulin resistance (Kim et al., 2013). When fed HFD, these mice showed higher glucose uptake during hyperinsulinemic-euglycemic clamps compared to HFD-fed WT mice, indicating that attenuation of skeletal muscle autophagy promoted insulin sensitivity in the context of overnutrition (Kim et al., 2013). A potential explanation for the enhanced insulin sensitivity in spite of marked skeletal muscle atrophy is the concomitant upregulation of FGF21. This myokine has pleiotropic insulin-sensitizing effects (such as enhanced beta-oxidation, increased energy expenditure, and WAT browning) that collectively confer protection from diet-induced insulin resistance (**Figure 3**; Kim et al., 2013). Contrary to the initial hypothesis that attenuation of skeletal muscle autophagy would promote insulin resistance, this study highlights the importance of inter-organ communication in determining the metabolic outcome of tissue-specific perturbations in autophagy. Nonetheless, muscle-specific insulin action was not directly examined, and, therefore it remains unresolved whether deficient autophagy induces impaired insulin signaling in muscle.

Contrasting with the above observations, others have shown that overactivation of skeletal muscle autophagy may afford protection against diet-induced insulin resistance (**Table 2**). In Beclin1[F121A] mice with constitutively active autophagy (described in the previous section), normal insulin signaling to

AKT in muscle was preserved during HFD, granting protection from diet-induced insulin resistance. This protective influence was attributed to a reduction in ER stress (Yamamoto et al., 2018) which, as mentioned before, can drive insulin resistance. Summarizing, whereas the duration of the HFD may determine the consequence on skeletal muscle autophagy, the effect of insulin to attenuate autophagy is preserved in HFD-fed mice otherwise afflicted by peripheral insulin resistance.

Muscle Cell Culture Models of Autophagy

Owing to the complex inter-organ communication networks that exist *in vivo*, as elegantly demonstrated by the above-described findings of Kim et al. (2013), cell culture models have been instrumental to discern the impact of autophagy on muscle intrinsic function. Interestingly, autophagic flux increases during C2C12 myoblast differentiation into myotubes. Resonating with the atrophy observed in *Atg7*-depleted mouse muscle described above, *Atg7* knockdown effectively blocked myoblast fusion and differentiation (McMillan and Quadrilatero, 2014). The consequence on insulin action was not explored.

Compared to animal studies, cell cultures also afford a simpler system to study the interrelation of autophagy and insulin action. In L6 skeletal muscle cells, transfection of dominant-negative ATG5K130R inhibited glucose uptake and impairs insulin signaling to IRS1 and AKT (Liu et al., 2015b). This work confirms that inhibition of autophagy is detrimental to insulin signaling in isolated skeletal muscle cells in absence of confounding contributions and signals from other tissues. We have shown that *Atg16l1* knockdown in L6 muscle cells markedly reduces the levels of the first target of the insulin receptor, IRS1. This phenotype was recapitulated in *Atg16l1*-knockout mouse embryonic fibroblasts, in which mechanistically we demonstrated proteasomal degradation of IRS1. Functionally, this was mediated by an E3 ubiquitin ligase complex composed of kelch-like 9 (KLHL9), KLHL13, and cullin 3 (CUL3) (Frendo-Cumbo et al., 2019). This complex now stands as a potential nodule connecting autophagy and insulin action beyond mTORC1.

Reciprocally to the reduction in insulin action upon alteration in autophagy, independent studies have found that insulin-resistant conditions in culture dysregulate autophagy. More specifically, high insulin/high glucose (HI/HG) treatment for 24 h provoked insulin resistance and impaired autophagy flux, both of which were relieved upon re-activation of autophagy and mitigation of ER stress by rapamycin treatment (Ahlstrom et al., 2017). Importantly, this effect was not observed in cells expressing the dominant-negative ATG5K130R, confirming that the restorative effects of autophagy activation on insulin sensitivity are autophagy-dependent. While this study did not examine whether insulin-mediated attenuation of autophagy was affected by HI/HG, treatment of L6 skeletal muscle myotubes with palmitate (a saturated fatty acid known to cause insulin resistance), prevented insulin-induced inhibition of autophagy at low doses (Ehrlicher et al., 2018).

In sum, findings in humans, mice and cell culture models identify that T2D and conditions known to induce insulin resistance (HFD feeding in mice, HI/HG and palmitate in cells) induce defects in skeletal muscle autophagy. However, whether these defects in autophagy in turn contribute to the development of insulin resistance is unclear: although muscle cell culture models of deficient autophagy display insulin resistance, mouse knockout models are complicated by inter-organ communication.

LIVER: ENERGY STORAGE AND GLUCOSE SUPPLIER

The liver is crucial for regulating whole-body glucose metabolism through a tightly regulated balance of glucose storage and release. Under fasted conditions and post-absorptively (between meals), the liver produces glucose through *de novo* gluconeogenesis (from amino acids and other intermediates) and glycogenolysis (glycogen breakdown). However, in conditions of nutrient plenty, insulin acts on liver hepatocytes to inhibit glucose production and promote lipid storage (**Figure 2**). During insulin resistance, insulin is unable to inhibit hepatic glucose production, and consequently blood glucose levels rise.

Studies in the liver and isolated hepatocytes have greatly contributed to our understanding of the significance of autophagy in metabolism. Hepatocytes were one of the first mammalian cell types in which autophagy was described and are the first cells in which the effects of insulin on inhibiting autophagy were characterized. The liver was also the first tissue in which lipophagy, the specific degradation of lipid droplets by autophagy, was described (Singh et al., 2009a). Under starvation conditions, autophagy is induced principally in the liver, which over a 2-day period leads to ~40% loss of liver protein in rodent models (Schworer et al., 1981; Mortimore et al., 1983; Ezaki et al., 2011). This upregulated hepatic autophagy is essential for the liver's role in maintaining blood glucose levels, as it regulates both gluconeogenesis (by producing amino acids used as precursors (Ezaki et al., 2011)) and glycogen breakdown (via glycophagy). Low circulating insulin levels are thought to be the primary driver of this process (Ezaki et al., 2011), removing inhibition of autophagy in hepatocytes. Much of this glucose is then secreted, maintaining blood glucose levels and providing energy to the rest of the body.

Given the intersection between autophagy and insulin signaling in regulating liver metabolism, it is especially compelling to speculate on the potential for changes in autophagy to contribute to the development of insulin resistance in this tissue. One such study by Ezquerro et al. (2019) described increased expression of *PIK3C3* in liver of T2D patients, while *ATG5*, *BECN1*, and *ATG7* gene expression and p62 protein content were unchanged. Interestingly, the LC3-II/LC3-I increased in prediabetic patients, but was unchanged in T2D patients compared to obese insulin-sensitive subjects (**Table 1**). This suggests that either enhanced autophagic flux or blunted lysosomal degradation of autophagosomes may occur in the liver of prediabetic patients. As all groups compared were obese, it is unclear whether obesity *per se* induces changes in hepatic autophagy (Ezquerro et al., 2019). However, further human

data examining the cause-effect relationship between deficient autophagy and insulin resistance in liver is lacking. This is likely due to the difficulty of evaluating autophagic flux in humans, as opposed to expression levels of autophagy genes, as well as to the invasive procedure required to extract liver samples from humans compared to the relative ease of sampling skeletal muscle and adipose tissue through superficial biopsies or from surgical material. Instead, rodent models form the basis of *in vivo* knowledge regarding autophagy regulation under conditions of insulin resistance.

HFD and genetic mouse models have been used to evaluate changes in autophagy in insulin resistant states (**Table 1**). When measured in the absence of lysosomal inhibitors, the LC3-II/LC3-I ratio and p62 content were unchanged in rats fed a HFD for 4 months (Ezquerro et al., 2016). However, autophagic flux (measured following *in vivo* treatment with chloroquine) decreased in the liver of *ob/ob* and HFD-fed mice, denoted by reduced LC3-II/LC3-I ratio, increased p62 accumulation and reduced autophagosome formation (Liu et al., 2009; Yang et al., 2010). Moreover, the expression of autophagy-related genes (*Vps34, Atg12, and Gabarapl1*) and of proteins LC3, Beclin 1, ATG5, and ATG7, was significantly lower compared to control mice, although gene expression of *Beclin1, Ulk2, Atg5, Sqstm1*, and *Atg7* was unaffected (Liu et al., 2009; Yang et al., 2010; Ezquerro et al., 2016). These features were associated with the development of insulin resistance and concomitant hyperinsulinemia. Causally, Liu et al. (2009) proposed that hyperinsulinemia is the main contributor to deficient autophagy, since treating mice with a PI3K inhibitor (LY294002) recovered defects in autophagic flux. Assuming that the hyperinsulinemia of *ob/ob* mice may have driven the altered autophagy, Yang et al. (2010) explored the effect of normalization of insulin levels using the pancreatic toxin streptozotocin (STZ). However, ATG7 levels were not restored, and instead the study suggested the elevated calpain 2 expression was responsible for ATG7 degradation, while autophagic flux was not measured.

To more precisely examine the consequence of the obesity-linked drop in ATG on insulin action, ATG7 was overexpressed in the liver of HFD and *ob/ob* mice. This treatment concomitantly improved insulin-stimulated phosphorylation of the hepatic insulin receptor and AKT, and reduced hepatic glucose production (Yang et al., 2010), ultimately improving skeletal muscle glucose uptake and whole-body insulin sensitivity. Mechanistically, ER stress and hepatic lipid accumulation, considered contributors to the development of hepatic insulin resistance, were curbed (Yang et al., 2010). Importantly, co-expression of dominant-negative ATG5 (ATG5K130R) that is unable to bind ATG12 and thus attenuates autophagic flux, abolished the beneficial effects of ATG7 on liver insulin signaling. These findings suggest that changes in autophagy are responsible for the fluctuations in insulin sensitivity upon changes in ATG7 expression.

Complementing this conclusion, hyperactivation of autophagy via whole-body expression of Beclin1[F121A] improved overall insulin sensitivity in HFD-fed mice, associated with reduced hepatic ER stress (Yamamoto et al., 2018). This study therefore supports the notion that the effects of autophagy on insulin sensitivity are mediated by the level of ER stress, and specifically that deficient autophagy promotes ER stress and subsequent insulin resistance.

Additional studies explored the effects of genetic attenuation of autophagy on insulin signaling (**Table 2**). Adenovirus-mediated ablation of *Atg7* in liver of mice lowered insulin-stimulated phosphorylation of the insulin receptor and AKT, accompanied by whole-body insulin resistance (**Figure 3**; Yang et al., 2010). However, contrasting findings were observed in liver-specific *Atg7* knockout mice, which displayed protection from diet-induced obesity and insulin resistance (Kim et al., 2013), although this study did not examine insulin signaling in the liver. The observed resistance to HFD-induced obesity and insulin resistance were associated with induction of FGF21, mirroring what was observed in muscle-specific *Atg7* knockout mice, as discussed in the previous section. Interestingly, liver-specific knockout of both *Atg7* and focal adhesion kinase family kinase-interacting protein of 200 kDa (*Fip200*) reduced starvation- and HFD-induced hepatic lipid accumulation, attributed to attenuation of the *de novo* lipogenic program in the liver (Kim et al., 2013; Ma et al., 2013). Thereby, the mice were protected from HFD induced hepatic steatosis. However, this finding remains controversial as others have shown augmented hepatic lipid accumulation in these liver-specific *Atg7* knockout mice following starvation, associated with defects in lipophagy – lipid droplet specific autophagy (Singh et al., 2009a). Therefore, it remains possible that defects in autophagy have an adverse impact on *de novo* lipogenesis in conditions that promote energy storage, reducing lipid accumulation and thereby the development of insulin resistance. Conversely, under catabolic conditions defects in autophagy prevent the rapid degradation of lipid droplets and release of lipids for energy provision, leading to an increase in lipid accumulation.

GENERAL LESSONS LEARNED

Insulin signaling and autophagy are a compelling representation of the homeostatic *yin* and *yang* between anabolic and catabolic processes. The antagonism between these two pathways is exemplified by the well described inhibition of autophagy by insulin signaling, as well as the numerous pathways that reciprocally regulate these processes (**Figure 4**). Central to this crosstalk is the mTORC1-ULK1 connection, which can be considered as a nexus between these pathways, along with FOXO1-directed transcriptional regulation. Moving forward, the levels, location and/or frequency of mTORC1 activation, coupled to its graded engagement of ULK1, may help define the crosstalk between these two processes.

The work presented herein examined consequences of altered autophagy on insulin signaling and further highlighted the complex cross regulation of these pathways (**Table 2**). Many studies in insulin-target tissues implicate defects in autophagy as potential contributors to the development of insulin resistance (**Table 1**). Therefore, attenuated autophagy may induce negative feedback inhibition of insulin signaling, overcoming the inhibitory action of insulin on autophagy.

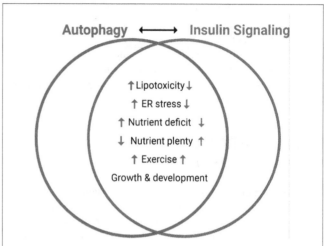

FIGURE 4 | Reciprocal regulation of autophagy and insulin signaling by various interventions and cellular states. The antagonism between autophagy and insulin signaling is a powerful representation of the homeostatic balance between catabolic and anabolic processes. Notably, autophagy and insulin signaling are reciprocally impacted by various stresses: lipotoxicity and ER stress induce insulin resistance, which independently promotes autophagy. Nutrient availability is a key regulator of both processes, with acute nutrient plenty promoting insulin secretion and thereby whole-body insulin action, and conversely starvation (nutrient deficit) inducing autophagy. Interestingly, exercise (not discussed here) promotes autophagy and insulin sensitivity in skeletal muscle and both processes are important in growth and development.

Important progress has been made to disclose the consequence of obesogenic and diabetic conditions on autophagy, and in turn the contribution of changes in autophagy to insulin resistance. However, our understanding of how deficient autophagy contributes to insulin resistance is incomplete and further examination is required in order to:

(a) Establish whether the autophagic process, as opposed to ATG expression alone, is in fact altered in T2D humans. To this end, Yang et al. (2010) provided the first evidence that defects in autophagic flux *per se* induces insulin resistance, rather than the loss of non-canonical functions of *Atg7*. More studies should complement examination of this involvement in the various specific-*Atg* knockout models discussed herein.

(b) Firmly establish if autophagic flux responds in a biphasic fashion during the development of insulin resistance. The studies analyzed support this possibility in aggregate, but the concept must be examined longitudinally in the same experimental system.

(c) Unravel the complete suite of molecular mechanisms through which deficient autophagy induces insulin resistance *in vivo*. In this regard, cell culture *Atg* gene-knockout models have already provided compelling evidence of how deficient autophagy induces insulin resistance (Yang et al., 2010; Liu et al., 2015b; Frendo-Cumbo et al., 2019). An important node of regulation, in addition to mTORC1-ULK1 is the control of IRS1 -life through the engagement of the ubiquitin-proteasomal machinery (Frendo-Cumbo et al., 2019). Superimposed on this direct molecular target are the indirect mechanisms of enhanced ER stress, inflammation and/or lipotoxicity, induced upon loss of autophagy and induce insulin resistance (**Figure 4**).

CONCLUSION

Our understanding of the crosstalk between autophagy and insulin action is mostly founded on investigations in adipose, muscle and liver of animal models, as well as cell culture models of these tissues. Future studies should clarify discrepant findings and important questions remain regarding the contribution of impairments in autophagy to the development of insulin resistance and T2D. Regardless of the mechanisms, it is clear that upregulating autophagy consistently improves insulin sensitivity (Yang et al., 2010; Pyo et al., 2013; Yamamoto et al., 2018).

Therefore, whether deficient autophagy is a cause or consequence of insulin resistance, or if it is in fact deficient in insulin resistance in humans, the therapeutic potential of autophagy induction to help treating insulin resistance and diabetes cannot be overlooked.

AUTHOR CONTRIBUTIONS

AK led the conception and design of the review. SF-C and VLT contributed to the design and wrote the first draft of the manuscript. All authors contributed to manuscript revision, read, and approved the submitted version.

ACKNOWLEDGMENTS

All figures were created with BioRender.com.

REFERENCES

Ahlstrom, P., Rai, E., Chakma, S., Cho, H. H., Rengasamy, P., and Sweeney, G. (2017). Adiponectin improves insulin sensitivity via activation of autophagic flux. *J. Mol. Endocrinol.* 59, 339–350. doi: 10.1530/JME-17-0096

Amitani, M., Asakawa, A., Amitani, H., and Inui, A. (2013). The role of leptin in the control of insulin-glucose axis. *Front. Neurosci.* 7:51. doi: 10.3389/fnins.2013. 00051

Cai, J., Pires, K. M., Ferhat, M., Chaurasia, B., Buffolo, M. A., Smalling, R., et al. (2018). Autophagy ablation in adipocytes induces insulin resistance and reveals roles for lipid peroxide and Nrf2 signaling in adipose-liver crosstalk. *Cell Rep.* 25, 1708–1717. doi: 10.1016/j.celrep.2018.10.040

Clemente-Postigo, M., Tinahones, A., Bekay, R., El Malagón, M. M., and Tinahones, F. J. (2020). The role of Autophagy in white adipose tissue function: implications for metabolic health. *Metabolites* 10, 1–30. doi: 10.3390/metabo10050179

Codogno, P., and Meijer, A. J. (2005). Autophagy and signaling: Their role in cell survival and cell death. *Cell Death Differ.* 12, 1509–1518. doi: 10.1038/sj.cdd. 4401751

DeFronzo, R. A., and Tripathy, D. (2009). Skeletal muscle insulin resistance is the primary defect in Type 2 Diabetes. *Diabetes Care* 32, S157–S163. doi: 10.2337/dc09-S302

Di Malta, C., Cinque, L., and Settembre, C. (2019). Transcriptional regulation of autophagy: mechanisms and diseases. *Front. Cell Dev. Biol.* 7:114. doi: 10.3389/fcell.2019.00114

Ehrlicher, S. E., Stierwalt, H. D., Newsom, S. A., and Robinson, M. M. (2018). Skeletal muscle autophagy remains responsive to hyperinsulinemia and hyperglycemia at higher plasma insulin concentrations in insulin-resistant mice. *Physiol. Rep.* 6:e13810. doi: 10.14814/phy2.13810

Ezaki, J., Matsumoto, N., Takeda-Ezaki, M., Komatsu, M., Takahashi, K., Hiraoka, Y., et al. (2011). Liver autophagy contributes to the maintenance of blood glucose and amino acid levels. *Autophagy* 7, 727–736. doi: 10.4161/auto.7.7. 15371

Ezquerro, S., Méndez-Giménez, L., Becerril, S., Moncada, R., Valentí, V., Catalán, V., et al. (2016). Acylated and desacyl ghrelin are associated with hepatic lipogenesis, β-oxidation and autophagy: Role in NAFLD amelioration after sleeve gastrectomy in obese rats. *Sci. Rep.* 6, 1–12. doi: 10.1038/srep39942

Ezquerro, S., Mocha, F., Frühbeck, G., Guzmán-Ruiz, R., Valentí, V., Mugueta, C., et al. (2019). Ghrelin reduces TNF-α-induced human hepatocyte apoptosis,

autophagy, and pyroptosis: role in obesity-associated NAFLD. *J. Clin. Endocrinol. Metab.* 104, 21–37. doi: 10.1210/jc.2018-01171

Ferhat, M., Funai, K., and Boudina, S. (2019). Autophagy in adipose tissue physiology and pathophysiology. *Antioxidants Redox Signal.* 31, 487–501. doi: 10.1089/ars.2018.7626

Frendo-Cumbo, S., Jaldin-Fincati, J. R., Coyaud, E., Laurent, E. M. N., Townsend, L. K., Tan, J. M. J., et al. (2019). Deficiency of the autophagy gene ATG16L1 induces insulin resistance through KLHL9/KLHL13/CUL3-mediated IRS1 degradation. *J. Biol. Chem.* 294, 16172–16185. doi: 10.1074/jbc.RA119.009110

Frontera, W. R., and Ochala, J. (2015). Skeletal muscle: a brief review of structure and function. *Calcif. Tissue Int.* 96, 183–195. doi: 10.1007/s00223-014-9915-y

Füllgrabe, J., Ghislat, G., Cho, D. H., and Rubinsztein, D. C. (2016). Transcriptional regulation of mammalian autophagy at a glance. *J. Cell Sci.* 129, 3059–3066. doi: 10.1242/jcs.188920

Goldstein, N., Haim, Y., Mattar, P., Hadadi-Bechor, S., Maixner, N., Kovacs, P., et al. (2019). Leptin stimulates autophagy/lysosome-related degradation of long-lived proteins in adipocytes. *Adipocyte* 8, 51–60. doi: 10.1080/21623945. 2019.1569447

Guilherme, A., Virbasius, J. V., Puri, V., and Czech, M. P. (2008). Adipocyte dysfunctions linking obesity to insulin resistance and type 2 diabetes. *Nat. Rev. Mol. Cell Biol.* 9, 367–377. doi: 10.1038/nrm2391

Haim, Y., Blüher, M., Slutsky, N., Goldstein, N., Klöting, N., Harman-Boehm, I., et al. (2015). Elevated autophagy gene expression in adipose tissue of obese humans: A potential non-cell-cycle-dependent function of E2F1. *Autophagy* 11, 2074–2088. doi: 10.1080/15548627.2015.1094597

He, C., Bassik, M. C., Moresi, V., Sun, K., Wei, Y., Zou, Z., et al. (2012). Exercise-induced BCL2-regulated autophagy is required for muscle glucose homeostasis. *Nature* 481, 511–515. doi: 10.1038/nature10758

Heilbronn, L. K., and Campbell, L. V. (2008). Adipose tissue macrophages, low grade inflammation and insulin resistance in human obesity. *Curr. Pharm. Des.* 14, 1225–1230. doi: 10.2174/138161208784246153

Heinitz, S., Gebhardt, C., Piaggi, P., Krüger, J., Heyne, H., Weiner, J., et al. (2019). Atg7 knockdown reduces chemerin secretion in murine adipocytes. *J. Clin. Endocrinol. Metab.* 104, 5715–5728. doi: 10.1210/jc.2018-01980

Hemmings, B. A., and Restuccia, D. F. (2012). PI3K-PKB/Akt Pathway. *Cold Spring Harb. Perspect. Biol.* 4:a011189. doi: 10.1101/cshperspect.a011189

Hotamisligil, G. S. (2010). Endoplasmic reticulum stress and the inflammatory basis of metabolic disease. *Cell* 140, 900–917. doi: 10.1016/j.cell.2010.02.034

Jung, C. H., Jun, C. B., Ro, S.-H., Kim, Y.-M., Otto, N. M., Cao, J., et al. (2009). ULK-Atg13-FIP200 complexes mediate mTOR signaling to the autophagy machinery. *Mol. Biol. Cell* 20, 1992–2003. doi: 10.1091/mbc.e08-12-1249

Jung, C. H., Seo, M., Otto, N. M., and Kim, D.-H. (2011). ULK1 inhibits the kinase activity of mTORC1 and cell proliferation. *Autophagy* 7, 1212–1221. doi: 10.4161/auto.7.10.16660

Kang, Y. H., Cho, M. H., Kim, J. Y., Kwon, M. S., Peak, J. J., Kang, S. W., et al. (2016). Impaired macrophage autophagy induces systemic insulin resistance in obesity. *Oncotarget* 7, 35577–35591. doi: 10.18632/oncotarget.9590

Kim, J., Kundu, M., Viollet, B., and Guan, K.-L. (2011). AMPK and mTOR regulate autophagy through direct phosphorylation of Ulk1. *Nat. Cell Biol.* 13, 132–141. doi: 10.1111/j.1743-6109.2008.01122

Kim, K. H., Jeong, Y. T., Oh, H., Kim, S. H., Cho, J. M., Kim, Y. N., et al. (2013). Autophagy deficiency leads to protection from obesity and insulin resistance by inducing Fgf21 as a mitokine. *Nat. Med.* 19, 83–92. doi: 10.1038/nm.3014

Klionsky, D. J., Abdel-Aziz, A. K., Abdelfatah, S., Abdellatif, M., Abdoli, A., Abel, S., et al. (2021). Guidelines for the use and interpretation of assays for monitoring autophagy (4th edition). *Autophagy* 17:382. doi: 10.1080/15548627.2020.1797280

Kovsan, J., Blüher, M., Tarnovscki, T., Klöting, N., Kirshtein, B., Madar, L., et al. (2011). Altered autophagy in human adipose tissues in obesity. *J. Clin. Endocrinol. Metab.* 96, 268–277. doi: 10.1210/jc.2010-1681

Kruse, R., Vind, B. F., Petersson, S. J., Kristensen, J. M., and Højlund, K. (2015). Markers of autophagy are adapted to hyperglycaemia in skeletal muscle in type 2 diabetes. *Diabetologia* 58, 2087–2095. doi: 10.1007/s00125-015-3654-0

Lee, S. B., Kim, S., Lee, J., Park, J., Lee, G., Kim, Y., et al. (2007). ATG1, an autophagy regulator, inhibits cell growth by negatively regulating S6 kinase. *EMBO Rep.* 8, 360–365. doi: 10.1038/sj.embor.7400917

Liu, H. Y., Han, J., Cao, S. Y., Hong, T., Zhuo, D., Shi, J., et al. (2009). Hepatic autophagy is suppressed in the presence of insulin resistance and hyperinsulinemia: inhibition of FoxO1-dependent expression of key autophagy genes by insulin. *J. Biol. Chem.* 284, 31484–31492. doi: 10.1074/jbc.M109.033936

Liu, K., Zhao, E., Ilyas, G., Lalazar, G., Lin, Y., Haseeb, M., et al. (2015a). Impaired macrophage autophagy increases the immune response in obese mice by promoting proinflammatory macrophage polarization. *Autophagy* 11, 271–284. doi: 10.1080/15548627.2015.1009787

Liu, Y., Palanivel, R., Rai, E., Park, M., Gabor, T. V., Scheid, M. P., et al. (2015b). Adiponectin stimulates autophagy and reduces oxidative stress to enhance insulin sensitivity during high-fat diet feeding in Mice. *Diabetes* 64, 36–48. doi: 10.2337/db14-0267

Loos, B., Du Toit, A., and Hofmeyr, J. H. S. (2014). Defining and measuring autophagosome flux - Concept and reality. *Autophagy* 10, 2087–2096. doi: 10.4161/15548627.2014.973338

Ma, D., Molusky, M. M., Song, J., Hu, C. R., Fang, F., Rui, C., et al. (2013). Autophagy deficiency by hepatic FIP200 deletion uncouples steatosis from liver injury in NAFLD. *Mol. Endocrinol.* 27, 1643–1654. doi: 10.1210/me.2013-1153

Maixner, N., Bechor, S., Vershinin, Z., Pecht, T., Goldstein, N., Haim, Y., et al. (2016). Transcriptional dysregulation of adipose tissue autophagy in obesity. *Physiology* 31, 270–282. doi: 10.1152/physiol.00048.2015

Mammucari, C., Milan, G., Romanello, V., Masiero, E., Rudolf, R., Del Piccolo, P., et al. (2007). FoxO3 controls autophagy in skeletal muscle in Vivo. *Cell Metab.* 6, 458–471. doi: 10.1016/j.cmet.2007.11.001

Masiero, E., Agatea, L., Mammucari, C., Blaauw, B., Loro, E., Komatsu, M., et al. (2009). Autophagy is required to maintain muscle mass. *Cell Metab.* 10, 507–515. doi: 10.1016/j.cmet.2009.10.008

McMillan, E. M., and Quadrilatero, J. (2014). Autophagy is required and protects against apoptosis during myoblast differentiation. *Biochem. J.* 462, 267–277. doi: 10.1042/BJ20140312

Meijer, A. J., and Codogno, P. (2008). Autophagy: A sweet process in diabetes. *Cell Metab.* 8, 275–276. doi: 10.1016/j.cmet.2008.09.001

Mizunoe, Y., Sudo, Y., Okita, N., Hiraoka, H., Mikami, K., Narahara, T., et al. (2017). Involvement of lysosomal dysfunction in autophagosome accumulation and early pathologies in adipose tissue of obese mice. *Autophagy* 13, 642–653. doi: 10.1080/15548627.2016.1274850

Møller, A. B., Kampmann, U., Hedegaard, J., Thorsen, K., Nordentoft, I., Vendelbo, M. H., et al. (2017). Altered gene expression and repressed markers of

autophagy in skeletal muscle of insulin resistant patients with type 2 diabetes. *Sci. Rep.* 7, 1–11. doi: 10.1038/srep43775

Mortimore, G. E., Hutson, N. J., and Surmacz, C. A. (1983). Quantitative correlation between proteolysis and macro- and microautophagy in mouse hepatocytes during starvation and refeeding. *Proc. Natl. Acad. Sci.* 80, 2179–2183. doi: 10.1073/pnas.80.8.2179

Müller, T. D., Lee, S. J., Jastroch, M., Kabra, D., Stemmer, K., Aichler, M., et al. (2013). p62 Links β-adrenergic input to mitochondrial function and thermogenesis. *J. Clin. Invest.* 123, 469–478. doi: 10.1172/JCI64209

Neel, B. A., Lin, Y., and Pessin, J. E. (2013). Skeletal muscle autophagy: A new metabolic regulator. *Trends Endocrinol. Metab.* 24, 635–643. doi: 10.1016/j.tem.2013.09.004

Nuñez, C. E., Rodrigues, V. S., Gomes, F. S., De Moura, R. F., Victorio, S. C., Bombassaro, B., et al. (2013). Defective regulation of adipose tissue autophagy in obesity. *Int. J. Obes.* 37, 1473–1480. doi: 10.1038/ijo.2013.27

Öst, A., Svensson, K., Ruishalme, I., Brännmark, C., Franck, N., Krook, H., et al. (2010). Attenuated mTOR signaling and enhanced autophagy in adipocytes from obese patients with Type 2 Diabetes. *Mol. Med.* 16, 235–246. doi: 10.2119/molmed.2010.00023

Pyo, J.-O., Yoo, S.-M., Ahn, H.-H., Nah, J., Hong, S.-H., Kam, T.-I., et al. (2013). Overexpression of Atg5 in mice activates autophagy and extends lifespan. *Nat. Commun.* 4:2300. doi: 10.1038/ncomms3300

Rashid, H.-O., Yadav, R. K., Kim, H.-R., and Chae, H.-J. (2015). ER stress: Autophagy induction, inhibition and selection. *Autophagy* 11, 1956–1977. doi: 10.1080/15548627.2015.1091141

Rodríguez, A., Gómez-Ambrosi, J., Catalán, V., Rotellar, F., Valentí, V., Silva, C., et al. (2012). The ghrelin O-Acyltransferase-Ghrelin system reduces TNF-α-Induced apoptosis and autophagy in human visceral adipocytes. *Diabetologia* 55, 3038–3050. doi: 10.1007/s00125-012-2671-5

Russell, R. C., Yuan, H.-X., and Guan, K.-L. (2014). Autophagy regulation by nutrient signaling. *Cell Res.* 24, 42–57. doi: 10.1038/cr.2013.166

Saely, C. H., Geiger, K., and Drexel, H. (2012). Brown versus white adipose tissue: a mini-review. *Gerontology* 58, 15–23. doi: 10.1159/000321319

Salvadó, L., Palomer, X., Barroso, E., and Vázquez-Carrera, M. (2015). Targeting endoplasmic reticulum stress in insulin resistance. *Trends Endocrinol. Metab.* 26, 438–448. doi: 10.1016/j.tem.2015.05.007

Sanchez, A. M. J., Csibi, A., Raibon, A., Cornille, K., Gay, S., Bernardi, H., et al. (2012). AMPK promotes skeletal muscle autophagy through activation of forkhead FoxO3a and interaction with Ulk1. *J. Cell. Biochem.* 113, 695–710. doi: 10.1002/jcb.23399

Schneider, J. L., and Cuervo, A. M. (2014). Autophagy and human disease: emerging themes. *Curr. Opin. Genet. Dev.* 26, 1–7. doi: 10.1016/j.gde.2014.04.003.Autophagy

Schworer, C. M., Shiffer, K. A., and Mortimore, G. E. (1981). Quantitative relationship between autophagy and proteolysis during graded amino acid deprivation in perfused rat liver. *J. Biol. Chem.* 256, 7652–7658. doi: 10.1016/s0021-9258(19)69010-1

Shibutani, S. T., and Yoshimori, T. (2014). A current perspective of autophagosome biogenesis. *Cell Res.* 24, 58–68. doi: 10.1038/cr.2013.159

Singh, R., Kaushik, S., Wang, Y., Xiang, Y., Novak, I., Komatsu, M., et al. (2009a). Autophagy regulates lipid metabolism. *Nature* 458, 1131–1135. doi: 10.1038/nature07976

Singh, R., Xiang, Y., Wang, Y., Baikati, K., Cuervo, A. M., Luu, Y. K., et al. (2009b). Autophagy regulates adipose mass and differentiation in mice. *J. Clin. Invest.* 119, 3329–3339. doi: 10.1172/JCI39228

Soussi, H., Reggio, S., Alili, R., Prado, C., Mutel, S., Pini, M., et al. (2015). DAPK2 downregulation associates with attenuated adipocyte autophagic clearance in human obesity. *Diabetes* 64, 3452–3463. doi: 10.2337/db14-1933

Tokarz, V. L., MacDonald, P. E., and Klip, A. (2018). The cell biology of systemic insulin function. *J. Cell Biol.* 217, 1–17. doi: 10.1083/jcb.201802095

Turpin, S. M., Ryall, J. G., Southgate, R., Darby, I., Hevener, A. L., Febbraio, M. A., et al. (2009). Examination of "lipotoxicity" in skeletal muscle of high-fat fed and ob/ ob mice. *J. Physiol.* 587, 1593–1605. doi: 10.1113/jphysiol.2008.166033

Winzell, M. S., and Ahren, B. (2004). The High-Fat Diet-Fed Mouse: A model for studying mechanisms and treatment of impaired glucose tolerance and type 2 diabetes. *Diabetes* 53, S215–S219. doi: 10.2337/diabetes.53.suppl_3.S215

Communication Between Autophagy and Insulin Action: At the Crux of Insulin Action-Insulin...

79

Wohlgemuth, S. E., Julian, D., Akin, D. E., Fried, J., Toscano, K., Leeuwenburgh, C., et al. (2007). Autophagy in the heart and liver during normal aging and calorie restriction. *Rejuvenation Res.* 10, 281–292. doi: 10.1089/rej.2006.0535

Xiong, X., Tao, R., DePinho, R. A., and Dong, X. C. (2012). The autophagy-related gene 14 (Atg14) is regulated by forkhead box O transcription factors and circadian rhythms and plays a critical role in hepatic autophagy and lipid metabolism. *J. Biol. Chem.* 287, 39107–39114. doi: 10.1074/jbc.M112.412569

Xu, P., Das, M., Reilly, J., and Davis, R. J. (2011). JNK regulates FoxO-dependent autophagy in neurons. *Genes Dev.* 25, 310–322. doi: 10.1101/gad.1984311

Yamamoto, S., Kuramoto, K., Wang, N., Situ, X., Priyadarshini, M., Zhang, W., et al. (2018). Autophagy differentially regulates insulin production and insulin sensitivity. *Cell Rep.* 23, 3286–3299. doi: 10.1016/j.celrep.2018.05.032

Yang, L., Li, P., Fu, S., Calay, E. S., Hotamisligil, G. S., Manuscript, A., et al. (2010). Defective hepatic autophagy in obesity promotes ER stress and causes insulin resistance. *Cell Metab.* 11, 467–478. doi: 10.1016/j.cmet.2010.04.005.Defective

Yoshii, S. R., and Mizushima, N. (2017). Monitoring and measuring autophagy. *Int. J. Mol. Sci.* 18, 1–13. doi: 10.3390/ijms18091865

Yoshizaki, T., Kusunoki, C., Kondo, M., Yasuda, M., Kume, S., Morino, K., et al. (2012). Autophagy regulates inflammation in adipocytes. *Biochem. Biophys. Res. Commun.* 417, 352–357. doi: 10.1016/j.bbrc.2011.11.114

Yu, L., Chen, Y., and Tooze, S. A. (2018). Autophagy pathway: Cellular and molecular mechanisms. *Autophagy* 14, 207–215. doi: 10.1080/15548627.2017.1378838

Zhang, Y., Goldman, S., Baerga, R., Zhao, Y., Komatsu, M., and Jin, S. (2009). Adipose-specific deletion of autophagy-related gene 7 (atg7) in mice reveals a role in adipogenesis. *Proc. Natl. Acad. Sci. U. S. A.* 106, 19860–19865. doi: 10.1073/pnas.0906048106

Zhao, J., Brault, J. J., Schild, A., Cao, P., Sandri, M., Schiaffino, S., et al. (2007). FoxO3 Coordinately activates protein degradation by the Autophagic/Lysosomal and proteasomal pathways in atrophying muscle cells. *Cell Metab.* 6, 472–483. doi: 10.1016/j.cmet.2007.11.004

5

Autophagy in Hepatic Steatosis

Vitor de Miranda Ramos, Alicia J. Kowaltowski and Pamela A. Kakimoto*

Departamento de Bioquímica, Instituto de Química, Universidade de São Paulo, São Paulo, Brazil

*Correspondence:
Pamela A. Kakimoto
pamela.kakimoto@gmail.com

Steatosis is the accumulation of neutral lipids in the cytoplasm. In the liver, it is associated with overeating and a sedentary lifestyle, but may also be a result of xenobiotic toxicity and genetics. Non-alcoholic fatty liver disease (NAFLD) defines an array of liver conditions varying from simple steatosis to inflammation and fibrosis. Over the last years, autophagic processes have been shown to be directly associated with the development and progression of these conditions. However, the precise role of autophagy in steatosis development is still unclear. Specifically, autophagy is necessary for the regulation of basic metabolism in hepatocytes, such as glycogenolysis and gluconeogenesis, response to insulin and glucagon signaling, and cellular responses to free amino acid contents. Also, genetic knockout models for autophagy-related proteins suggest a critical relationship between autophagy and hepatic lipid metabolism, but some results are still ambiguous. While autophagy may seem necessary to support lipid oxidation in some contexts, other evidence suggests that autophagic activity can lead to lipid accumulation instead. This structured literature review aims to critically discuss, compare, and organize results over the last 10 years regarding rodent steatosis models that measured several autophagy markers, with genetic and pharmacological interventions that may help elucidate the molecular mechanisms involved.

Keywords: liver, steatosis, autophagy, rodent models, review

INTRODUCTION

Liver steatosis refers to the accumulation of neutral lipids within organelles called lipid droplets (LDs) located in the hepatocyte cytoplasm. Currently, non-alcoholic fatty liver disease (NAFLD), an umbrella term used to define different conditions in which LDs are present in more than 5% of the hepatocyte and are associated with metabolic diseases (Godoy-Matos et al., 2020) has attracted growing interest. NAFLD is categorized by histological grading of liver biopsies, considering the presence and extension of steatosis, hepatocyte ballooning, and inflammation. Non-alcoholic fatty liver (NAFL) refers to simple steatosis, while non-alcoholic steatohepatitis (NASH) requires hepatocyte ballooning and inflammation (Kleiner et al., 2005; Jahn et al., 2019). Fibrosis may be present in NASH and indicates a more critical scenario that can evolve to irreversible cirrhosis and hepatocellular carcinoma (Loomba and Adams, 2019). There are no approved treatments for NAFLD, and liver transplantation is increasingly necessary for its irreversible consequences (Younossi, 2019).

Notably, NAFLD is widely heterogeneous among patients, and only a small fraction (about 20% of NASH) will develop cirrhosis and liver-derived complications. It is still unclear why. The disease's pathogenesis was once defined as the result of "two hits": first lipid accumulation in the hepatocyte, followed by secondary injury caused by inflammation or oxidative stress, for instance (Day and James, 1998). Over the last 20 years other researchers revisited this hypothesis, more consensually proposing that multiple hits, in parallel, may cause NASH (Tilg and Moschen, 2010; Tilg et al., 2020). Mechanistically, the literature consensus is that steatosis can lead to injury, but injury itself, e.g., inflammation, can also lead to steatosis. In 2018, an international expert consensus defined that Metabolic Associated Fatty Liver Disease (MAFLD) is a more appropriate acronym to define steatosis associated with metabolic dysfunction. It considers more universal environmental, metabolic, and genetic factor influences for each patient. This may help to destigmatize patients (due to presumed culpability of "alcoholic" vs. "non-alcoholic"), classify the variants of the disease better, and further improve therapeutic strategies (Eslam et al., 2020).

Indeed, different environmental and genetic factors are known to trigger the development of NAFL and NASH, and mechanisms responsible for the progression of the disease are still being elucidated. At the cellular level, multiple organelles and cellular functions have been found to be impaired. The resulting disorders may be turning point events in NAFLD progression and aggravation, and include endoplasmic reticulum (ER) stress, lysosomal dysfunction, mitochondrial dysfunction, oxidative stress, and impaired autophagy (Lian et al., 2020). Of particular interest, autophagy is a major mechanism controlling liver metabolism, not only as a nutrient stress rescue pathway, but also in physiological responses to fasting-feeding cycles (Ueno and Komatsu, 2017).

There are three types of autophagy: (1) macroautophagy, in which the autophagosome is formed and sequesters cellular components for degradation in lysosomes, (2) microautophagy, in which small parts of cytoplasm are directly sequestered and degraded by endosomes and lysosomes, and (3) chaperone-mediated autophagy, in which proteins containing the KFERQ motif are targeted toward direct degradation in lysosomes. In this review, we will focus on macroautophagy, and call it "autophagy" from now on.

In lipid metabolism, autophagy has been found to regulate both the degradation and formation of LDs (Kwanten et al., 2014). Singh et al. (2009) first characterized the relationship between degradation of lipids and autophagy activation, and coined this process "lipophagy.". They suggest that basal autophagy regulates triglyceride (TG) content in the liver and is important for lipid mobilization during fasting. On the other hand, Shibata et al. (2009, 2010) showed that microtubule-associated protein 1 light chain 3 (LC3), a crucial autophagy protein, is involved in LD formation. Moreover, autophagy during NAFLD is found to be either active or impaired in many studies using similar models. Thus, the contribution of autophagic activity toward lipid metabolism and, consequently, for steatosis development is still a matter of intense debate in the literature.

In this review, we aimed to evaluate the last 10 years of literature results about steatosis rodent models that measured several autophagy markers, with genetic and pharmacological interventions, in a structured manner. We prepared our tables

and focus article lists by searching for "autophagy AND liver AND (nafld OR obesity)" in Scopus and Pubmed, followed by double-blind exclusion in Rayyan QCRI (Ouzzani et al., 2016). We also excluded reviews, experiments not performed in rodents, and papers published in languages other than English. We retrieved all original papers evaluating autophagy markers in steatosis and summarized them by the type of model and results obtained on steatosis and autophagic markers measured in the liver. Our aim was to identify and discuss molecular mechanisms behind the following questions: (1) How is autophagy affected by steatosis? (2) Which molecular pathways of autophagic flux are mainly targeted? (3) Is there a difference in autophagic participation in chronic nutritional overload and fasting-induced steatosis? (4) How can pharmacological interventions and autophagy knockout models help elucidate the interplay between autophagic flux and steatosis?

DIET-INDUCED STEATOSIS MODELS

Diets Enriched in Fat

Diets containing more than 30% of energy from fat are considered high-fat diets (HFDs) and models of diet-induced obesity (DIO) and liver steatosis (Jahn et al., 2019). Carbohydrate sources are usually substituted by fat from lard or vegetable oils, and protein is kept around 15–20%. HFDs are widely variable in composition and may be described under other names reflecting quantities of sucrose, fructose, and/or cholesterol, e.g., "high-fat/high-sucrose," "high-fat/high-cholesterol," "Western diet," etc. As a NAFLD model, HFDs containing just excessive fat promote NAFL, but induce NASH only after a long period of feeding (>1 year). Other strategies are used to speed up NASH development, by adding cholesterol and fructose directly to the food, as in the Western Diet, adding fructose and/or sucrose to the water, or using a chemical "disease catalyzer" such as carbon tetrachloride, in low doses (Tsuchida et al., 2018; Boland et al., 2019; Jahn et al., 2019).

We summarized the main diets retrieved from our search (**Table 1**), but others exist in the literature. A point of concern is that many authors compare HFDs to chow diets, which we and others do not advise (Hariri and Thibault, 2010; Lai et al., 2014; Kakimoto and Kowaltowski, 2016; Preguiça et al., 2020). The source and quantity of ingredients can vary profoundly between chow diets and nutrient-defined diets, compromising metabolic outcome comparisons. The best control diets are purified, containing the same ingredients normalized

TABLE 1 | Diets used to induce steatosis and their components.

Name	% fat	% sucrose	% fructose	% added cholesterol
High-fat diet (HFD)	>30 ≤60	≤10	0	≥0 ≤2
High-fat/high-sucrose diet	>30 ≤60	>10 <45	0	≥0 ≤2
Western diet	~40	0	>30	≥0 ≤2

by total calorie content, changing quantity and not quality, and keeping micronutrients, proteins, and fibers in the same proportions. Notably, manufacturers suggest adequate matching controls for each intervention in open-access databases. In addition to care with control diets, it should be noted that, while these dietary/sedentary models for DIO/steatosis have advantages, they do not necessarily resemble human NAFLD at the molecular level. Each model's limitations has been thoroughly discussed elsewhere (Friedman et al., 2018; Jahn et al., 2019; Preguiça et al., 2020).

Figure 1 shows compiled information from our search considering the percentage of energy from fat, duration of the dietary intervention, and levels of lipidated LC3 and p62/sequestosome-1 (SQSTM-1), detected by SDS-PAGE and Western blots, compared to animals fed chow or LFD. Both proteins are widely used as monitors of autophagy activation/flux in the literature; LC3-II is the molecular signature of autophagosome formation, and binds to p62, favoring cargo capture for degradation (Pankiv et al., 2007). We highlight that comparisons must be interpreted with caution, as thoroughly discussed by Klionsky et al. (2021).

Excluding papers that involved genetic interventions (**Supplementary Table 1**), our study compiled 56 papers and 59 comparisons (papers are listed in **Supplementary Table 1**). We did not include publications in this structured analysis that omitted percentages from fat, duration of the diet, and the status of steatosis. We found that HFD promoted steatosis in virtually all studies, most of which were performed in male C57BL/6 mice fed 60% energy from fat. Animals were fed for 1–184 weeks; 17 ± 22 weeks on average. In general, authors suggest impaired autophagic flux occurs in HFD, accompanied by lipid accumulation. We find that LC3-II levels varied widely even under similar setups, while p62 is mostly accumulated in animals fed 60% energy from fat, and unchanged or reduced when fat content was lower than 60%.

The smaller number of papers using genetically-modified mice and HFD are summarized in **Supplementary Table 2**. We added information comparing with same genotype mice fed chow or LFD. Out of 14 publications, 9 still developed steatosis. The remaining 5 did not report more lipid accumulation over the control counterpart. Curiously, levels of LC3-II and p62 are mostly unchanged by these interventions.

Studies without genetic interventions (**Supplementary Table 1**) vary widely in the duration of the HFD-feeding, but autophagic flux seems to be compromised after 6 weeks, when steatosis is already settled. Some experimental designs are useful to find differences in the models and elucidate the mechanism behind autophagic flux alteration. Hsu et al., 2016, followed steatosis, ER stress, autophagy, and apoptosis markers from 2 to 16 weeks of HFD (45% of fat, 20% of sucrose as energy sources). In comparison to chow, lipid accumulation was always identified, while AMPK (adenosine monophosphate-activated protein kinase) phosphorylation increased at 4 and 8 weeks, and fell at 16 weeks. Total LC3-II was increased at 8 weeks and its ratio to LC3-I increased at 16 weeks. PERK (protein kinase R-like endoplasmic reticulum kinase) phosphorylation was reduced at all time points tested, while cleaved caspase 12 was increased

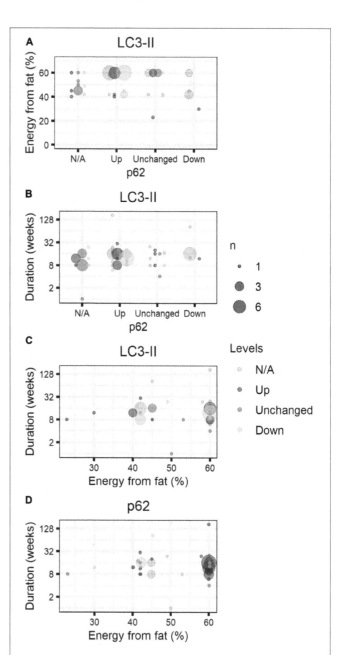

FIGURE 1 | HFD papers. Number of journal articles (*n*) describing diet fat content (in percentage of energy), duration of the intervention, and LC3-II and p62 protein levels in the liver in comparison to control groups (chow or LFD), normalized by a housekeeping protein. LC3-II and p62 were estimated by the authors through SDS-PAGE Western blots and described semi-quantitatively or qualitatively. The size of the circle corresponds to the total number of articles with the same description. Colors refer to LC3-II **(A–C)** or p62 **(D)** qualitative status. [gray = N/A (not available), blue = Up, orange = Unchanged, yellow = Down].

only at 2 and 4 weeks, and PARP (poly ADP-ribose polymerase) at 8 weeks (Hsu et al., 2016). While other markers were not assessed, from this data it seems lipid accumulation and unfolded protein response (UPR) activation occur first, and autophagy flux is probably increased at 8 weeks, after AMPK activation. Similar findings were observed in the spontaneous OVE26 diabetic mice, but over 5–8 months (Zhang Q. et al., 2015). Accordingly, high-fat fed rats submitted to sleeve gastrectomy showed significant TG reduction, and lower markers of ER stress and UPR activation, accompanied by increased β-oxidation, AMPK and autophagic activation (Ezquerro et al., 2016, 2020). Similar changes were found using roux-en-Y gastric bypass interventions (He et al., 2015; Ma et al., 2020). ER stress and UPR activation are common findings in the steatotic liver of rodents and humans, and many targets have been suggested as possible points of intervention for NAFLD treatment (Lebeaupin et al., 2018).

To evaluate the effect of type (not quantity) of fats on liver steatosis and autophagy markers, Wang M.-E. et al. (2017) formulated a diet analogous to the Research Diets D12492 (60% energy from fat, containing soybean oil and lard as fat sources), but substituting about half of the lard for coconut oil. This yields a higher proportion of medium-chain fatty acids (MCFA) in comparison to long-chain fatty acids (LCFA) (Wang M.-E. et al., 2017). The MCFA-enriched diet promoted similar results to LCFA regarding body weight gain, increased fasting glycemia, and liver steatosis, but to a lesser extent. Animals showed reduced staining with Sirius Red and collagen, suggesting less fibrosis in the MCFA groups. While both diets increased the content of LC3-II, only the LCFA-enriched diet accumulated p62 and increased ER stress markers. The authors conclude that MCFA may alleviate autophagic flux impairment produced by HFD. Consistently, markers of lipotoxicity-induced autophagy impairment in *in vitro* studies could be modulated by increasing the content of MCFA to LCFA in the lipid mix. This may be associated with LCFA-induced expression of RUBICON, a negative regulator of autophagosome fusion to lysosomes, described as a possible regulatory node of autophagy impairment and steatosis induced by HFD (Tanaka et al., 2016).

Methionine-Choline Deficient Diets

The methionine-choline deficient (MCD) diet is another popular model to quickly induce NASH in rodents (Santhekadur et al., 2018). The rationale is that choline deficiency compromises the export of lipids by the liver, while increasing uptake, and thus promoting accumulation in the cytoplasm (Rinella et al., 2008). MCD diets are usually enriched in sucrose and can vary in the percentage of energy from fat (10–60%). After about 4 weeks of feeding, animals develop steatosis, inflammation, fibrosis, and extensive liver damage. Although it promotes hepatic histology similar to human NASH, the model is dissimilar to most human disease presentations, as animals lose weight and do not become insulin resistant (Friedman et al., 2018). Machado et al. (2015) described that 8 weeks of MCD diet, compared to 16-week Western Diet, promoted severe liver damage, inflammation and fibrosis, but accumulated fewer triglycerides. On the other hand, Western Diet promoted weight gain, more extensive triglyceride accumulation, insulin resistance, and dyslipidemia. The authors suggest that the MCD diet is a reasonable model for liver injury and evolution of NASH, but the Western Diet is more appropriate to study NAFLD and its consequences for other tissues. Since human NAFLD is slowly progressive and will evolve to NASH only in a minority of patients, the MCD diet remains a harsh, but complementary, study model.

We summarized all papers in our search using the MCD diet as a NASH model that evaluated steatosis, LC3-II and/or p62, and compared it to an LFD or chow diet (**Table 2**). The time course of MCD diet feeding varied from 1.5 to 10 weeks. Most of the studies, except one in male BALB/c mice, were performed in male C57BL/6 mice. Consistently, the MCD diet promoted steatosis and p62 accumulation in all studies. LC3-II was unchanged (1 out of 18 comparisons), increased (12/18), or decreased (5/18). Most authors concluded that autophagic flux is compromised in MCD diet-fed animals. Notably, Wang et al. (2018) found LC3-II and p62 levels increased at 3-weeks of MCD in both C57BL/6 and obese *db/db* mice. HFD promoted similar results at 12 weeks. The authors suggest, by combining many animal and cell lineage models of steatosis, that autophagic flux impairment is a typical result of deficient lysosomal acidification induced by ER stress and asparagine accumulation. The same group described impaired autophagolysosome formation and acidification, mediated by upregulation of the C-X-C motif chemokine 10, using HFHC and MCD as steatosis models (Zhang et al., 2017). Similarly, Tang et al. (2020) promoted steatosis using HFD, the MCD diet, and cell models, and found decreased autophagic flux due to deficient autophagolysosome formation, which the authors ascribe to increased synthesis of osteopontin (OPN). The neutralization of OPN restored autophagic flux and reduced triglyceride accumulation.

ER stress is commonly observed in lipid overload/lipotoxicity models, and many authors suggest it is the upstream signal of reduced autophagic flux (González-Rodríguez et al., 2014). Interestingly, Hernández-Alvarez et al. (2019) recently described that the mitofusin-2 (Mfn2) binds to phosphatidylserine and is responsible for phospholipid shuttling between ER and mitochondria to produce phosphatidylethanolamine and phosphatidylcholine. Human NASH patients and MCD- and HFD-fed mice have reduced Mfn2 content and aberrant lipid metabolism. Preventing ER stress normalized inflammation and fibrosis markers, but not lipid metabolism (Hernández-Alvarez et al., 2019). While reduced Mfn2 has been strongly associated with impaired autophagic flux in many cell types and tissues (Muñoz et al., 2013; Sebastián et al., 2016), cellular lipid composition and mitochondrial phosphatidylethanolamine synthesis are known to be essential for full autophagic activation (Koga et al., 2010; Thomas et al., 2018). Since phosphatidylethanolamine is incorporated into LC3-I by ATG3 and ATG7 ("ATG" denotes autophagy related proteins), reduced availability in NASH patients may also be a player in impaired autophagic flux.

From these studies comparing many steatosis models, we suggest that steatosis and autophagy flux impairment in the liver may be dissociated from systemic glucose homeostasis and adiposity, and converge as a cellular responses to lipid accumulation *per se*.

Leptin and Leptin Receptor Deficient Mice

Leptin (*ob/ob*) and leptin receptor (*db/db*) deficient mice are obesity models with spontaneous mutations resulting in lack

TABLE 2 | MCD model.

References	Strain	Duration of MCD (weeks),% energy from fat, catalog	LC3-II/housekeeping	p62/housekeeping
			(vs. Chow or LFD)	
Ji et al., 2015	C57BL/6	4	Up	Up
Machado et al., 2015	C57BL/6	8, 20%, MP Biomedicals, #960439	Down	N/A
Xie et al., 2015	BALB/c	1.5	Up	N/A
Chen et al., 2016	C57BL/6	10	Down	Up
Zhang X. et al., 2016	C57BL/6	4	Up	Up
Zhang X. et al., 2016	C57BL/6 CXCR3 KO	4	Up	Up
Zhang et al., 2017	C57BL/6	4	Up	Up
Lee et al., 2018	C57BL/6	4, 30%	Up	Up
Wang et al., 2018	C57BL/6	3	Up	Up
Wang et al., 2018	db/db	3	Up	Up
Cruces-Sande et al., 2018	C57BL/6	4, 10%, Envigo, TD. 90262	Unchanged	Up
Zheng Y. et al., 2018	C57BL/6	3, 10%	Up	Unchanged
Zeng et al., 2018	C57BL/6	5	Down	Up
Wu C. et al., 2018	C57BL/6	4	Down	Up
Veskovic et al., 2019	C57BL/6	6	Up	Up
Chen et al., 2019	db/db	4	Up	Up
Li et al., 2019a	C57BL/6	4, 21%, Research Diets, A02082002B	Down	Up
Tang et al., 2020	C57BL/6	8	Up	Up

Articles using MCD as a NASH model, describing intervention duration, liver steatosis, LC3-II and p62 protein in the liver in comparison to control groups (chow or LFD), normalized by a housekeeping protein. LC3-II and p62 were obtained by the authors through SDS-PAGE Western blots and described semi-quantitatively or qualitatively. All experiments observed increases lipid accumulation in the liver. All animals were male mice (N/A, not available).

of leptin signaling. These animals are hyperphagic and have severe body weight gain at early ages (Wang B. et al., 2014). An interesting aspect when comparing ob/ob and db/db animals to dietary models is that, usually, hyperphagia models are fed with chow diets, containing most of the energy from carbohydrates, and not fat. Obesity is thus the result of hypercaloric ingestion and lack of leptin signaling. The animals spontaneously develop hyperinsulinemia, dyslipidemia, and liver steatosis. A critique of these models is that obese humans become hyperleptinemic and typically leptin-resistant over time (Wang B. et al., 2014).

In **Table 3**, we summarized our search for papers that evaluated steatosis, lipidated LC3 and/or p62 concomitantly and compared WT mice and ob/ob or db/db mice as a NAFLD model. All mice used were male from 7 to 22 weeks of age and developed steatosis with chow diets. Like the other obesity and NAFLD models, p62 is accumulated in all papers that measured it (5/5). LC3-II is increased in half the publications, while the other half is decreased (3/6). Overall, autophagic flux is impaired.

Two of these studies found that increased sirtuin 1 (SIRT1) expression could restore autophagic flux in db/db and ob/ob mice (Huang et al., 2017; Hong et al., 2018). Both models have decreased SIRT1 protein levels compared to WT. Through different pharmacological interventions, i.e., ginsenoside Rb2, erythropoietin, or resveratrol, authors found that AMPK activation and increased levels of SIRT1 both increase autophagic flux and reduce steatosis. In another study, ob/ob mice under calorie restriction or metformin treatment showed increased SIRT1 levels and autophagic flux, as well as reduced steatosis in comparison to *ad libitum* fed animals. *In vitro* experiments

suggest a mechanism independent of AMPK of SIRT1-dependent autophagy activation for metformin, which remains to be clarified (Song et al., 2015).

Adenosine monophosphate-activated protein kinase signaling is a central hub in the liver, controlling glycogen and lipid metabolism (González et al., 2020). Its activation counteracts mTOR (mechanistic target of rapamycin kinase) signaling by increasing autophagic flux through the phosphorylation of ULK1 (unc-51 like autophagy activating kinase 1) in Ser317 e Ser777 (Kim et al., 2011), while SIRT1 is known to deacetylate many

TABLE 3 | Leptin and leptin-receptor deficient mice.

References	Genetics	Final age (weeks)	LC3-II/ housekeeping	p62/ housekeeping
			(vs. WT)	
Liu et al., 2015	ob/ob	14	Up	N/A
Hong et al., 2018	ob/ob	14	Down	Up
Zheng W. et al., 2018	ob/ob	12	Down	N/A
Yang et al., 2020	ob/ob	9	Up	Up
Kim et al., 2016	db/db	22	N/A	Up
Huang et al., 2017	db/db	10	Down	Up
Matsumoto et al., 2019	db/db	7	Up	Up

Articles using leptin- or leptin receptor-deficient mice, describing intervention duration, and LC3-II and p62 protein in the liver in comparison to control groups (WT mice), normalized by a housekeeping protein. LC3-II and p62 were obtained by the authors through SDS-PAGE Western blots and described semi-quantitatively or qualitatively. All experiments observed increases in lipid accumulation in the liver. All animals were male mice (N/A, not available).

autophagy proteins, and to be a downstream target of adipose tissue triglyceride lipase (ATGL) induction of lipophagy in the liver (Lee et al., 2008; Sathyanarayan et al., 2017). Furthermore, melatonin and berberine effects on autophagy activation and reduced steatosis were also observed to be SIRT1-dependent in mice under HFD with intact leptin signaling, as confirmed in liver-specific knockouts (Sun et al., 2018; Stacchiotti et al., 2019). Resveratrol is defined as a SIRT1 activator and is described by many authors to increase autophagic flux and alleviate steatosis in many rodent models, including HFD, MCD, and genetic interventions thought to relieve ER stress and inflammation (Li et al., 2014; Ji et al., 2015; Zhang Y. et al., 2015; Ding et al., 2017; Milton-Laskibar et al., 2018). The similar contributions of SIRT1 activation in different models suggest a common point of intervention in steatosis development and subsequent resolution. However, some clinical trials did not observe significant reduction of steatosis upon 12 weeks of treatment (Kantartzis et al., 2018; Farzin et al., 2020), a finding that is still under debate regarding the effects of overdosage and treatment length (Fogacci et al., 2018).

Mechanisms of Autophagy Impairment in NAFLD

Why NAFLD models lead to impaired autophagy is still debated. Several mechanisms leading to dysfunction of late steps in the autophagic process, such as decreased lysosomal function and autophagosome-lysosome fusion, have been proposed. Interestingly, different literature results suggest that these steps may be impaired as a consequence of ER-stress in NAFLD models. Wang et al. (2018) demonstrated that cellular responses to ER stress promote increased levels of asparagine, leading to decreased lysosome acidification in animals fed MCD or HFHC diets as well as hepatocyte cultures treated with MCD. Moreover, in vitro studies by Miyagawa et al. (2016) demonstrated that palmitate-induced ER-stress supports impaired autophagosome-lysosome fusion in hepatic cells, as this was attenuated by co-treatment with chemical chaperone. Curiously, lysosome acidification and function were not altered by palmitate. These studies may suggest that, although all NAFLD models culminate in autophagic impairment, specific mechanisms could be favored under each condition. This has also been suggested by other authors based on different responses of autophagy markers comparing HFD with high sucrose and HFHS diets (Simoes et al., 2020). In addition to these evidences, the UPR and autophagy have recently been shown to share common regulatory pathways. The spliced form of XBP1 (sXBP1), a transcription factor necessary for UPR activation, binds to the promoter region and activates the expression of transcription factor EB (TFEB). This interaction is reduced in steatotic hepatic tissue (Zhang et al., 2020). TFEB is the main transcription factor that binds to the CLEAR regulatory motif and promotes expression of an array of lysosomal and autophagic genes (Napolitano and Ballabio, 2016). Thus, downregulation of TFEB expression may not only lead to decreased lysosome biogenesis and activity, but also affect overall autophagy activation. Along with ER-stress-derived mechanisms, obesogenic diets were shown to promote iNOS localization at the lysosome surface, causing nitric oxide stress, impaired lysosomal function and decreased TFEB activation (Qian et al., 2019). Finally, autophagosome-lysosome fusion may also be suppressed by RUBICON, a BECLIN-1 interacting protein, which was shown to be upregulated in the hepatic tissue of mice fed HFD, and to contribute toward NAFLD progression (Matsunaga et al., 2009; Zhong et al., 2009; Tanaka et al., 2016).

Changes in AMPK and mTORC1 activity are also suggested to mediate impaired autophagy during NAFLD. Recent findings suggest that upregulation of CD36, a protein that facilitates fatty acid uptake in hepatocytes, leads to inhibition of autophagy initiation in fatty livers, through the AMPK/ULK1/BECLIN-1 pathway (Li et al., 2019b; Samovski and Abumrad, 2019). In fact, liver-specific AMPK activation was shown to counteract steatosis development during obesity by different mechanisms, including autophagy activation (Garcia et al., 2019). Bariatric surgery in rodents, for instance, improves steatosis while increasing AMPK and decreasing mTORC1 activation (Ezquerro et al., 2016; Ma et al., 2020). Moreover, increased cytosolic acetyl-CoA derived from peroxisomal β-oxidation present in the liver of HFD fed animals was shown to promote mTOR localization at the lysosome surface, increasing ULK1 phosphorylation by mTORC1 and inhibiting autophagy (He et al., 2020). Although AMPK and mTORC1 are known regulators of autophagy initiation by activation/inhibition of the ULK1/2 complex, both are important modulators of lysosome function, and, therefore, of late steps of the autophagic process (reviewed by Carroll and Dunlop, 2017). For instance, activation of mTORC1 at the lysosome surface is known to phosphorylate TFEB, promoting its cytosolic localization. In contrast, decreased lysosome-derived amino acids, promoted either by nutrient deprivation or by lysosomal dysfunction, can inhibit mTORC1 activity, causing TFEB dephosphorylation and translocation to the nucleus. Conversely, TFEB activation can upregulate lysosomal activity and restore mTORC1 activation (Napolitano and Ballabio, 2016; Zhang et al., 2018). This feedback signaling is known to oscillate in the hepatic tissue and is directly related to steatosis development, while disruptions in favor of mTORC1 activation can exacerbate NAFLD progression (Zhang et al., 2018). mTORC1 activation in NAFLD models may also inhibit autophagosome-lysosome fusion by inactivating PACER protein, a mediator of autolysosome formation (Cheng et al., 2019). Importantly, mTOR activity can also be regulated by AMPK status. Even though AMPK activity can modulate lysosome function by regulating TFEB activation, V-ATPase activity, and calcium transport in different physiological or pathological contexts (McGuire and Forgac, 2018; Bonam et al., 2019; Fernandez-Mosquera et al., 2019; Deus et al., 2020), to the best of our knowledge the participation of similar mechanisms in NAFLD models has not yet been further explored.

Chronic lipid exposure can also lead to altered Ca^{2+} signaling in different tissues, promoting dysregulation of metabolic signals during obesity (Fu et al., 2011; Guney et al., 2020). Increased cytoplasmic Ca^{2+} concentration, decreased ER Ca^{2+} levels and store-operated-calcium-entry (SOCE) are reported in steatotic hepatocytes and are known to contribute toward NAFLD progression (Arruda et al., 2017; Ali et al., 2019). Calcium is an important regulator of autophagic activity (Filippi-Chiela et al., 2016; Bootman et al., 2018). In fact, treatment of obese mice with calcium channel blockers rescued abnormal cytoplasmatic Ca^{2+} levels in hepatocytes and restored impaired autophagosome-lysosome fusion (Park et al., 2014). Additionally, decreased levels of ATG7 protein in steatotic livers are shown to be related to calpain proteolytic activity (Yang et al., 2010). Together, these results indicate that altered Ca^{2+} signaling can affect different steps of autophagy regulation during NAFLD progression and may represent an important signaling hub in this context.

Finally, altered lipid availability during obesity is also thought to contribute toward autophagy impairment. To that end, Koga et al. (2010) demonstrated that *in vitro* and *in vivo* lipid overload can impair autophagosome-lysosome fusion due to altered lipid composition in both membranes. Phospholipid availability is also known to modulate autophagosome formation (reviewed by Hsu and Shi, 2017; Soto-Avellaneda and Morrison, 2020), which may be a contributing factor toward decreased autophagic activity during NAFLD.

In general terms, dysfunction at the later steps of autophagy pathways leads to accumulation of autophagic vesicles and, therefore, of lipidated LC3. Conversely, decreased autophagy initiation or impaired autophagosome formation leads to lower autophagosome content and decreased LC3-II. In our summary of autophagic markers in NAFLD models, we observed a high variability of LC3-II levels between studies, mostly found either increased or decreased. This corroborates evidence showing that impairment of autophagic activity can occur at different steps of autophagy regulation during NAFLD development. A summary of mechanisms discussed here is represented in **Figure 2**.

AUTOPHAGY MACHINERY INTERVENTIONS

Autophagic Pharmacological Interventions

In this section we analyzed all articles from our search that evaluated the effects of known pharmacological modulators of autophagy on hepatic steatosis. The results are summarized in **Table 4**. Data is divided according to experimental design, separating pharmacological interventions administered during diet feeding, at the end of the diet, or after. Overall, we analyzed 27 experiments from 17 different studies in rodent models of diet-induced hepatic steatosis that administered rapamycin as an autophagy activator or chloroquine and 3-methyladenine (3-MA) as inhibitors. Importantly, some experiments evaluated the effects of autophagic modulators alone or in combination with other interventions (named co-interventions). In summary, 18 experiments (from 14 studies) showed a negative correlation between autophagy and steatosis levels, meaning that steatosis was up- or downregulated in the presence of an autophagy inhibitor or activator, respectively. Eight experiments did not present changes in steatosis levels, and one showed a positive correlation, meaning an increase in steatosis after autophagy activation.

With the exception of one study, all experiments that chronically administered rapamycin to animals during the period of diet feeding showed an improvement in steatosis outcome, suggesting that autophagy activation during the development of NAFLD counteracts TG accumulation in hepatocytes. Of note, the experiment showing a positive correlation between rapamycin administration and steatosis was performed with a co-intervention of branched chain amino acids (BCAA) to mice fed a HFD, which was shown by the authors to severely increase liver injury and to reduce hepatic TG levels, but to increase free fatty acids (FFA) and lipotoxicity; rapamycin reversed these effects (Zhang F. et al., 2016). In agreement with the protective role of autophagy, chronic chloroquine or 3-MA administration with HFD increased steatosis levels compared to HFD alone, or even inhibited the protective effect of other co-interventions.

An interesting study by Zhang et al. (2018) evaluated the effects of acute chloroquine administration to mice before analyzing hepatic TGs and LDs at different time points of HFD feeding. They showed that autophagy inhibition by chloroquine only increased steatosis levels after 10 weeks of HF feeding, without significant effects earlier (3 weeks) or later (16 weeks). These results suggest that autophagic degradation of LDs by lipophagy may not be essential at the initial periods of NAFLD development, but participation may increase with time. Also, decreased lipophagic activity after 16 weeks is probably associated with impaired autophagic flux, which is more evident at this time point compared to 10 weeks. This time course is in agreement with the study from Yang et al. (2010) showing that ATG7 levels are unchanged after 7 weeks of HFD, but decreased after 16 weeks, and virtually absent after 22 weeks.

When evaluating the effects of rapamycin as a therapeutic intervention after HFD feeding, 2 out of 3 studies reported decreased hepatic steatosis, while one did not observe any changes. The main difference that we could observe between these studies was that both reports with an improved outcome administered rapamycin for at least 12 weeks after the diet, while the study without effects only submitted the animals to 2 weeks of treatment. It is therefore possible that therapeutic effects of rapamycin on hepatic steatosis require longer treatment periods. However, we cannot exclude the fact that other experimental differences between the studies may also contribute toward divergent outcomes. In this context, results with autophagy inhibitors administered after HFD feeding were controversial. Two different studies from the same group that administered chloroquine for 6 or 12 weeks after initial 12 weeks of HFD feeding did not observe any changes in steatosis levels (He et al., 2016a,b). In contrast, chronic exposure of 3-MA to rats after 8 weeks of HFD feeding lead to increased steatotic outcome (Zhou and Ye, 2018). Also, chloroquine administration to mice fed HFD for the same time period reversed the protective effects of the co-intervention (Sun et al., 2015). While literature data seems inconclusive, it is possible that inhibition of autophagy after NAFLD development may only upregulate steatosis if autophagic activity is not already fully compromised.

In conclusion, data from pharmacological interventions indicates that modulation of autophagic activity starting at early points of HFD administration is more successful in modifying

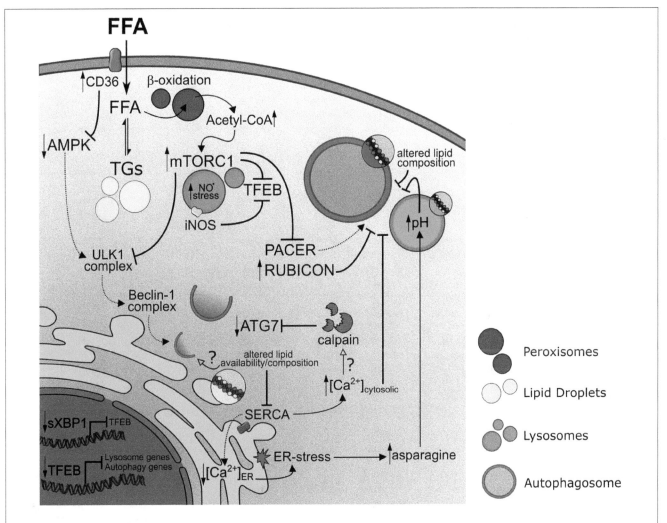

FIGURE 2 | Autophagy impairment in NAFLD models. References to the mechanism represented above are discussed in Section "Mechanisms of Autophagy Impairment in NAFLD" of this manuscript. Longer arrows indicate activation mechanisms, while doted lines or full lines indicate downregulated or upregulated pathways, respectively. Crossed lines indicate inhibitory mechanisms. Small arrows pointing up or down indicate increased or decreased levels/activity, respectively. Unfilled arrows along with question marks indicate hypothetical mechanisms. FFA, free fat acids; TGs, triglycerides; NO·, nitric oxide; ER, endoplasmic reticulum.

the final levels of steatosis, clearly indicating a close relationship between autophagy and NAFLD development. However, when administration occurs at later points of the diet or even after it, results are more susceptible to variations and may be a result of differences in NAFLD development or in duration of the pharmacological intervention.

Autophagic Genetic Interventions

In this section we analyzed all the articles found in our search that used genetic interventions to either stimulate or suppress autophagy in mouse livers and concomitantly measured hepatosteatosis outcome. The rundown of results obtained is presented in **Tables 5–7** and divided into nutrient overload, fasting, or control steatosis models.

Nutritional Overload Models

Within nutrient overload steatosis models (**Table 5**), 13 different experiments were analyzed from 9 manuscripts which genetically

modulated the expression of ATG7, ATG4B, ATG14, TFEB, FIP200, and ULK1. Five experiments (from 4 manuscripts) downregulated autophagic activity and observed increased steatosis outcome, while another 4 upregulated autophagic genes and observed decreased steatosis outcome. These were all assigned here as a negative correlation between autophagy and steatosis. In contrast, 3 other interventions (from 2 manuscripts) downregulated autophagic activity and showed a concomitant decrease in liver steatosis levels after diet, which were assigned as a positive correlation. Finally, one experiment downregulated autophagy and did not observe changes in steatosis after HFD.

Autophagy dysfunction in NAFLD models is well reported in the literature and is thought to be an important hallmark of steatosis worsening (Singh et al., 2009; Wang et al., 2018; Wu W. K. K. et al., 2018; Li et al., 2019b; Lian et al., 2020). Changes in autophagic flux are also observed in humans diagnosed with NAFL and NASH (González-Rodríguez et al., 2014) and prediabetic obese patients (Ezquerro et al., 2019).

TABLE 4 | Pharmacological intervention on autophagy.

	Animal	Diet (fat concentration, duration)	Pharmacological intervention	Time point of intervention	Duration of intervention	Co-intervention	Autophagy modulation (up/down)	Steatosis outcome (up/down)	Correlation (+/0/−)
Chang et al., 2009b	KK/HlJ	HFD (67%, 10 weeks)	Rapamycin	During diet	Last 6 weeks	No	Up	Down	−
Wang C. et al., 2014	C57BL/6J	HFD (60%, 14 weeks)	Rapamycin	During diet	14 weeks	No	Up	Down	−
Zhang F. et al., 2016	C57BL/6J	HFD (60%, 12 weeks)	Rapamycin	During diet	12 weeks	BCAA	Up	Up	+
Chen et al., 2016	C57BL/6J	MCD (10 weeks)	Rapamycin	During diet	10 weeks	No	Up	Down	−
Ren et al., 2019	C57BL/6	HFD (not described, 6 weeks)	Rapamycin	During diet	6 weeks	Hypoxia	Up	Down	−
Lu et al., 2020	C57BL/6J, male and females	ApoEKO + HFD (not described, 8 weeks)	Rapamycin	During diet	8 weeks	No	Up	Down	−
Zhao et al., 2020	C57BL/6J	HFD (60%, 13 weeks)	Rapamycin	During diet	Last 8 weeks	No	Up	Down	−
Chen et al., 2016	C57BL/6J	MCD (10 weeks)	Chloroquine	During diet	10 weeks	No	Down	Up	−
Zeng et al., 2018	C57BL/6	MCD (5 weeks)	Chloroquine	During diet	5 weeks	Acetylshikonin	Down	Up	−
Ren et al., 2019	C57BL/6	HFD (not described, 6 weeks)	3-MA	During diet	6 weeks	Hypoxia	Down	Up	−
Lin et al., 2013	C57BL/6	HFD (60% calories, 12 weeks)	Rapamycin	End of diet	Acute – before sacrifice	No	Up	Down	−
Lin et al., 2013	C57BL/6	HFD (60% calories, 12 weeks)	Chloroquine	End of diet	Acute – before sacrifice	No	Down	Up	−
Zhang et al., 2018	C57BL/6J, male and female	HFD (60%, 3 weeks)	Chloroquine	End of diet	Acute – before sacrifice	No	Down	Unchanged	0
Zhang et al., 2018	C57BL/6J, male and female	HFD (60%, 10 weeks)	Chloroquine	End of diet	Acute – before sacrifice	No	Down	Up	−
Zhang et al., 2018	C57BL/6J, male and female	HFD (60%, 16 weeks)	Chloroquine	End of diet	Acute – before sacrifice	No	Down	Unchanged	0
Tong et al., 2016	db/db	Regular chow	Chloroquine	Not applied	3 days	No	Down	Unchanged	0
Tong et al., 2016	db/db	Regular chow	Chloroquine	Not applied	3 days	GW501516	Down	Up	−
Zhu et al., 2020	C57BL/6J	HFD (60%, 12 weeks)	3-MA	End of diet	Last 2 weeks	Nrg4	Down	Up	−
Chang et al., 2009a	C57BL/6J	HFD (67%, 20 week)	Rapamycin	After diet	16 weeks	No	Up	Down	−
Zhou and Ye, 2018	Sprague-Dawley	HFD (45%, 8 week) + STZ	Rapamycin	After diet	12 weeks	No	Up	Down	−
Tu et al., 2020	Sprague-Dawley	HFD (60%, 6 weeks)	Rapamycin	After diet	2 weeks	No	Up	Unchanged	0
Sun et al., 2015	C57BL/6	HFD (not described, 8 weeks)	Chloroquine	After diet	6 weeks	NaHS	Down	Up	−
He et al., 2016a	C57BL/6	HFD (60%, 12 weeks)	Chloroquine	After diet	6 weeks	No	Down	Unchanged	0
He et al., 2016a	C57BL/6	HFD (60%, 12 weeks)	Chloroquine	After diet	6 weeks	Berberine chloride	Down	Unchanged	0
He et al., 2016b	C57BL/6	HFD (60%, 12 weeks)	Chloroquine	After diet	12 weeks	No	Down	Unchanged	0
He et al., 2016b	C57BL/6	HFD (60%, 12 weeks)	Chloroquine	After diet	12 weeks	Liraglutide	Down	Unchanged	0
Zhou and Ye, 2018	Sprague-Dawley	HFD (45%, 8 week) + STZ	3-MA	After diet	12 weeks	No	Down	Up	−

Articles using pharmacological interventions in the autophagy process in comparison to control groups (vehicle), normalized by a housekeeping protein. LC3-II and p62 were measured by the authors through SDS-PAGE Western blots and described semi-quantitatively or qualitatively. All but two studies used male animals. Positive correlation = steatosis is up, and autophagy is up OR steatosis is down, and autophagy is down; negative correlation = steatosis is up, and autophagy is down OR steatosis is down, and autophagy is up.

Autophagic degradation of LDs (lipophagy) is commonly thought necessary for TG turnover and FFA β-oxidation, which prevents lipotoxicity and further progression of the disease (Singh and Cuervo, 2011; Carotti et al., 2020). Thus, models with impaired autophagy activation are expected to accumulate more TGs in hepatocytes after an obesogenic diet, while activation of autophagy should prevent or improve this outcome. In agreement, autophagy-deficient *Atg4b*-null and *Tfeb*-Li KO mice exposed to different models of diet-induced steatosis presented increased hepatic TGs compared to WT

TABLE 5 | Autophagy protein genetic interventions and obesity models.

References	Animal	Fat (% energy from fat), duration (weeks). Other information about diet	Genetic intervention	Autophagic target	Autophagy modulation (up/down)	Steatosis outcome (up/down)	Correlation (+/0/−)
Yang et al., 2010	ob/ob mice	regular chow diet	adenoviral-Atg7 overexpression	ATG7	Up	Down	−
Kim et al., 2013	C57BL/6J	60%, 13	Atg7 f/f; Alb-Cre mice (Atg7-Li KO)	ATG7	Down	Down	+
Byun et al., 2020	C57BL/6 + Ad-Jmjd3	60%, 8	adenoviral-Atg7 shRNA	ATG7	Down	Up	−
Fernández et al., 2017	C57Bl6/129 Sv	42%, 8	Atg4b-null mice	ATG4B	Down	Up	−
Fernández et al., 2017	C57Bl6/129 Sv	30% sucrose	Atg4b-null mice	ATG4B	Down	Up	−
Xiong et al., 2012	C57BL/6J	60%, 12	adenoviral-Atg14 overexpression	ATG14	Up	Down	−
Settembre et al., 2013	C57BL/6	42%, 12	TcfebloxP/loxP; Alb-Cre mice (Tfeb-Li KO)	TFEB	Down	Up	−
Settembre et al., 2013	C57BL/6	42%, 12	adenoviral-TFEB overexpression	TFEB	Up	Down	−
Zhang et al., 2018	C57BL/6J	60%, 16	adenoviral-TFEB overexpression	TFEB	Up	Down	−
Ma et al., 2013	C57BL/6J	60%, 5, fed	Fip200 f/f; Alb-Cre mice (Fip200-Li KO)	FIP200	Down	Unchanged	0
Ma et al., 2013	C57BL/6J	60%, 5, fasted	Fip200 f/f; Alb-Cre mice (Fip200-Li KO)	FIP200	Down	Down	+
Ma et al., 2013	C57BL/6J	60%, 5, fasted	Fip200 f/f; adeno-Cre injection (Fip200-conditional KO)	FIP200	Down	Down	+
Li et al., 2014	C57BL/6J	45%, 12	Heterozygous Ulk1-KO mice (Ulk1 +/−)	ULK1	Down	Up	−

Articles using genetic interventions in the autophagy machinery and obesity models to promote steatosis, describing the diet fat content, intervention duration, liver steatosis, and LC3-II and p62 protein in levels in the liver in comparison to control groups (WT), normalized by a housekeeping protein. LC3-II and p62 were measured by the authors through SDS-PAGE Western blots and described semi-quantitatively or qualitatively. All animals were male mice. Positive correlation = steatosis is up, and autophagy is up OR steatosis is down, and autophagy is down; Negative correlation = steatosis is up, and autophagy is down OR steatosis is down, and autophagy is up.

TABLE 6 | Autophagy protein genetic interventions and fasting.

References	Animal	Fasting period (hours)	Genetic intervention	Autophagic target	Autophagy modulation (up/down)	Steatosis outcome (up/down)	Correlation (+/0/−)
Singh et al., 2009	C57BL/6	24	Atg7 f/f; Alb-Cre mice (Atg7-Li KO)	ATG7	Down	Up	−
Shibata et al., 2009	not described	12, 24	Atg7 f/f; Alb-Cre mice (Atg7-Li KO)	ATG7	Down	Down	+
Kim et al., 2013	C57BL/6J	24	Atg7 f/f; Alb-Cre mice (Atg7-Li KO)	ATG7	Down	Down	+
Kwanten et al., 2014	C57BL/6J	24	Atg7 f/f; Alb-Cre mice (Atg7-Li KO)	ATG7	Down	Down	+
Takahashi et al., 2020	C57BL/6	24	Atg7 f/f; Alb-Cre mice (Atg7-Li KO)	ATG7	Down	Down	+
Saito et al., 2019	C57BL/6	not described	Atg7 f/f; Alb-Cre mice (Atg7-Li KO)	ATG7	Down	Down	+
Takagi et al., 2016	C57BL/6J	36	Atg5 f/f; Alb-Cre mice (Atg5-Li KO)	ATG5	Down	Down	+
Li et al., 2018	C57BL/6J	16	Atg5 f/f; Alb-Cre mice (Atg5-Li KO)	ATG5	Down	Down	+
Takahashi et al., 2020	C57BL/6	6-48	Atg5 f/f;Mx1-Cre (Atg5-Li conditional KO)	ATG5	Down	Down	+
Settembre et al., 2013	C57BL/6	24	TcfebloxP/loxP; Alb-Cre mice (Tfeb-Li KO)	TFEB	Down	Up	−
Ma et al., 2013	C57BL/6J	16	Fip200 f/f; Alb-Cre mice (Fip200-Li KO)	FIP200	Down	Down	+

Articles using genetic interventions in the autophagy machinery and fasting models to promote steatosis, describing fasting duration, liver steatosis, and LC3-II and p62 protein in levels in the liver in comparison to control groups (fed), normalized by a housekeeping protein. LC3-II and p62 levels were determined through SDS-PAGE Western blots in the manuscripts and described semi-quantitatively or qualitatively. All animals were male mice. Positive correlation = steatosis is up, and autophagy is up OR steatosis is down, and autophagy is down; Negative correlation = steatosis is up, and autophagy is down OR steatosis is down, and autophagy is up.

(Settembre et al., 2013; Fernández et al., 2017). Also, experiments that overexpressed ATG7 in adult *ob/ob* mice (Yang et al., 2010), that overexpressed ATG14 in mice fed a HFD (Xiong et al., 2012), or that overexpressed TFEB in the livers of adult C57BL/6 mice before (Settembre et al., 2013) and even after 12 weeks of HFD (Zhang et al., 2018) all found decreased hepatic TG content, corroborating the idea that reactivation of autophagy in NAFLD can be a strategy to improve steatosis and other associated metabolic dysfunctions. In line with this, Byun et al. (2020) showed that adenoviral-mediated expression

TABLE 7 | Autophagy protein genetic interventions plus chow or LFD diets.

References	Animal	Age at the end (weeks)	Genetic intervention	Autophagic target	Autophagy modulation (up/down)	Steatosis outcome (up/down)	Correlation (+/0/−)
Singh et al., 2009	C57BL/6	16	*Atg7* f/f; Alb-Cre mice (*Atg7*-Li KO)	ATG7	Down	Up	−
Yang et al., 2010	C57BL/6	14	adenoviral-*Atg7*shRNA	ATG7	Down	Up	−
Settembre et al., 2013	C57BL/6	not described	*Atg7* f/f; adeno-Alb-Cre injection (*Atg7*-Li conditional KO)	ATG7	Down	Up	−
Takahashi et al., 2020	C57BL/6	5	*Atg7* f/f; Alb-Cre mice (*Atg7*-Li KO)	ATG7	Down	Unchanged	0
Byun et al., 2020	C57BL/6 + Ad-Jmjd3	12	adenoviral-*Atg7*shRNA	ATG7	Down	Up	−
Fernández et al., 2017	C57Bl6/129 Sv	16	*Atg4b*-null mice	ATG4	Down	Unchanged	0
Xiong et al., 2012	C57BL/6J	12	adenoviral-Atg14 shRNA	ATG14	Down	Up	−
Ma et al., 2013	C57BL/6J	not described	Fip200 f/f; Alb-Cre mice (Fip200-Li KO)	FIP200	Down	Unchanged	0

Articles using genetic interventions in the autophagy machinery to promote steatosis, describing liver steatosis, and LC3-II and p62 protein in levels in the liver in comparison to control groups (WT), normalized by a housekeeping protein. LC3-II and p62 levels were measured by the authors through SDS-PAGE Western blots and described semi-quantitatively or qualitatively. All animals were male mice. Positive correlation = steatosis is up, and autophagy is up OR steatosis is down, and autophagy is down; Negative correlation = steatosis is up, and autophagy is down OR steatosis is down, and autophagy is up.

of the JMJD3 protein decreases hepatosteatosis induced by HFD in a mechanism dependent on ATG7 expression. This effect is abolished by *Atg7* KD, further indicating that autophagic activity counteracts lipid accumulation in NAFLD models (Byun et al., 2020).

While modulating ATG7 expression in adult obese mice showed a negative correlation with steatosis development, an experiment using mice born with depleted hepatic ATG7 showed the opposite effect. *Atg7* f/f; Alb-Cre (*Atg7*-Li KO) mice that were fed a HFD showed apparent lower accumulation of LDs in the liver (Kim et al., 2013). In agreement, early depletion of FIP200 in the liver of mice fed a HFD did not alter hepatic TG levels in animals in the fed state, even though it promoted impaired autophagic flux. In HFD-fed animals when fasted, early and late depletion of FIP200 decreased TG content compared to WT under the same conditions (Ma et al., 2013), suggesting that impaired autophagy can prevent lipid accumulation in certain contexts. Interestingly, FIP200 is part of an initiation complex in autophagy machinery, interacting with ULK1/2 to regulate the induction of autophagosome formation (Chen and Klionsky, 2011). However, the authors suggest that FIP200 may have other regulatory roles in autophagy, as they had an unexpected observation of accumulated LC3-II in KO animals, indicative of impaired late autophagy machinery rather than initiation. To support this, heterozygous *Ulk1*-KO mice (*Ulk1*±) fed a HFD showed opposite effects, increasing lipid accumulation in hepatocytes in comparison to WT animals (Li et al., 2014).

Although the majority of analyzed articles point to a protective role of autophagy in steatosis promoted by nutrient overload, there are conflicting data in the literature that cannot be overlooked. Comparing differences in experimental models and designs for each study can help unveil possible issues that may contribute toward this divergence. For instance, FIP200 and ATG7 are required for autophagy initiation and expansion phases meaning that Li-KO animals for these genes have virtually total hepatic autophagy impairment. These animals develop hepatomegaly with changes in hepatic structure (Komatsu et al., 2005; Kim et al., 2013; Ma et al., 2013), while showing decreased or unchanged accumulation of lipids upon dietary intervention. In contrast, *Atg4b*-null, *Tfeb*-Li KO, and *Atg7* KD by shRNA

interventions, which were found to promote increased lipid accumulation, only partially compromise autophagy activation, which may be sufficient to keep basal autophagic functions in the liver. In fact, *Tfeb*-Li KO animals do not present significant liver histological changes compared to WT animals (Settembre et al., 2013). Therefore, time and type of genetic intervention as well as animal genetic background may contribute to apparent differences in literature data. Additionally, duration of diet stimulus may be a contributing factor. For example, Ma et al., 2013 did not observe changes in steatosis levels of *Fip200*-KO compared to WT animals after 5 weeks of diet without fasting stimulation. Since most of the articles ranged from 8 to 16 weeks of diet, the duration performed in this study may not be sufficient to observe the contribution of autophagy in hepatic steatosis, which is apparently more evident around 10 weeks, according to Zhang et al., 2018.

Fasting Models

Within fasting-induced steatosis models, we analyzed 11 experiments from 10 manuscripts that used genetic liver-specific KO models for ATG7, ATG5, TFEB, and FIP200 (**Table 6**). From these 11 experiments, 9 showed a positive correlation between autophagic activity and steatosis levels, meaning that KO animals showed lower TGs levels in the livers after fasting compared to WT. Two out of 11 experiments showed a negative correlation, where an increase in TG levels was observed in fasted KO animals.

When analyzing both experiments that showed a negative correlation, one evaluated the effects of ATG7 and the other of TFEB depletion. While results with *Atg7*-Li KO seem conflicting, TFEB genetic modulation experiments in the literature are apparently more consistent toward a protective role against steatosis. TFEB translocation to the nucleus is known to be necessary during fasting stimulus to promote the expression of genes related to lysosomal biogenesis, autophagic machinery and lysosome-autophagosome fusion (Settembre et al., 2013). Interestingly, TFEB activation by fasting may also increase lipid catabolism by upregulation of genes related to mitochondrial biogenesis and β-oxidation through transcriptional regulation of PGC1α (peroxisome proliferative activated receptor gamma coactivator 1 alpha), and PPARα (peroxisome proliferator activated receptor alpha). However, it was unclear if these effects were dependent or independent of canonical autophagy, since TFEB overexpression was not able to restore normal lipid levels in animals with ATG7 hepatic depletion in the fed condition. It is therefore possible that TFEB has a transcriptional regulatory role in lipid metabolism during fasting that differs from other autophagy-mediated regulations.

During prolonged starvation periods, autophagy is activated in hepatocytes, and is necessary for liver physiological adaptation (Takagi et al., 2016; Ruan et al., 2017; Ueno and Komatsu, 2017). LD numbers and size also increase as a strategy to avoid FFA lipotoxicity with higher lipid mobilization. However, the role for autophagy in fasting-induced steatosis remains ambiguous. LC3 was shown to associate with LDs during fasting. Two different roles can be attributed to this translocation. First, autophagosomes may form in LDs to engulf them, in order to promote the breakage of TGs by lysosomal lipases and release FFA for β-oxidation (lipophagy) (Singh et al., 2009). Second, autophagy machinery may be necessary for LD biogenesis during fasting (Shibata et al., 2009, 2010). Therefore, autophagy activation during fasting may have a double catabolic and anabolic regulatory participation in lipid metabolism.

In our search, 9 out of 10 experiments with genetic KO of proteins related to autophagy initiation (FIP200) and autophagosome expansion (ATG7 and ATG5) demonstrated lack of liver adaptation to fasting relative to lipid accumulation, favoring the anabolic role of autophagy. Different reasons may lead to reduced lipid contents in hepatocytes. FFA oxidation may be increased in autophagy-deficient animals, however, this is less likely since these animals probably accumulate damaged mitochondria due to impaired mitophagy, as has been reported in some models (Kwanten et al., 2014). Additionally, either TG or LD biosynthesis may be impaired, or liver export of lipids through VLDLs (very low-density lipoprotein) could be increased.

Different signaling pathways have been recently proposed to participate in this effect. Komatsu's group published interesting data from two studies demonstrating that autophagy regulates the levels of NCoR1 (nuclear receptor co-repressor 1), a suppressor of LXRα (liver receptor X alpha) and PPARα transcription factors that, in turn, regulate the expression of genes related to lipogenesis and β-oxidation, respectively. Mice with impaired autophagy displayed NCoR1 accumulation and downregulation of genes associated with both TG synthesis and FFA oxidation. Thus, the authors suggest that autophagy-deficient models have hampered TG biosynthesis and overall lipid mobilization necessary for tissue adaptation to fasting (Saito et al., 2019; Takahashi et al., 2020). In fact, hepatocyte accumulation of lipids and FFA oxidation is necessary for ketogenesis increment during fasting (Rui, 2014), and both are compromised in autophagy-KO mice (Takagi et al., 2016). In agreement, Kim et al. (2013) also found that genes related to de novo FFA and TG synthesis were downregulated in Atg7-Li KO mice. The same study also found that KO mice had lower adipose tissue mass, which is the main source of lipids during fasting. Decreased fat mass was probably due to increased circulating FGF21, which promoted adipose tissue

browning and increased systemic FFA oxidation. Therefore, endocrine changes in autophagy Li-KO mice may also contribute to the observed effects. Finally, another study suggested that impaired fasting-induced steatosis in Atg5-Li KO mice is not related to changes in de novo lipid biogenesis or β-oxidation levels, but rather to increased activation of NRF2 (nuclear factor erythroid 2–related factor 2), since double-knockout animals for ATG5 and NRF2 had restored phenotypes (Li et al., 2018).

Although results in the literature seem contradictory, clearly autophagy machinery is necessary for liver lipid metabolism adaptation to fasting. Mechanistically, the catabolic role of autophagy through degradation of LDs does not seem to be as evident in fasting-induced steatosis models as observed in nutrient-overload models, since almost all studies showed impaired accumulation of lipids in autophagy-deficient animals. Instead, the autophagic process appears to be part of a complex signaling network that may involve LD biogenesis and transcriptional regulation of metabolic pathways important to respond to physiological changes.

Control Models

In this section we analyzed the effects of autophagic genetic interventions in animals without any steatotic stimulation, to discuss the regulation of basal lipid metabolism by autophagy. We located 8 different experiments from 8 manuscripts, of which 4 showed negative correlation between autophagy modulation and steatosis outcome and 4 showed no alterations in steatosis (**Table 7**).

When analyzing the experiments targeting ATG7, we observe that similar genetic models showed divergent outcomes in the literature. For example, two different studies that infected mice with adenoviral-Atg7 shRNA observed either increased or unchanged steatotic outcome in the basal physiological state (Yang et al., 2010; Byun et al., 2020). Similar data is present with Atg7-Li KO animals: one study shows higher hepatic lipid accumulation and another shows no alterations (Singh et al., 2009; Takahashi et al., 2020). Interestingly, we find that the duration of experiments may be an important contributing factor. For instance, Yang et al. (2010) analyzed the hepatic tissue at a shorter time (7–10 days) after Ad-Atg7 shRNA infection compared to Byun et al. (2020) (4 weeks). The age of Atg7-Li KO mice at the end of the study was also lower in work by Takahashi et al. (2020) (5 weeks) compared to the study by Singh et al. (2009) (16 weeks). Therefore, we speculate that longer periods of ATG7 downregulation may be necessary to observe changes in hepatic lipid accumulation in the basal state. Although this might be relevant, several other features involving differences in genetic background and changes in environmental or experimental conditions may be equally responsible for literature divergence. In addition to the controversial results promoted by ATG7 modulation, other studies with depletion of ATG4B or FIP200 did not observe any changes in steatosis levels in the basal state compared to wild-type animals, while knockdown of ATG14 led to increased steatosis.

Overall, the effects of genetic modulation of autophagic genes on basal liver lipid metabolism are highly divergent in the literature. This suggests that the interplay between autophagy and liver lipid metabolism under normal physiological conditions is not a straightforward process. Instead, the interaction is context-dependent.

Further Considerations

Over the past 10 years, different studies have been trying to elucidate the role of the autophagic process in lipid metabolism. Since then, many controversial ideas have emerged and are still being investigated. Autophagy machinery can apparently play different roles in hepatocyte lipid mobilization, regulating either catabolic or anabolic pathways, depending on context (Zechner et al., 2017). In our compilation of literature data, most studies indicated that inhibiting autophagy (pharmacologically or genetically) in NAFLD models increases steatosis. Likewise, promoting autophagic activity (pharmacologically or genetically), either during or after model development, improves steatosis outcome by decreasing lipid accumulation in hepatocytes. This is in line with the proposal that autophagic activity is necessary for lipid degradation during overnutrition-induced steatosis.

Interestingly, although there is still some conflicting data, this scenario is the opposite for fasting-induced steatosis models. In this context, most data using autophagy-deficient mice demonstrated an impaired capacity for lipid accumulation in response to fasting stimulus. Although it is tempting to hypothesize that autophagy's role in steatosis development may vary according to the source of stimulation, it is possible that this apparent difference between NAFLD and fasting models found in our research comes from differences in the strategies used for autophagy modulation as well. For instance, studies investigating nutritional overload steatosis covered a greater variety of strategies, such as pharmacological inhibition/activation, genetic knockdown, knockout or overexpression of autophagic pathways. Conversely, all the results from the studies in the fasting group were from genetic knockout models. Additionally, only two studies investigated the effect of autophagy modulation on NAFLD and fasting steatosis within their work and both found similar outcomes, irrespective of the steatotic stimulus.

Even so, *in vitro* studies may help understand how the participation of autophagy in lipid metabolism can be modulated. For instance, inhibition of autophagy in hepatocytes and other mammalian cells treated with oleic acid leads to LD accumulation (Singh et al., 2009; Li et al., 2018), indicating that lipophagy is activated in this model. In contrast, autophagy is not necessary for LD degradation during acute amino acid starvation with HBSS in mammalian cells. Instead, autophagic degradation of organelles during HBSS starvation releases FFAs, that are converted to TGs in a protective mechanism dependent on DGAT1 activity, supporting LD formation (Rambold et al., 2015; Nguyen et al., 2017). Interestingly, lipophagy participation was observed during serum starvation, in media containing glucose and amino acids (Rambold et al., 2015). This suggests that lipophagy can be regulated by nutrient availability. In fact, different metabolites can regulate autophagy during fasting. Decreased amino acid levels after prolonged fasting inhibit mTORC1 activity and promote autophagy (Ueno and Komatsu, 2017). In contrast, fasting-induced increments in cytosolic acetyl-CoA derived from

peroxisomal β-oxidation support mTORC1 activation, inhibiting autophagy/lipophagy (He et al., 2020). Curiously, recent data published as a pre-print suggests that mTORC1 activity may have differential roles in the regulation of autophagy and lipophagy, depending on its subcellular localization. The authors proposed that phosphorylation of Plin3 by mTORC1 at the surface of LDs is necessary for FIP200 and ATG16 recruitment to the organelle during oleic acid activation of lipophagy (Garcia-Macia et al., 2019). Based on this evidence, we speculate that amino acid availability may be necessary to support mTORC1 activity promoting autophagic machinery recruitment to LDs, allowing the participation of lipophagy in LD turnover. Conversely, lower amino acid concentrations during starvation, or even during prolonged fasting, may decrease lipophagy activation by similar mechanisms, while other lipolysis pathways can occur. New evidence on lipophagy mechanisms and its co-regulation with neutral lipolysis pathway are emerging fast (recently reviewed by Zechner et al., 2017; Schulze and McNiven, 2019; Shin, 2020), along with crosstalk signaling between autophagy and LDs (reviewed by Ogasawara et al., 2020), and will certainly help clarify current questions in the field.

The protective role of autophagy against steatosis development in NAFLD models is mainly associated with TG hydrolysis by lipophagy activation (Carotti et al., 2020). However, it is possible that autophagic activity may affect lipid metabolism directly or indirectly by different mechanisms. For instance, autophagy is necessary for mitochondrial quality control, and proper mitochondrial function is important for FA oxidation. In fact, mitophagy also counteracts NAFLD progression (Glick et al., 2012; Ma et al., 2013). Also, many genetic autophagy modulation models showed alterations in the expression of genes related to lipid biosynthesis and/or degradation (Yang et al., 2010; Kim et al., 2013; Ma et al., 2013), suggesting that transcriptional regulation of lipid metabolism by autophagic activity is also important. However, the mechanism supporting it is less clear in the context of diet-induced steatosis models compared to recent findings with fasting-induced steatosis (Saito et al., 2019; Takahashi et al., 2020). Finally, genetic autophagy modulation can promote changes in peripheral lipid metabolism even in liver-specific models (Kim et al., 2013; Settembre et al., 2013), which may also contribute toward hepatic steatosis levels. Taken together, these findings bring an additional layer, beyond lipophagy stimulation, to the discussion regarding the mechanism of autophagic activation in NAFLD models. Importantly, we highlight that although autophagic activation improved hepatic steatosis in most studies, chronic treatment with rapamycin may be detrimental to adipose tissue function and promote glucose intolerance (Houde et al., 2010; Paschoal et al., 2017; Wang Y. et al., 2017), which makes it a controversial NAFLD therapy.

Regarding the anabolic role of autophagy, there is still poor evidence if autophagic machinery can act directly on LD formation sites, but it is possible that proteins from the LC3/GABARAP family can play a role in the formation of this organelle, as for other ER-derived vesicles (Schaaf et al., 2016). Until now, different indirect mechanisms are proposed to explain autophagy participation in LD formation, involving transcriptional regulation of TG synthesis (Takahashi et al., 2020), regulation of NRF2 activity (Li et al., 2018), and endocrine regulation of FFA supply by the adipose tissue (Kim et al., 2013).

Recently, there is growing evidence of lysosome-dependent mechanisms of lipid metabolism regulation that do not involve autophagosome formation. Besides lipolysis facilitation by chaperon-mediated autophagy (Kaushik and Cuervo, 2015), lysosomes can form contact sites with LDs that mediate direct transfer of lipid content to the lysosome lumen, especially during nutrient deprivation conditions (Schulze et al., 2020). Additionally, a new SQSTM1-mediated autophagy-independent lysosomal degradation (SMAILD) pathway has been proposed to degrade SCAP (SREBF chaperone) proteins, necessary for the regulation of transcription factors related to lipid biosynthesis, while pharmacological activation of this pathway reduced hepatic steatosis (Zheng et al., 2020). These new discoveries corroborate the fact that a *Tfeb* Li-KO study showed different outcomes compared to other autophagic KO models during fasting-induced steatosis.

AUTOPHAGY MARKERS

Autophagy is a very dynamic process within the cell. Moreover, the balance between autophagosome formation and degradation may quickly change in response to metabolic and environmental stimuli, adapting the flux to cellular necessities. This creates a challenge to correctly measure and interpret data that reflects changes in autophagic activity, especially in animal models. In our summary of literature results, most of the studies relied on the evaluation of LC3 forms and p62/SQSTM1 protein levels. To a lesser extent, changes in the levels of BECLIN-1 and ATG proteins were also measured in NAFLD models. Finally, a few studies also used electron microscopy or LC3 imaging (by immunofluorescence, IF or immunohistochemistry, IHC) as a method to measure autophagosome numbers. The participation of commonly used markers in the general autophagy pathway is illustrated in **Figure 3**. The overall summary of each marker and changes observed after steatosis is described in **Table 8**.

From all markers measured, p62 levels were the most consistent. From 88 studies, 72 found them increased in the livers of NAFLD models compared to control, while 16 found levels either decreased or unchanged. P62/SQSTM1 is most known as an adaptor that mediates the degradation of sequestered cargo through autophagy. It normally functions by binding to polyubiquitinated targets that in turn are delivered to autophagic digestion through p62 and LC3-II interaction. Thus, its levels are expected to correlate inversely with autophagic activity, since p62 itself is degraded within autophagolysosomes (Long et al., 2017). However, to evaluate p62 mRNA along with protein results is recommended in order to assist in data interpretation, once p62 can be intensively regulated at the transcriptional level (Klionsky et al., 2021). In the context of NAFLD, p62 is thought to accumulate in hepatocytes because of decreased autophagic flux. In severe cases, p62 can aggregate with insoluble

protein inclusions known as Mallory-Denk bodies (MDBs). The observation of MDBs in hepatocytes is commonly associated with poor prognosis in NASH patients and correlates with proinflammatory M1-polarization of macrophages within liver biopsies (Zatloukal et al., 2007; Fukushima et al., 2018). Of note, a few articles opted to measure changes in insoluble and soluble fractions of p62, as an indication of protein aggregates (Park et al., 2014; Cho et al., 2018), which may be more indicated when studying NASH models. Additionally, other studies analyzed p62 phosphorylation levels at Ser403 as a marker, which is known to be an important step for the degradation of ubiquitinated proteins and protein aggregates (Matsumoto et al., 2011; Klionsky et al., 2021). Interestingly, p62 aggregation induced by lipotoxicity is dependent on its phosphorylation by TBK1 (TANK Binding kinase 1) at the same residue, while inhibition of this kinase prevented the formation of ubiquitin-p62 aggregates in mouse NASH models (Cho et al., 2018). In addition to its role in autophagic protein degradation, p62 has been proposed to participate in a Parkin-independent mitophagy mechanism that counteracts liver damage during NAFLD (Yamada et al., 2018). Regarding its role in lipid metabolism, it is not clear whether p62 acts directly as an adaptor that targets LDs to autophagic degradation, although there is data indicating it is present on the surface of the LDs and required for lipophagy (reviewed by Roberts and Olzmann, 2020). Finally, p62 is an important connector of autophagy and other cellular protective pathways. Its activity is known to promote NRF2 activation by competitively interacting with Keap1 through its KIR region and to promote its autophagic degradation, releasing NRF2 from the cytosol and allowing its nuclear translocation (Long et al., 2017). This mechanism is dependent on its phosphorylation at serine 349 (Ichimura et al., 2013; Sánchez-Martín et al., 2019). In turn, NRF2 itself is known to promote p62 expression, leading to a feedback loop against cellular stress (Jain et al., 2010; Taniguchi et al., 2016). Importantly, p62-dependent activation of NRF2 plays an important role against lipotoxicity in hepatocytes (Park et al., 2015; Lee et al., 2020). Moreover, accumulation of p62 due to impaired autophagic activity may lead to sustained activation of NRF2, which is a hallmark of many tumorigenic processes, including hepatocellular carcinoma (Taniguchi et al., 2016). Thus, the p62-NRF2 axis may be an important effector connecting impaired autophagy and NAFLD progression toward carcinoma.

Differently from p62 results, LC3-II levels presented significant variation. When compared to housekeeping proteins (mostly β-actin), we observed that 30 studies out of 74 found increased LC3-II levels, 34 found it decreased, and 10 found it unchanged. Similar proportions were obtained in studies that measured LC3-II in relation to LC3-I (LC3-II/I ratio). Importantly, many experts advise against LC3-II comparisons to LC3-I, mainly because immunoreactivity tends to be different between both forms, thus their variations in blots are therefore not proportional, which may complicate result interpretation (Mizushima and Yoshimori, 2007; Bonam et al., 2020; Klionsky et al., 2021). While LC3-II levels correlate with autophagosome numbers in the cell, changes observed in this marker cannot support conclusions regarding the

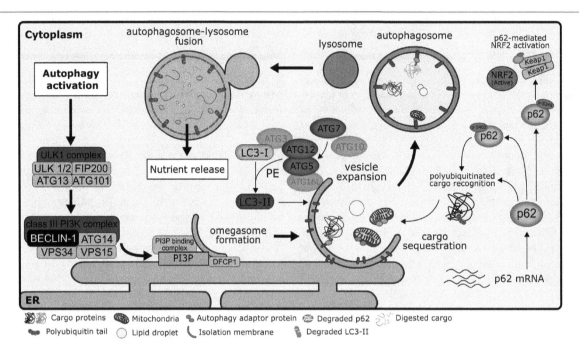

FIGURE 3 | Overview of autophagy pathways in mammalian cells. Common autophagy markers and their participation in autophagic machinery, as discussed in Section "Autophagy Markers." Signaling pathways that culminate in autophagy induction commonly lead to the activation of ULK1 kinase complex, promoting its localization at autophagy initiation sites near the endoplasmic reticulum (ER). ULK1 complex activity regulates the activation of the class III phosphatidylinositol 3-kinase (PI3K) complex, consisting of class III PI3K, VPS34, and other interacting proteins, including BECLIN-1. This complex is responsible for the production of phosphatidylinositol 3-phosphate (PI3P) at the site of early isolation membrane formation, which is essential for the nucleation step in the autophagic pathway. PI3P acts as a signaling molecule that recruits the double FYVE containing protein 1 (DFCP1) and other PI3P-binding proteins that promote the omegasome formation. At the expansion step, the autophagy-related protein 7 (ATG7) functions as an E1-like enzyme that catalyzes the conjugation of ATG12 to ATG5 in collaboration with the E2-like activity of ATG10. ATG12-ATG5 interacts with ATG16L at the vesicle membrane, marking the lipidation site. Microtubule-associated proteins 1A/1B light chain (LC3) at its mature form (LC3-I) are conjugated to phosphatidylethanolamine (PE) through the combined activity of ATG7 (E1-like enzyme), ATG3 (E2-like enzyme) and ATG12-ATG5 (E3 ligase enzyme). LC3 conjugated to PE (named LC3-II) is located at the autophagosome membrane and is important for the expansion and completion of the isolation membrane. P62/sequestosome-1 (named p62) works as an autophagy adaptor that recognizes polyubiquitinated cargos that will be sequestered for autophagic degradation due to their interaction with LC3-II. P62 phosphorylation at serine 403 (p-S403) increases affinity for polyubiquitinated targets and is promoted during autophagy activation. P62 phosphorylation at serine 349 (p-S349) is important for its competitive interaction with KEAP1 protein, promoting the activation of the NRF2 transcription factor, important during non-alcoholic liver disease (NALFD) development. Other autophagy adaptors besides p62 may participate during cargo recognition of selective autophagy. After autophagosome closure, the autophagic pathway proceeds with the formation of the autolysosome. The autophagosome external membrane fuses with the lysosome, releasing lysosome acidic hydrolases into the autophagosome lumen, and promoting cargo digestion. Importantly, LC3-II and p62 present within the autolysosome are also degraded in this process.

TABLE 8 | Autophagy markers.

	LC3-II (WB)	LC3 II/I (WB)	LC3 imaging (IF or IHC)	p62	Beclin-1	Atg5	Atg7	Atg12	EM (autophagosome)
Up	30	20	14	72	12	7	5	2	10
Down	34	20	7	7	14	5	13	1	4
Unchanged	10	4	1	9	3	1	2	1	0
Total	74	44	22	88	29	13	20	4	14

Markers and changes observed after steatosis is established.

intensity of autophagic activity if analyzed alone, because autophagosome levels in the cell are a sum of formation and degradation rates, and LC3-II changes can indicate variations in both processes. This is exemplified by the fact that about half of the studies found it either increased or decreased in NAFLD models, while most reached the conclusion of impaired autophagic activity. To that end, many studies measured autophagic flux *in vivo* by comparing animals that were injected with lysosome inhibitors a few hours before sacrifice to untreated animals within the same group. In addition, multiple methodological strategies may be used in parallel to complement the limitations of a single analysis or marker, allowing better interpretation of changes in autophagy dynamics *in vivo* (Bonam et al., 2020; Klionsky et al., 2021).

Importantly, autophagic flux can vary greatly in the hepatic tissue in physiological states with circadian cycles and periods after feeding (Ma et al., 2011; Martinez-Lopez et al., 2017; Toledo et al., 2018). Thus, control for these variables is an important concern during *in vivo* analysis of autophagy and may also be a source of variability within and between studies.

Similar to LC3-II findings, other markers related to autophagy initiation and autophagosome formation machinery also presented increased variability. For example, BECLIN-1 levels were found increased in 12 out of 29 studies, decreased in 14 and unchanged in 3. BECLIN-1 is a protein part of the VPS34 complex that functions downstream of ULK-1 in the autophagy initiation cascade. Its phosphorylation is known to be necessary to activate VPS34 and VPS15 kinase activity, increasing local production of phosphatidylinositol-3-phosphate and inducing the formation and expansion of the phagophore (Zachari and Ganley, 2017). Although autophagy can be initiated through BECLIN-1-independent mechanisms (Klionsky et al., 2021), after the induction of phagophore formation, membrane expansion and completion steps require LC3-I conjugation to phosphatidylethanolamine (LC3-II), a process that is dependent on the ATG5-ATG12 complex and ATG7 activity (reviewed by Chen and Klionsky, 2011; Ueno and Komatsu, 2017; Clarke and Simon, 2019). Thus, measuring the levels of these proteins can be indicative of the capacity to induce autophagosome formation and to activate autophagy. Interestingly, we observed that alterations in the levels of BECLIN-1 and ATG7 correlated

with alterations in LC3-II levels in the studies that analyzed both markers concomitantly, as would be expected. All studies that found decreased BECLIN-1 or decreased ATG7 also found lower LC3-II levels (or LC3-II/I ratios). Conversely, 3 out of 4 and 9 out of 11 studies that found increased ATG7 or BECLIN-1 also found increased LC3-II, respectively. Mechanistically, the expression of these proteins can be regulated by important transcription factors that act in a manner sensitive to metabolic states in the hepatic tissue, such as TFEB and PPARα (Lee et al., 2014; Napolitano and Ballabio, 2016). In addition, protease activity may also have a contribution, as has been shown for calpain-mediated degradation of ATG7 in obesity (Yang et al., 2010).

Due to the specificity of each protein in the autophagic signaling cascade, we highlight the fundamental necessity to evaluate different markers simultaneously to reach better conclusions regarding alterations in autophagic activity. To that end, many methods to measure autophagy during *in vivo* experiments are being developed and will certainly contribute to improving our knowledge.

AUTHOR CONTRIBUTIONS

VR and PK performed conceptualization and data curation. VR, PK, and AK contributed to funding and writing. All authors contributed to the article and approved the submitted version.

REFERENCES

Ali, E. S., Rychkov, G. Y., and Barritt, G. J. (2019). Deranged hepatocyte intracellular Ca2+ homeostasis and the progression of non-alcoholic fatty liver disease to hepatocellular carcinoma. *Cell Calcium* 82:102057. doi: 10.1016/j.ceca.2019.102057

Arruda, A. P., Pers, B. M., Parlakgul, G., Güney, E., Goh, T., Cagampan, E., et al. (2017). Defective STIM-mediated store operated Ca2+ entry in hepatocytes leads to metabolic dysfunction in obesity. *ELife* 6:e29968. doi: 10.7554/eLife.29968

Boland, M. L., Oró, D., Tølbøl, K. S., Thrane, S. T., Nielsen, J. C., Cohen, T. S., et al. (2019). Towards a standard diet-induced and biopsy-confirmed mouse model of non-alcoholic steatohepatitis: impact of dietary fat source. *World J. Gastroenterol.* 25, 4904–4920. doi: 10.3748/wjg.v25.i33.4904

Bonam, S. R., Bayry, J., Tschan, M. P., and Muller, S. (2020). Progress and challenges in the use of MAP1LC3 as a legitimate marker for measuring dynamic autophagy in vivo. *Cells* 9:1321. doi: 10.3390/cells9051321

Bonam, S. R., Wang, F., and Muller, S. (2019). Lysosomes as a therapeutic target. *Nat. Rev. Drug Discov.* 18, 923–948. doi: 10.1038/s41573-019-0036-1

Bootman, M. D., Chehab, T., Bultynck, G., Parys, J. B., and Rietdorf, K. (2018). The regulation of autophagy by calcium signals: do we have a consensus? *Cell Calcium* 70, 32–46. doi: 10.1016/j.ceca.2017.08.005

Byun, S., Seok, S., Kim, Y.-C., Zhang, Y., Yau, P., Iwamori, N., et al. (2020). Fasting-induced FGF21 signaling activates hepatic autophagy and lipid degradation via JMJD3 histone demethylase. *Nat. Commun.* 11:807. doi: 10.1038/s41467-020-14384-z

Carotti, S., Aquilano, K., Zalfa, F., Ruggiero, S., Valentini, F., Zingariello, M., et al. (2020). Lipophagy impairment is associated with disease progression in NAFLD. *Front. Physiol.* 11:850. doi: 10.3389/fphys.2020.00850

Carroll, B., and Dunlop, E. A. (2017). The lysosome: a crucial hub for AMPK and mTORC1 signalling. *Biochem. J.* 474, 1453–1466. doi: 10.1042/BCJ20160780

Chang, G.-R., Chiu, Y.-S., Wu, Y.-Y., Chen, W.-Y., Liao, J.-W., Chao, T.-H., et al. (2009a). Rapamycin protects against high fat diet–induced obesity in C57BL/6J mice. *J. Pharmacol. Sci.* 109, 496–503. doi: 10.1254/jphs.08215FP

Chang, G.-R., Wu, Y.-Y., Chiu, Y.-S., Chen, W.-Y., Liao, J.-W., Hsu, H.-M., et al. (2009b). Long-term administration of rapamycin reduces adiposity, but impairs glucose tolerance in high-fat diet-fed KK/HlJ mice. *Basic Clin. Pharmacol. Toxicol.* 105, 188–198. doi: 10.1111/j.1742-7843.2009.00427.x

Chen, R., Wang, Q., Song, S., Liu, F., He, B., and Gao, X. (2016). Protective role of autophagy in methionine-choline deficient diet-induced advanced nonalcoholic steatohepatitis in mice. *Eur. J. Pharmacol.* 770, 126–133. doi: 10.1016/j.ejphar.2015.11.012

Chen, X., Chan, H., Zhang, L., Liu, X., Ho, I. H. T., Zhang, X., et al. (2019). The phytochemical polydatin ameliorates non-alcoholic steatohepatitis by restoring lysosomal function and autophagic flux. *J. Cell. Mol. Med.* 23, 4290–4300. doi: 10.1111/jcmm.14320

Chen, Y., and Klionsky, D. J. (2011). The regulation of autophagy – unanswered questions. *J. Cell Sci.* 124, 161–170. doi: 10.1242/jcs.064576

Cheng, X., Ma, X., Zhu, Q., Song, D., Ding, X., Li, L., et al. (2019). Pacer is a mediator of mTORC1 and GSK3-TIP60 signaling in regulation of autophagosome maturation and lipid metabolism. *Mol. Cell* 73, 788–802.e7. doi: 10.1016/j.molcel.2018.12.017

Cho, C., Park, H., Ho, A., Semple, I. A., Kim, B., Jang, I., et al. (2018). Lipotoxicity induces hepatic protein inclusions through TANK binding kinase 1–mediated p62/sequestosome 1 phosphorylation. *Hepatology* 68, 1331–1346. doi: 10.1002/hep.29742

Clarke, A. J., and Simon, A. K. (2019). Autophagy in the renewal, differentiation and homeostasis of immune cells. *Nat. Rev. Immunol.* 19, 170–183. doi: 10.1038/s41577-018-0095-2

Cruces-Sande, M., Vila-Bedmar, R., Arcones, A. C., González-Rodríguez, Á, Rada, P., Gutiérrez-de-Juan, V., et al. (2018). Involvement of G protein-coupled receptor kinase 2 (GRK2) in the development of non-alcoholic steatosis and steatohepatitis in mice and humans. *Biochim. Biophys. Acta Mol. Basis Dis.* 1864, 3655–3667. doi: 10.1016/j.bbadis.2018.09.027

Day, C. P., and James, O. F. W. (1998). Steatohepatitis: a tale of two "hits"? *Gastroenterology* 114, 842–845. doi: 10.1016/S0016-5085(98)70599-2

Deus, C. M., Yambire, K. F., Oliveira, P. J., and Raimundo, N. (2020). Mitochondria–lysosome crosstalk: from physiology to neurodegeneration. *Trends in Mol. Med.* 26, 71–88. doi: 10.1016/j.molmed.2019.10.009

Ding, S., Jiang, J., Zhang, G., Bu, Y., Zhang, G., and Zhao, X. (2017). Resveratrol and caloric restriction prevent hepatic steatosis by regulating SIRT1-autophagy pathway and alleviating endoplasmic reticulum stress in high-fat diet-fed rats. *PLoS One* 12:e0183541. doi: 10.1371/journal.pone.0183541

Eslam, M., Sanyal, A. J., George, J., Sanyal, A., Neuschwander-Tetri, B., Tiribelli, C., et al. (2020). MAFLD: a consensus-driven proposed nomenclature for metabolic associated fatty liver disease. *Gastroenterology* 158, 1999–2014.e1. doi: 10.1053/j.gastro.2019.11.312

Ezquerro, S., Becerril, S., Tuero, C., Méndez-Giménez, L., Mocha, F., Moncada, R., et al. (2020). Role of ghrelin isoforms in the mitigation of hepatic inflammation, mitochondrial dysfunction, and endoplasmic reticulum stress after bariatric surgery in rats. *Int. J. Obes.* 44, 475–487. doi: 10.1038/s41366-019-0420-2

Ezquerro, S., Méndez-Giménez, L., Becerril, S., Moncada, R., Valentí, V., Catalán, V., et al. (2016). Acylated and desacyl ghrelin are associated with hepatic lipogenesis, β-oxidation and autophagy: role in NAFLD amelioration after sleeve gastrectomy in obese rats. *Sci. Rep.* 6:39942. doi: 10.1038/srep39942

Ezquerro, S., Mocha, F., Frühbeck, G., Guzmán-Ruiz, R., Valentí, V., Mugueta, C., et al. (2019). Ghrelin reduces TNF-α–induced human hepatocyte apoptosis, autophagy, and pyroptosis: role in obesity-associated NAFLD. *J. Clin. Endocrinol. Metab.* 104, 21–37. doi: 10.1210/jc.2018-01171

Farzin, L., Asghari, S., Rafraf, M., Asghari-Jafarabadi, M., and Shirmohammadi, M. (2020). No beneficial effects of resveratrol supplementation on atherogenic risk factors in patients with nonalcoholic fatty liver disease. *Int. J. Vitam. Nutr. Res.* 90, 279–289. doi: 10.1024/0300-9831/a000528

Fernández, ÁF., Bárcena, C., Martínez-García, G. G., Tamargo-Gómez, I., Suárez, M. F., Pietrocola, F., et al. (2017). Autophagy counteracts weight gain, lipotoxicity and pancreatic β-cell death upon hypercaloric pro-diabetic regimens. *Cell Death Dis.* 8:e2970. doi: 10.1038/cddis.2017.373

Fernandez-Mosquera, L., Yambire, K. F., Couto, R., Pereyra, L., Pabis, K., Ponsford, A. H., et al. (2019). Mitochondrial respiratory chain deficiency inhibits lysosomal hydrolysis. *Autophagy* 15, 1572–1591. doi: 10.1080/15548627.2019.1586256

Filippi-Chiela, E. C., Viegas, M. S., Thomé, M. P., Buffon, A., Wink, M. R., and Lenz, G. (2016). Modulation of autophagy by calcium signalosome in human disease. *Mol. Pharmacol.* 90, 371–384. doi: 10.1124/mol.116.105171

Fogacci, F., Banach, M., and Cicero, A. F. G. (2018). Resveratrol effect on patients with non-alcoholic fatty liver disease: a matter of dose and treatment length. *Diabetes Obes. Metab.* 20, 1798–1799. doi: 10.1111/dom.13324

Friedman, S. L., Neuschwander-Tetri, B. A., Rinella, M., and Sanyal, A. J. (2018). Mechanisms of NAFLD development and therapeutic strategies. *Nat. Med.* 24, 908–922. doi: 10.1038/s41591-018-0104-9

Fu, S., Yang, L., Li, P., Hofmann, O., Dicker, L., Hide, W., et al. (2011). Aberrant lipid metabolism disrupts calcium homeostasis causing liver endoplasmic reticulum stress in obesity. *Nature* 473, 528–531. doi: 10.1038/nature09968

Fukushima, H., Yamashina, S., Arakawa, A., Taniguchi, G., Aoyama, T., Uchiyama, A., et al. (2018). Formation of p62-positive inclusion body is associated with macrophage polarization in non-alcoholic fatty liver disease: aggregation of p62 and macrophages. *Hepatol. Res.* 48, 757–767. doi: 10.1111/hepr.13071

Garcia, D., Hellberg, K., Chaix, A., Wallace, M., Herzig, S., Badur, M. G., et al. (2019). Genetic liver-specific AMPK activation protects against diet-induced obesity and NAFLD. *Cell Rep.* 26, 192–208.e6. doi: 10.1016/j.celrep.2018.12.036

Garcia-Macia, M., Santos-Ledo, A., Leslie, J., Paish, H., Watson, A., Borthwick, L., et al. (2019). mTORC1-Plin3 pathway is essential to activate lipophagy and protects against hepatosteatosis. *bioRxiv* 812990. doi: 10.1101/812990

Glick, D., Zhang, W., Beaton, M., Marsboom, G., Gruber, M., Simon, M. C., et al. (2012). BNIP3 regulates mitochondrial function and lipid metabolism in the liver. *Mol. Cell. Biol.* 32, 2570–2584. doi: 10.1128/MCB.00167-12

Godoy-Matos, A. F., Silva Júnior, W. S., and Valerio, C. M. (2020). NAFLD as a continuum: from metabolic syndrome and diabetes. *Diabetol. Metab. Syndr.* 12:60. doi: 10.1186/s13098-020-00570-y

González, A., Hall, M. N., Lin, S.-C., and Hardie, D. G. (2020). AMPK and TOR: the Yin and Yang of cellular nutrient sensing and growth control. *Cell Metab.* 31, 472–492. doi: 10.1016/j.cmet.2020.01.015

González-Rodríguez, Á, Mayoral, R., Agra, N., Valdecantos, M. P., Pardo, V., Miquilena-Colina, M. E., et al. (2014). Impaired autophagic flux is associated with increased endoplasmic reticulum stress during the development of NAFLD. *Cell Death Dis.* 5:e1179. doi: 10.1038/cddis.2014.162

Guney, E., Arruda, A. P., Parlakgul, G., Cagampan, E., Min, N., Lee, Y., et al. (2020). Aberrant Ca2+ homeostasis in adipocytes links inflammation to metabolic dysregulation in obesity. *bioRxiv* 10.1101/2020.10.28.360008

Hariri, N., and Thibault, L. (2010). High-fat diet-induced obesity in animal models. *Nutr. Res. Rev.* 23, 270–299. doi: 10.1017/S0954422410000168

He, A., Chen, X., Tan, M., Chen, Y., Lu, D., Zhang, X., et al. (2020). Acetyl-CoA derived from hepatic peroxisomal β-oxidation inhibits autophagy and promotes steatosis via mTORC1 activation. *Mol. Cell* 79, 30–42.e4. doi: 10.1016/j.molcel.2020.05.007

He, B., Liu, L., Yu, C., Wang, Y., and Han, P. (2015). Roux-en-Y gastric bypass reduces lipid overaccumulation in liver by upregulating hepatic autophagy in obese diabetic rats. *Obes. Surg.* 25, 109–118. doi: 10.1007/s11695-014-1342-7

He, Q., Mei, D., Sha, S., Fan, S., Wang, L., and Dong, M. (2016a). ERK-dependent mTOR pathway is involved in berberine-induced autophagy in hepatic steatosis. *J. Mol. Endocrinol.* 57, 251–260. doi: 10.1530/JME-16-0139

He, Q., Sha, S., Sun, L., Zhang, J., and Dong, M. (2016b). GLP-1 analogue improves hepatic lipid accumulation by inducing autophagy via AMPK/mTOR pathway. *Biochem. Biophys. Res. Commun.* 476, 196–203. doi: 10.1016/j.bbrc.2016.05.086

Hernández-Alvarez, M. I., Sebastián, D., Vives, S., Ivanova, S., Bartoccioni, P., Kakimoto, P., et al. (2019). Deficient endoplasmic reticulum-mitochondrial phosphatidylserine transfer causes liver disease. *Cell* 177, 881–895.e17. doi: 10.1016/j.cell.2019.04.010

Hong, T., Ge, Z., Meng, R., Wang, H., Zhang, P., Tang, S., et al. (2018). Erythropoietin alleviates hepatic steatosis by activating SIRT1-mediated autophagy. *Biochim. Biophys. Acta Mol. Cell Biol. Lipids* 1863, 595–603. doi: 10.1016/j.bbalip.2018.03.001

Houde, V. P., Brule, S., Festuccia, W. T., Blanchard, P. G., Bellmann, K., Deshaies, Y., et al. (2010). Chronic rapamycin treatment causes glucose intolerance and hyperlipidemia by upregulating hepatic gluconeogenesis and impairing lipid deposition in adipose tissue. *Diabetes* 59, 1338–1348. doi: 10.2337/db09-1324

Hsu, H.-C., Liu, C.-H., Tsai, Y.-C., Li, S.-J., Chen, C.-Y., Chu, C.-H., et al. (2016). Time-dependent cellular response in the liver and heart in a dietary-induced obese mouse model: the potential role of ER stress and autophagy. *Eur. J. Nutr.* 55, 2031–2043. doi: 10.1007/s00394-015-1017-8

Hsu, P., and Shi, Y. (2017). Regulation of autophagy by mitochondrial phospholipids in health and diseases. *Biochim. Biophys. Acta Mol. Cell Biol. Lipids* 1862, 114–129. doi: 10.1016/j.bbalip.2016.08.003

Huang, Q., Wang, T., Yang, L., and Wang, H.-Y. (2017). Ginsenoside Rb2 alleviates hepatic lipid accumulation by restoring autophagy via induction of Sirt1 and activation of AMPK. *Int. J. Mol. Sci.* 18:1063. doi: 10.3390/ijms18051063

Ichimura, Y., Waguri, S., Sou, Y., Kageyama, S., Hasegawa, J., Ishimura, R., et al. (2013). Phosphorylation of p62 activates the Keap1-Nrf2 pathway during selective autophagy. *Mol. Cell* 51, 618–631. doi: 10.1016/j.molcel.2013.08.003

Jahn, D., Kircher, S., Hermanns, H. M., and Geier, A. (2019). Animal models of NAFLD from a hepatologist's point of view. *Biochim. Biophys. Acta Mol. Basis Dis.* 1865, 943–953. doi: 10.1016/j.bbadis.2018.06.023

Jain, A., Lamark, T., Sjøttem, E., Bowitz Larsen, K., Atesoh Awuh, J., Øvervatn, A., et al. (2010). p62/SQSTM1 is a target gene for transcription factor NRF2 and creates a positive feedback loop by inducing antioxidant response element-driven gene transcription. *J. Biol. Chem.* 285, 22576–22591. doi: 10.1074/jbc.M110.118976

Ji, G., Wang, Y., Deng, Y., Li, X., and Jiang, Z. (2015). Resveratrol ameliorates hepatic steatosis and inflammation in methionine/choline-deficient diet-induced steatohepatitis through regulating autophagy. *Lipids Health Dis.* 14:134. doi: 10.1186/s12944-015-0139-6

Kakimoto, P. A., and Kowaltowski, A. J. (2016). Effects of high fat diets on rodent liver bioenergetics and oxidative imbalance. *Redox Biol.* 8, 216–225. doi: 10.1016/j.redox.2016.01.009

Kantartzis, K., Fritsche, L., Bombrich, M., Machann, J., Schick, F., Staiger, H., et al. (2018). Effects of resveratrol supplementation on liver fat content in overweight and insulin-resistant subjects: a randomized, double-blind, placebo-controlled clinical trial. *Diabetes Obes. Metab.* 20, 1793–1797. doi: 10.1111/dom.13268

Kaushik, S., and Cuervo, A. M. (2015). Degradation of lipid droplet-associated proteins by chaperone-mediated autophagy facilitates lipolysis. *Nat. Cell Biol.* 17, 759–770. doi: 10.1038/ncb3166

Kim, J., Kundu, M., Viollet, B., and Guan, K.-L. (2011). AMPK and mTOR regulate autophagy through direct phosphorylation of Ulk1. *Nat. Cell Biol.* 13, 132–141. doi: 10.1038/ncb2152

Kim, K. E., Jung, Y., Min, S., Nam, M., Heo, R. W., Jeon, B. T., et al. (2016). Caloric restriction of db/db mice reverts hepatic steatosis and body weight with divergent hepatic metabolism. *Sci. Rep.* 6:30111. doi: 10.1038/srep30111

Kim, K. H., Jeong, Y. T., Oh, H., Kim, S. H., Cho, J. M., Kim, Y.-N., et al. (2013). Autophagy deficiency leads to protection from obesity and insulin resistance by inducing Fgf21 as a mitokine. *Nat. Med.* 19, 83–92. doi: 10.1038/nm.3014

Kleiner, D. E., Brunt, E. M., Natta, M. V., Behling, C., Contos, M. J., Cummings, O. W., et al. (2005). Design and validation of a histological scoring system for nonalcoholic fatty liver disease. *Hepatology* 41, 1313–1321. doi: 10.1002/hep.20701

Klionsky, D. J., Abdel-Aziz, A. K., Abdelfatah, S., Abdellatif, M., Abdoli, A., Abel, S., et al. (2021). Guidelines for the use and interpretation of assays for monitoring autophagy, 4th Edn. *Autophagy*. 1–382. doi: 10.1080/15548627.2020.1797280 [Epub ahead of print]

Koga, H., Kaushik, S., and Cuervo, A. M. (2010). Altered lipid content inhibits autophagic vesicular fusion. *FASEB J.* 24, 3052–3065. doi: 10.1096/fj.09-144519

Komatsu, M., Waguri, S., Ueno, T., Iwata, J., Murata, S., Tanida, I., et al. (2005). Impairment of starvation-induced and constitutive autophagy in Atg7-deficient mice. *J. Cell Biol.* 169, 425–434. doi: 10.1083/jcb.200412022

Kwanten, W. J., Martinet, W., Michielsen, P. P., and Francque, S. M. (2014). Role of autophagy in the pathophysiology of nonalcoholic fatty liver disease: a controversial issue. *World J. Gastroenterol.* 20, 7325–7338. doi: 10.3748/wjg.v20.i23.7325

Lai, M., Chandrasekera, P. C., and Barnard, N. D. (2014). You are what you eat, or are you? The challenges of translating high-fat-fed rodents to human obesity and diabetes. *Nutr. Diabetes* 4:e135. doi: 10.1038/nutd.2014.30

Lebeaupin, C., Vallée, D., Hazari, Y., Hetz, C., Chevet, E., and Bailly-Maitre, B. (2018). Endoplasmic reticulum stress signalling and the pathogenesis of non-alcoholic fatty liver disease. *J. Hepatol.* 69, 927–947. doi: 10.1016/j.jhep.2018.06.008

Lee, E. S., Kwon, M.-H., Kim, H. M., Woo, H. B., Ahn, C. M., and Chung, C. H. (2020). Curcumin analog CUR5–8 ameliorates nonalcoholic fatty liver disease in mice with high-fat diet-induced obesity. *Metabolism* 103:154015. doi: 10.1016/j.metabol.2019.1634015

Lee, I. H., Cao, L., Mostoslavsky, R., Lombard, D. B., Liu, J., Bruns, N. E., et al. (2008). A role for the NAD-dependent deacetylase Sirt1 in the regulation of autophagy. *Proc. Natl. Acad. Sci. U.S.A.* 105, 3374–3379. doi: 10.1073/pnas.0712145105

Lee, J. M., Wagner, M., Xiao, R., Kim, K. H., Feng, D., Lazar, M. A., et al. (2014). Nutrient-sensing nuclear receptors coordinate autophagy. *Nature* 516, 112–115. doi: 10.1038/nature13961

Lee, S., Nam, K.-H., Seong, J. K., and Ryu, D.-Y. (2018). Molybdate attenuates lipid accumulation in the livers of mice fed a diet deficient in methionine and choline. *Biol. Pharm. Bull.* 41, 1203–1210. doi: 10.1248/bpb.b18-00020

Li, L., Hai, J., Li, Z., Zhang, Y., Peng, H., Li, K., et al. (2014). Resveratrol modulates autophagy and NF-κB activity in a murine model for treating non-alcoholic fatty liver disease. *Food Chem. Toxicol.* 63, 166–173. doi: 10.1016/j.fct.2013.08.036

Li, Y., Chao, X., Yang, L., Lu, Q., Li, T., Ding, W.-X., et al. (2018). Impaired fasting-induced adaptive lipid droplet biogenesis in liver-specific Atg5-deficient mouse liver is mediated by persistent nuclear factor-like 2 activation. *Am. J. Pathol.* 188, 1833–1846. doi: 10.1016/j.ajpath.2018.04.015

Li, Y., Li, X., Wang, Y., Shen, C., and Zhao, C. (2019a). Metformin alleviates inflammatory response in non-alcoholic steatohepatitis by restraining signal

transducer and activator of transcription 3-mediated autophagy inhibition in vitro and in vivo. *Biochem. Biophys. Res. Commun.* 513, 64–72. doi: 10.1016/j.bbrc.2019.03.077

Li, Y., Yang, P., Zhao, L., Chen, Y., Zhang, X., Zeng, S., et al. (2019b). CD36 plays a negative role in the regulation of lipophagy in hepatocytes through an AMPK-dependent pathway. *J. Lipid Res.* 60, 844–855. doi: 10.1194/jlr.M090969

Lian, C.-Y., Zhai, Z.-Z., Li, Z.-F., and Wang, L. (2020). High fat diet-triggered non-alcoholic fatty liver disease: a review of proposed mechanisms. *Chem. Biol. Interact.* 330:109199. doi: 10.1016/j.cbi.2020.109199

Lin, C.-W., Zhang, H., Li, M., Xiong, X., Chen, X., Chen, X., et al. (2013). Pharmacological promotion of autophagy alleviates steatosis and injury in alcoholic and non-alcoholic fatty liver conditions in mice. *J. Hepatol.* 58, 993–999. doi: 10.1016/j.jhep.2013.01.011

Liu, M., Xu, L., Yin, L., Qi, Y., Xu, Y., Han, X., et al. (2015). Potent effects of dioscin against obesity in mice. *Sci. Rep.* 5:7973. doi: 10.1038/srep07973

Long, M., Li, X., Li, L., Dodson, M., Zhang, D. D., and Zheng, H. (2017). Multifunctional p62 effects underlie diverse metabolic diseases. *Trends Endocrinol. Metab.* 28, 818–830. doi: 10.1016/j.tem.2017.09.001

Loomba, R., and Adams, L. A. (2019). The 20% rule of NASH progression: the natural history of advanced fibrosis and cirrhosis caused by NASH. *Hepatology* 70, 1885–1888. doi: 10.1002/hep.30946

Lu, W., Mei, J., Yang, J., Wu, Z., Liu, J., Miao, P., et al. (2020). ApoE deficiency promotes non-alcoholic fatty liver disease in mice via impeding AMPK/mTOR mediated autophagy. *Life Sci.* 252:117601. doi: 10.1016/j.lfs.2020.117601

Ma, D., Molusky, M. M., Song, J., Hu, C.-R., Fang, F., Rui, C., et al. (2013). Autophagy deficiency by hepatic FIP200 deletion uncouples steatosis from liver injury in NAFLD. *Mol. Endocrinol.* 27, 1643–1654. doi: 10.1210/me.2013-1153

Ma, D., Panda, S., and Lin, J. D. (2011). Temporal orchestration of circadian autophagy rhythm by C/EBPβ: C/EBPβ regulates circadian autophagy rhythm. *EMBO J.* 30, 4642–4651. doi: 10.1038/emboj.2011.322

Ma, N., Ma, R., Tang, K., Li, X., and He, B. (2020). Roux-en-Y gastric bypass in obese diabetic rats promotes autophagy to improve lipid metabolism through mTOR/p70S6K signaling pathway. *J. Diabetes Res.* 2020:4326549. doi: 10.1155/2020/4326549

Machado, M. V., Michelotti, G. A., Xie, G., Almeida Pereira, T., de Almeida, T. P., Boursier, J., et al. (2015). Mouse models of diet-induced nonalcoholic steatohepatitis reproduce the heterogeneity of the human disease. *PLoS One* 10:e0127991. doi: 10.1371/journal.pone.0127991

Martinez-Lopez, N., Tarabra, E., Toledo, M., Garcia-Macia, M., Sahu, S., Coletto, L., et al. (2017). System-wide benefits of intermeal fasting by autophagy. *Cell Metab.* 26, 856–871.e5. doi: 10.1016/j.cmet.2017.09.020

Matsumoto, G., Wada, K., Okuno, M., Kurosawa, M., and Nukina, N. (2011). Serine 403 phosphorylation of p62/SQSTM1 regulates selective autophagic clearance of ubiquitinated proteins. *Mol. Cell* 44, 279–289. doi: 10.1016/j.molcel.2011.07.039

Matsumoto, Y., Yoshizumi, T., Toshima, T., Takeishi, K., Fukuhara, T., Itoh, S., et al. (2019). Ectopic localization of autophagosome in fatty liver is a key factor for liver regeneration. *Organogenesis* 15, 24–34. doi: 10.1080/15476278.2019.1633872

Matsunaga, K., Saitoh, T., Tabata, K., Omori, H., Satoh, T., Kurotori, N., et al. (2009). Two Beclin 1-binding proteins, Atg14L and Rubicon, reciprocally regulate autophagy at different stages. *Nat. Cell Biol.* 11, 385–396. doi: 10.1038/ncb1846

McGuire, C. M., and Forgac, M. (2018). Glucose starvation increases V-ATPase assembly and activity in mammalian cells through AMP kinase and phosphatidylinositide 3-kinase/Akt signaling. *J. Biol. Chem.* 293, 9113–9123. doi: 10.1074/jbc.RA117.001327

Milton-Laskibar, I., Aguirre, L., Etxeberria, U., Milagro, F. I., Martínez, J. A., and Portillo, M. P. (2018). Involvement of autophagy in the beneficial effects of resveratrol in hepatic steatosis treatment. A comparison with energy restriction. *Food Funct.* 9, 4207–4215. doi: 10.1039/c8fo00930a

Miyagawa, K., Oe, S., Honma, Y., Izumi, H., Baba, R., and Harada, M. (2016). Lipid-induced endoplasmic reticulum stress impairs selective autophagy at the step of autophagosome-lysosome fusion in hepatocytes. *Am. J. Pathol.* 186, 1861–1873. doi: 10.1016/j.ajpath.2016.03.003

Mizushima, N., and Yoshimori, T. (2007). How to interpret LC3 immunoblotting. *Autophagy* 3, 542–545. doi: 10.4161/auto.4600

Muñoz, J. P., Ivanova, S., Sánchez-Wandelmer, J., Martínez-Cristóbal, P., Noguera, E., Sancho, A., et al. (2013). Mfn2 modulates the UPR and mitochondrial function via repression of PERK. *EMBO J.* 32, 2348–2361. doi: 10.1038/emboj. 2013.168

Napolitano, G., and Ballabio, A. (2016). TFEB at a glance. *J. Cell Sci.* 129, 2475–2481. doi: 10.1242/jcs.146365

Nguyen, T. B., Louie, S. M., Daniele, J. R., Tran, Q., Dillin, A., Zoncu, R., et al. (2017). DGAT1-dependent lipid droplet biogenesis protects mitochondrial function during starvation-induced autophagy. *Dev. Cell* 42, 9–21.e5. doi: 10. 1016/j.devcel.2017.06.003

Ogasawara, Y., Tsuji, T., and Fujimoto, T. (2020). Multifarious roles of lipid droplets in autophagy – target, product, and what else? *Semin. Cell Dev. Biol.* 108, 47–54. doi: 10.1016/j.semcdb.2020.02.013

Ouzzani, M., Hammady, H., Fedorowicz, Z., and Elmagarmid, A. (2016). Rayyan—a web and mobile app for systematic reviews. *Syst. Rev.* 5:210. doi: 10.1186/s13643-016-0384-4

Pankiv, S., Clausen, T. H., Lamark, T., Brech, A., Bruun, J.-A., Outzen, H., et al. (2007). p62/SQSTM1 binds directly to Atg8/LC3 to facilitate degradation of ubiquitinated protein aggregates by autophagy. *J. Biol. Chem.* 282, 24131–24145. doi: 10.1074/jbc.M702824200

Park, H.-W., Park, H., Semple, I. A., Jang, I., Ro, S.-H., Kim, M., et al. (2014). Pharmacological correction of obesity-induced autophagy arrest using calcium channel blockers. *Nat. Commun.* 5:4834. doi: 10.1038/ncomms5834

Park, J. S., Kang, D. H., Lee, D. H., and Bae, S. H. (2015). Concerted action of p62 and Nrf2 protects cells from palmitic acid-induced lipotoxicity. *Biochem. Biophys. Res. Commun.* 466, 131–137. doi: 10.1016/j.bbrc.2015.08.120

Paschoal, V. A., Amano, M. T., Belchior, T., Magdalon, J., Chimin, P., Andrade, M. L., et al. (2017). mTORC1 inhibition with rapamycin exacerbates adipose tissue inflammation in obese mice and dissociates macrophage phenotype from function. *Immunobiology* 222, 261–271. doi: 10.1016/j.imbio.2016.09.014

Preguiça, I., Alves, A., Nunes, S., Fernandes, R., Gomes, P., Viana, S. D., et al. (2020). Diet-induced rodent models of obesity-related metabolic disorders—a guide to a translational perspective. *Obes. Rev.* 21:e13081. doi: 10.1111/obr. 13081

Qian, Q., Zhang, Z., Li, M., Savage, K., Cheng, D., Rauckhorst, A. J., et al. (2019). Hepatic lysosomal iNOS activity impairs autophagy in obesity. *Cell. Mol. Gastroenterol. Hepatol.* 8, 95–110. doi: 10.1016/j.jcmgh.2019.03.005

Rambold, A. S., Cohen, S., and Lippincott-Schwartz, J. (2015). Fatty acid trafficking in starved cells: regulation by lipid droplet lipolysis, autophagy, and mitochondrial fusion dynamics. *Dev. Cell* 32, 678–692. doi: 10.1016/j.devcel. 2015.01.029

Ren, H., Wang, D., Zhang, L., Kang, X., Li, Y., Zhou, X., et al. (2019). Catalpol induces autophagy and attenuates liver steatosis in ob/ob and high-fat diet-induced obese mice. *Aging* 11, 9461–9477. doi: 10.18632/aging.102396

Rinella, M. E., Elias, M. S., Smolak, R. R., Fu, T., Borensztajn, J., and Green, R. M. (2008). Mechanisms of hepatic steatosis in mice fed a lipogenic methionine choline-deficient diet. *J. Lipid Res.* 49, 1068–1076. doi: 10.1194/jlr.M800042-JLR200

Roberts, M. A., and Olzmann, J. A. (2020). Protein quality control and lipid droplet metabolism. *Annu. Rev. Cell Dev. Biol.* 36, 115–139. doi: 10.1146/annurev-cellbio-031320-101827

Ruan, H.-B., Ma, Y., Torres, S., Zhang, B., Feriod, C., Heck, R. M., et al. (2017). Calcium-dependent O-GlcNAc signaling drives liver autophagy in adaptation to starvation. *Genes Dev.* 31, 1655–1665. doi: 10.1101/gad.305441.117

Rui, L. (2014). Energy metabolism in the liver. *Compr. Physiol.* 4, 177–197. doi: 10.1002/cphy.c130024

Saito, T., Kuma, A., Sugiura, Y., Ichimura, Y., Obata, M., Kitamura, H., et al. (2019). Autophagy regulates lipid metabolism through selective turnover of NCoR1. *Nat. Commun.* 10:1567. doi: 10.1038/s41467-019-08829-3

Samovski, D., and Abumrad, N. A. (2019). Regulation of lipophagy in NAFLD by cellular metabolism and CD36. *J. Lipid Res.* 60, 755–757. doi: 10.1194/jlr. C093674

Sánchez-Martín, P., Saito, T., and Komatsu, M. (2019). p62/ SQSTM 1: 'Jack of all trades' in health and cancer. *FEBS J.* 286, 8–23. doi: 10.1111/febs.14712

Santhekadur, P. K., Kumar, D. P., and Sanyal, A. J. (2018). Preclinical models of non-alcoholic fatty liver disease. *J. Hepatol.* 68, 230–237. doi: 10.1016/j.jhep. 2017.10.031

Sathyanarayan, A., Mashek, M. T., and Mashek, D. G. (2017). ATGL promotes autophagy/lipophagy via SIRT1 to control hepatic lipid droplet catabolism. *Cell Rep.* 19, 1–9. doi: 10.1016/j.celrep.2017.03.026

Schaaf, M. B. E., Keulers, T. G., Vooijs, M. A., and Rouschop, K. M. A. (2016). LC3/GABARAP family proteins: autophagy-(un)related functions. *FASEB J.* 30, 3961–3978. doi: 10.1096/fj.201600698R

Schulze, R. J., Krueger, E. W., Weller, S. G., Johnson, K. M., Casey, C. A., Schott, M. B., et al. (2020). Direct lysosome-based autophagy of lipid droplets in hepatocytes. *Proc. Natl. Acad. Sci. U. S. A.* 117, 32443–32452. doi: 10.1073/pnas. 2011442117

Schulze, R. J., and McNiven, M. A. (2019). Lipid droplet formation and lipophagy in fatty liver disease. *Semin. Liver Dis.* 39, 283–290. doi: 10.1055/s-0039-168 5524

Sebastián, D., Sorianello, E., Segalés, J., Irazoki, A., Ruiz-Bonilla, V., Sala, D., et al. (2016). Mfn2 deficiency links age-related sarcopenia and impaired autophagy to activation of an adaptive mitophagy pathway. *EMBO J.* 35, 1677–1693. doi: 10.15252/embj.201593084

Settembre, C., De Cegli, R., Mansueto, G., Saha, P. K., Vetrini, F., Visvikis, O., et al. (2013). TFEB controls cellular lipid metabolism through a starvation-induced autoregulatory loop. *Nat. Cell Biol.* 15, 647–658. doi: 10.1038/ncb2718

Shibata, M., Yoshimura, K., Furuya, N., Koike, M., Ueno, T., Komatsu, M., et al. (2009). The MAP1-LC3 conjugation system is involved in lipid droplet formation. *Biochem. Biophys. Res. Commun.* 382, 419–423. doi: 10.1016/j.bbrc. 2009.03.039

Shibata, M., Yoshimura, K., Tamura, H., Ueno, T., Nishimura, T., Inoue, T., et al. (2010). LC3, a microtubule-associated protein1A/B light chain3, is involved in cytoplasmic lipid droplet formation. *Biochem. Biophys. Res. Commun.* 393, 274–279. doi: 10.1016/j.bbrc.2010.01.121

Shin, D. W. (2020). Lipophagy: molecular mechanisms and implications in metabolic disorders. *Mol. Cells* 43, 686–693.

Simoes, I. C. M., Karkucinska-Wieckowska, A., Janikiewicz, J., Szymanska, S., Pronicki, M., Dobrzyn, P., et al. (2020). Western diet causes obesity-induced nonalcoholic fatty liver disease development by differentially compromising the autophagic response. *Antioxidants* 9:995. doi: 10.3390/antiox9100995

Singh, R., and Cuervo, A. M. (2011). Autophagy in the cellular energetic balance. *Cell Metab.* 13, 495–504. doi: 10.1016/j.cmet.2011.04.004

Singh, R., Kaushik, S., Wang, Y., Xiang, Y., Novak, I., Komatsu, M., et al. (2009). Autophagy regulates lipid metabolism. *Nature* 458, 1131–1135. doi: 10.1038/nature07976

Song, Y. M., Lee, Y., Kim, J.-W., Ham, D.-S., Kang, E.-S., Cha, B. S., et al. (2015). Metformin alleviates hepatosteatosis by restoring SIRT1-mediated autophagy induction via an AMP-activated protein kinase-independent pathway. *Autophagy* 11, 46–59. doi: 10.4161/15548627.2014.984271

Soto-Avellaneda, A., and Morrison, B. E. (2020). Signaling and other functions of lipids in autophagy: a review. *Lipids Health Dis.* 19:214. doi: 10.1186/s12944-020-01389-2

Stacchiotti, A., Grossi, I., García-Gómez, R., Patel, G., Salvi, A., Lavazza, A., et al. (2019). Melatonin effects on non-alcoholic fatty liver disease are related to microRNA-34a-5p/Sirt1 axis and autophagy. *Cells* 8:1053. doi: 10.3390/cells8091053

Sun, L., Zhang, S., Yu, C., Pan, Z., Liu, Y., Zhao, J., et al. (2015). Hydrogen sulfide reduces serum triglyceride by activating liver autophagy via the AMPK-mTOR pathway. *Am. J. Physiol. Endocrinol. Metab.* 309, E925–E935. doi: 10.1152/ajpendo.00294.2015

Sun, Y., Xia, M., Yan, H., Han, Y., Zhang, F., Hu, Z., et al. (2018). Berberine attenuates hepatic steatosis and enhances energy expenditure in mice by inducing autophagy and fibroblast growth factor 21: berberine regulates hepatic steatosis and energy metabolism. *Br. J. Pharmacol.* 175, 374–387. doi: 10.1111/bph.14079

Takagi, A., Kume, S., Kondo, M., Nakazawa, J., Chin-Kanasaki, M., Araki, H., et al. (2016). Mammalian autophagy is essential for hepatic and renal ketogenesis during starvation. *Sci. Rep.* 6:18944. doi: 10.1038/srep18944

Takahashi, S., Sou, Y.-S., Saito, T., Kuma, A., Yabe, T., Sugiura, Y., et al. (2020). Loss of autophagy impairs physiological steatosis by accumulation of NCoR1. *Life Sci. Alliance* 3:e201900513. doi: 10.26508/lsa.201900513

Tanaka, S., Hikita, H., Tatsumi, T., Sakamori, R., Nozaki, Y., Sakane, S., et al. (2016). Rubicon inhibits autophagy and accelerates hepatocyte apoptosis and lipid accumulation in nonalcoholic fatty liver disease in mice. *Hepatology* 64, 1994–2014. doi: 10.1002/hep.28820

Tang, M., Jiang, Y., Jia, H., Patpur, B. K., Yang, B., Li, J., et al. (2020). Osteopontin acts as a negative regulator of autophagy accelerating lipid accumulation during the development of nonalcoholic fatty liver disease. *Artif. Cells Nanomed. Biotechnol.* 48, 159–168. doi: 10.1080/21691401.2019.1699822

Taniguchi, K., Yamachika, S., He, F., and Karin, M. (2016). p62/SQSTM1-Dr. Jekyll and Mr. Hyde that prevents oxidative stress but promotes liver cancer. *FEBS Lett.* 590, 2375–2397. doi: 10.1002/1873-3468.12301

Thomas, H. E., Zhang, Y., Stefely, J. A., Veiga, S. R., Thomas, G., Kozma, S. C., et al. (2018). Mitochondrial complex I activity is required for maximal autophagy. *Cell Rep.* 24, 2404–2417.e8. doi: 10.1016/j.celrep.2018.07.101

Tilg, H., Adolph, T. E., and Moschen, A. R. (2020). Multiple parallel hits hypothesis in NAFLD – revisited after a decade. *Hepatology* 73, 833–842. doi: 10.1002/hep.31518

Tilg, H., and Moschen, A. R. (2010). Evolution of inflammation in nonalcoholic fatty liver disease: the multiple parallel hits hypothesis. *Hepatology* 52, 1836–1846. doi: 10.1002/hep.24001

Toledo, M., Batista-Gonzalez, A., Merheb, E., Aoun, M. L., Tarabra, E., Feng, D., et al. (2018). Autophagy regulates the liver clock and glucose metabolism by degrading CRY1. *Cell Metab.* 28, 268–281.e4. doi: 10.1016/j.cmet.2018.05.023

Tong, W., Ju, L., Qiu, M., Xie, Q., Chen, Y., Shen, W., et al. (2016). Liraglutide ameliorates non-alcoholic fatty liver disease by enhancing mitochondrial architecture and promoting autophagy through the SIRT1/SIRT3-FOXO3a pathway: liraglutide cures NAFLD by mitochondrial administration. *Hepatol. Res.* 46, 933–943. doi: 10.1111/hepr.12634

Tsuchida, T., Lee, Y. A., Fujiwara, N., Ybanez, M., Allen, B., Martins, S., et al. (2018). A simple diet- and chemical-induced murine NASH model with rapid progression of steatohepatitis, fibrosis and liver cancer. *J. Hepatol.* 69, 385–395. doi: 10.1016/j.jhep.2018.03.011

Tu, G., Dai, C., Qu, H., Wang, Y., and Liao, B. (2020). Role of exercise and rapamycin on the expression of energy metabolism genes in liver tissues of rats fed a high-fat diet. *Mol. Med. Rep.* 22, 2932–2940. doi: 10.3892/mmr.2020.11362

Ueno, T., and Komatsu, M. (2017). Autophagy in the liver: functions in health and disease. *Nat. Rev. Gastroenterol. Hepatol.* 14, 170–184. doi: 10.1038/nrgastro.2016.185

Veskovic, M., Mladenovic, D., Milenkovic, M., Tosic, J., Borozan, S., Gopcevic, K., et al. (2019). Betaine modulates oxidative stress, inflammation, apoptosis, autophagy, and Akt/mTOR signaling in methionine-choline deficiency-induced fatty liver disease. *Eur. J. Pharmacol.* 848, 39–48. doi: 10.1016/j.ejphar.2019.01.043

Wang, B., Charukeshi Chandrasekera, P., and Pippin, J. J. (2014). Leptin- and leptin receptor-deficient rodent models: relevance for human type 2 diabetes. *Curr. Diabetes Rev.* 10, 131–145. doi: 10.2174/1573399810666140508121012

Wang, C., Yan, Y., Hu, L., Zhao, L., Yang, P., Moorhead, J. F., et al. (2014). Rapamycin-mediated CD36 translational suppression contributes to alleviation of hepatic steatosis. *Biochem. Biophys. Res. Commun.* 447, 57–63. doi: 10.1016/j.bbrc.2014.03.103

Wang, M.-E., Singh, B. K., Hsu, M.-C., Huang, C., Yen, P. M., Wu, L.-S., et al. (2017). Increasing dietary medium-chain fatty acid ratio mitigates high-fat diet-induced non-alcoholic steatohepatitis by regulating autophagy. *Sci. Rep.* 7:13999. doi: 10.1038/s41598-017-14376-y

Wang, X., Zhang, X., Chu, E. S. H., Chen, X., Kang, W., Wu, F., et al. (2018). Defective lysosomal clearance of autophagosomes and its clinical implications in nonalcoholic steatohepatitis. *FASEB J.* 32, 37–51. doi: 10.1096/fj.201601393R

Wang, Y., He, Z., and Li, X. (2017). Chronic rapamycin treatment improved metabolic phenotype but inhibited adipose tissue browning in high-fat diet-fed C57BL/6J mice. *Biol. Pharm. Bull.* 40, 1352–1360. doi: 10.1248/bpb.b16-00946

Wu, C., Jing, M., Yang, L., Jin, L., Ding, Y., Lu, J., et al. (2018). Alisol A 24-acetate ameliorates nonalcoholic steatohepatitis by inhibiting oxidative stress and stimulating autophagy through the AMPK/mTOR pathway. *Chem. Biol. Interact.* 291, 111–119. doi: 10.1016/j.cbi.2018.06.005

Wu, W. K. K., Zhang, L., and Chan, M. T. V. (2018). "Autophagy, NAFLD and NAFLD-related HCC," in *Obesity, Fatty Liver and Liver Cancer Advances in Experimental Medicine and Biology*, ed. J. Yu (Singapore: Springer Singapore), 127–138. doi: 10.1007/978-981-10-8684-7_10

Xie, F., Jia, L., Lin, M., Shi, Y., Yin, J., Liu, Y., et al. (2015). ASPP2 attenuates triglycerides to protect against hepatocyte injury by reducing autophagy in a cell and mouse model of non-alcoholic fatty liver disease. *J. Cell. Mol. Med.* 19, 155–164. doi: 10.1111/jcmm.12364

Xiong, X., Tao, R., DePinho, R. A., and Dong, X. C. (2012). The autophagy-related Gene 14 (Atg14) is regulated by forkhead box o transcription factors

and circadian rhythms and plays a critical role in hepatic autophagy and lipid metabolism. *J. Biol. Chem.* 287, 39107–39114. doi: 10.1074/jbc.M112.412569

Yamada, T., Murata, D., Adachi, Y., Itoh, K., Kameoka, S., Igarashi, A., et al. (2018). Mitochondrial stasis reveals p62-mediated ubiquitination in parkin-independent mitophagy and mitigates nonalcoholic fatty liver disease. *Cell Metab.* 28, 588–604. doi: 10.1016/j.cmet.2018.06.014

Yang, L., Li, P., Fu, S., Calay, E. S., and Hotamisligil, G. S. (2010). Defective hepatic autophagy in obesity promotes ER stress and causes insulin resistance. *Cell Metab.* 11, 467–478. doi: 10.1016/j.cmet.2010.04.005

Yang, S., Qu, Y., Zhang, H., Xue, Z., Liu, T., Yang, L., et al. (2020). Hypoglycemic effects of polysaccharides from Gomphidiaceae rutilus fruiting bodies and their mechanisms. *Food Funct.* 11, 424–434. doi: 10.1039/C9FO02283J

Younossi, Z. M. (2019). Non-alcoholic fatty liver disease – a global public health perspective. *J. Hepatol.* 70, 531–544. doi: 10.1016/j.jhep.2018.10.033

Zachari, M., and Ganley, I. G. (2017). The mammalian ULK1 complex and autophagy initiation. *Essays Biochem.* 61, 585–596. doi: 10.1042/EBC20170021

Zatloukal, K., French, S. W., Stumptner, C., Strnad, P., Harada, M., Toivola, D. M., et al. (2007). From Mallory to Mallory–Denk bodies: what, how and why? *Exp. Cell Res.* 313, 2033–2049. doi: 10.1016/j.yexcr.2007.04.024

Zechner, R., Madeo, F., and Kratky, D. (2017). Cytosolic lipolysis and lipophagy: two sides of the same coin. *Nat. Rev. Mol. Cell Biol.* 18, 671–684. doi: 10.1038/nrm.2017.76

Zeng, J., Zhu, B., and Su, M. (2018). Autophagy is involved in acetylshikonin ameliorating non-alcoholic steatohepatitis through AMPK/mTOR pathway. *Biochem. Biophys. Res. Commun.* 503, 1645–1650. doi: 10.1016/j.bbrc.2018.07.094

Zhang, F., Zhao, S., Yan, W., Xia, Y., Chen, X., Wang, W., et al. (2016). Branched chain amino acids cause liver injury in obese/diabetic mice by promoting adipocyte lipolysis and inhibiting hepatic autophagy. *EBioMedicine* 13, 157–167. doi: 10.1016/j.ebiom.2016.10.013

Zhang, H., Yan, S., Khambu, B., Ma, F., Li, Y., Chen, X., et al. (2018). Dynamic MTORC1-TFEB feedback signaling regulates hepatic autophagy, steatosis and liver injury in long-term nutrient oversupply. *Autophagy* 14, 1779–1795. doi: 10.1080/15548627.2018.1490850

Zhang, Q., Li, Y., Liang, T., Lu, X., Zhang, C., Liu, X., et al. (2015). ER stress and autophagy dysfunction contribute to fatty liver in diabetic mice. *Int. J. Biol. Sci.* 11, 559–568. doi: 10.7150/ijbs.10690

Zhang, X., Han, J., Man, K., Li, X., Du, J., Chu, E. S. H., et al. (2016). CXC chemokine receptor 3 promotes steatohepatitis in mice through mediating inflammatory cytokines, macrophages and autophagy. *J. Hepatol.* 64, 160–170. doi: 10.1016/j.jhep.2015.09.005

Zhang, X., Wu, W. K., Xu, W., Man, K., Wang, X., Han, J., et al. (2017). C-X-C motif chemokine 10 impairs autophagy and autolysosome formation in non-alcoholic steatohepatitis. *Theranostics* 7, 2822–2836. doi: 10.7150/thno.19068

Zhang, Y., Chen, M., Zhou, Y., Yi, L., Gao, Y., Ran, L., et al. (2015). Resveratrol improves hepatic steatosis by inducing autophagy through the cAMP signaling pathway. *Mol. Nutr. Food Res.* 59, 1443–1457. doi: 10.1002/mnfr.201500016

Zhang, Z., Qian, Q., Li, M., Shao, F., Ding, W.-X., Lira, V. A., et al. (2020). The unfolded protein response regulates hepatic autophagy by sXBP1-mediated activation of TFEB. *Autophagy* 1–15. doi: 10.1080/15548627.2020.1788889 [Epub ahead of print]

Zhao, R., Zhu, M., Zhou, S., Feng, W., and Chen, H. (2020). Rapamycin-loaded mPEG-PLGA nanoparticles ameliorate hepatic steatosis and liver injury in non-alcoholic fatty liver disease. *Front. Chem.* 8:407. doi: 10.3389/fchem.2020.00407

Zheng, W., Zhou, J., Song, S., Kong, W., Xia, W., Chen, L., et al. (2018). Dipeptidyl-peptidase 4 inhibitor sitagliptin ameliorates hepatic insulin resistance by modulating inflammation and autophagy in ob/ob mice. *Int. J. Endocrinol.* 2018:8309723. doi: 10.1155/2018/8309723

Zheng, Y., Wang, M., Zheng, P., Tang, X., and Ji, G. (2018). Systems pharmacology-based exploration reveals mechanisms of anti-steatotic effects of Jiang Zhi Granule on non-alcoholic fatty liver disease. *Sci. Rep.* 8:13681. doi: 10.1038/s41598-018-31708-8

Zheng, Z.-G., Zhu, S.-T., Cheng, H.-M., Zhang, X., Cheng, G., Thu, P. M., et al. (2020). Discovery of a potent SCAP degrader that ameliorates HFD-induced obesity, hyperlipidemia and insulin resistance via an autophagy-independent lysosomal pathway. *Autophagy* 1–22. doi: 10.1080/15548627.2020.1757955 [Epub ahead of print]

Zhong, Y., Wang, Q. J., Li, X., Yan, Y., Backer, J. M., Chait, B. T., et al. (2009). Distinct regulation of autophagic activity by Atg14L and Rubicon associated with Beclin 1–phosphatidylinositol-3-kinase complex. *Nat. Cell Biol.* 11, 468–476. doi: 10.1038/ncb1854

Zhou, W., and Ye, S. (2018). Rapamycin improves insulin resistance and hepatic steatosis in type 2 diabetes rats through activation of autophagy: effect of

rapamycin on insulin resistance. *Cell Biol. Int.* 42, 1282–1291. doi: 10.1002/cbin. 11015

Zhu, B., Mei, W., Jiao, T., Yang, S., Xu, X., Yu, H., et al. (2020). Neuregulin 4 alleviates hepatic steatosis via activating AMPK/mTOR-mediated autophagy in aged mice fed a high fat diet. *Eur. J. Pharmacol.* 884:173350. doi: 10.1016/j. ejphar.2020.173350

6

Liraglutide Alleviates Hepatic Steatosis by Activating the TFEB-Regulated Autophagy-Lysosomal Pathway

Yunyun Fang[1†], Linlin Ji[1†], Chaoyu Zhu[1], Yuanyuan Xiao[1], Jingjing Zhang[2], Junxi Lu[1], Jun Yin[1,3]* and Li Wei[1]*

[1] Shanghai Key Laboratory of Diabetes Mellitus, Department of Endocrinology and Metabolism, Shanghai Diabetes Institute, Shanghai Clinical Center for Diabetes, Shanghai Key Clinical Center for Metabolic Disease, Shanghai Jiao Tong University Affiliated Sixth People's Hospital, Shanghai, China, [2] National Demonstration Center for Experimental Fisheries Science Education, Shanghai Ocean University, Shanghai, China, [3] Department of Endocrinology and Metabolism, Shanghai Eighth People's Hospital, Shanghai, China

*Correspondence:
Jun Yin
yinjun@sjtu.edu.cn
Li Wei
weili63@hotmail.com

[†] These authors have contributed equally to this work

Liraglutide, a glucagon-like peptide-1 receptor agonist (GLP-1RA), has been demonstrated to alleviate non-alcoholic fatty liver disease (NAFLD). However, the underlying mechanism has not been fully elucidated. Increasing evidence suggests that autophagy is involved in the pathogenesis of hepatic steatosis. In this study, we examined whether liraglutide could alleviate hepatic steatosis through autophagy-dependent lipid degradation and investigated the underlying mechanisms. Herein, the effects of liraglutide on NAFLD were evaluated in a high-fat diet (HFD)-induced mouse model of NAFLD as well as in mouse primary and HepG2 hepatocytes exposed to palmitic acid (PA). The expression of the GLP-1 receptor (GLP-1R) was measured in vivo and in vitro. Oil red O staining was performed to detect lipid accumulation in hepatocytes. Electron microscopy was used to observe the morphology of autophagic vesicles and autolysosomes. Autophagic flux activity was measured by infecting HepG2 cells with mRFP-GFP-LC3 adenovirus. The roles of GLP-1R and transcription factor EB (TFEB) in autophagy-lysosomal activation were explored using small interfering RNA. Liraglutide treatment alleviated hepatic steatosis in vivo and in vitro. In models of hepatic steatosis, microtubule-associated protein 1B light chain-3-II (LC3-II) and SQSTM1/P62 levels were elevated in parallel to blockade of autophagic flux. Liraglutide treatment restored autophagic activity by improving lysosomal function. Furthermore, treatment with autophagy inhibitor chloroquine weakened liraglutide-induced autophagy activation and lipid degradation. TFEB has been identified as a key regulator of lysosome biogenesis and autophagy. The protein levels of nuclear TFEB and its downstream targets CTSB and LAMP1 were decreased in hepatocytes treated with PA, and these decreases were reversed by liraglutide treatment. Knockdown of TFEB expression compromised the effects of liraglutide on lysosome biogenesis and hepatic lipid accumulation. Mechanistically, GLP-1R expression was decreased in HFD mouse livers as well as PA-stimulated hepatocytes, and liraglutide treatment reversed the downregulation of GLP-1R expression *in vivo* and *in vitro*. Moreover, GLP-1R inhibition could mimic the effect of the TFEB downregulation-mediated decrease in lysosome biogenesis. Thus, our findings suggest that liraglutide attenuated hepatic steatosis via restoring autophagic flux, specifically the GLP-1R-TFEB-mediated autophagy-lysosomal pathway.

Keywords: non-alcoholic fatty liver disease, liraglutide, autophagy-lysosome, lysosomal biogenesis, TFEB

INTRODUCTION

Non-alcoholic fatty liver disease (NAFLD), characterized by excessive triglyceride (TG) accumulation in the liver, is commonly associated with insulin resistance, obesity, diabetes, and cardiovascular disease (Arab et al., 2018). Currently, the prevalence of NAFLD is estimated to be approximately 10–35% in the general population, making it the most common liver disease worldwide (Vernon et al., 2011). Thus, there is an urgent need to develop new preventive and therapeutic strategies to alleviate NAFLD.

Liraglutide, a glucagon-like peptide-1 receptor agonist (GLP-1RA), exhibits beneficial effects on weight loss, cardiovascular function, and NAFLD in addition to its glucose-lowering effect, especially in patients with obesity (Drucker, 2018; Muller et al., 2019). Previous studies suggested that liraglutide could alleviate high-fat diet (HFD)−induced hepatic lipid accumulation in a weight loss-independent manner (Lyu et al., 2020). However, the mechanism underlying the effects of liraglutide on NAFLD remains unclear.

Autophagy is an important lysosome-mediated process for the degradation of cellular components, including damaged organelles and misfolded proteins, for the maintenance of intracellular energy homeostasis (Yang and Klionsky, 2010). Increasing evidence has demonstrated that autophagy is necessary for regulating lipid metabolism because lipid droplets are degraded through lipophagy (Singh et al., 2009; Cui et al., 2020). Disruption of autophagy might therefore contribute to the aggravation of hepatic lipid accumulation (Wu et al., 2020). Recent studies revealed that liraglutide could alleviate hepatic steatosis, reduce oxidative stress, and activate autophagy (Tong et al., 2016). However, the exact mechanisms underlying these effects have not been fully elucidated.

Lysosomes are organelles involved in the process of intracellular substrate degradation through autophagosome-lysosome fusion and play a critical role in regulating autophagic flux and lipid droplet clearance. Normally, lysosomal lipid degradation capacity depends on a sufficient number of lysosomes and the activation of acid hydrolase enzymes (Sinha et al., 2014; Pi et al., 2019). Transcription factor EB (TFEB),

a key member of the microphthalmia family (MiT/TFE), has been identified as a key regulator of lysosome biogenesis and autophagy (Medina et al., 2011). Under normal conditions, TFEB is inactive and in the cytosol, whereas fasting and stress conditions induce its dephosphorylation-mediated activation and subsequent nuclear translocation. TFEB activation upon nuclear translocation may promote lysosomal biogenesis and substrate degradation (Zhang et al., 2018). Recently, TFEB has emerged as a key regulator of the lysosomal degradation of lipid droplets (Su et al., 2018). Moreover, deficient lysosomal clearance, resulting from reduced lysosome quantity and hydrolytic enzyme activity, was implicated in the development of NAFLD (Wang et al., 2019). These findings highlight a potential role of TFEB in the treatment of NAFLD via the promotion of autophagy-dependent lipid degradation. However, whether TFEB mediates the beneficial effect of liraglutide on hepatic autophagic flux and lipid degradation remains unclear.

In this study, we assessed the effects of liraglutide on hepatic steatosis and investigated the underlying molecular mechanisms. Our results revealed that autophagy activation mediated the effect of liraglutide in decreasing hepatic steatosis. Moreover, liraglutide activated autophagic flux and lipid degradation via the GLP-1R-TFEB-mediated autophagy-lysosomal pathway.

MATERIALS AND METHODS

Animal Treatment

Eight-week-old C57BL/6J mice weighting 23–28 g were purchased from the Model Animal Research Center of Nanjing University. All animals were maintained in a specific pathogen-free barrier facility under a 12 h light/dark cycle. After a week of adaptation, the mice were randomly divided into two groups ($n = 10$). They were fed a normal chow diet (D12450J, Research Diets) or HFD (D12492, Research Diets) for 18 weeks. The mice were then intraperitoneally administered either liraglutide (400 μg/kg/day, Novo Nordisk, Denmark) or equivoluminal 0.9% saline for another 4 weeks. Body weight was measured weekly, and food intake was recorded every 3 days. All animal procedures were conducted according to the guidelines for Experimental Animal Research.

Glucose Tolerance Test and Insulin Tolerance Test

The intraperitoneal glucose tolerance test (IPGTT) and insulin tolerance test (ITT) were performed to evaluate glucose tolerance

Abbreviations: GLP-1RA, glucagon-like peptide-1 receptor agonist; NAFLD, non-alcoholic fatty liver disease; GLP-1R, glucagon-like peptide-1 receptor; PA, palmitic acid; TFEB, transcription factor EB; siRNA, small interfering RNA; LC3-II, microtubule-associated protein 1B light chain-3-II; HFD, high-fat diet; IGPTT, intraperitoneal glucose tolerance test; ITT, insulin tolerance test; TG, serum triglycerides; TC, total cholesterol; LDL-C, low-density lipoprotein cholesterol; ALT, alanine transferase; AST, aspartic acid transaminase; FBS, fetal bovine serum; OA, oleic acid.

and insulin sensitivity after 4 weeks liraglutide treatment. For IPGTT, the mice were intraperitoneally injected with glucose (2 g/kg body weight) after overnight fasting. For ITT, the mice were fasted for 6 h and injected with insulin (Humulin R, Eli Lilly and Company) at a concentration of 1 U/kg body weight. Blood glucose was monitored with a glucometer (Roche, Switzerland) at regular intervals (0, 15, 30, 60, 90, and 120 min).

Biochemical and Lipid accumulation Measurements

The mice were sacrificed after an overnight fast. Serum triglyceride (TG), total cholesterol (TC), low-density lipoprotein cholesterol (LDL-C), alanine aminotransferase (ALT), and aspartic acid transaminase (AST) levels were examined using an automatic biochemistry analyzer (Rayto Technologies, China). The TG and TC of liver tissues and hepatocytes were measured using an Enzymatic Assay Kit (Applygen Technologies, China; Nanjing Jiancheng, China) according to the manufacturer's protocol.

Histopathological Analysis

Fresh liver specimens were fixed with 4% paraformaldehyde and embedded in paraffin. Paraffin sections were stained with H&E according to a standard procedure (Chang et al., 2010). Images were captured using a light microscope (Leica Microsystems, Germany).

Oil Red O Staining and BODIPY 493/503 Staining

To assess hepatic steatosis, liver tissues were embedded in optimum cutting temperature and immediately frozen in liquid nitrogen. Frozen liver sections were stained with Oil Red O (O0625, Sigma-Aldrich) according to the manufacturer's instructions. For in vitro studies, the hepatocytes were washed twice with phosphate-buffered saline and fixed in 4% paraformaldehyde for 30 min. Fixed cells were stained with Oil Red O solution for 0.5–1 h and gently washed with 60% isopropanol. Three images per sample were captured using a light microscope (Leica Microsystems, Germany). Lipid droplets were also detected by labeling with the BODIPY 493/503 (D3922, Invitrogen, United States) lipid dye. The images were obtained using a confocal microscope (Carl Zeiss, Germany).

Electron Microscopy

Autophagic vacuoles and autolysosomes were observed using an electron microscope (Olympus, Japan). Fresh liver tissue pieces were fixed with 2.5% glutaraldehyde, dehydrated in a graded ethanol series, and embedded in Epon 812 (Electron Microscopy Sciences, United States).

Cell Culture and Treatments

Human hepatoma HepG2 cells were obtained from the Type Culture Collection of the Chinese Academy of Sciences (Shanghai, China). Murine primary hepatocytes were isolated from male C57BL/6J mice (8 weeks old) using the collagenase

IV perfusion technique as previously described (Seglen, 1976; Klaunig et al., 1981). All cells were cultured in DMEM/HIGH GLUCOSE medium containing 10% fetal bovine serum (FBS) and 1% penicillin-streptomycin (Gibco, United States) in a 5% CO_2 incubator at 37°C. To establish a lipid-loaded cell model mimicking NAFLD in vitro, palmitic acid (PA, P9767, Sigma-Aldrich) was added to the culture medium at a final concentration of 0.2–0.6 μM. For in vitro experiments, cells were incubated in serum-free medium overnight and were then treated with or without liraglutide (S8256, Selleck Chemicals; 100–500 nM) in serum-free media containing PA or vehicle for 24 h. To examine the effect of liraglutide on hepatic autophagic flux, chloroquine (CQ, C6628, Sigma Aldrich; 50 μM), a classical autophagy inhibitor that blocks the fusion of autophagosomes with lysosomes, was added to the medium for 4–6 h as a negative control. To investigate the TFEB-mediated effects of liraglutide on lysosome biogenesis and autophagy, HepG2 cells were transfected with small interfering RNA (siRNA) targeted against TFEB (Genepharma, China) for 48 h using Lipofectamine 2000 (Thermo Fisher Scientific, United States). The siRNA sequences used are as follows: sense 5'-GACGAAGGUUCAACAUCAATT-3' and antisense 5'-UUGAUGUUGAACCUUCGUCTT-3'. To further investigate the mechanism of TFEB nuclear translocation, HepG2 cells were transfected with GLP-1R plasmid (Hanbio Biotechnology, China) and small interfering RNA (siRNA) targeted against GLP-1R (Genepharma, China). The siRNA sequences used were as follows: sense 5'-GGACCAGGAACUCCAACAUTT-3' and antisense 5'-AUGUUGGAGUUCCUGGUCCTT-3'.

Western Blot and Immunofluorescence Analysis

Total protein from liver tissue and hepatocytes was extracted with RIPA Lysis Buffer (P0013B, Beyotime, China) at 4°C. Nuclear and cytoplasmic fractions were separated for analysis of TFEB translocation using a commercial kit (78835, Thermo Fisher Scientific, United States) according to the manufacturer's instructions. Protein samples (20–30 μg) were separated using SDS-PAGE (Bio-Rad Laboratories, United States) and transferred to PVDF membranes (Millipore Corporation, United States). The membranes were blocked with 5% skimmed milk and incubated with primary antibody for 12 h followed by incubation with horseradish peroxidase-conjugated secondary antibodies. Primary antibodies against LC3A/B (1:1,000, 12741), Beclin1 (1:1,000, 3495), Atg5 (1:1,000, 12994), Atg7 (1:1,000, 8558), GAPDH (1:1,000, 2118s), cathepsin B (1:1,000, 31718), p62 (1:1,000, 5114s), and β-actin (1:1,000, 4970s) were obtained from Cell Signaling Technology (United States). Antibodies against lysosome-associated membrane protein 1 (LAMP1) (1:1,000, sc-20011) and SIRT1 (1:1,000, sc-15404) were from Santa Cruz Biotechnology, and the anti-TFEB (1:2,000, A303-673A) antibody was from Bethyl Laboratories (United States). The antibody against GLP-1R (1:1,000, ab39072) was from Abcam (United Kingdom). Membrane signals were detected using an enhanced chemiluminescence method (Thermo Fisher Scientific, United States). The band intensities were quantitated using ImageJ software. For immunofluorescence, cells were fixed with 4% paraformaldehyde for 15 min at 37°C. After fixation, the cells were permeabilized with 0.25% Triton X-100 for 15 min, blocked with 2% BSA for 30 min, and then incubated with an anti-TFEB antibody (1: 100, MAB9170-100, R&D Systems, United States) overnight at 4°C. The next day, cells were stained with a secondary antibody for 1 h and DAPI for 5 min. Immunofluorescence was visualized using a fluorescent microscope (Leica Microsystems, Germany).

Analysis of Autophagic Flux

For autophagic flux measurement, human hepatoma HepG2 cells were transfected with adenovirus harboring mRFP-GFP-LC3 (Hanbio Biotechnology, China). The cells were then treated with 0.4 μM PA, liraglutide, or CQ for 24 h. After treatment, yellow and red puncta were detected using a confocal microscope (Carl Zeiss, Germany).

Statistical Analysis

The data are expressed as the mean ± standard error of the mean (SEM). Unpaired two-tailed t-tests were used for intergroup comparisons. One-way analysis of variance with post hoc Bonferroni tests was performed for comparisons between multiple groups.

RESULTS

Liraglutide Improves Systemic Glucose and Lipid Homeostasis in HFD-Fed Mice

To explore the beneficial effect of liraglutide on hepatic lipid accumulation, C57BL/6 mice were fed a HFD or chow diet for 18 weeks and were then administered liraglutide (400 μg/kg/day) or saline for another 4 weeks. From the 4th week of intervention, HFD-fed mice exhibited a higher body weight than control mice, which was the case until the end of the experiment (**Figure 1A**). Liraglutide treatment significantly decreased body weight in HFD-fed mice (**Figure 1B[[AQ11]]**). Total food intake was decreased in both liraglutide-treated controls and HFD-fed mice (**Figure 1D**). Further, although liraglutide treatment induced a transient reduction of food intake during the first 2 weeks, no significant differences were found between the HFD groups treated with or without liraglutide during 3–4 weeks (**Supplementary Figure S1**). In addition, GTT and ITT indicated that liraglutide alleviated glucose intolerance and insulin resistance in HFD-fed mice (**Figures 1E,F**). However, no significant differences were observed in GTT results between these groups after blood glucose was adjusted as a% of initial glucose (**Supplementary Figures S2A,B**). Regarding systemic lipid metabolism, as shown in **Figures 1G-I**, the serum levels of TG, TC, and LDL-C in HFD-fed mice were decreased by liraglutide treatment. Taken together, these results suggest that liraglutide reduced body weight and restored systemic glucose and lipid homeostasis in diet-induced obese mice.

Liraglutide Mitigates HFD-Induced Hepatic Steatosis and Liver Injury

Since liraglutide improved systemic lipid homeostasis, we further investigated its effects on HFD-induced hepatic steatosis. H&E and Oil red O staining revealed that liraglutide treatment visibly attenuated HFD-induced hepatic lipid accumulation, with a reduced number of intracellular lipid droplets and ballooning hepatocytes (**Figure 2A**). Consistent with these changes, liver weight and hepatic TG content in HFD mice were significantly higher than those in chow diet-fed mice. Liraglutide also decreased liver weight and hepatic TG accumulation in HFD-fed mice. No significant differences were observed in TC content between these groups (**Figures 2B–D**). Biochemical analysis revealed that elevated serum ALT and AST levels in HFD group mice were clearly decreased by liraglutide (**Figures 2E,F**). Collectively, these results indicated that liraglutide exerted its hepatoprotective effects by alleviating hepatic steatosis and liver injury.

Liraglutide Attenuates PA-Induced Lipid Accumulation in vitro

To confirm whether liraglutide could alleviate hepatic lipid accumulation in vitro, primary mouse hepatocytes and HepG2 cells were employed. As shown in **Figures 3A,E**, lipid accumulation was significantly increased in both PA-stimulated primary mouse hepatocytes and HepG2 cells, an effect which was suppressed by co-incubation with liraglutide. Liraglutide treatment also significantly decreased intracellular TG content in these cell models (**Figures 3C,G**). However, no significant differences were observed in TC content (**Figures 3D,H**). Our results revealed that liraglutide directly reduced hepatic steatosis in vitro.

Liraglutide Induces Autophagy in HFD Mice

To explore whether liraglutide alleviated hepatic steatosis in HFD mice by activating autophagy, EM was performed. We observed large numbers of lipid droplets and autophagosome-like vesicles in the livers of HFD mice. These vesicles might derive from the sequestration of small lipid droplets or a portion of large lipid droplets, suggestive of lipid-laden autophagosomes. In contrast, virtually no lipid droplets were observed in liver sections from liraglutide-treated HFD mice, as intracellular lipids were engulfed and degraded within the autolysosome compartment (**Figures 4A–C**). Western blot revealed that the levels of autophagy indicators Atg7 and Beclin1 were lower in HFD mice, while those of LC3-II and autophagic selective substrate SQSTM1/p62 were significantly higher, indicating a blockade of autophagy-lysosomal degradation. Liraglutide treatment restored HFD-inhibited autophagy by increasing the protein expression of Atg7 and Beclin1 (**Figures 4D,E**) and decreasing the expression of LC3-II and p62 (**Figures 4F,G**). These findings suggest that hepatic steatosis impaired autophagy degradation,

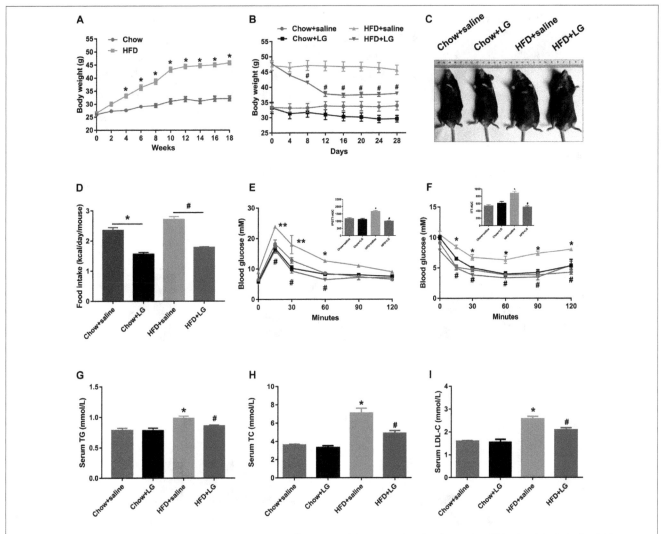

FIGURE 1 | Liraglutide improves systemic glucose and lipid metabolism in HFD mice. **(A)** Body weight before intervention. **(B)** Body weight during liraglutide treatment. **(C)** Representative photos of chow diet- and HFD-fed mice treated with liraglutide (400 μg/kg) or saline daily for 4 weeks. **(D)** Food intake (kcal/day/mouse). **(E,F)** IPGTT and ITT results were obtained after liraglutide treatment. AUC: the area under the curve. **(G–I)** Serum triglycerides (TG), cholesterol (TC), and LDL-C levels. The data are expressed as mean ± SEM; $n = 3$–5. *$P < 0.01$, **$P < 0.05$ vs. Chow + saline group; #$P < 0.01$ vs. HFD + saline group.

while liraglutide alleviated lipid accumulation by promoting autophagy-lysosomal–dependent lipid degradation.

Liraglutide Attenuates PA-Induced Lipid Accumulation by Enhancing Autophagic Flux

To further explore the mechanism underlying the liraglutide-mediated alleviation of hepatic steatosis via autophagic flux activation, primary mouse hepatocytes were isolated and incubated with free fatty acids. An increase in LC3-II and p62 levels was observed in hepatocytes after PA treatment, whereas oleic acid (OA) had no effect on the expression of these proteins (**Supplementary Figure S3A**). Furthermore, the expression of LC3-II and p62 increased in PA-stimulated primary mouse hepatocytes in a dose-dependent manner (**Supplementary Figure S1B**). However, the increase was

reversed by liraglutide, indicating that liraglutide alleviated the PA–triggered dysfunction of autolysosomal degradation (**Figure 5A**). Moreover, HepG2 cells were infected with mRFP-GFP-LC3 adenovirus to confirm whether liraglutide could promote autophagic flux (**Figures 5B,C**). When an Ad-mRFP-GFP-LC3 construct is used, GFP fluorescence only indicates autophagosomes, since it can be easily quenched in the acidic pH of autolysosomes. However, mRFP detects both autophagosomes and autolysosomes, since it is more stable under acidic conditions. Using this approach, we observed that the ratio of mRFP to GFP signals was significantly decreased in PA-stimulated HepG2 cells, suggesting the accumulation of non-acidic autophagosomes. In liraglutide–treated cells, more mRFP signals were observed, indicating that autophagic flux was enhanced without impeding autophagosome-lysosome fusion/or autolysosome function. In addition, blocking fusion by CQ weakened the liraglutide-increased ratio of mRFP to GFP signals.

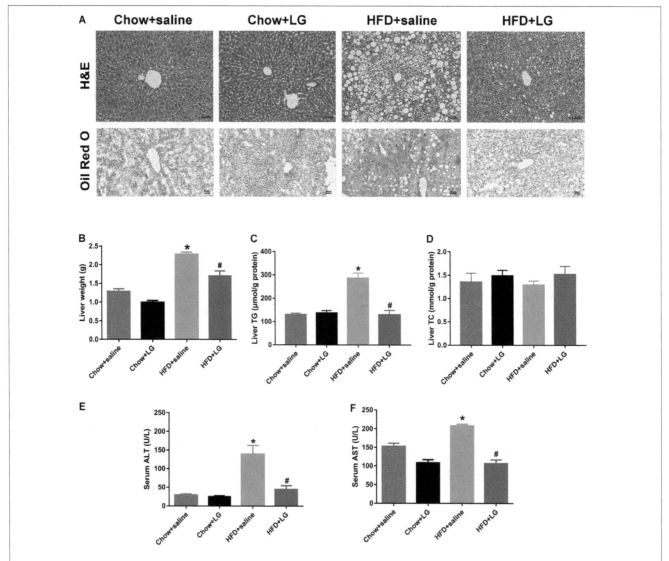

FIGURE 2 | Liraglutide attenuates hepatic steatosis and liver injury in HFD mice. **(A)** H&E and Oil red O staining of liver tissue (scale bars = 50 μm). **(B)** Liver weight (g). **(C,D)** Liver TG and TC levels. **(E,F)** Serum ALT and AST levels. The data are expressed as mean ± SEM; n = 3–5. *P < 0.01 vs. Chow + saline group; #P < 0.01 vs. HFD + saline group.

We then investigated whether liraglutide-induced autophagy was involved in its beneficial effect on lipid accumulation. As shown in **Figures 5D,E**, liraglutide treatment decreased BODIPY 493/503 fluorescence intensity and intracellular TG content in primary hepatocytes. However, these improvements were significantly diminished with CQ. Together, our results indicate that liraglutide alleviated hepatic steatosis partially by promoting the autophagy-lysosomal pathway.

Liraglutide Stimulates Lysosome Biogenesis by Inducing TFEB Translocation

Given that TFEB plays a critical role in the regulation of autophagy and lysosome biogenesis, we evaluated whether liraglutide alleviated steatosis by promoting

TFEB-dependent lysosome biogenesis *in vivo* and *in vitro*. Upon its dephosphorylation and nuclear translocation, TFEB activates lysosome-associated gene transcription. Thus, we used subcellular fractionation to confirm its localization. Western blot revealed that nuclear TFEB and its downstream target CTSB were remarkably decreased in the livers of HFD-fed mice, and these decreases were reversed by liraglutide treatment. In contrast, LAMP1 expression was increased, possibly due to a compensatory response for autophagy inhibition (**Figure 6A**). Consistently, we observed that liraglutide promoted TFEB nuclear translocation and enhanced CTSB and LAMP1 expression in PA–stimulated HepG2 cells (**Figures 6C,D**). In addition, immunofluorescent results revealed that liraglutide increased the ratio of nuclear to cytosolic TFEB in HepG2 cells (**Figure 6B**). Overall, these findings suggest that

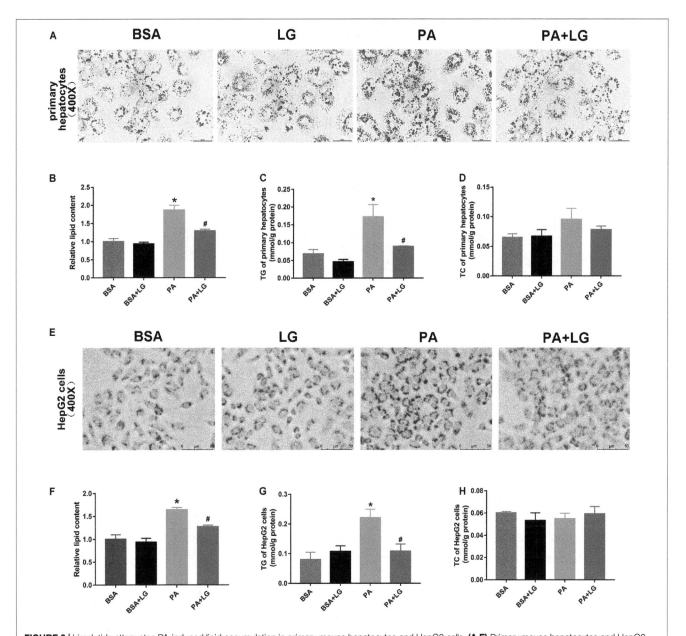

FIGURE 3 | Liraglutide attenuates PA-induced lipid accumulation in primary mouse hepatocytes and HepG2 cells. **(A,E)** Primary mouse hepatocytes and HepG2 cells were co-incubated with PA and liraglutide for 24 h. Lipid accumulation was assessed by Oil red O staining (scale bars = 50 μm). **(B,F)** Relative lipid content. **(C,G)** Hepatocyte TG content. **(D,H)** Hepatocyte TC content. The data are expressed as mean ± SEM; $n = 3$. *$P < 0.05$ vs. BSA group; #$P < 0.05$ vs. PA group.

liraglutide stimulated lysosome biogenesis by inducing TFEB nuclear translocation.

Liraglutide Attenuates PA-Induced Lipid Accumulation by Activating TFEB-Mediated Lysosome Biogenesis

To explore whether TFEB was responsible for the beneficial effects of liraglutide on lysosome biogenesis and lipid accumulation in hepatocytes, a TFEB siRNA (siTFEB) was used to silence TFEB in HepG2 cells. Results showed that TFEB downregulation decreased the expression of CTSB and LAMP1 in liraglutide-treated HepG2 cells (**Figure 7A**). In

addition, decreased BODIPY 493/503 fluorescence intensity and TG content with liraglutide treatment in HepG2 cells were not observed under TFEB knockdown (**Figures 7B,C**). Our results demonstrate that TFEB plays a critical role in lysosome biogenesis and mediates the beneficial effect of liraglutide on PA-induced intracellular lipid accumulation.

Liraglutide Activates TFEB and Its Downstream Targets Through GLP-1R

To evaluate whether GLP-1R was involved in the action of liraglutide, the GLP-1R protein levels in livers and hepatocytes were detected by western blotting. GLP1-R expression was

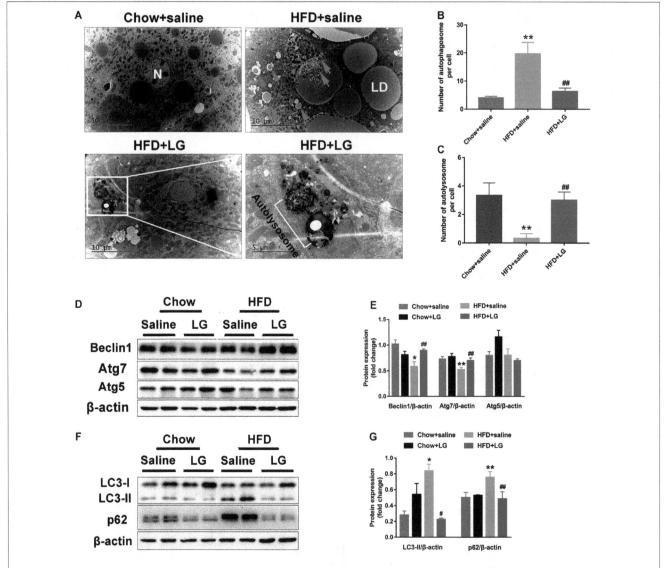

FIGURE 4 | Liraglutide activates autophagy in HFD-fed mice. **(A)** Representative electron microscopy images of autophagic vacuoles in the liver. Orange arrows indicate autophagic vacuoles (partly containing lipid droplets). Boxed area indicates autolysosome. High magnification of boxed areas in the liraglutide treatment group is presented on the right (scale bars = 10, 5 μm). N, nucleus; LD, lipid droplet; arrows, autophagosome; white box, autolysosome. **(B)** Quantitative analysis of number of autophagosomes per cell. **(C)** Quantitative analysis of number of autolysosomes per cell. **(D,E)** Expression of autophagy-associated proteins Atg5, Atg7, and Beclin1 in livers of HFD-fed mice analyzed by western blot. **(F,G)** Expression of autophagy-associated proteins LC3-II and autophagic selective substrate p62 in livers of HFD-fed mice analyzed by western blot. The data are expressed as mean ± SEM; $n = 3$. *$P < 0.01$, **$P < 0.05$ vs. Chow + saline group; #$P < 0.01$ ##$P < 0.05$ vs. HFD + saline group.

significantly decreased in HFD mouse livers and PA—stimulated hepatocytes. Further, liraglutide treatment reversed the downregulation of GLP-1R expression *in vivo* and *in vitro* (**Figures 8A–C**). To further investigate whether GLP-1R mediated the effect of liraglutide on TFEB-induced lysosome biogenesis, a GLP-1R siRNA (siGLP-1R) was used to silence GLP-1R in HepG2 cells. Results revealed that the downregulation of GLP-1R decreased the expression of TFEB and its downstream targets CTSB and LAMP1 in liraglutide-treated HepG2 cells (**Figure 8D**). Simultaneously, a GLP-1R plasmid was used to overexpress GLP-1R in HepG2 cells. GLP-1R overexpression enhanced the TFEB-mediated increase of CTSB and LAMP1

expression in PA-treated HepG2 cells (**Figure 8E**). Taken together, our results suggest that liraglutide upregulates TFEB and its downstream target proteins through GLP-1R.

DISCUSSION

In this study, we examined the beneficial effect of liraglutide on hepatic steatosis in HFD-fed mice and hepatocytes. Our results demonstrated that liraglutide alleviated hepatic lipid accumulation through activation of the autophagy-lysosomal pathway. Further, we found that, through GLP-1R activation,

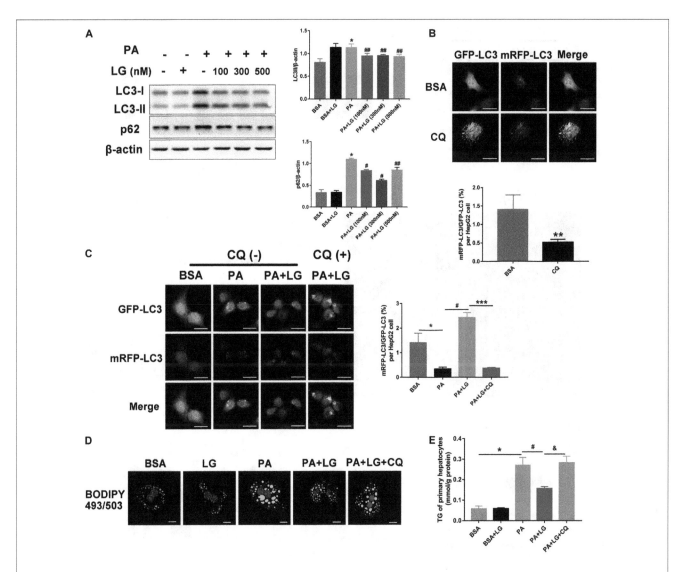

FIGURE 5 | Liraglutide attenuates lipid accumulation by enhancing autophagic flux *in vitro*. **(A)**. Primary mouse hepatocytes were co-incubated with PA and different concentrations of liraglutide for 24 h. Expression of LC3-II and p62 was analyzed by western blot. **(B)**. Evaluation of autophagic flux in Ad-mRFP-GFP-LC3-infected cells with or without CQ treatment. **(C)**. After Ad-mRFP-GFP-LC3 infection, HepG2 cells were pretreated with PA and liraglutide for 20 h, followed by 4 h of co-treatment with 50 μM of CQ. The ratio of mRFP to GFP per cell (n = 10) was calculated (scale bars = 20 μm). **(D)** Lipid droplets were detected by labeling with lipid dye BODIPY 493/503 (green) in primary mouse hepatocytes treated with or without liraglutide and CQ. Nuclei were stained with DAPI (blue) (scale bars = 10 μm). **(E)** Intracellular TG content was measured. The data are expressed as mean ± SEM. *P < 0.01, **P < 0.05 vs. BSA group; ***P < 0.01 vs. PA + LG group; #P < 0.01, ##P < 0.05 vs. PA group; &P < 0.01 vs. PA + LG group.

liraglutide promoted the nuclear translocation of TFEB as well as the expression of its targets CTSB and LAMP1, associated with lysosomal biogenesis and the autophagosome-lysosomal pathway. The increased nuclear translocation of TFEB reduced lipid accumulation in hepatocytes (**Figure 9**).

As novel potential therapeutic agents for NAFLD, GLP-1RAs were reported to reduce hepatic lipid accumulation (Wu et al., 2019). Further, clinical trial results revealed that liraglutide decreased liver fat content and body weight in patients with type 2 diabetes and NAFLD (Petit et al., 2017). GLP-1RAs also attenuated lipid accumulation in the livers of various animal models (Zheng et al., 2017; Kalavalapalli et al., 2019). These findings were consistent with our results, which indicated that

liraglutide significantly decreased liver lipid content as well as plasma TG, ALT, and AST in HFD-fed mice. Another report described a number of effects for GLP-1RAs, including increased postprandial insulin secretion, decreased appetite, and enhanced weight loss (Armstrong et al., 2016). Previous studies suggested that the beneficial effect of GLP-1RAs on weight loss is mainly attributed to the inhibition of food intake, especially for short-term interventions (Kanoski et al., 2011; Wei et al., 2015). A recent research on exendin-4 treatment in mice revealed a decrease in food intake during the first 2 weeks, which disappeared from 2 to 8 weeks (Xu et al., 2016). Consistently, in our study, we observed that the transient reduction in food intake vanished in the last 2 weeks of liraglutide treatment. Thus,

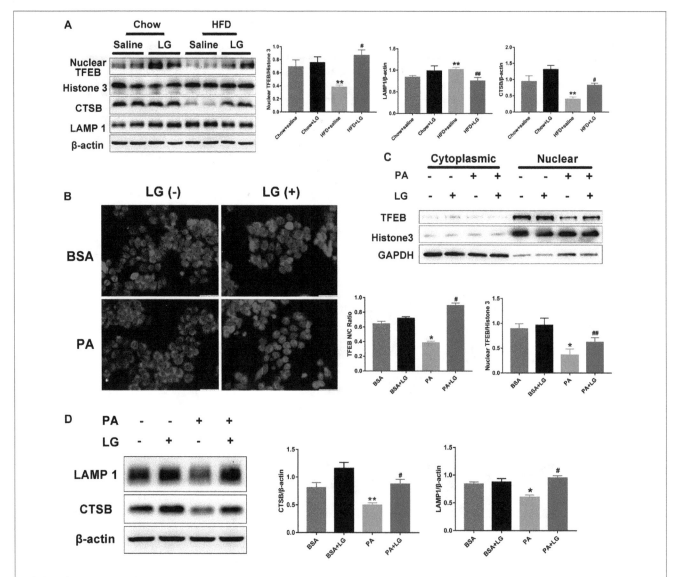

FIGURE 6 | Liraglutide stimulates lysosome biogenesis by inducing TFEB nuclear translocation. **(A)** Expression of nuclear TFEB, CTSB, and LAMP1 in the livers of HFD-fed mice treated with or without liraglutide. Relative expression levels were normalized to β-actin and Histone 3 levels. **(B)** HepG2 cells were co-incubated with or without PA and liraglutide for 24 h. After fixation, immunofluorescence staining was performed for TFEB localization (scale bars = 50 μm). **(C)** Western blot detection of cytoplasm and nuclear TFEB expression in HepG2 cells treated with or without liraglutide. Relative expression levels were normalized to GAPDH and Histone 3 levels, respectively. **(D)** Western blot detection of CTSB and LAMP1 expression in HepG2 cells. The data are expressed as mean ± SEM; $n = 3$. $^{*}P < 0.01$, $^{**}P < 0.05$ vs. BSA group; $^{#}P < 0.01$, $^{##}P < 0.05$ vs. PA group.

we speculated that the weight loss resulting from GLP-1RAs was not entirely dependent on the reduced food intake during long-term administration. Moreover, we investigated the expression of GLP-1R. Interestingly, liraglutide treatment reversed the down-regulation of GLP-1R expression in both *in vivo* and *in vitro* NAFLD models. Therefore, the systemic metabolic effects of GLP-1RAs might be attributed to a combination of the above-described mechanisms (Zhou et al., 2019; Mantovani et al., 2020).

Autophagy is important for the maintenance of cellular metabolism and energy homeostasis. Accumulating evidence has indicated that defective autophagy contributes to the aggravation of hepatic steatosis (Miyagawa et al., 2016; Chu et al., 2019). Normally, autophagy is supposed to break down lipid droplets

through the lipophagy degradation pathway (Martinez-Lopez and Singh, 2015). A previous study found that GLP-1RA-induced autophagy could remove excess lipid droplets and thus alleviate lipotoxicity (Yu et al., 2019). Moreover, exendin-4 protected hepatocytes and reduced steatosis via autophagy, in turn reducing endoplasmic reticulum stress-related hepatocyte apoptosis (Sharma et al., 2011). However, the mechanism underlying this upregulation of autophagy is unclear. A previous study in mice demonstrated that GLP-1RAs alleviated lipid accumulation through activation of AMPK/mTOR-dependent autophagy, a classic autophagy pathway (He et al., 2016). In the current work, EM examination revealed a large number of lipid droplets surrounded or partly engulfed by autophagosome-like

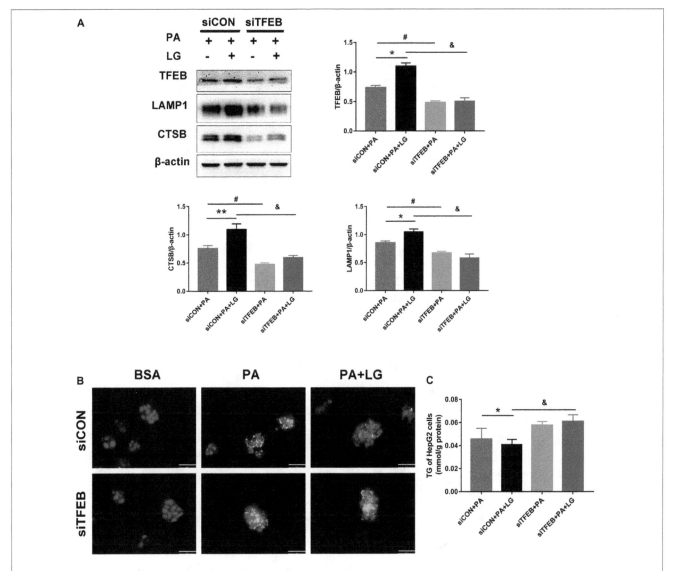

FIGURE 7 | TFEB knockdown weakens the effects of liraglutide on lysosome biogenesis and lipid accumulation. **(A)** Western blot detection of TFEB and its downstream targets CTSB and LAMP1 in HepG2 cells expressing TFEB-siRNA or control-siRNA. Relative expression levels were normalized to β-actin levels. **(B)** Lipid droplets in HepG2 cells treated with TFEB-siRNA or control-siRNA were detected via labeling with the lipid dye BODIPY 493/503 (green). Nuclei were stained with DAPI (scale bars = 50 μm). **(C)** The TG content of HepG2 cells. The data are expressed as the mean ± SEM; $n = 3$. $*P < 0.01$, $**P < 0.05$ and $^{\#}P < 0.01$ vs. siCON + PA group; $^{\&}P < 0.01$ vs. siCON + PA + LG group.

vesicles in the livers of HFD mice. Further, instead of these lipid droplets, lipid-laden autolysosomes were observed following liraglutide treatment. Consistently, the levels of autophagosome formation marker LC3−II and autophagic substrate p62 decreased after treatment with liraglutide. Thus, we inferred that liraglutide restored HFD-inhibited autophagy, perhaps in an autophagy-lysosomal pathway-dependent manner.

Autophagy is a dynamic process. As the terminal stage of autophagic flux, lysosomes fuse with autophagosomes, followed by lysosomal degradation and cellular lipid clearance (Chao et al., 2018a). Defective lysosomal biogenesis and clearance impair autophagic flux, leading to intracellular lipid accumulation during the development of NAFLD (Chao et al., 2018b). Previous studies found that HFD disrupted lysosomal biogenesis

in hepatocytes, which was associated with lipid degradation (Pi et al., 2019). We employed lysosomal inhibitor CQ to further investigate autophagy-lysosomal pathway involvement and found that liraglutide stimulated autophagic flux, as demonstrated by a reduction in autophagosome accumulation indicated by mRFP-GFP-LC3. In addition, the liraglutide-mediated attenuation of lipid accumulation in PA-stimulated HepG2 cells was significantly compromised following CQ treatment. Importantly, this is the first work to demonstrate that liraglutide activates the autophagy-lysosomal pathway to alleviate hepatic lipid accumulation.

MiT−TFE subfamily members, including MITF, TFE3, and TFEB, positively regulate lysosomal biogenesis. Among these transcription factors, TFEB enhances lipid metabolism

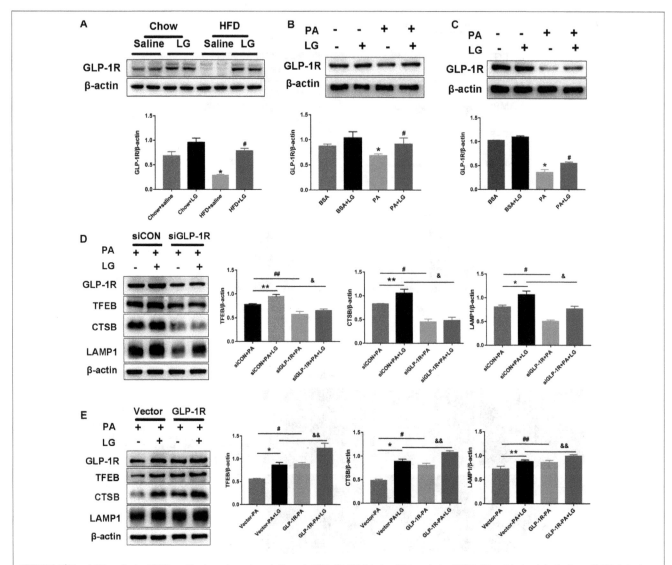

FIGURE 8 | Liraglutide activates TFEB and its downstream targets through GLP-1R. **(A)** Western blot analysis of GLP-1R protein levels in the liver of HFD-fed mice treated with or without liraglutide. Relative expression levels were normalized to β-actin levels. **(B,C)** Western blot detection of GLP-1R in primary mouse hepatocytes and HepG2 cells treated with or without liraglutide. **(D)** Western blot detection of GLP-1R, TFEB, and its downstream targets CTSB and LAMP1 in HepG2 cells transfected with TFEB-siRNA or control-siRNA. **(E)** Western blot detection of GLP-1R, TFEB, and its downstream targets CTSB and LAMP1 in HepG2 cells with or without GLP-1R overexpression. The data are expressed as the mean ± SEM; $n = 3$. *$P < 0.01$, **$P < 0.05$ vs. Chow + saline group or BSA group or siCON + PA group or Vector-PA group; #$P < 0.01$,##$P < 0.05$ vs. HFD + saline group or PA group or siCON + PA group or Vector-PA group; &$P < 0.01$, &&$P < 0.05$ vs. siCON + PA + LG group or Vector-PA + LG group.

by regulating genes that encode lysosome biogenesis- and lipolysis-related factors (Napolitano and Ballabio, 2016). Under nutrient-depleted conditions, TFEB was activated by an autoregulatory feedback loop and subsequently regulated cellular lipid catabolism (Settembre et al., 2013). Recent studies have revealed that TFEB nuclear translocation was promoted by pharmacologically activating the AMPK pathway and eventually alleviated hepatic steatosis in HFD-fed mice (Chen et al., 2019). In addition, TFEB regulated multiple steps of lipid metabolism, such as lipid recruitment and degradation, as well as fatty acid oxidation (Li et al., 2016; Evans et al., 2019). However, the exact influence of liraglutide on TFEB-mediated lysosomal biogenesis had not been studied previously. Our study firstly

revealed that liraglutide activated autophagic flux by inducing TFEB nuclear translocation and increasing the expression of its downstream targets CTSB and LAMP1. After silencing TFEB, the liraglutide-mediated promotion of lysosome biogenesis and alleviation of hepatic steatosis were attenuated. Moreover, we found that silencing of GLP-1R could mimic the effects TFEB downregulation in decreasing lysosome biogenesis, whereas its overexpression increased TFEB activation and the expression of its downstream targets CTSB and LAMP1, indicating that GLP-1R mediated the effect of liraglutide in promoting lysosome biogenesis. Therefore, we speculated that liraglutide activates the autophagy-lysosomal pathway to reduce hepatic lipid accumulation through GLP-1R-mediated TFEB activation.

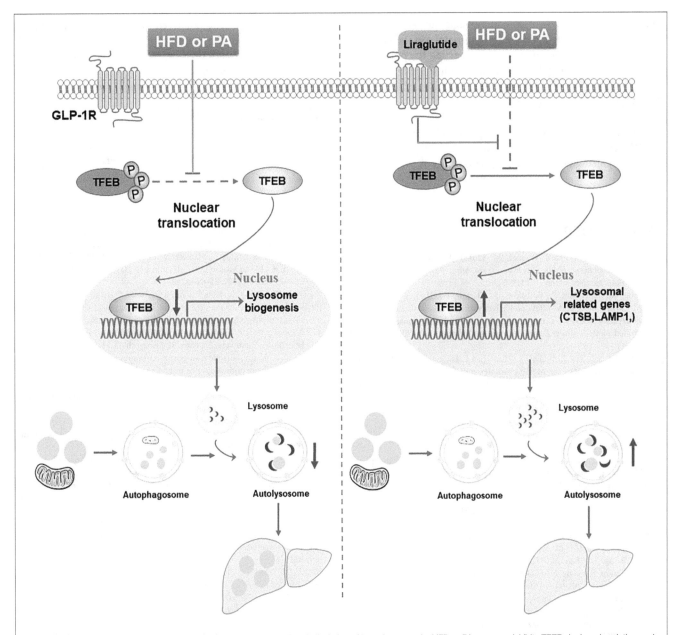

FIGURE 9 | Schematic diagram of the mechanism of liraglutide-mediated alleviation of hepatic steatosis. HFD or PA exposure inhibits TFEB dephosphorylation and nuclear translocation. TFEB regulates lysosomal biogenesis and function. The blocking of TFEB nuclear translocation leads to autophagic flux impairment and subsequently aggravates hepatic steatosis. Liraglutide, a GLP-1R agonist, alleviates hepatic steatosis through enhancing autophagic flux. Mechanistically, liraglutide activates TFEB and its downstream targets through activation of GLP-1R.

In response to nutrients, GLP-1RAs were also found to alleviate liver steatosis through the upregulation of SIRT1 expression, activating the AMPK pathway and inhibiting SREBP-1c expression (Xu et al., 2014). Moreover, data from recent studies demonstrated that AMPK/SIRT1 pathway activation could upregulate the expression of various autophagy-related genes (Song et al., 2015; Huang et al., 2017). For instance, SIRT1 deacetylation could induce autophagy in an autophagy protein 5-dependent manner (Sun et al., 2018). In the current work, we

found that liraglutide decreased SIRT1 expression in PA-treated primary mouse hepatocytes (**Supplementary Figure S4C**). However, the opposite results were observed in mice, which requires further investigation.

CONCLUSION

In conclusion, our study reveals that liraglutide attenuates hepatic steatosis via activation of autophagic flux, especially the GLP-1R-TFEB-mediated autophagy-lysosomal pathway. These findings provide a novel mechanism supporting the potential of GLP-1RAs as promising therapeutic agents for NAFLD.

ETHICS STATEMENT

The animal study was reviewed and approved by Animal Ethical and Welfare Committee of Shanghai Sixth People's Hospital Affiliated to Shanghai Jiao Tong University School.

JZ and JL collected and analyzed the data. YF interpreted the results and wrote the manuscript. LW and JY contributed to manuscript read and revision. All authors have read and approved the submitted version.

AUTHOR CONTRIBUTIONS

YF and LW designed the study. YF and LJ carried out the experimental work. CZ and YX assisted in performing research.

REFERENCES

Arab, J. P., Arrese, M., and Trauner, M. (2018). Recent insights into the pathogenesis of nonalcoholic fatty liver disease. *Annu. Rev. Pathol.* 13, 321–350. doi: 10.1146/annurev-pathol-020117-043617

Armstrong, M. J., Gaunt, P., Aithal, G. P., Barton, D., Hull, D., Parker, R., et al. (2016). Liraglutide safety and efficacy in patients with non-alcoholic steatohepatitis (LEAN): a multicentre, double-blind, randomised, placebo-controlled phase 2 study. *Lancet* 387, 679–690. doi: 10.1016/S0140-6736(15)00803-X

Chang, X., Yan, H., Fei, J., Jiang, M., Zhu, H., Lu, D., et al. (2010). Berberine reduces methylation of the MTTP promoter and alleviates fatty liver induced by a high-fat diet in rats. *J. Lipid Res.* 51, 2504–2515. doi: 10.1194/jlr.M001958

Chao, X., Ni, H. M., and Ding, W. X. (2018a). Insufficient autophagy: a novel autophagic flux scenario uncovered by impaired liver TFEB-mediated lysosomal biogenesis from chronic alcohol-drinking mice. *Autophagy* 14, 1646–1648. doi: 10.1080/15548627.2018.1489170

Chao, X., Wang, S., Zhao, K., Li, Y., Williams, J. A., Li, T., et al. (2018b). Impaired TFEB-mediated lysosome biogenesis and autophagy promote chronic ethanol-induced liver injury and steatosis in mice. *Gastroenterology* 155, 865–879. doi: 10.1053/j.gastro.2018.05.027

Chen, X., Chan, H., Zhang, L., Liu, X., Ho, I., Zhang, X., et al. (2019). The phytochemical polydatin ameliorates non-alcoholic steatohepatitis by restoring lysosomal function and autophagic flux. *J. Cell. Mol. Med.* 23, 4290–4300. doi: 10.1111/jcmm.14320

Chu, Q., Zhang, S., Chen, M., Han, W., Jia, R., Chen, W., et al. (2019). Cherry Anthocyanins Regulate NAFLD by Promoting Autophagy Pathway. *Oxidat. Med. Cell. Longev.* 2019, 1–16. doi: 10.1155/2019/4825949

Cui, W., Sathyanarayan, A., Lopresti, M., Aghajan, M., Chen, C., and Mashek, D. G. (2020). Lipophagy-derived fatty acids undergo extracellular efflux via lysosomal exocytosis. *Autophagy* [Epub ahead of print]. doi: 10.1080/15548627.2020.1728097

Drucker, D. J. (2018). Mechanisms of action and therapeutic application of glucagon-like peptide-1. *Cell Metab.* 27, 740–756. doi: 10.1016/j.cmet.2018.03.001

Evans, T. D., Zhang, X., Jeong, S. J., He, A., Song, E., Bhattacharya, S., et al. (2019). TFEB drives PGC-1alpha expression in adipocytes to protect against diet-induced metabolic dysfunction. *Sci. Signal.* 12:eaau2281. doi: 10.1126/scisignal.aau2281

He, Q., Sha, S., Sun, L., Zhang, J., and Dong, M. (2016). GLP-1 analogue improves hepatic lipid accumulation by inducing autophagy via AMPK/mTOR pathway. *Biochem. Biophys. Res. Commun.* 476, 196–203. doi: 10.1016/j.bbrc.2016.05.086

Huang, Q., Wang, T., Yang, L., and Wang, H. Y. (2017). Ginsenoside rb2 alleviates hepatic lipid accumulation by restoring autophagy via induction of sirt1 and activation of AMPK. *Int. J. Mol. Sci.* 18:1063. doi: 10.3390/ijms18051063

Kalavalapalli, S., Bril, F., Guingab, J., Vergara, A., Garrett, T. J., Sunny, N. E., et al. (2019). Impact of exenatide on mitochondrial lipid metabolism in mice with nonalcoholic steatohepatitis. *J. Endocrinol.* 241, 293–305. doi: 10.1530/JOE-19-0007

Kanoski, S. E., Fortin, S. M., Arnold, M., Grill, H. J., and Hayes, M. R. (2011). Peripheral and central GLP-1 receptor populations mediate the anorectic effects of peripherally administered GLP-1 receptor agonists, liraglutide and exendin-4. *Endocrinology* 152, 3103–3112. doi: 10.1210/en.2011-0174

Klaunig, J. E., Goldblatt, P. J., Hinton, D. E., Lipsky, M. M., Chacko, J., and Trump, B. F. (1981). Mouse liver cell culture. I. Hepatocyte isolation. *In Vitro* 17, 913–925. doi: 10.1007/BF02618288

Li, X., Zhang, X., Zheng, L., Kou, J., Zhong, Z., Jiang, Y., et al. (2016). Hypericin-mediated sonodynamic therapy induces autophagy and decreases lipids in THP-1 macrophage by promoting ROS-dependent nuclear translocation of TFEB. *Cell Death Dis.* 7:e2527. doi: 10.1038/cddis.2016.433

Lyu, J., Imachi, H., Fukunaga, K., Sato, S., Kobayashi, T., Dong, T., et al. (2020). Role of ATP-binding cassette transporter A1 in suppressing lipid accumulation by glucagon-like peptide-1 agonist in hepatocytes. *Mol. Metab.* 34, 16–26. doi: 10.1016/j.molmet.2019.12.015

Mantovani, A., Byrne, C. D., Scorletti, E., Mantzoros, C. S., and Targher, G. (2020). Efficacy and safety of anti-hyperglycaemic drugs in patients with non-alcoholic fatty liver disease with or without diabetes: an updated systematic review of randomized controlled trials. *Diabetes Metab.* [Epub ahead of print]. doi: 10.1016/j.diabet.2019.12.007

Martinez-Lopez, N., and Singh, R. (2015). Autophagy and lipid droplets in the liver. *Annu. Rev. Nutr.* 35, 215–237. doi: 10.1146/annurev-nutr-071813-105336

Medina, D. L., Fraldi, A., Bouche, V., Annunziata, F., Mansueto, G., Spampanato, C., et al. (2011). Transcriptional activation of lysosomal exocytosis promotes cellular clearance. *Dev. Cell.* 21, 421–430. doi: 10.1016/j.devcel.2011.07.016

Miyagawa, K., Oe, S., Honma, Y., Izumi, H., Baba, R., and Harada, M. (2016). Lipid-induced endoplasmic reticulum stress impairs selective autophagy at the step of autophagosome-lysosome fusion in hepatocytes. *Am. J. Pathol.* 186, 1861–1873. doi: 10.1016/j.ajpath.2016.03.003

Muller, T. D., Finan, B., Bloom, S. R., D'Alessio, D., Drucker, D. J., Flatt, P. R., et al. (2019). Glucagon-like peptide 1 (GLP-1). *Mol. Metab.* 30, 72–130. doi: 10.1016/j.molmet.2019.09.010

Napolitano, G., and Ballabio, A. (2016). TFEB at a glance. *J. Cell. Sci.* 129, 2475–2481. doi: 10.1242/jcs.146365

Petit, J. M., Cercueil, J. P., Loffroy, R., Denimal, D., Bouillet, B., Fourmont, C., et al. (2017). Effect of liraglutide therapy on liver fat content in patients with inadequately controlled type 2 diabetes: the Lira-NAFLD study. *J. Clin. Endocrinol. Metab.* 102, 407–415. doi: 10.1210/jc.2016-2775

Pi, H., Liu, M., Xi, Y., Chen, M., Tian, L., Xie, J., et al. (2019). Long-term exercise prevents hepatic steatosis: a novel role of FABP1 in regulation of autophagy-lysosomal machinery. *FASEB J.* 33, 11870–11883. doi: 10.1096/fj.201900812R

Seglen, P. O. (1976). Preparation of isolated rat liver cells. *Methods Cell Biol.* 13, 29–83. doi: 10.1016/s0091-679x(08)61797-5

Settembre, C., De Cegli, R., Mansueto, G., Saha, P. K., Vetrini, F., Visvikis, O., et al. (2013). TFEB controls cellular lipid metabolism through a starvation-induced autoregulatory loop. *Nat. Cell. Biol.* 15, 647–658. doi: 10.1038/ncb2718

Sharma, S., Mells, J. E., Fu, P. P., Saxena, N. K., and Anania, F. A. (2011). GLP-1 analogs reduce hepatocyte steatosis and improve survival by enhancing the unfolded protein response and promoting macroautophagy. *PLoS One* 6:e25269. doi: 10.1371/journal.pone.0025269

Singh, R., Kaushik, S., Wang, Y., Xiang, Y., Novak, I., Komatsu, M., et al. (2009). Autophagy regulates lipid metabolism. *Nature* 458, 1131–1135. doi: 10.1038/nature07976

Sinha, R. A., Farah, B. L., Singh, B. K., Siddique, M. M., Li, Y., Wu, Y., et al. (2014). Caffeine stimulates hepatic lipid metabolism by the autophagy-lysosomal pathway in mice. *Hepatology* 59, 1366–1380. doi: 10.1002/hep.26667

Song, Y. M., Lee, Y. H., Kim, J. W., Ham, D. S., Kang, E. S., Cha, B. S., et al. (2015). Metformin alleviates hepatosteatosis by restoring SIRT1-mediated autophagy induction via an AMP-activated protein kinase-independent pathway. *Autophagy* 11, 46–59. doi: 10.4161/15548627.2014.984271

Su, H., Li, Y., Hu, D., Xie, L., Ke, H., Zheng, X., et al. (2018). Procyanidin B2 ameliorates free fatty acids-induced hepatic steatosis through regulating TFEB-mediated lysosomal pathway and redox state. *Free Radic. Biol. Med.* 126, 269–286. doi: 10.1016/j.freeradbiomed.2018.08.024

Sun, Y., Xia, M., Yan, H., Han, Y., Zhang, F., Hu, Z., et al. (2018). Berberine attenuates hepatic steatosis and enhances energy expenditure in mice by inducing autophagy and fibroblast growth factor 21. *Br. J. Pharmacol.* 175, 374–387. doi: 10.1111/bph.14079

Tong, W., Ju, L., Qiu, M., Xie, Q., Chen, Y., Shen, W., et al. (2016). Liraglutide ameliorates non-alcoholic fatty liver disease by enhancing mitochondrial architecture and promoting autophagy through the SIRT1/SIRT3-FOXO3a pathway. *Hepatol. Res.* 46, 933–943. doi: 10.1111/hepr.12634

Vernon, G., Baranova, A., and Younossi, Z. M. (2011). Systematic review: the epidemiology and natural history of non-alcoholic fatty liver disease and non-alcoholic steatohepatitis in adults. *Aliment. Pharmacol. Ther.* 34, 274–285. doi: 10.1111/j.1365-2036.2011.04724.x

Wang, Y., Zhao, H., Li, X., Wang, Q., Yan, M., Zhang, H., et al. (2019). Formononetin alleviates hepatic steatosis by facilitating TFEB-mediated lysosome biogenesis and lipophagy. *J. Nutr. Biochem.* 73:108214. doi: 10.1016/j.jnutbio.2019.07.005

Wei, Q., Li, L., Chen, J. A., Wang, S. H., and Sun, Z. L. (2015). Exendin-4 improves thermogenic capacity by regulating fat metabolism on brown adipose tissue in mice with diet-induced obesity. *Ann. Clin. Lab. Sci.* 45, 158–165.

Wu, K., Zhao, T., Hogstrand, C., Xu, Y., Ling, S., Chen, G., et al. (2020). FXR-mediated inhibition of autophagy contributes to FA-induced TG accumulation and accordingly reduces FA-induced lipotoxicity. *Cell Commun. Signal.* 18:47. doi: 10.1186/s12964-020-0525-1

Wu, Y. R., Shi, X. Y., Ma, C. Y., Zhang, Y., Xu, R. X., and Li, J. J. (2019). Liraglutide improves lipid metabolism by enhancing cholesterol efflux associated with ABCA1 and ERK1/2 pathway. *Cardiovasc. Diabetol.* 18:146. doi: 10.1186/s12933-019-0954-6

Xu, F., Li, Z., Zheng, X., Liu, H., Liang, H., Xu, H., et al. (2014). SIRT1 mediates the effect of GLP-1 receptor agonist exenatide on ameliorating hepatic steatosis. *Diabetes* 63, 3637–3646. doi: 10.2337/db14-0263

Xu, F., Lin, B., Zheng, X., Chen, Z., Cao, H., Xu, H., et al. (2016). GLP-1 receptor agonist promotes brown remodelling in mouse white adipose tissue through SIRT1. *Diabetologia* 59, 1059–1069. doi: 10.1007/s00125-016-3896-5

Yang, Z., and Klionsky, D. J. (2010). Mammalian autophagy: core molecular machinery and signaling regulation. *Curr. Opin. Cell Biol.* 22, 124–131. doi: 10.1016/j.ceb.2009.11.014

Yu, X., Hao, M., Liu, Y., Ma, X., Lin, W., Xu, Q., et al. (2019). Liraglutide ameliorates non-alcoholic steatohepatitis by inhibiting NLRP3 inflammasome and pyroptosis activation via mitophagy. *Eur. J. Pharmacol.* 864:172715. doi: 10.1016/j.ejphar.2019.172715

Zhang, H., Yan, S., Khambu, B., Ma, F., Li, Y., Chen, X., et al. (2018). Dynamic MTORC1-TFEB feedback signaling regulates hepatic autophagy, steatosis and liver injury in long-term nutrient oversupply. *Autophagy* 14, 1779–1795. doi: 10.1080/15548627.2018.1490850

Zheng, X., Xu, F., Liang, H., Cao, H., Cai, M., Xu, W., et al. (2017). SIRT1/HSF1/HSP pathway is essential for exenatide-alleviated, lipid-induced hepatic endoplasmic reticulum stress. *Hepatology* 66, 809–824. doi: 10.1002/hep.29238

Zhou, J. Y., Poudel, A., Welchko, R., Mekala, N., Chandramani-Shivalingappa, P., Rosca, M. G., et al. (2019). Liraglutide improves insulin sensitivity in high fat diet induced diabetic mice through multiple pathways. *Eur. J. Pharmacol.* 861:172594. doi: 10.1016/j.ejphar.2019.172594

7

Relationship Between Autophagy and Metabolic Syndrome Characteristics in the Pathogenesis of Atherosclerosis

Jing Xu[1,2], Munehiro Kitada[1,3]*, Yoshio Ogura[1] and Daisuke Koya[1,3]

[1] Department of Diabetology and Endocrinology, Kanazawa Medical University, Uchinada, Japan, [2] Department of Endocrinology and Metabolism, The Affiliated Hospital of Guizhou Medical University, Guiyang, China, [3] Division of Anticipatory Molecular Food Science and Technology, Medical Research Institute, Kanazawa Medical University, Uchinada, Japan

*Correspondence:
Munehiro Kitada
kitta@kanazawa-med.ac.jp

Atherosclerosis is the main cause of mortality in metabolic-related diseases, including cardiovascular disease and type 2 diabetes (T2DM). Atherosclerosis is characterized by lipid accumulation and increased inflammatory cytokines in the vascular wall, endothelial cell and vascular smooth muscle cell dysfunction and foam cell formation initiated by monocytes/macrophages. The characteristics of metabolic syndrome (MetS), including obesity, glucose intolerance, dyslipidemia and hypertension, may activate multiple mechanisms, such as insulin resistance, oxidative stress and inflammatory pathways, thereby contributing to increased risks of developing atherosclerosis and T2DM. Autophagy is a lysosomal degradation process that plays an important role in maintaining cellular metabolic homeostasis. Increasing evidence indicates that impaired autophagy induced by MetS is related to oxidative stress, inflammation, and foam cell formation, further promoting atherosclerosis. Basal and mild adaptive autophagy protect against the progression of atherosclerotic plaques, while excessive autophagy activation leads to cell death, plaque instability or even plaque rupture. Therefore, autophagic homeostasis is essential for the development and outcome of atherosclerosis. Here, we discuss the potential role of autophagy and metabolic syndrome in the pathophysiologic mechanisms of atherosclerosis and potential therapeutic drugs that target these molecular mechanisms.

Keywords: autophagy, inflammation, oxidative stress, atherosclerosis, metabolic syndrome, type 2 diabetes

INTRODUCTION

Atherosclerosis is the main cause of mortality and morbidity in metabolic-related diseases, including cardiovascular disease (CVD) and type 2 diabetes mellitus (T2DM) (Weber and Noels, 2011; Barquera et al., 2015; Schneider et al., 2016). The formation of atherosclerotic plaques is divided into four stages: fatty streaks, atheromatous plaques, complicated atheromatous plaques and clinical complications (Hassanpour et al., 2019). Rupture of plaques may lead to an acute occlusion of artery, myocardial infarction or stroke. Three types of cells, endothelial cells (ECs), vascular smooth muscle cells (VSMCs) and monocytes/macrophages, participate in the development of plaques. Lipids and multiple inflammatory cytokines accumulate in the vascular wall. Monocytes migrate to the endothelium of blood vessels, enter into the inner membrane then proliferate and differentiate into macrophages. In this process, monocytes combine with lipoproteins to form foam cells. In smooth muscle cells (SMCs), with the secretion of fibrous elements, the accumulation of fatty streaks and the production of extracellular matrix, plaques develop and increase in size gradually. When macrophages and SMCs die, the necrotic core of the lesion rich in lipid will be formed. Meanwhile, matrix metalloproteinases and neovascularization secreted by macrophages weaken the stability of fibrous plaques. Once plaque rupture, the recruitment of platelets will be initiated to form thrombus (Lusis, 2000; Glass and Witztum, 2001; Hassanpour et al., 2019).

Metabolic syndrome (MetS) is defined as a series of chronic metabolic disorders. Although the details and criteria of the definition differ among different associations, such as the World Health Organization (WHO) (Alberti and Zimmet, 1998), the European Group for the Study of Insulin Resistance (EGIR) (Balkau and Charles, 1999), the National Cholesterol Education Program's Adult Treatment Panel III (NCEP: ATP III) (Expert Panel on Detection et al., 2001) and the International Diabetes Federation (IDF) (Alberti et al., 2006), the essential characteristics include obesity, glucose intolerance, dyslipidemia and hypertension (Eckel et al., 2005; McCracken et al., 2018) (**Table 1**). These characteristics of MetS may contribute to insulin resistance, oxidative stress, inflammation and endothelial dysfunction, which are pivotal mechanisms associated with the pathogenesis of atherosclerosis. Therefore, the regulation of MetS is essential for preventing the progression of atherosclerosis.

Autophagy is a lysosomal degradation process that plays an important role in maintaining cellular metabolic homeostasis. Previous studies have demonstrated that impaired autophagy is associated with metabolic disorders such as T2DM and MetS via inflammatory pathways and various metabolic stresses (Xu et al., 2016; Kitada et al., 2017; Turkmen, 2017). Autophagy exerts both protective and detrimental effects on cardiovascular disorders. In the progression of atherosclerotic plaques, basal and adaptive autophagy may reduce oxidative stress, inflammation and lipid accumulation and delay the formation of plaques. However, excessive autophagy may cause cell death and plaque instability (Kitada et al., 2016; Luo et al., 2016; Zhu et al., 2017). Therefore, maintaining autophagic homeostasis in cells may be a therapeutic strategy for the treatment of atherosclerosis.

In this review, we discuss the role of autophagy and MetS characteristics in the pathogenesis of atherosclerosis and potential therapeutic drugs that target these molecular mechanisms.

METABOLIC SYNDROME CHARACTERISTICS AND THE FORMATION OF ATHEROSCLEROTIC PLAQUES

The prevalence of MetS is increasing worldwide. In the nearly an decade from 2003 to 2012, the overall prevalence of MetS increased by 1.2% (from 32.9 to 34.7%) in the United States based on the NCEP: ATP III criterion (Aguilar et al., 2015). According to a systematic review summarizing 18 studies, despite differences in methodology, diagnostic criteria and the ages of subjects, nearly 1/5th of the adult population or more are affected by MetS, with a particular increase in prevalence in the Asia-Pacific region (Ranasinghe et al., 2017). A cross-sectional study involving 109,551 Chinese adults showed that MetS was closely related to CVD, especially when MetS was defined by the NCEP: ATP III criteria (Li et al., 2019). The characteristics of MetS, including obesity, glucose intolerance, dyslipidemia and hypertension, may contribute to insulin resistance/hyperinsulinemia, the activation of oxidative stress, the accumulation of proinflammatory cytokines, endothelial dysfunction and other pathological mechanisms. These changes may lead to the pathogenesis of atherosclerosis (Eckel et al., 2005).

Obesity

Obesity is a chronic inflammatory disorder characterized by the accumulation of both visceral and subcutaneous fat. Mechanisms of obesity-induced atherosclerosis may involve insulin resistance, an imbalance of adipokines, oxidative stress, inflammation and endothelial dysfunction (Nigro et al., 2006; Lovren et al., 2015) (**Figure 1A**).

Insulin signaling plays a pivotal role in activating nitric oxide (NO), a vasodilator and antiatherogenic agent, to maintain endothelial function (Zeng and Quon, 1996; Zeng et al., 2000). Typically, insulin binds to the insulin receptor, resulting in tyrosine phosphorylation of insulin receptor substrate-1/2 (IRS-1/IRS-2) and the activation of phosphatidylinositol 3-kinase (PI3K) and protein kinase B (Akt), subsequently augmenting glucose transport and other metabolic processes (Di Pino and DeFronzo, 2019). The administration of endothelin-1 (ET-1), a vasoconstrictor, leads to insulin resistance, as characterized by a decrease in IRS-1 protein levels and suppressed PI3K/Akt activation in rat skeletal muscle (Wilkes et al., 2003) and adipocytes (Ishibashi et al., 2001), further promoting increased vasoconstriction and atherogenesis. In obese conditions, adipose tissue, liver, and skeletal muscle are considered key organs associated with insulin resistance (McArdle et al., 2013). Circulating free fatty acids (FFAs) are released from adipose tissue. In the liver, FFAs increase the production of hepatic glucose and triglycerides (TGs) and induce the secretion of very low-density lipoproteins (VLDLs), which are atherogenic. In skeletal muscle, FFAs reduce insulin sensitivity by inhibiting PI3K activation. Increasing FFAs induces pancreatic insulin secretion, resulting in compensatory hyperinsulinemia and exacerbating insulin resistance (Eckel et al., 2005; McCracken et al., 2018). Moreover, FFA-induced hyperinsulinemia stimulates the mitogen-activated protein kinase (MAPK) pathway and increases reactive oxygen species (ROS) levels and proinflammatory and prothrombotic mediator production via nicotinamide adenine dinucleotide phosphate (NADPH) oxidase stimulation, linking insulin resistance, oxidative stress and inflammation (Satish et al., 2019).

Adipose tissue is the main source of anti-inflammatory and proinflammatory adipokines. Imbalances in these adipokines may contribute to insulin resistance and endothelial dysfunction,

TABLE 1 | Definitions of metabolic syndrome.

Characteristics	WHO 1999	EGIR 1999	NCEP: ATP III 2001	IDF 2006
Basic elements	Glucose intolerance, IGT or diabetes mellitus and/or insulin resistance **plus 2 or more of the following**:	Plasma insulin concentration >75th percentile of non-diabetic patients **plus 2 or more of the following:**	**3 or more of the following:**	Central obesity **plus any 2 of the following:**
Obesity	Waist-to-hip ratio of 0.90 (men) or 0.85 (women) and/or BMI > 30 kg/m^2	Waist circumference > 94 cm (men) or 80 cm (women)	Waist circumference > 102 cm (men) or 88 cm (women)	Waist circumference* (ethnicity specific) or BMI > 30 kg/m^2
Fasting plasma glucose	Impaired fasting glucose	≥6.1 mmol/l (110 mg/dl) but non-diabetic	≥5.6 mmol/l (100 mg/dl)	≥5.6 mmol/l (100 mg/dl) or previously diagnosed T2DM
Dyslipidemia	TG ≥ 1.7 mmol/l (150 mg/dl); HDL-C < 0.9 mmol/l (35 mg/dl) (men) or <1.0 mmol/l (39 mg/dl) (women)	TG ≥ 1.7 mmol/l (150 mg/dl) or on treatment; HDL-C < 1.0 mmol/l (39 mg/dl) (men and women)	TG ≥ 1.7 mmol/l (150 mg/dl) HDL-C < 1.7 mmol/l (40 mg/dl) (men); <1.29 mmol/l (50 mg/dl) (women)	TG ≥ 1.7 mmol/l (150 mg/dl) or on treatment HDL-C < 1.03 mmol/l (40 mg/dl) (men) of <1.29 mmol/l (50 mg/dl) (women) or on treatment
Hypertension	≥140/90 mmHg	≥140/90 mmHg	Systolic ≥ 130 mmHg or diastolic ≥ 85 mmHg	Systolic ≥ 130 mmHg or diastolic ≥ 85 mmHg or on treatment
Others	Urinary albumin excretion rate ≥ 20 μg/min or albumin/creatinine ≥ 20 mg/g			

*Waist circumference: for European populations, >94 cm (men) and >80 cm (women); for South Asian, Chinese and Japanese populations, >90 cm (men) and >80 cm (women); for ethnic South and Central American populations, use the South Asian data; and for sub-Saharan African, Eastern Mediterranean and Middle Eastern (Arab) populations, use the European data.

leading to atherosclerosis (Lovren et al., 2015). Previous research has shown that resistin, a proinflammatory adipokine, can induce the expression of inflammatory cytokines such as tumor necrosis factor-α (TNF-α) and interleukin-12 (IL-12) in macrophages in a nuclear factor-κB (NF-κB)-dependent manner to promote foam cell formation (Silswal et al., 2005). Moreover, resistin increases the expression of vascular cell adhesion molecule-1 (VCAM-1), monocyte chemoattractant protein (MCP-1) and ET-1 in ECs (Verma et al., 2003). These link resistin to obesity-induced atherosclerosis. Another important adipokine is leptin. Obese individuals exhibit enhanced circulating leptin levels but fail to increase energy expenditure and reduce food intake due to leptin resistance. Two mouse models are widely used to study diabetes- and obesity-associated atherosclerosis: ob/ob mice, which have a mutation in the leptin-encoding gene, and db/db mice, which encode the leptin receptor (Wu and Huan, 2007). Leptin can also stimulate the production of proinflammatory cytokines (Francisco et al., 2018). Adiponectin is an anti-inflammatory adipokine that can directly upregulate insulin sensitivity (Kadowaki et al., 2006; Yamauchi and Kadowaki, 2013). Adiponectin can directly stimulate the production of NO via PI3K-dependent pathways in ECs to mediate vasodilator actions (Chen et al., 2003). In ApoE$^{-/-}$ mice, adiponectin attenuated serum TC, TG and LDL-C levels induced by a high-fat diet, reduced the gene expression of TNF-α, interleukin-6 (IL-6), and VCAM-1, suppressed the activation of the NF-κB pathway, and ultimately inhibited the formation of atherosclerotic plaques (Wang et al., 2016). Another study showed that the association of adiponectin with T-cadherin can protect against neointima proliferation and atherosclerosis (Fujishima et al., 2017).

In both obese human and mouse models, elevated levels of FFAs and fat accumulation increase systemic oxidative stress (Furukawa et al., 2004; Hansel et al., 2004). Oxidative stress results from an imbalance between the production of ROS and antioxidant defenses (Le Lay et al., 2014). In obese mice and adipocytes, increased ROS production is due to an increase in NADPH oxidase. Treatment with NADPH oxidase inhibitors reduces ROS production (Hansel et al., 2004). Elevated ROS can induce nuclear translocation of the NF-κB p65 subunit, activating downstream inflammatory genes and increasing the expression of intercellular adhesion molecule-1 (ICAM-1) and VCAM-1 in ECs (Jayakumar et al., 2014; Medda et al., 2015). Another important oxidative biomolecule is oxidized low-density lipoprotein (oxLDL), which is also elevated in obese individuals (Srikanthan et al., 2016). Oxidation induced by oxLDL can activate IκB kinase (IKK)/NF-κB and c-Jun N-terminal kinase (JNK), leading to endothelial cell death and dysfunction, which contribute to the development of atherosclerosis (Valente et al., 2014).

Obesity is considered a chronic low-grade inflammation (Saltiel and Olefsky, 2017). Multiple inflammatory cytokines, such as TNF-α, IL-6 and C-reactive protein (CRP), are overproduced in adipose tissue, ECs and macrophages in obese humans and in mouse models (Wellen and Hotamisligil, 2005; Coelho et al., 2013). Chronic activation of the NF-κB pathway in ECs upregulates the levels of inflammation-related genes, such as ICAM-1, VCAM-1, and MCP-1, and proinflammatory cytokines, such as TNF-α, IL-6 and IL-1β, further leading to endothelial dysfunction (Kitada et al., 2016). In addition, inflammasome-mediated processes are important in the development of atherosclerosis (De Nardo and Latz, 2011; Lu and Kakkar, 2014). During obesity, the circulating FFAs palmitate and ceramide lead to the activation of the nucleotide-binding oligomerization domain-like receptor family pyrin domain containing 3 (NLRP3) inflammasome (De Nardo and Latz, 2011). Then, NLRP3 activates the production of the

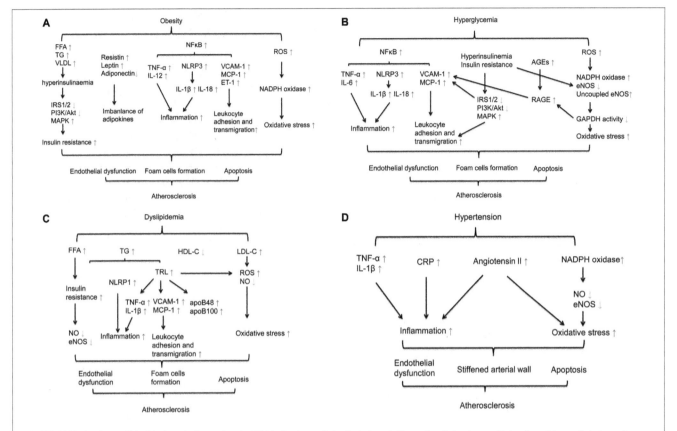

FIGURE 1 | Mechanisms of MetS-induced atherosclerosis. **(A)** Mechanisms of obesity-induced atherosclerosis involvement in insulin resistance, imbalanced adipokines, oxidative stress, and inflammation. **(B)** Mechanisms of hyperglycemia-induced atherosclerosis involvement in inflammation, insulin resistance, the activation of AGEs and oxidative stress. **(C)** Mechanisms of dyslipidemia-induced atherosclerosis involvement in insulin resistance, inflammation and oxidative stress. **(D)** Mechanisms of hypertension-induced atherosclerosis involvement in inflammation, the renin angiotensin system and oxidative stress.

mature forms of IL-1β and IL-18, which participate in insulin resistance (Stienstra et al., 2010; Vandanmagsar et al., 2011; Wen et al., 2011) and accelerate atherosclerotic progression (Satish and Agrawal, 2020).

Glucose Intolerance

Clinical studies have demonstrated that hyperglycemia is a major predictor of atherosclerosis in both diabetic and non-diabetic subjects (Zhang et al., 2006; Nagareddy et al., 2013; Gan et al., 2019). High glucose (HG) may damage arterial cells and play an important role in the progression of atherogenesis. The mechanisms of HG-induced atherosclerosis may involve interactions among insulin resistance, inflammation, advanced glycation end products (AGEs) and oxidative stress, ultimately leading to endothelial dysfunction (**Figure 1B**).

Insulin resistance is a characteristic feature of T2DM and is usually accompanied by compensatory hyperinsulinemia (Roden and Shulman, 2019). Under diabetic conditions, insulin signaling is impaired at the level of IRS-1, leading to decreased glucose transport and metabolism, impaired endothelial nitric oxide synthase (eNOS) activation and endothelial dysfunction. With increasing concentrations of glucose, the PI3K/Akt pathway is suppressed, leading to proliferative dysfunction in ECs (Varma et al., 2005). Moreover, the MAPK pathway

is activated by compensatory hyperinsulinemia, subsequently inducing the expression of VCAM-1 and monocyte adhesion. Insulin resistance suppresses the PI3K/Akt pathway and induces the MAPK pathway to promote endothelial dysfunction and proatherosclerotic events in ECs (Madonna et al., 2004; Di Pino and DeFronzo, 2019).

Another mechanism of HG-induced plaque formation involves activation of the inflammatory/inflammasome pathway. The endothelium is sensitive to changes in glucose concentrations. HG promotes leukocyte adhesion to endothelial cells, which is an initial step in atherogenesis. In human aortic endothelial cells, short-term HG incubation (no more than 12 h) may increase the levels of some adhesion molecules, such as VCAM-1 and MCP-1, via protein kinase C (PKC) and/or NF-κB pathway activation (Piga et al., 2007; Azcutia et al., 2010). These adhesion molecules facilitate monocyte adhesion to ECs, and monocytes differentiate into intimal macrophages and accelerate fatty streak formation. Moreover, monocytes incubated in HG exhibit increased expression of cytokines such as IL-1β and IL-6 (Dasu et al., 2007). NLRP3 inflammasome activation is elevated in type 2 diabetic patients (Lee et al., 2013; Chen et al., 2019) and diabetic rodent models (Luo et al., 2014; Hou et al., 2020). Excessive activation of NLRP3 is associated with cardiac inflammation (Luo et al., 2014). The NLRP3 inflammasome also promotes the secretion of mature IL-1β and IL-18 to initiate the recruitment of inflammatory cytokines, leading to atherothrombosis (Satish and Agrawal, 2020). NF-κB can promote the transcription of NLRP3, pro-IL-1β, and pro-IL-18 in the vascular endothelial cells of diabetic rats. Inhibition of NF-κB reduces activation of the NLRP3 inflammasome and mature IL-1β in HG-treated H9c2 cells, which are heart myoblasts, ameliorating cardiac inflammation, apoptosis and fibrosis (Luo et al., 2014).

HG-induced AGEs are also key proatherogenic mediators in diabetes (Bornfeldt and Tabas, 2011). AGE-modified proteins and lipoproteins can bind to and activate their receptors, such as receptor for AGEs (RAGE). RAGE is expressed in ECs and promotes VCAM-1 expression (Harja et al., 2009). Deletion of RAGE attenuates leukocyte recruitment and protects against atherosclerosis by reducing oxidative stress and decreasing the expression of proinflammatory markers, including NF-κB p65, VCAM-1, and MCP-1, in diabetic ApoE$^{(-/-)}$ mice (Soro-Paavonen et al., 2008).

HG-mediated oxidative stress has been shown to accelerate the progression of atherosclerosis (Giacco and Brownlee, 2010; Katakami, 2018). In the context of diabetes, mitochondria exhibit increased ROS production due to impaired electron transport and ROS scavenging (Xu J. et al., 2020). In mitochondria, ROS activate NADPH oxidases, uncouple eNOS, amplify the production of ROS and reduce GAPDH activity. Inhibition of GAPDH activity increases the expression of RAGE and activates the PKC pathway, which links oxidative stress, RAGE and inflammation and contributes to atherosclerosis (Schaffer et al., 2012; Shah and Brownlee, 2016).

Dyslipidemia

Dyslipidemia in MetS is closely related to obesity and is characterized by hypertriglyceridemia, low levels of high-density lipoprotein cholesterol (HDL-C) and high levels of low-density lipoprotein cholesterol (LDL-C) (Eckel et al., 2005). Accumulating evidence has demonstrated that hypertriglyceridemia is strongly associated with increased risk of atherosclerosis (Do et al., 2013; Jørgensen et al., 2013; Thomsen et al., 2014). The accumulation of toxic lipid metabolites in muscle, liver, adipocytes and arterial tissues contributes to insulin resistance and endothelial dysfunction and accelerates atherosclerosis. With increases in circulating FFAs released from adipose tissue and transported into the liver, hepatic TG synthesis increases. Hypertriglyceridemia is also a reflection of insulin resistance (Eckel et al., 2005). TG-rich lipoproteins (TRLs) of hepatic origin, such as apolipoprotein B (apoB) 48 and apoB 100, are related to atherosclerosis and are found in plaques (Pal et al., 2003). Dyslipidemia-induced atherosclerosis may be related to multiple mechanisms, including insulin resistance (as mentioned in the obesity section), elevated ROS, and inflammation, leading to endothelial dysfunction (Peng et al., 2017).

Endogenous NO is a signaling molecule that has antiatherosclerotic effects. NO inhibition by excess ROS is the main cause of endothelial dysfunction (Higashi et al., 2009; Bruno et al., 2018). FFAs and TRLs can stimulate intracellular ROS production and cause cellular injury and death in human aortic endothelial cells (Wang et al., 2009). TG accumulation is also related to macrophage oxidative stress, which elevates mitochondrial ROS generation, further promoting foam cell formation (Rosenblat et al., 2012).

Multiple studies have suggested that oxidized FFAs stimulate inflammatory cytokines (Wang et al., 2009; Gower et al., 2011). TRLs upregulate the endothelial expression of ICAM-1 and VCAM-1, facilitate the monocyte infiltration and enhance the endothelial inflammation (Wang et al., 2013). TRL remnants can induce endothelial cell apoptosis and vascular injury by increasing the secretion of cytokines such as IL-1β and TNF-α (Shin et al., 2004). Elevated TG and VLDL were related to arterial inflammation through the NLRP1 inflammasome activation in ECs (Bleda et al., 2016). Low HDL-C is closely related to oxidative stress and insulin resistance (Hansel et al., 2004), which results in endothelial dysfunction through lipotoxicity (Satish et al., 2019) (**Figure 1C**).

Hypertension

Blood pressure (BP) levels are strongly correlated with visceral obesity and insulin resistance (Aboonabi et al., 2019). Under insulin resistance/hyperinsulinemia, ET-1 can suppress insulin-induced Akt activation in VSMCs to exacerbate the development of hypertension and atherosclerosis (Lin et al., 2015). Increased systolic BP levels may stiffen the arterial wall and accelerate the progression of atherosclerosis (Mulè et al., 2014; Aboonabi et al., 2019). Hypertension is associated with oxidative stress, increased NADPH oxidase activity, the inactivation of NO, and the downregulation of NO synthase (NOS) isoforms, leading to endothelial dysfunction (Furukawa et al., 2004). Inflammatory cytokines are also pivotal mediators. Increased serum levels of CRP (Sesso et al., 2003), monocyte TNF-α secretion, and serum IL-6 concentrations were reported in patients with hypertension, suggesting a close association between inflammation and hypertension. Moreover, the renin angiotensin system (RAS) plays a major physiological role in endothelial dysfunction and vascular inflammation (Montezano et al., 2014). Studies have demonstrated that angiotensin (Ang) II accelerates the development of atherosclerosis in apoE$^{-/-}$ mice (Daugherty et al., 2000; Weiss et al., 2001). An *in vitro* study also showed that Ang II can induce oxidative stress, inflammation and mitochondrial damage in human umbilical vein endothelial cells (HUVECs), leading to apoptosis and endothelial cell senescence (Dang et al., 2018) (**Figure 1D**).

AUTOPHAGY IN ATHEROSCLEROSIS

Autophagy is a cellular pathway involved in protein and organelle degradation to maintain cellular metabolic homeostasis (Mizushima et al., 2008). Autophagic dysfunction is closely associated with cancer, neurodegeneration and aging-related diseases such as obesity, diabetes and cardiovascular disorders (Mizushima et al., 2008; Rubinsztein et al., 2011; Kobayashi and Liang, 2015; Kitada et al., 2017). The role of autophagy in atherosclerosis is controversial. On one hand, multiple studies have demonstrated a protective effect of maintaining basal autophagy in atherosclerosis (Kim and Lee, 2014; Nussenzweig et al., 2015; Kim et al., 2018). Characteristics of MetS contribute to impaired autophagy, leading to accumulation of cytotoxic aggregates, dysfunctional organelles (Zhang et al., 2018) and present within the atherosclerotic plaque (Lavandero et al., 2015). Drugs targeting mammalian target of rapamycin (mTOR) signaling showed an effect of stabilizing plaques via repairing impaired autophagy (Ma et al., 2016). On the other hand, although autophagy is critical for maintaining cellular homeostasis under various stress conditions, excessive autophagy may induce autophagy-dependent cell death (Liu and Levine, 2015). MetS-induced reactive ROS, oxidized lipids and inflammation seem to be related to impaired or excessive autophagy activation, contributing to damage to the vascular wall and the development of atherosclerosis.

Regulatory Mechanisms of Autophagy

Autophagy occurs at a basal level and is highly inducible by starvation and other stresses to increase the number of autophagosomes. Autophagosomes enclose misfolded proteins or damaged organelles and then fuse with lysosomes to form autophagolysosomes (Mizushima and Komatsu, 2011). During these processes, multiple autophagy-related genes (Atgs) and proteins are involved (Gatica et al., 2015). Atg1 and microtubule-associated protein 1A/1B-light chain 3 (LC3) are widely regarded as critical markers of autophagy initiation. The conversion of LC3-I to LC3-II causes the formation of autophagolysosomes, and nucleoporin p62 (p62) facilitates the docking of cargo to the cell membrane (Nussenzweig et al., 2015; Hassanpour et al., 2019). The regulatory mechanism of autophagy is closely related to nutritional status. Under conditions of overnutrition or the effects of insulin, class I PI3K is induced to activate mTOR and mTOR complex 1 (mTORC1), thus inhibiting the activation of Atg1. In conditions of nutrient insufficiency, the Class III PI3K-beclin1 complex is triggered to promote the assembly of the Atg12-Atg5-Atg16L complex and Atg8/LC3 and then stimulate autophagosome formation (Shao et al., 2016). In the pathogenesis of atherosclerosis, cavelin-1, a marker protein for caveolar organelles, is involved in the regulation of autophagy. After the formation of phagophore through both mTOR and PI3K pathways, the complex of phagophore and Atg5-Atg12-Atg16 combine with caveolin-1, then interact with LC3 to promote autophagosome formation and facilitate caveolin-1 degradation (Hou et al., 2021). Caveloin-1 deficiency showed elevated Atg7, beclin1 and LC3-II, which indicated an increasing of autophagic activity and atheroprotection (Wu Z. et al., 2019). Characteristics of MetS including glucose (Bai et al., 2020) and dyslipidemia (Chen et al., 2018) inhibited the formation of autophagosomes via activating caveolin-1. Therefore, autophagy may have a close association with the characteristics of MetS and play a key role in the pathogenesis of atherosclerosis (**Figure 2A**).

Autophagy in ECs

Endothelial cells are an effective, permeable barrier between circulating blood and tissues (Zhu et al., 2017). MetS-induced autophagy dysregulation has been identified as a critical factor in endothelial dysfunction and atherosclerosis.

LDL can suppress endothelial autophagy by activating the PI3K/Akt/mTOR pathway in ECs (Zhu L. et al., 2019). In addition, ox-LDL can inhibit autophagic flux by suppressing the Sirtuin 1 (SIRT 1)/forkhead box protein O1 (FoxO1) pathway to promote apoptosis and adhesion molecule expression in ECs (Wang et al., 2019; Wu Q. et al., 2019). A previous study showed that basal autophagy in ECs induced endothelial eNOS expression and NO bioavailability to maintain endothelial function (Fetterman et al., 2016). Autophagy decreases oxidative stress and inhibits the expression of inflammatory cytokines, including MCP-1 and IL-8. Moreover, inefficient autophagy promotes inflammation and apoptosis and contributes to the development of atherosclerotic plaques in ECs. Impaired autophagy (via Atg3 siRNA) suppresses eNOS phosphorylation and NO production and induces ROS accumulation and inflammatory cytokine production (Bharath et al., 2014). Our previous study also showed that autophagy defects in ECs induced IL-6-dependent endothelial-to-mesenchymal transition and organ fibrosis (Takagaki et al., 2020). High glucose-induced caveolin-1 enhanced LDL transcytosis via autophagic degradation pathway (Bai et al., 2020) and attenuated autophagic flux in response to proatherogenic cytokines (Zhang X. et al., 2020), while caveolin-1 silencing induced autophagy in Human ECs (Bai et al., 2020). This evidence indicates that basal autophagy is a key regulator of oxidant-antioxidant balance and inflammatory-anti-inflammatory balance in ECs.

However, excessive autophagy may mediate cell death in ECs and lead to plaque instability (Martinet and De Meyer, 2009). A previous study indicated that elevated ROS generation caused by oxLDL could induce excessive autophagy characterized by increases in LC3, beclin-1 and Atg5 and apoptosis in ECs, which is a proatherosclerotic characteristic (Ding et al., 2012). Additionally, other research showed that elevated ROS (Shen et al., 2013) and oxLDL (Peng et al., 2014) initiated autophagy in human ECs in an atherosclerotic environment (**Figure 2B**).

Autophagy in VSMCs

Abnormalities, death and proliferation in VSMCs participate in the formation and instability of atherosclerotic plaques (Zhang Y. Y. et al., 2020), even lead to vascular neointimal hyperplasia, a central pathogenetic event of post-percutaneous coronary intervention (PCI) restenosis (Zhu and Zhang, 2018). Autophagy is crucial for VSMC function, survival and the development of neointimal hyperplasia in post-PCI restenosis (Zhu and Zhang, 2018). The deficiency of autophagy in VSMCs accelerates cell senescence and promotes diet-induced atherogenesis (Grootaert et al., 2015). The characteristics of MetS have complicated effects on autophagic activity in VSMCs. Previous studies demonstrated that atherosclerotic lesions were markedly increased in high-fat diet-fed ApoE$^{-/-}$ mice and mice with VSMC-specific Atg7 deletion compared with ApoE$^{-/-}$ control mice (Masuyama et al., 2018; Osonoi et al., 2018; Nahapetyan et al., 2019). Modest concentrations of oxLDL (10–40 μg/ml) (Ding et al., 2013) and excess free cholesterol (Xu et al., 2010) enhanced autophagy in VSMCs, as characterized by elevated levels of beclin-1, LC3-II, and

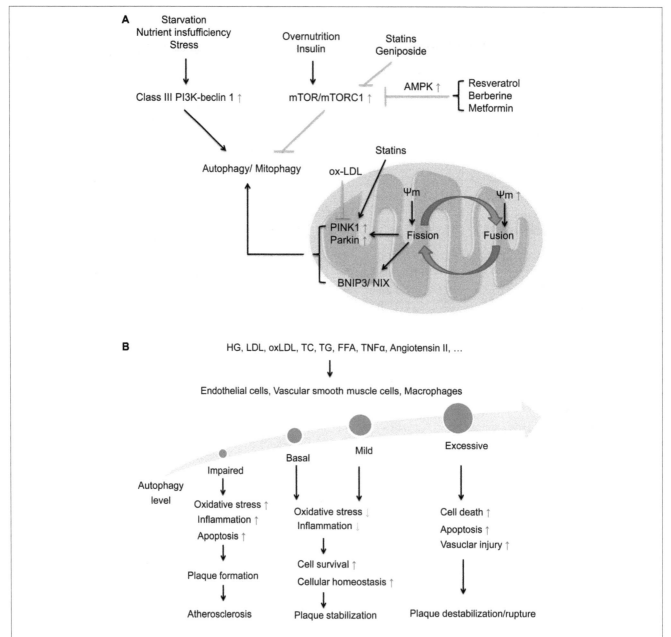

FIGURE 2 | Regulation of autophagy and autophagy levels in different types of cells involved in the progression of atherosclerosis. **(A)** Regulation of autophagy in different states via two major signaling pathways: the inductive pathway mediated by Class-III PI3K-beclin1 signaling and the inhibitory pathway mediated by Class I PI3K-mTOR signaling. Some compounds, such as resveratrol, berberine, metformin, statins and geniposide, may activate autophagy by suppressing the mTOR signaling pathway. Damaged mitochondria are eliminated by mitophagy through the accumulation of PINK1/Parkin pathway and BNIP3/NIX pathway on the mitochondrial surface. With changes in mitochondrial membrane potential (Ψm), this process is coordinated with mitochondrial fusion and fission process. Ox-LDL inhibited PINK1/Parkin then impaired mitophagy and stains activate Parkin-dependent mitophagy. **(B)** Basal and mild adaptive autophagy suppresses oxidative stress and inflammation and increases cell survival and cellular homeostasis to protect against the progression of atherosclerotic plaques, while impaired and excessive autophagy activation leads to increased oxidative stress and inflammation, cell death, and apoptosis, further contributing to plaque instability and rupture.

Atg5. Induced autophagy is considered a cellular survival mechanism to prevent the death of VSMCs. All these evidence indicate that basal and modest autophagic activity in VSMCs is a protective mechanism against cell death and maintains plaque stability.

In contrast, excessively activated autophagy may result in VSMC death and plaque destabilization. Severe oxidative stress

or inflammation stimulates excessive autophagy. TNF-α induces the expression of LC3-II and beclin1 via the JNK/Akt pathway, leading to VSMC death (Jia et al., 2006). In addition, Ang II increases the production of ROS, increases the levels of LC3-II and beclin-1 and decreases Sequestosome 1 (SQSTM1)/p62 to promote autophagosome formation in rat vascular SMCs, which may also be detrimental (Yu et al., 2014) (**Figure 2B**).

Autophagy in Macrophages

Macrophages play pivotal roles in all stages of atherosclerosis. During the formation of atherosclerotic plaques, monocytes in the bone marrow are stimulated by MetS conditions, such as elevated TC and LDL, to enter the blood circulation. Circulating monocytes move into the subendothelium of vessel walls and differentiate into macrophages, subsequently turning into foam cells that are filled with oxLDL (Tabas and Bornfeldt, 2016).

The suppression of autophagy in macrophages may lead to apoptosis and plaque destabilization. Macrophage Atg5 deficiency increases apoptosis and oxidative stress in fat-fed LDL receptor-knockout mice and promotes plaque necrosis (Liao et al., 2012). Macrophage-specific Atg5-knockout mice exhibit increased p62 levels and decreased LC3 levels, which are characteristic of autophagy deficiency. Moreover, Atg5-null macrophages secrete IL-1β, leading to inflammasome activation and increased plaques (Razani et al., 2012). Another study demonstrated that macrophage autophagy could be induced by Akt inhibitors, mTOR inhibitors and mTOR-siRNA, while PI3K inhibitors had the opposite effect, which indicates that activating autophagy of macrophage via the inhibition of the PI3K/Akt/mTOR pathway can stabilize vulnerable atherosclerotic plaques (Zhai et al., 2014). This evidence suggests an atheroprotective role for basal autophagy in macrophages.

However, excessive autophagy may also lead to autophagic death in macrophages via poorly understood type II programmed cell death, which further exacerbates the inflammatory response (Liu and Levine, 2015; Hassanpour et al., 2019). Future studies are necessary to identify the detrimental role of autophagy in macrophages (**Figure 2B**).

Mitophagy

Mitochondrial dynamics, including mitochondrial fusion, fission, biogenesis and mitochonial autophagy (mitophagy) can be regulated by the characteristics of MetS (Vásquez-Trincado et al., 2016). Cells selectively remove dysfunctional and damaged organelles via mitophagy. Briefly, the process of mitophagy is mainly regulated by PTEN-induced kinase 1 (PINK1) and Parkin proteins. Damaged mitochondria are eliminated by mitophagy through the accumulation of PINK1 and Parkin on the mitochondrial surface. With changes in mitochondrial membrane potential (Ψm), this process is coordinated with mitochondrial fusion and fission process. Pro-apoptotic BH3-only domain protein (BNIP3) and NIX are also involved in the selective mitochondrial clearance (Ashrafi and Schwarz, 2013; Vásquez-Trincado et al., 2016) (**Figure 2A**). Deregulation of mitophagy leads to accumulation of dysfunctional and damaged mitochondria, results in the overload of ROS, depletion of adenosine triphosphate (ATP) and apoptosis of cardiomyocytes, which may lead to the pathogenesis of CVD including atherosclerosis (Chistiakov et al., 2018; Morciano et al., 2020).

The molecular mechanism mediating mitophagy in the pathogenesis of atherosclerosis may involve mitochondrial fission, accumulation of PINK1 and the recruitment of Parkin to mitochondria. Multiple studies demonstrated that

characteristics of MetS, especially obesity and dyslipidemia impaired mitochondrial dynamic and mitophagy. Ox-LDL decreased mitochondrial aldehyde dehydrogenase 2 (ALDH2) via ROS-mediated VSMCs senescence (Zhu H. et al., 2019), caused endothelial apoptosis via inhibiting fusion and mitophagy (Zheng and Lu, 2020). Ox-LDL inhibited PINK1 and Parkin then impaired mitophagy flux, which leads to VSMC apoptosis (Swiader et al., 2016). Moreover, another research showed that SIRT3/FOXO3a/parkin pathway in macrophages is a potential target for suppressing NLRP3 inflammasome activation to attenuate plaque size and vulnerability (Ma et al., 2018).

PHARMACOLOGICAL INTERVENTIONS IN THE TREATMENT OF ATHEROSCLEROSIS

Based on the effects of MetS characteristics and autophagy on the pathogenesis of atherosclerosis, we suggest that targeted autophagy therapy may be an effective and promising strategy for atherosclerosis treatment. At present, many drugs for the treatment of MetS have additional benefits on autophagy regulation to protect against atherosclerosis. The underlying mechanisms of these drugs are related to the inhibition of the mTOR signaling pathway, oxidative stress, inflammation or hyperlipidemia (**Figure 2A** and **Table 2**).

Resveratrol

Resveratrol, an activator of 5'-adenosine monophosphate-activated protein kinase (AMPK), is a polyphenolic phytoalexin that occurs naturally in many plant parts and products. Resveratrol has been verified to have antidiabetic (Kitada et al., 2011; Szkudelski and Szkudelska, 2015) and cardiovascular benefits (Bonnefont-Rousselot, 2016). Resveratrol treatment results in a decrease in the size and density of atherosclerotic plaques and a reduction in layer thickness in a rabbit model (Wang et al., 2005). Resveratrol prevents high-fat/sucrose diet-induced central arterial wall inflammation and stiffening in a monkey model (Mattison et al., 2014). In addition to directly activating autophagy by inhibiting mTOR (Sanches-Silva et al., 2020), the underlying mechanisms include the indirect activation of autophagy via anti-inflammatory and antioxidant effects. Resveratrol is the most well-known compound that stimulates members of the sirtuin family. Our previous research showed that sirtuin 1 (SIRT1) inactivation induces inflammation through NF-κB activation and dysregulates autophagy via mTOR/AMPK pathways in THP-1 cells, a human monocyte cell line (Takeda-Watanabe et al., 2012), which indicated the relationship between autophagy impairment and inflammation. Another *in vitro* study showed that resveratrol enhanced autophagic flux and promoted ox-LDL degradation in HUVECs (Zhang et al., 2016) and macrophages (Liu B. et al., 2014) via the upregulation of SIRT1. Resveratrol also attenuates EC inflammation by inducing autophagy in part via the activation of the AMPK/SIRT1 pathway (Chen et al., 2013) and SIRT1/FoxO1 pathway (Wu Q. et al., 2019). Moreover, resveratrol can promote autophagosome

TABLE 2 | Antiatherosclerotic compounds and mechanisms.

Compounds	Mechanisms of autophagy induction	Primary functions	Antiatherosclerotic effects
Resveratrol	AMPK activation, mTOR inhibition, anti-inflammation, antioxidation, SIRT1 activation	AMPK activation	Decreases the size and density of atherosclerotic plaques, reduces the layer thickness (Wang et al., 2005)
Metformin	AMPK activation, mTOR inhibition, anti-inflammation, antioxidation, anti-hyperlipidemia	Anti-hyperglycemia	Reduces monocyte-to-macrophage differentiation (Vasamsetti et al., 2015), promotes cholesterol efflux, attenuates plaque formation, and decreases atherosclerotic lesion areas (Luo et al., 2017)
Statins	mTOR inhibition, anti-inflammation	Anti-hyperlipidemia	Plaques stabilization (Bea et al., 2002; Rodriguez et al., 2017), reduces infarct size (Andres et al., 2014)
Berberine	AMPK activation, mTOR inhibition, anti-inflammation, antioxidation, anti-hyperlipidemia	AMPK activation	Inhibition of inflammation in macrophages (Fan et al., 2015)
Geniposide	mTOR inhibition	Anti-inflammation	Decreases the size of atherosclerotic plaques (Xu Y. L. et al., 2020)

formation characterized by LC3 production and p62 degradation and suppress palmitic acid-induced ROS to attenuate endothelial oxidative injury in HUVECs (Zhou et al., 2019).

Metformin

Metformin is the recommended first-line treatment for T2DM. Beyond its antidiabetic effects, the benefits of metformin on MetS and cardiovascular diseases have also been confirmed (Zhou et al., 2018). As an inducer of AMPK, the underlying mechanisms of metformin may contribute to stimulating autophagy via the AMPK pathway and exert anti-inflammatory, antihyperlipidemic and antioxidant effects.

Metformin can directly activate AMPK and then suppress the mTOR pathway to induce autophagy and inhibit atherosclerosis (You et al., 2020). An *in vitro* study showed that metformin inhibits IL-1β, IL-6, and IL-8 in ECs, VSMCs, and macrophages by blocking the PI3K-Akt/NF-κB pathway (Isoda et al., 2006). In addition, metformin reduces monocyte-to-macrophage differentiation and attenuates Ang II-induced atherosclerotic plaque formation in ApoE$^{-/-}$ mice by decreasing AMPK activity to suppress the phosphorylation of signal transducer and activator of transcription 3 (STAT3) (Vasamsetti et al., 2015). Given its antihyperlipidemic effects, metformin protects against ox-LDL-induced lipid uptake and apoptosis in macrophage (Huangfu et al., 2018), prevents TC uptake during oxidative

stress-induced atherosclerosis (Gopoju et al., 2018). Combination therapy with metformin and atorvastatin decreased the atherosclerotic lesion areas in rabbits fed a high-cholesterol diet. In macrophages, this cotreatment promoted cholesterol efflux to achieve antiatherosclerotic benefits (Luo et al., 2017). In terms of antioxidant effects, metformin reduces NADPH oxidase and increases antioxidative enzymes such as superoxide dismutase (SOD), glutathione peroxidase and catalase in cultured human monocytes/macrophages, which alter the oxidative status of macrophages and increases antioxidative activity (Bułdak et al., 2016).

Statins

Statins are the cornerstone for the prevention of atherosclerotic cardiovascular disease (Rodriguez et al., 2017). Statins exert stabilizing effects on vulnerable atherosclerotic plaques in both clinical research (Rodriguez et al., 2017) and animal models (Bea et al., 2002). Beyond the hypolipidemic effects, stains are considered autophagy inducers via mTOR inhibition, mediating anti-inflammatory elements to protect against atherosclerosis (Mizuno et al., 2011; Martinet et al., 2014). In macrophages, atorvastatin inhibits LPS-induced inflammatory factors such as IL-1β and TNF-α by enhancing autophagy through the Akt/mTOR signaling pathway (Han et al., 2018). In VSMCs, atorvastatin protects against transforming growth factor-β1 (TGF-β1)-induced calcification by stimulating autophagy (Liu D. et al., 2014). Moreover, atorvastatin can reverse the endothelial cell dysfunction induced by Ang II (Dang et al., 2018). Simvastatin, another kind of statin, inhibits the mTOR pathway to increase autophagy (Wei et al., 2013) and activates Parkin-dependent mitophagy (Andres et al., 2014) in cardiomyocytes. This evidence highlights the role of statins in the treatment of atherosclerosis.

Natural Products

Similar to resveratrol, berberine, an extract of Coptis, exhibits antioxidant, anti-inflammatory, and antihyperlipidemic effects (Tillhon et al., 2012). A previous study showed that berberine suppressed ox-LDL-induced inflammation and increased the conversion from LC3-I to LC3-II in macrophages through the activation of the AMPK/mTOR pathway (Fan et al., 2015).

Geniposide, an extract of *Gardenia jasminoides Ellis,* shows antioxidant and anti-inflammatory effects (Fu et al., 2012). Previous study demonstrated that geniposide decreased the size of atherosclerotic plaques, inhibited the progression of atherosclerosis in high fat diet-fed ApoE$^{-/-}$ mice. The potential mechanism may contribute to the reinforce of macrophage autophagy by inhibiting the triggering receptor expressed on myeloid cell 2 (TREM2)/mTOR signaling (Xu Y. L. et al., 2020).

CONCLUSION

The characteristics of MetS are closely related to oxidative stress, inflammation, insulin resistance, and imbalanced adipokines and are responsible for both impaired and excessive autophagy. Autophagy homeostasis is the key regulator of MetS-induced atherosclerosis. Dysregulation of autophagy induced by MetS contributes to endothelial dysfunction, monocyte/macrophage migration and adhesion that lead to the progression of atherosclerosis. Basal and mild adaptive autophagy protect against the progression of atherosclerotic plaques, while impaired autophagy or excessive autophagy activation induced by MetS is related to oxidative stress, inflammation, apoptosis, and foam cell formation, contributing to plaque instability or even plaque rupture. Presently, multiple drugs used to treat MetS have been indicated to regulate autophagy beyond their fundamental effects. Given the double-edged sword effect of autophagy, precise control of autophagy should be considered a potential therapeutic strategy in the prevention and treatment of atherosclerosis.

AUTHOR CONTRIBUTIONS

JX contributed to drafting and writing the article. MK, YO, and DK contributed to the discussion of the review. All authors revised the manuscript critically for important intellectual content and approved the final version to be published. MK is responsible for the integrity of the content.

REFERENCES

Aboonabi, A., Meyer, R. R., and Singh, I. (2019). The association between metabolic syndrome components and the development of atherosclerosis. *J. Hum. Hypertens.* 33, 844–855. doi: 10.1038/s41371-019-0273-0

Aguilar, M., Bhuket, T., Torres, S., Liu, B., and Wong, R. J. (2015). Prevalence of the metabolic syndrome in the United States, 2003-2012. *JAMA* 313, 1973–1974. doi: 10.1001/jama.2015.4260

Alberti, K. G., Zimmet, P., and Shaw, J. (2006). Metabolic syndrome–a new world-wide definition. A consensus statement from the international diabetes federation. *Diabet. Med.* 23, 469–480. doi: 10.1111/j.1464-5491.2006.01858.x

Alberti, K. G., and Zimmet, P. Z. (1998). Definition, diagnosis and classification of diabetes mellitus and its complications. Part 1: diagnosis and classification of diabetes mellitus provisional report of a WHO consultation. *Diabet. Med.* 15, 539–553. doi: 10.1002/(sici)1096-9136(199807)15:7<539::aid-dia668>3.0.co;2-s

Andres, A. M., Hernandez, G., Lee, P., Huang, C., Ratliff, E. P., Sin, J., et al. (2014). Mitophagy is required for acute cardioprotection by simvastatin. *Antioxid. Redox Signal.* 21, 1960–1973. doi: 10.1089/ars.2013.5416

Ashrafi, G., and Schwarz, T. L. (2013). The pathways of mitophagy for quality control and clearance of mitochondria. *Cell Death Differ.* 20, 31–42. doi: 10.1038/cdd.2012.81

Azcutia, V., Abu-Taha, M., Romacho, T., Vázquez-Bella, M., Matesanz, N., Luscinskas, F. W., et al. (2010). Inflammation determines the pro-adhesive properties of high extracellular d-glucose in human endothelial cells in vitro and rat microvessels in vivo. *PLoS One* 5:e10091. doi: 10.1371/journal.pone.0010091

Bai, X., Yang, X., Jia, X., Rong, Y., Chen, L., Zeng, T., et al. (2020). CAV1-CAVIN1-LC3B-mediated autophagy regulates high glucose-stimulated LDL transcytosis. *Autophagy* 16, 1111–1129. doi: 10.1080/15548627.2019.1659613

Balkau, B., and Charles, M. A. (1999). Comment on the provisional report from the WHO consultation. European Group for the Study of Insulin Resistance (EGIR). *Diabet. Med.* 16, 442–443. doi: 10.1046/j.1464-5491.1999.00059.x

Barquera, S., Pedroza-Tobías, A., Medina, C., Hernández-Barrera, L., Bibbins-Domingo, K., Lozano, R., et al. (2015). Global overview of the epidemiology of atherosclerotic cardiovascular disease. *Arch. Med. Res.* 46, 328–338. doi: 10.1016/j.arcmed.2015.06.006

Bea, F., Blessing, E., Bennett, B., Levitz, M., Wallace, E. P., and Rosenfeld, M. E. (2002). Simvastatin promotes atherosclerotic plaque stability in apoE-deficient mice independently of lipid lowering. *Arterioscler. Thromb. Vasc. Biol.* 22, 1832–1837. doi: 10.1161/01.atv.0000036081.01231.16

Bharath, L. P., Mueller, R., Li, Y., Ruan, T., Kunz, D., Goodrich, R., et al. (2014). Impairment of autophagy in endothelial cells prevents shear-stress-induced increases in nitric oxide bioavailability. *Can. J. Physiol. Pharmacol.* 92, 605–612. doi: 10.1139/cjpp-2014-0017

Bleda, S., de Haro, J., Varela, C., Ferruelo, A., and Acin, F. (2016). Elevated levels of triglycerides and vldl-cholesterol provoke activation of nlrp1 inflammasome in endothelial cells. *Int. J. Cardiol.* 220, 52–55. doi: 10.1016/j.ijcard.2016.06.193

Bonnefont-Rousselot, D. (2016). Resveratrol and cardiovascular diseases. *Nutrients* 8:250. doi: 10.3390/nu8050250

Bornfeldt, K. E., and Tabas, I. (2011). Insulin resistance, hyperglycemia, and atherosclerosis. *Cell Metab.* 14, 575–585. doi: 10.1016/j.cmet.2011.07.015

Bruno, R. M., Masi, S., Taddei, M., Taddei, S., and Virdis, A. (2018). Essential hypertension and functional microvascular ageing. *High Blood Press Cardiovasc. Prev.* 25, 35–40. doi: 10.1007/s40292-017-0245-9

Bułdak, Ł., Łabuzek, K., Bułdak, R. J., Machnik, G., Bołdys, A., Basiak, M., et al. (2016). Metformin reduces the expression of NADPH oxidase and increases the expression of antioxidative enzymes in human monocytes/macrophages cultured in vitro. *Exp. Ther. Med.* 11, 1095–1103. doi: 10.3892/etm.2016.2977

Chen, H., Montagnani, M., Funahashi, T., Shimomura, I., and Quon, M. J. (2003). Adiponectin stimulates production of nitric oxide in vascular endothelial cells. *J. Biol. Chem.* 278, 45021–45026. doi: 10.1074/jbc.M307878200

Chen, K., Feng, L., Hu, W., Chen, J., Wang, X., Wang, L., et al. (2019). Optineurin inhibits NLRP3 inflammasome activation by enhancing mitophagy of renal tubular cells in diabetic nephropathy. *FASEB J.* 33, 4571–4585. doi: 10.1096/fj.201801749RRR

Chen, M. L., Yi, L., Jin, X., Liang, X. Y., Zhou, Y., Zhang, T., et al. (2013). Resveratrol attenuates vascular endothelial inflammation by inducing autophagy through the cAMP signaling pathway. *Autophagy* 9, 2033–2045. doi: 10.4161/auto.26336

Chen, Z., Nie, S. D., Qu, M. L., Zhou, D., Wu, L. Y., Shi, X. J., et al. (2018). The autophagic degradation of Cav-1 contributes to PA-induced apoptosis and inflammation of astrocytes. *Cell Death Dis.* 9:771. doi: 10.1038/s41419-018-0795-3

Chistiakov, D. A., Shkurat, T. P., Melnichenko, A. A., Grechko, A. V., and Orekhov, A. N. (2018). The role of mitochondrial dysfunction in cardiovascular disease: a brief review. *Ann. Med.* 50, 121–127. doi: 10.1080/07853890.2017.1417631

Coelho, M., Oliveira, T., and Fernandes, R. (2013). Biochemistry of adipose tissue: an endocrine organ. *Arch. Med. Sci.* 9, 191–200. doi: 10.5114/aoms.2013.33181

Dang, H., Song, B., Dong, R., and Zhang, H. (2018). Atorvastatin reverses the dysfunction of human umbilical vein endothelial cells induced by angiotensin II. *Exp. Ther. Med.* 16, 5286–5297. doi: 10.3892/etm.2018.6846

Dasu, M. R., Devaraj, S., and Jialal, I. (2007). High glucose induces IL-1beta expression in human monocytes: mechanistic insights. *Am. J. Physiol. Endocrinol. Metab.* 293, E337–E346. doi: 10.1152/ajpendo.00718.2006

Daugherty, A., Manning, M. W., and Cassis, L. A. (2000). Angiotensin II promotes atherosclerotic lesions and aneurysms in apolipoprotein E-deficient mice. *J. Clin. Invest.* 105, 1605–1612. doi: 10.1172/jci7818

De Nardo, D., and Latz, E. (2011). NLRP3 inflammasomes link inflammation and metabolic disease. *Trends Immunol.* 32, 373–379. doi: 10.1016/j.it.2011.05.004

Di Pino, A., and DeFronzo, R. A. (2019). Insulin resistance and atherosclerosis: implications for insulin-sensitizing agents. *Endocr. Rev.* 40, 1447–1467. doi: 10.1210/er.2018-00141

Ding, Z., Wang, X., Khaidakov, M., Liu, S., Dai, Y., and Mehta, J. L. (2012). Degradation of heparan sulfate proteoglycans enhances oxidized-LDL-mediated autophagy and apoptosis in human endothelial cells. *Biochem. Biophys. Res. Commun.* 426, 106–111. doi: 10.1016/j.bbrc.2012.08.044

Ding, Z., Wang, X., Schnackenberg, L., Khaidakov, M., Liu, S., Singla, S., et al. (2013). Regulation of autophagy and apoptosis in response to ox-LDL in vascular smooth muscle cells, and the modulatory effects of the microRNA hsa-let-7 g. *Int. J. Cardiol.* 168, 1378–1385. doi: 10.1016/j.ijcard.2012.12.045

Do, R., Willer, C. J., Schmidt, E. M., Sengupta, S., Gao, C., Peloso, G. M., et al. (2013). Common variants associated with plasma triglycerides and risk for coronary artery disease. *Nat. Genet.* 45, 1345–1352. doi: 10.1038/ng.2795

Eckel, R. H., Grundy, S. M., and Zimmet, P. Z. (2005). The metabolic syndrome. *Lancet* 365, 1415–1428. doi: 10.1016/s0140-6736(05)66378-7

Expert Panel on Detection, Evaluation, and Treatment of High Blood Cholesterol in Adults (2001). Executive summary of the third report of The National Cholesterol Education Program (NCEP) expert panel on detection, evaluation, and treatment of high blood cholesterol in adults (Adult Treatment Panel III). *JAMA.* 285, 2486–2497. doi: 10.1001/jama.285.19.2486

Fan, X., Wang, J., Hou, J., Lin, C., Bensoussan, A., Chang, D., et al. (2015). Berberine alleviates ox-LDL induced inflammatory factors by up-regulation of autophagy via AMPK/mTOR signaling pathway. *J. Transl. Med.* 13:92. doi: 10.1186/s12967-015-0450-z

Fetterman, J. L., Holbrook, M., Flint, N., Feng, B., Bretón-Romero, R., Linder, E. A., et al. (2016). Restoration of autophagy in endothelial cells from patients with diabetes mellitus improves nitric oxide signaling. *Atherosclerosis* 247, 207–217. doi: 10.1016/j.atherosclerosis.2016.01.043

Francisco, V., Pino, J., Gonzalez-Gay, M. A., Mera, A., Lago, F., Gómez, R., et al. (2018). Adipokines and inflammation: is it a question of weight? *Br. J. Pharmacol.* 175, 1569–1579. doi: 10.1111/bph.14181

Fu, Y., Liu, B., Liu, J., Liu, Z., Liang, D., Li, F., et al. (2012). Geniposide, from Gardenia jasminoides Ellis, inhibits the inflammatory response in the primary mouse macrophages and mouse models. *Int. Immunopharmacol.* 14, 792–798. doi: 10.1016/j.intimp.2012.07.006

Fujishima, Y., Maeda, N., Matsuda, K., Masuda, S., Mori, T., Fukuda, S., et al. (2017). Adiponectin association with T-cadherin protects against neointima proliferation and atherosclerosis. *FASEB J.* 31, 1571–1583. doi: 10.1096/fj.201601064R

Furukawa, S., Fujita, T., Shimabukuro, M., Iwaki, M., Yamada, Y., Nakajima, Y., et al. (2004). Increased oxidative stress in obesity and its impact on metabolic syndrome. *J. Clin. Invest.* 114, 1752–1761. doi: 10.1172/jci21625

Gan, W., Bragg, F., Walters, R. G., Millwood, I. Y., Lin, K., Chen, Y., et al. (2019). Genetic predisposition to Type 2 diabetes and risk of subclinical atherosclerosis and cardiovascular diseases among 160,000 chinese adults. *Diabetes* 68, 2155–2164. doi: 10.2337/db19-0224

Gatica, D., Chiong, M., Lavandero, S., and Klionsky, D. J. (2015). Molecular mechanisms of autophagy in the cardiovascular system. *Circ. Res.* 116, 456–467. doi: 10.1161/circresaha.114.303788

Giacco, F., and Brownlee, M. (2010). Oxidative stress and diabetic complications. *Circ. Res.* 107, 1058–1070. doi: 10.1161/circresaha.110.223545

Glass, C. K., and Witztum, J. L. (2001). Atherosclerosis. The road ahead. *Cell* 104, 503–516. doi: 10.1016/s0092-8674(01)00238-0

Gopoju, R., Panangipalli, S., and Kotamraju, S. (2018). Metformin treatment prevents SREBP2-mediated cholesterol uptake and improves lipid homeostasis during oxidative stress-induced atherosclerosis. *Free Radic. Biol. Med.* 118, 85–97. doi: 10.1016/j.freeradbiomed.2018.02.031

Gower, R. M., Wu, H., Foster, G. A., Devaraj, S., Jialal, I., Ballantyne, C. M., et al. (2011). CD11c/CD18 expression is upregulated on blood monocytes during hypertriglyceridemia and enhances adhesion to vascular cell adhesion molecule-1. *Arterioscler. Thromb. Vasc. Biol.* 31, 160–166. doi: 10.1161/atvbaha.110.215434

Grootaert, M. O., da Costa Martins, P. A., Bitsch, N., Pintelon, I., De Meyer, G. R., Martinet, W., et al. (2015). Defective autophagy in vascular smooth muscle cells accelerates senescence and promotes neointima formation and atherogenesis. *Autophagy* 11, 2014–2032. doi: 10.1080/15548627.2015.1096485

Han, F., Xiao, Q. Q., Peng, S., Che, X. Y., Jiang, L. S., Shao, Q., et al. (2018). Atorvastatin ameliorates LPS-induced inflammatory response by autophagy via AKT/mTOR signaling pathway. *J. Cell. Biochem.* 119, 1604–1615. doi: 10.1002/jcb.26320

Hansel, B., Giral, P., Nobecourt, E., Chantepie, S., Bruckert, E., Chapman, M. J., et al. (2004). Metabolic syndrome is associated with elevated oxidative stress and dysfunctional dense high-density lipoprotein particles displaying impaired antioxidative activity. *J. Clin. Endocrinol. Metab.* 89, 4963–4971. doi: 10.1210/jc.2004-0305

Harja, E., Chang, J. S., Lu, Y., Leitges, M., Zou, Y. S., Schmidt, A. M., et al. (2009). Mice deficient in PKCbeta and apolipoprotein E display decreased atherosclerosis. *FASEB. J.* 23, 1081–1091. doi: 10.1096/fj.08-120345

Hassanpour, M., Rahbarghazi, R., Nouri, M., Aghamohammadzadeh, N., Safaei, N., and Ahmadi, M. (2019). Role of autophagy in atherosclerosis: foe or friend? *J. Inflamm. (Lond.)* 16:8. doi: 10.1186/s12950-019-0212-4

Higashi, Y., Noma, K., Yoshizumi, M., and Kihara, Y. (2009). Endothelial function and oxidative stress in cardiovascular diseases. *Circ. J.* 73, 411–418. doi: 10.1253/circj.cj-08-1102

Hou, K., Li, S., Zhang, M., and Qin, X. (2021). Caveolin-1 in autophagy: a potential therapeutic target in atherosclerosis. *Clin. Chim. Acta* 513, 25–33. doi: 10.1016/j.cca.2020.11.020

Hou, Y., Lin, S., Qiu, J., Sun, W., Dong, M., Xiang, Y., et al. (2020). NLRP3 inflammasome negatively regulates podocyte autophagy in diabetic nephropathy. *Biochem. Biophys. Res. Commun.* 521, 791–798. doi: 10.1016/j.bbrc.2019.10.194

Huangfu, N., Wang, Y., Cheng, J., Xu, Z., and Wang, S. (2018). Metformin protects against oxidized low density lipoprotein-induced macrophage apoptosis and inhibits lipid uptake. *Exp. Ther. Med.* 15, 2485–2491. doi: 10.3892/etm.2018.5704

Ishibashi, K. I., Imamura, T., Sharma, P. M., Huang, J., Ugi, S., and Olefsky, J. M. (2001). Chronic endothelin-1 treatment leads to heterologous desensitization of insulin signaling in 3T3-L1 adipocytes. *J. Clin. Invest.* 107, 1193–1202. doi: 10.1172/jci11753

Isoda, K., Young, J. L., Zirlik, A., MacFarlane, L. A., Tsuboi, N., Gerdes, N., et al. (2006). Metformin inhibits proinflammatory responses and nuclear factor-kappaB in human vascular wall cells. *Arterioscler. Thromb. Vasc. Biol.* 26, 611–617. doi: 10.1161/01.atv.0000201938.78044.75

Jayakumar, T., Chang, C. C., Lin, S. L., Huang, Y. K., Hu, C. M., Elizebeth, A. R., et al. (2014). Brazilin ameliorates high glucose-induced vascular inflammation via inhibiting ROS and CAMs production in human umbilical vein endothelial cells. *Biomed. Res. Int.* 2014:403703. doi: 10.1155/2014/403703

Jia, G., Cheng, G., Gangahar, D. M., and Agrawal, D. K. (2006). Insulin-like growth factor-1 and TNF-alpha regulate autophagy through c-jun N-terminal kinase and Akt pathways in human atherosclerotic vascular smooth cells. *Immunol. Cell. Biol.* 84, 448–454. doi: 10.1111/j.1440-1711.2006.01454.x

Jørgensen, A. B., Frikke-Schmidt, R., West, A. S., Grande, P., Nordestgaard, B. G., and Tybjærg-Hansen, A. (2013). Genetically elevated non-fasting triglycerides and calculated remnant cholesterol as causal risk factors for myocardial infarction. *Eur. Heart J.* 34, 1826–1833. doi: 10.1093/eurheartj/ehs431

Kadowaki, T., Yamauchi, T., Kubota, N., Hara, K., Ueki, K., and Tobe, K. (2006). Adiponectin and adiponectin receptors in insulin resistance, diabetes, and the metabolic syndrome. *J. Clin. Invest.* 116, 1784–1792. doi: 10.1172/jci29126

Katakami, N. (2018). Mechanism of development of atherosclerosis and cardiovascular disease in diabetes mellitus. *J. Atheroscler. Thromb.* 25, 27–39. doi: 10.5551/jat.RV17014

Kim, J., Lim, Y. M., and Lee, M. S. (2018). The role of autophagy in systemic metabolism and human-type diabetes. *Mol. Cells* 41, 11–17. doi: 10.14348/molcells.2018.2228

Kim, K. H., and Lee, M. S. (2014). Autophagy–a key player in cellular and body metabolism. *Nat. Rev. Endocrinol.* 10, 322–337. doi: 10.1038/nrendo.2014.35

Kitada, M., Kume, S., Imaizumi, N., and Koya, D. (2011). Resveratrol improves oxidative stress and protects against diabetic nephropathy through normalization of Mn-SOD dysfunction in AMPK/SIRT1-independent pathway. *Diabetes* 60, 634–643. doi: 10.2337/db10-0386

Kitada, M., Ogura, Y., and Koya, D. (2016). The protective role of Sirt1 in vascular tissue: its relationship to vascular aging and atherosclerosis. *Aging (Albany NY)* 8, 2290–2307. doi: 10.18632/aging.101068

Kitada, M., Ogura, Y., Monno, I., and Koya, D. (2017). Regulating autophagy as a therapeutic target for diabetic nephropathy. *Curr. Diab. Rep.* 17:53. doi: 10.1007/s11892-017-0879-y

Kobayashi, S., and Liang, Q. (2015). Autophagy and mitophagy in diabetic cardiomyopathy. *Biochim. Biophys. Acta* 1852, 252–261. doi: 10.1016/j.bbadis.2014.05.020

Lavandero, S., Chiong, M., Rothermel, B. A., and Hill, J. A. (2015). Autophagy in cardiovascular biology. *J. Clin. Invest.* 125, 55–64. doi: 10.1172/jci73943

Le Lay, S., Simard, G., Martinez, M. C., and Andriantsitohaina, R. (2014). Oxidative stress and metabolic pathologies: from an adipocentric point of view. *Oxid. Med. Cell Longev.* 2014:908539. doi: 10.1155/2014/908539

Lee, H. M., Kim, J. J., Kim, H. J., Shong, M., Ku, B. J., and Jo, E. K. (2013). Upregulated NLRP3 inflammasome activation in patients with type 2 diabetes. *Diabetes* 62, 194–204. doi: 10.2337/db12-0420

Li, W., Song, F., Wang, X., Wang, D., Chen, D., Yue, W., et al. (2019). Relationship between metabolic syndrome and its components and cardiovascular disease in middle-aged and elderly Chinese population: a national cross-sectional survey. *BMJ Open* 9:e027545. doi: 10.1136/bmjopen-2018-027545

Liao, X., Sluimer, J. C., Wang, Y., Subramanian, M., Brown, K., Pattison, J. S., et al. (2012). Macrophage autophagy plays a protective role in advanced atherosclerosis. *Cell Metab.* 15, 545–553. doi: 10.1016/j.cmet.2012.01.022

Lin, Y. J., Juan, C. C., Kwok, C. F., Hsu, Y. P., Shih, K. C., Chen, C. C., et al. (2015). Endothelin-1 exacerbates development of hypertension and atherosclerosis in modest insulin resistant syndrome. *Biochem. Biophys. Res. Commun.* 460, 497–503. doi: 10.1016/j.bbrc.2015.03.017

Liu, B., Zhang, B., Guo, R., Li, S., and Xu, Y. (2014). Enhancement in efferocytosis of oxidized low-density lipoprotein-induced apoptotic RAW264.7 cells through Sirt1-mediated autophagy. *Int. J. Mol. Med.* 33, 523–533. doi: 10.3892/ijmm.2013.1609

Liu, D., Cui, W., Liu, B., Hu, H., Liu, J., Xie, R., et al. (2014). Atorvastatin protects vascular smooth muscle cells from TGF-β1-stimulated calcification by inducing autophagy via suppression of the β-catenin pathway. *Cell. Physiol. Biochem.* 33, 129–141. doi: 10.1159/000356656

Liu, Y., and Levine, B. (2015). Autosis and autophagic cell death: the dark side of autophagy. *Cell Death Differ.* 22, 367–376. doi: 10.1038/cdd.2014.143

Lovren, F., Teoh, H., and Verma, S. (2015). Obesity and atherosclerosis: mechanistic insights. *Can. J. Cardiol.* 31, 177–183. doi: 10.1016/j.cjca.2014.11.031

Lu, X., and Kakkar, V. (2014). Inflammasome and atherogenesis. *Curr. Pharm. Des.* 20, 108–124. doi: 10.2174/13816128113199990586

Luo, B., Li, B., Wang, W., Liu, X., Xia, Y., Zhang, C., et al. (2014). NLRP3 gene silencing ameliorates diabetic cardiomyopathy in a type 2 diabetes rat model. *PLoS One* 9:e104771. doi: 10.1371/journal.pone.0104771

Luo, F., Guo, Y., Ruan, G. Y., Long, J. K., Zheng, X. L., Xia, Q., et al. (2017). Combined use of metformin and atorvastatin attenuates atherosclerosis in rabbits fed a high-cholesterol diet. *Sci. Rep.* 7:2169. doi: 10.1038/s41598-017-02080-w

Luo, Y., Lu, S., Zhou, P., Ai, Q. D., Sun, G. B., and Sun, X. B. (2016). Autophagy: an exposing therapeutic target in atherosclerosis. *J. Cardiovasc. Pharmacol.* 67, 266–274. doi: 10.1097/fjc.0000000000000342

Lusis, A. J. (2000). Atherosclerosis. *Nature* 407, 233–241. doi: 10.1038/35025203

Ma, M., Song, L., Yan, H., Liu, M., Zhang, L., Ma, Y., et al. (2016). Low dose tunicamycin enhances atherosclerotic plaque stability by inducing autophagy. *Biochem. Pharmacol.* 100, 51–60. doi: 10.1016/j.bcp.2015.11.020

Ma, S., Chen, J., Feng, J., Zhang, R., Fan, M., Han, D., et al. (2018). Melatonin ameliorates the progression of atherosclerosis via mitophagy activation and NLRP3 inflammasome inhibition. *Oxid. Med. Cell Longev.* 2018:9286458. doi: 10.1155/2018/9286458

Madonna, R., Pandolfi, A., Massaro, M., Consoli, A., and De Caterina, R. (2004). Insulin enhances vascular cell adhesion molecule-1 expression in human cultured endothelial cells through a pro-atherogenic pathway mediated by p38 mitogen-activated protein-kinase. *Diabetologia* 47, 532–536. doi: 10.1007/s00125-004-1330-x

Martinet, W., De Loof, H., and De Meyer, G. R. Y. (2014). mTOR inhibition: a promising strategy for stabilization of atherosclerotic plaques. *Atherosclerosis* 233, 601–607. doi: 10.1016/j.atherosclerosis.2014.01.040

Martinet, W., and De Meyer, G. R. (2009). Autophagy in atherosclerosis: a cell survival and death phenomenon with therapeutic potential. *Circ. Res.* 104, 304–317. doi: 10.1161/circresaha.108.188318

Masuyama, A., Mita, T., Azuma, K., Osonoi, Y., Nakajima, K., Goto, H., et al. (2018). Defective autophagy in vascular smooth muscle cells enhances atherosclerotic plaque instability. *Biochem. Biophys. Res. Commun.* 505, 1141–1147. doi: 10.1016/j.bbrc.2018.09.192

Mattison, J. A., Wang, M., Bernier, M., Zhang, J., Park, S. S., Maudsley, S., et al. (2014). Resveratrol prevents high fat/sucrose diet-induced central arterial wall inflammation and stiffening in nonhuman primates. *Cell Metab.* 20, 183–190. doi: 10.1016/j.cmet.2014.04.018

McArdle, M. A., Finucane, O. M., Connaughton, R. M., McMorrow, A. M., and Roche, H. M. (2013). Mechanisms of obesity-induced inflammation and insulin resistance: insights into the emerging role of nutritional strategies. *Front. Endocrinol. (Lausanne)* 4:52. doi: 10.3389/fendo.2013.00052

McCracken, E., Monaghan, M., and Sreenivasan, S. (2018). Pathophysiology of the metabolic syndrome. *Clin. Dermatol.* 36, 14–20. doi: 10.1016/j.clindermatol.2017.09.004

Medda, R., Lyros, O., Schmidt, J. L., Jovanovic, N., Nie, L., Link, B. J., et al. (2015). Anti inflammatory and anti angiogenic effect of black raspberry extract on human esophageal and intestinal microvascular endothelial cells. *Microvasc. Res.* 97, 167–180. doi: 10.1016/j.mvr.2014.10.008

Mizuno, Y., Jacob, R. F., and Mason, R. P. (2011). Inflammation and the development of atherosclerosis. *J. Atheroscler. Thromb.* 18, 351–358. doi: 10.5551/jat.7591

Mizushima, N., and Komatsu, M. (2011). Autophagy: renovation of cells and tissues. *Cell* 147, 728–741. doi: 10.1016/j.cell.2011.10.026

Mizushima, N., Levine, B., Cuervo, A. M., and Klionsky, D. J. (2008). Autophagy fights disease through cellular self-digestion. *Nature* 451, 1069–1075. doi: 10.1038/nature06639

Montezano, A. C., Nguyen Dinh Cat, A., Rios, F. J., and Touyz, R. M. (2014). Angiotensin II and vascular injury. *Curr. Hypertens. Rep.* 16:431. doi: 10.1007/s11906-014-0431-2

Morciano, G., Patergnani, S., Bonora, M., Pedriali, G., Tarocco, A., Bouhamida, E., et al. (2020). Mitophagy in cardiovascular diseases. *J. Clin. Med.* 9:892. doi: 10.3390/jcm9030892

Mulè, G., Calcaterra, I., Nardi, E., Cerasola, G., and Cottone, S. (2014). Metabolic syndrome in hypertensive patients: an unholy alliance. *World J. Cardiol.* 6, 890–907. doi: 10.4330/wjc.v6.i9.890

Nagareddy, P. R., Murphy, A. J., Stirzaker, R. A., Hu, Y., Yu, S., Miller, R. G., et al. (2013). Hyperglycemia promotes myelopoiesis and impairs the resolution of atherosclerosis. *Cell Metab.* 17, 695–708. doi: 10.1016/j.cmet.2013.04.001

Nahapetyan, H., Moulis, M., Grousset, E., Faccini, J., Grazide, M. H., Mucher, E., et al. (2019). Altered mitochondrial quality control in Atg7-deficient VSMCs promotes enhanced apoptosis and is linked to unstable atherosclerotic plaque phenotype. *Cell Death Dis.* 10:119. doi: 10.1038/s41419-019-1400-0

Nigro, J., Osman, N., Dart, A. M., and Little, P. J. (2006). Insulin resistance and atherosclerosis. *Endocr. Rev.* 27, 242–259. doi: 10.1210/er.2005-0007

Nussenzweig, S. C., Verma, S., and Finkel, T. (2015). The role of autophagy in vascular biology. *Circ. Res.* 116, 480–488. doi: 10.1161/circresaha.116.303805

Osonoi, Y., Mita, T., Azuma, K., Nakajima, K., Masuyama, A., Goto, H., et al. (2018). Defective autophagy in vascular smooth muscle cells enhances cell death and atherosclerosis. *Autophagy* 14, 1991–2006. doi: 10.1080/15548627.2018.1501132

Pal, S., Semorine, K., Watts, G. F., and Mamo, J. (2003). Identification of lipoproteins of intestinal origin in human atherosclerotic plaque. *Clin. Chem. Lab. Med.* 41, 792–795. doi: 10.1515/cclm.2003.120

Peng, J., Luo, F., Ruan, G., Peng, R., and Li, X. (2017). Hypertriglyceridemia and atherosclerosis. *Lipids Health Dis.* 16:233. doi: 10.1186/s12944-017-0625-0

Peng, N., Meng, N., Wang, S., Zhao, F., Zhao, J., Su, L., et al. (2014). An activator of mTOR inhibits oxLDL-induced autophagy and apoptosis in vascular endothelial cells and restricts atherosclerosis in apolipoprotein E−/− mice. *Sci. Rep.* 4:5519. doi: 10.1038/srep05519

Piga, R., Naito, Y., Kokura, S., Handa, O., and Yoshikawa, T. (2007). Short-term high glucose exposure induces monocyte-endothelial cells adhesion and transmigration by increasing VCAM-1 and MCP-1 expression in human aortic endothelial cells. *Atherosclerosis* 193, 328–334. doi: 10.1016/j.atherosclerosis.2006.09.016

Ranasinghe, P., Mathangasinghe, Y., Jayawardena, R., Hills, A. P., and Misra, A. (2017). Prevalence and trends of metabolic syndrome among adults in the asia-pacific region: a systematic review. *BMC Public Health* 17:101. doi: 10.1186/s12889-017-4041-1

Razani, B., Feng, C., Coleman, T., Emanuel, R., Wen, H., Hwang, S., et al. (2012). Autophagy links inflammasomes to atherosclerotic progression. *Cell Metab.* 15, 534–544. doi: 10.1016/j.cmet.2012.02.011

Roden, M., and Shulman, G. I. (2019). The integrative biology of type 2 diabetes. *Nature* 576, 51–60. doi: 10.1038/s41586-019-1797-8

Rodriguez, F., Maron, D. J., Knowles, J. W., Virani, S. S., Lin, S., and Heidenreich, P. A. (2017). Association between intensity of statin therapy and mortality in patients with atherosclerotic cardiovascular disease. *JAMA Cardiol.* 2, 47–54. doi: 10.1001/jamacardio.2016.4052

Rosenblat, M., Volkova, N., Paland, N., and Aviram, M. (2012). Triglyceride accumulation in macrophages upregulates paraoxonase 2 (PON2) expression via ROS-mediated JNK/c-Jun signaling pathway activation. *Biofactors* 38, 458–469. doi: 10.1002/biof.1052

Rubinsztein, D. C., Marino, G., and Kroemer, G. (2011). Autophagy and aging. *Cell* 146, 682–695. doi: 10.1016/j.cell.2011.07.030

Saltiel, A. R., and Olefsky, J. M. (2017). Inflammatory mechanisms linking obesity and metabolic disease. *J. Clin. Invest.* 127, 1–4. doi: 10.1172/jci92035

Sanches-Silva, A., Testai, L., Nabavi, S. F., Battino, M., Pandima Devi, K., Tejada, S., et al. (2020). Therapeutic potential of polyphenols in cardiovascular diseases: regulation of mTOR signaling pathway. *Pharmacol. Res.* 152:104626. doi: 10.1016/j.phrs.2019.104626

Satish, M., and Agrawal, D. K. (2020). Atherothrombosis and the NLRP3 inflammasome – endogenous mechanisms of inhibition. *Transl. Res.* 215, 75–85. doi: 10.1016/j.trsl.2019.08.003

Satish, M., Saxena, S. K., and Agrawal, D. K. (2019). Adipokine dysregulation and insulin resistance with atherosclerotic vascular disease: metabolic syndrome or independent sequelae? *J. Cardiovasc. Transl. Res.* 12, 415–424. doi: 10.1007/s12265-019-09879-0

Schaffer, S. W., Jong, C. J., and Mozaffari, M. (2012). Role of oxidative stress in diabetes-mediated vascular dysfunction: unifying hypothesis of diabetes revisited. *Vascul. Pharmacol.* 57, 139–149. doi: 10.1016/j.vph.2012.03.005

Schneider, A. L., Kalyani, R. R., Golden, S., Stearns, S. C., Wruck, L., Yeh, H. C., et al. (2016). Diabetes and prediabetes and risk of hospitalization: the Atherosclerosis Risk in Communities (ARIC) study. *Diabetes Care* 39, 772–779. doi: 10.2337/dc15-1335

Sesso, H. D., Buring, J. E., Rifai, N., Blake, G. J., Gaziano, J. M., and Ridker, P. M. (2003). C-reactive protein and the risk of developing hypertension. *JAMA* 290, 2945–2951. doi: 10.1001/jama.290.22.2945

Shah, M. S., and Brownlee, M. (2016). Molecular and cellular mechanisms of cardiovascular disorders in diabetes. *Circ. Res.* 118, 1808–1829. doi: 10.1161/circresaha.116.306923

Shao, B. Z., Han, B. Z., Zeng, Y. X., Su, D. F., and Liu, C. (2016). The roles of macrophage autophagy in atherosclerosis. *Acta Pharmacol. Sin.* 37, 150–156. doi: 10.1038/aps.2015.87

Shen, W., Tian, C., Chen, H., Yang, Y., Zhu, D., Gao, P., et al. (2013). Oxidative stress mediates chemerin-induced autophagy in endothelial cells. *Free Radic. Biol. Med.* 55, 73–82. doi: 10.1016/j.freeradbiomed.2012.11.011

Shin, H. K., Kim, Y. K., Kim, K. Y., Lee, J. H., and Hong, K. W. (2004). Remnant lipoprotein particles induce apoptosis in endothelial cells by NAD(P)H oxidase-mediated production of superoxide and cytokines via lectin-like oxidized low-density lipoprotein receptor-1 activation: prevention by cilostazol. *Circulation* 109, 1022–1028. doi: 10.1161/01.cir.0000117403.64398.53

Silswal, N., Singh, A. K., Aruna, B., Mukhopadhyay, S., Ghosh, S., and Ehtesham, N. Z. (2005). Human resistin stimulates the pro-inflammatory cytokines TNF-alpha and IL-12 in macrophages by NF-kappaB-dependent pathway. *Biochem. Biophys. Res. Commun.* 334, 1092–1101. doi: 10.1016/j.bbrc.2005.06.202

Soro-Paavonen, A., Watson, A. M., Li, J., Paavonen, K., Koitka, A., Calkin, A. C., et al. (2008). Receptor for advanced glycation end products (RAGE) deficiency attenuates the development of atherosclerosis in diabetes. *Diabetes* 57, 2461–2469. doi: 10.2337/db07-1808

Srikanthan, K., Feyh, A., Visweshwar, H., Shapiro, J. I., and Sodhi, K. (2016). Systematic review of metabolic syndrome biomarkers: a panel for early detection, management, and risk stratification in the West Virginian population. *Int. J. Med. Sci.* 13, 25–38. doi: 10.7150/ijms.13800

Stienstra, R., Joosten, L. A., Koenen, T., van Tits, B., van Diepen, J. A., van den Berg, S. A., et al. (2010). The inflammasome-mediated caspase-1 activation controls adipocyte differentiation and insulin sensitivity. *Cell Metab.* 12, 593–605. doi: 10.1016/j.cmet.2010.11.011

Swiader, A., Nahapetyan, H., Faccini, J., D'Angelo, R., Mucher, E., Elbaz, M., et al. (2016). Mitophagy acts as a safeguard mechanism against human vascular

smooth muscle cell apoptosis induced by atherogenic lipids. *Oncotarget* 7, 28821–28835. doi: 10.18632/oncotarget.8936

Szkudelski, T., and Szkudelska, K. (2015). Resveratrol and diabetes: from animal to human studies. *Biochim. Biophys. Acta* 1852, 1145–1154. doi: 10.1016/j.bbadis.2014.10.013

Tabas, I., and Bornfeldt, K. E. (2016). Macrophage phenotype and function in different stages of atherosclerosis. *Circ. Res.* 118, 653–667. doi: 10.1161/circresaha.115.306256

Takagaki, Y., Lee, S. M., Dongqing, Z., Kitada, M., Kanasaki, K., and Koya, D. (2020). Endothelial autophagy deficiency induces IL6 – dependent endothelial mesenchymal transition and organ fibrosis. *Autophagy* 16, 1905–1914. doi: 10.1080/15548627.2020.1713641

Takeda-Watanabe, A., Kitada, M., Kanasaki, K., and Koya, D. (2012). SIRT1 inactivation induces inflammation through the dysregulation of autophagy in human THP-1 cells. *Biochem. Biophys. Res. Commun.* 427, 191–196. doi: 10.1016/j.bbrc.2012.09.042

Thomsen, M., Varbo, A., Tybjærg-Hansen, A., and Nordestgaard, B. G. (2014). Low nonfasting triglycerides and reduced all-cause mortality: a mendelian randomization study. *Clin. Chem.* 60, 737–746. doi: 10.1373/clinchem.2013.219881

Tillhon, M., Guamán Ortiz, L. M., Lombardi, P., and Scovassi, A. I. (2012). Berberine: new perspectives for old remedies. *Biochem. Pharmacol.* 84, 1260–1267. doi: 10.1016/j.bcp.2012.07.018

Turkmen, K. (2017). Inflammation, oxidative stress, apoptosis, and autophagy in diabetes mellitus and diabetic kidney disease: the four horsemen of the apocalypse. *Int. Urol. Nephrol.* 49, 837–844. doi: 10.1007/s11255-016-1488-4

Valente, A. J., Irimpen, A. M., Siebenlist, U., and Chandrasekar, B. (2014). OxLDL induces endothelial dysfunction and death via TRAF3IP2: inhibition by HDL3 and AMPK activators. *Free Radic. Biol. Med.* 70, 117–128. doi: 10.1016/j.freeradbiomed.2014.02.014

Vandanmagsar, B., Youm, Y. H., Ravussin, A., Galgani, J. E., Stadler, K., Mynatt, R. L., et al. (2011). The NLRP3 inflammasome instigates obesity-induced inflammation and insulin resistance. *Nat. Med.* 17, 179–188. doi: 10.1038/nm.2279

Varma, S., Lal, B. K., Zheng, R., Breslin, J. W., Saito, S., Pappas, P. J., et al. (2005). Hyperglycemia alters PI3k and Akt signaling and leads to endothelial cell proliferative dysfunction. *Am. J. Physiol. Heart Circ. Physiol.* 289, H1744–H1751. doi: 10.1152/ajpheart.01088.2004

Vasamsetti, S. B., Karnewar, S., Kanugula, A. K., Thatipalli, A. R., Kumar, J. M., and Kotamraju, S. (2015). Metformin inhibits monocyte-to-macrophage differentiation via AMPK-mediated inhibition of STAT3 activation: potential role in atherosclerosis. *Diabetes* 64, 2028–2041. doi: 10.2337/db14-1225

Vásquez-Trincado, C., García-Carvajal, I., Pennanen, C., Parra, V., Hill, J. A., Rothermel, B. A., et al. (2016). Mitochondrial dynamics, mitophagy and cardiovascular disease. *J. Physiol.* 594, 509–525. doi: 10.1113/jp271301

Verma, S., Li, S. H., Wang, C. H., Fedak, P. W., Li, R. K., Weisel, R. D., et al. (2003). Resistin promotes endothelial cell activation: further evidence of adipokine-endothelial interaction. *Circulation* 108, 736–740. doi: 10.1161/01.cir.0000084503.91330.49

Wang, L., Gill, R., Pedersen, T. L., Higgins, L. J., Newman, J. W., and Rutledge, J. C. (2009). Triglyceride-rich lipoprotein lipolysis releases neutral and oxidized FFAs that induce endothelial cell inflammation. *J. Lipid. Res.* 50, 204–213. doi: 10.1194/jlr.M700505-JLR200

Wang, X., Chen, Q., Pu, H., Wei, Q., Duan, M., Zhang, C., et al. (2016). Adiponectin improves NF-κB-mediated inflammation and abates atherosclerosis progression in apolipoprotein E-deficient mice. *Lipids Health Dis.* 15:33. doi: 10.1186/s12944-016-0202-y

Wang, Y., Che, J., Zhao, H., Tang, J., and Shi, G. (2019). Paeoniflorin attenuates oxidized low-density lipoprotein-induced apoptosis and adhesion molecule expression by autophagy enhancement in human umbilical vein endothelial cells. *J. Cell. Biochem.* 120, 9291–9299. doi: 10.1002/jcb.28204

Wang, Y. I., Bettaieb, A., Sun, C., DeVerse, J. S., Radecke, C. E., Mathew, S., et al. (2013). Triglyceride-rich lipoprotein modulates endothelial vascular cell adhesion molecule (VCAM)-1 expression via differential regulation of endoplasmic reticulum stress. *PLoS One* 8:e78322. doi: 10.1371/journal.pone.0078322

Wang, Z., Zou, J., Cao, K., Hsieh, T. C., Huang, Y., and Wu, J. M. (2005). Dealcoholized red wine containing known amounts of resveratrol suppresses atherosclerosis in hypercholesterolemic rabbits without affecting plasma lipid levels. *Int. J. Mol. Med.* 16, 533–540.

Weber, C., and Noels, H. (2011). Atherosclerosis: current pathogenesis and therapeutic options. *Nat. Med.* 17, 1410–1422. doi: 10.1038/nm.2538

Wei, Y. M., Li, X., Xu, M., Abais, J. M., Chen, Y., Riebling, C. R., et al. (2013). Enhancement of autophagy by simvastatin through inhibition of Rac1-mTOR signaling pathway in coronary arterial myocytes. *Cell. Physiol. Biochem.* 31, 925–937. doi: 10.1159/000350111

Weiss, D., Kools, J. J., and Taylor, W. R. (2001). Angiotensin II-induced hypertension accelerates the development of atherosclerosis in apoE-deficient mice. *Circulation* 103, 448–454. doi: 10.1161/01.cir.103.3.448

Wellen, K. E., and Hotamisligil, G. S. (2005). Inflammation, stress, and diabetes. *J. Clin. Invest.* 115, 1111–1119. doi: 10.1172/jci25102

Wen, H., Gris, D., Lei, Y., Jha, S., Zhang, L., Huang, M. T., et al. (2011). Fatty acid-induced NLRP3-ASC inflammasome activation interferes with insulin signaling. *Nat. Immunol.* 12, 408–415. doi: 10.1038/ni.2022

Wilkes, J. J., Hevener, A., and Olefsky, J. (2003). Chronic endothelin-1 treatment leads to insulin resistance in vivo. *Diabetes* 52, 1904–1909. doi: 10.2337/diabetes.52.8.1904

Wu, K. K., and Huan, Y. (2007). Diabetic atherosclerosis mouse models. *Atherosclerosis* 191, 241–249. doi: 10.1016/j.atherosclerosis.2006.08.030

Wu, Q., Hu, Y., Jiang, M., Wang, F., and Gong, G. (2019). Effect of autophagy regulated by sirt1/foxo1 pathway on the release of factors promoting thrombosis from vascular endothelial cells. *Int. J. Mol. Sci.* 20:4132. doi: 10.3390/ijms20174132

Wu, Z., Huang, C., Xu, C., Xie, L., Liang, J. J., Liu, L., et al. (2019). Caveolin-1 regulates human trabecular meshwork cell adhesion, endocytosis, and autophagy. *J. Cell. Biochem.* 120, 13382–13391. doi: 10.1002/jcb.28613

Xu, J., Kitada, M., and Koya, D. (2020). The impact of mitochondrial quality control by Sirtuins on the treatment of type 2 diabetes and diabetic kidney disease. *Biochim. Biophys. Acta Mol. Basis Dis.* 1866:165756. doi: 10.1016/j.bbadis.2020.165756

Xu, K., Yang, Y., Yan, M., Zhan, J., Fu, X., and Zheng, X. (2010). Autophagy plays a protective role in free cholesterol overload-induced death of smooth muscle cells. *J. Lipid Res.* 51, 2581–2590. doi: 10.1194/jlr.M005702

Xu, Y., Zhou, Q., Xin, W., Li, Z., Chen, L., and Wan, Q. (2016). Autophagy downregulation contributes to insulin resistance mediated injury in insulin receptor knockout podocytes in vitro. *PeerJ* 4:e1888. doi: 10.7717/peerj.1888

Xu, Y. L., Liu, X. Y., Cheng, S. B., He, P. K., Hong, M. K., Chen, Y. Y., et al. (2020). Geniposide enhances macrophage autophagy through downregulation of TREM2 in atherosclerosis. *Am. J. Chin. Med.* 48, 1821–1840. doi: 10.1142/s0192415x20500913

Yamauchi, T., and Kadowaki, T. (2013). Adiponectin receptor as a key player in healthy longevity and obesity-related diseases. *Cell Metab.* 17, 185–196. doi: 10.1016/j.cmet.2013.01.001

You, G., Long, X., Song, F., Huang, J., Tian, M., Xiao, Y., et al. (2020). Metformin activates the AMPK-mTOR pathway by modulating lncRNA TUG1 to induce autophagy and inhibit atherosclerosis. *Drug Des. Devel. Ther.* 14, 457–468. doi: 10.2147/dddt.s233932

Yu, K. Y., Wang, Y. P., Wang, L. H., Jian, Y., Zhao, X. D., Chen, J. W., et al. (2014). Mitochondrial KATP channel involvement in angiotensin II-induced autophagy in vascular smooth muscle cells. *Basic Res. Cardiol.* 109:416. doi: 10.1007/s00395-014-0416-y

Zeng, G., Nystrom, F. H., Ravichandran, L. V., Cong, L. N., Kirby, M., Mostowski, H., et al. (2000). Roles for insulin receptor, PI3-kinase, and Akt in insulin-signaling pathways related to production of nitric oxide in human vascular endothelial cells. *Circulation* 101, 1539–1545. doi: 10.1161/01.cir.101.13.1539

Zeng, G., and Quon, M. J. (1996). Insulin-stimulated production of nitric oxide is inhibited by wortmannin. Direct measurement in vascular endothelial cells. *J. Clin. Invest.* 98, 894–898. doi: 10.1172/jci118871

Zhai, C., Cheng, J., Mujahid, H., Wang, H., Kong, J., Yin, Y., et al. (2014). Selective inhibition of PI3K/Akt/mTOR signaling pathway regulates autophagy of macrophage and vulnerability of atherosclerotic plaque. *PLoS One* 9:e90563. doi: 10.1371/journal.pone.0090563

Zhang, X., Ramírez, C. M., Aryal, B., Madrigal-Matute, J., Liu, X., Diaz, A., et al. (2020). Cav-1 (Caveolin-1) deficiency increases autophagy in the endothelium and attenuates vascular inflammation and atherosclerosis. *Arterioscler. Thromb. Vasc. Biol.* 40, 1510–1522. doi: 10.1161/atvbaha.120.314291

Zhang, Y., Cao, X., Zhu, W., Liu, Z., Liu, H., Zhou, Y., et al. (2016). Resveratrol enhances autophagic flux and promotes Ox-LDL degradation in HUVECs via upregulation of SIRT1. *Oxid. Med. Cell. Longev.* 2016:7589813. doi: 10.1155/2016/7589813

Zhang, Y., Whaley-Connell, A. T., Sowers, J. R., and Ren, J. (2018). Autophagy as an emerging target in cardiorenal metabolic disease: from pathophysiology to management. *Pharmacol. Ther.* 191, 1–22. doi: 10.1016/j.pharmthera.2018.06.004

Zhang, Y. F., Hong, J., Zhan, W. W., Li, X. Y., Gu, W. Q., Yang, Y. S., et al. (2006). Hyperglycaemia after glucose loading is a major predictor of preclinical atherosclerosis in nondiabetic subjects. *Clin. Endocrinol. (Oxf.)* 64, 153–157. doi: 10.1111/j.1365-2265.2005.02440.x

Zhang, Y. Y., Shi, Y. N., Zhu, N., Wang, W., Deng, C. F., Xie, X. J., et al. (2020). Autophagy: a killer or guardian of vascular smooth muscle cells. *J. Drug Target* 28, 449–455. doi: 10.1080/1061186x.2019.1705312

Zheng, J., and Lu, C. (2020). Oxidized LDL causes endothelial apoptosis by inhibiting mitochondrial fusion and mitochondria autophagy. *Front. Cell. Dev. Biol.* 8:600950. doi: 10.3389/fcell.2020.600950

Zhou, J., Massey, S., Story, D., and Li, L. (2018). Metformin: an old drug with new applications. *Int. J. Mol. Sci.* 19:2863. doi: 10.3390/ijms19102863

Zhou, X., Yang, J., Zhou, M., Zhang, Y., Liu, Y., Hou, P., et al. (2019). Resveratrol attenuates endothelial oxidative injury by inducing autophagy via the activation of transcription factor EB. *Nutr. Metab. (Lond.)* 16:42. doi: 10.1186/s12986-019-0371-6

Zhu, H., Wang, Z., Dong, Z., Wang, C., Cao, Q., Fan, F., et al. (2019). Aldehyde dehydrogenase 2 deficiency promotes atherosclerotic plaque instability through accelerating mitochondrial ROS-mediated vascular smooth muscle cell senescence. *Biochim. Biophys. Acta Mol. Basis Dis.* 1865, 1782–1792. doi: 10.1016/j.bbadis.2018.09.033

Zhu, H., and Zhang, Y. (2018). Life and death partners in Post-PCI restenosis: apoptosis, autophagy, and the cross-talk between them. *Curr. Drug Targets* 19, 1003–1008. doi: 10.2174/1389450117666160625072521

Zhu, L., Wu, G., Yang, X., Jia, X., Li, J., Bai, X., et al. (2019). Low density lipoprotein mimics insulin action on autophagy and glucose uptake in endothelial cells. *Sci. Rep.* 9:3020. doi: 10.1038/s41598-019-39559-7

Zhu, Y. N., Fan, W. J., Zhang, C., Guo, F., Li, W., Wang, Y. F., et al. (2017). Role of autophagy in advanced atherosclerosis (Review). *Mol. Med. Rep.* 15, 2903–2908. doi: 10.3892/mmr.2017.6403

8

Metabolic Syndrome Triggered by Fructose Diet Impairs Neuronal Function and Vascular Integrity in ApoE-KO Mouse Retinas: Implications of Autophagy Deficient Activation

María C. Paz[1,2†], Pablo F. Barcelona[1,2], Paula V. Subirada[1,2], Magali E. Ridano[1,2†], Gustavo A. Chiabrando[1,2], Claudia Castro[3] and María C. Sánchez[1,2*]

[1] Departamento de Bioquímica Clínica, Facultad de Ciencias Químicas, Universidad Nacional de Córdoba, Córdoba, Argentina, [2] Centro de Investigaciones en Bioquímica Clínica e Inmunología, Consejo Nacional de Investigaciones Científicas y Técnicas, Córdoba, Argentina, [3] Instituto de Medicina y Biología Experimental de Cuyo, Consejo Nacional de Investigaciones Científicas y Técnicas, Facultad de Ciencias Médicas, Universidad Nacional de Cuyo, Mendoza, Argentina

*Correspondence:
María C. Sánchez
csanchez@fcq.unc.edu.ar

Metabolic syndrome is a disorder characterized by a constellation of clinical findings such as elevated blood glucose, hyperinsulinemia, dyslipidemia, hypertension, and obesity. A positive correlation has been found between metabolic syndrome or its components and retinopathy, mainly at microvascular level, in patients without a history of diabetes. Here, we extend the investigations beyond the vascular component analyzing functional changes as well as neuronal and glial response in retinas of Apolipoprotein E knockout (ApoE-KO) mice fed with 10% w/v fructose diet. Given that autophagy dysfunction is implicated in retinal diseases related to hyperglycemia and dyslipidemia, the activation of this pathway was also analyzed. Two months of fructose intake triggered metabolic derangements in ApoE-KO mice characterized by dyslipidemia, hyperglycemia and hyperinsulinemia. An increased number of TUNEL positive cells, in addition to the ganglion cell layer, was observed in the inner nuclear layer in retina. Vascular permeability, evidenced by albumin–Evans blue leakage and extravasation of albumin was also detected. Furthermore, a significant decrease of the glial fibrillary acidic protein expression was confirmed by Western blot analysis. Absence of both Müller cell gliosis and pro-angiogenic response was also demonstrated. Finally, retinas of ApoE-KO FD mice showed defective autophagy activation as judged by LC3B mRNA and p62 protein levels correlating with the increased cell death. These results demonstrated that FD induced in ApoE-KO mice biochemical alterations compatible with metabolic syndrome associated with neuronal impairment and mild vascular alterations in the retina.

Keywords: metabolic parameters, non-proliferative retinopathy, functional retinal changes, neurodegeneration, vascular permeability, cellular processes

INTRODUCTION

Metabolic Syndrome (MetS) is a complex disorder of metabolism considered a global epidemic that involves a high socio-economic cost (Sherling et al., 2017). This syndrome defined as a constellation of metabolic abnormalities including elevated blood glucose, hyperinsulinemia, dyslipidemia, hypertension and obesity (Schwartz and Reaven, 2006) affects approximately 20–25% of the adult population (Ibrahim et al., 2019). Individuals with MetS have two to threefold risk of developing cardiovascular disease and fivefold risk of developing type 2 Diabetes Mellitus (DM) (Wild et al., 2004). In this sense, deleterious effects of MetS extend beyond the heart affecting other organs such as the retina (Thierry et al., 2015; Zarei et al., 2017), doubling the number of people with visual impairment. Accumulating evidences, stemming from clinical and experimental research have shown that, in addition to the vascular component, neurons and glial cells are also affected in retinopathies and their dysfunction may contribute to disease progression (Dorrell et al., 2010; Liu et al., 2010; Fu et al., 2015). Although, type 2 DM is frequently associated with MetS, this syndrome can also occur as an isolated entity, which provides an opportunity to study the early retinal consequences of systemic metabolic changes. While diagnosis of DM has clear-cut definitions, many patients experience before the onset of frank diabetes a series of biochemical alterations which affect the cardiovascular and metabolic condition (Forouhi et al., 2007; Nathan et al., 2007), contributing the latter to development of retinopathy (Mbata et al., 2017). The association of MetS and retinopathy in patients without a history of diabetes has been researched, mainly at vascular level, in a number of studies (Wong et al., 2004; Keenan et al., 2009; Peng et al., 2010; Liu et al., 2015). However, little is known about the functional retinal changes, neuroglial response and molecular mechanisms involved. Even though numerous animal models of MetS have been established (Wong et al., 2016) further investigations of its deleterious consequences on retina are still necessary. In this study, we hypothesized that a combination of genetic condition plus carbohydrate-rich diet would be sufficient to induce MetS and retinal damage. Specifically, ApoE-KO mice spontaneously hypercholesterolemic were fed with a diet supplemented with 10% of fructose (FD), an important and pervasive sweetener in Western diets that produces impaired glucose tolerance and increases the blood triglyceride concentrations (Tappy and Rosset, 2019). In this *in vivo* model of MetS, we characterized the effects of metabolic derangement on retinal function over time and analyzed the vascular, neuronal and glial alterations.

Abbreviations: ApoE-KO, apolipoprotein E knockout; AUC, area under the curve; BRB, blood retinal barrier; CQ, chloroquine; DM, Diabetes Mellitus; ERG, electroretinogram; FD, fructose diet; GCL, Ganglion cell layer; GFAP, glial fibrilar acid protein; GS, glutamine synthase; GSA-IB4, Griffonia Simplicifolia Isolectin-B4; HIF, hypoxia inducible factor; HDL, high-density lipoproteins; LDL, low-density lipoproteins; ILM, inner limitant membrane; INL, inner nuclear layer; IPGTT, intraperitoneal glucose tolerance test; LC3B, microtubule-associated proteins 1A/1B light chain 3B; MetS, Metabolic Syndrome; MGCs, Müller glial cells; ND, normal diet; ONL, outer nuclear layer; TUNEL, terminal deoxynucleotidyltransferase biotin dUTP nick end labeling; VEGF, vascular endothelial growth factor; VLDL, very low density lipoproteins; IDL, intermediate density lipoproteins.

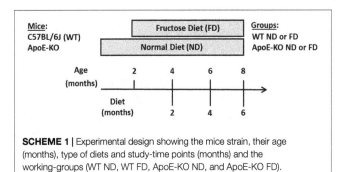

SCHEME 1 | Experimental design showing the mice strain, their age (months), type of diets and study-time points (months) and the working-groups (WT ND, WT FD, ApoE-KO ND, and ApoE-KO FD).

Finally, given that autophagy deregulation is implicated in many retinal pathologies related to hyperglycemia and dyslipidemia (Meng et al., 2017), we investigated if this cellular homeostatic mechanism (Kim et al., 2008; Rodriguez-Muela et al., 2012; Wen et al., 2019) was activated in FD-fed ApoE-KO mice, once retinal abnormalities were detected.

MATERIALS AND METHODS

Mouse Model

Male C57BL/6J wild type (WT) and Apolipoprotein E-deficient (ApoE-KO) mice on C57BL/6J background (The Jackson Laboratories, Bar Harbor, ME, United States), 8 weeks of age (20–22 g), were used for this study. Mice were maintained under standard laboratory conditions of temperature (22 ± 1°C) and light (12-h light/12-h dark cycle) with free access to food and water. Mice were randomly divided in the following groups: WT mice fed either a normal diet (ND) with free access to tap water (WT ND) or fructose diet (WT FD) receiving 10% (w/v) D (−) fructose p.a. (Biopack, Argentina) in drinking water. Additional group of age-matched ApoE-KO mice were given a ND (ApoE-KO ND) or fructose diet (ApoE-KO FD). All experimental groups received a standard commercial mice chow. Fructose solution was replaced every 2 days. Mice were sacrificed at three time points: 2, 4, and 6 months of feeding (**Scheme 1**). Whole eyes or retinas of sacrificed mice were collected and processed for Western blot, Real-Time PCR (qRT-PCR), immunohistochemistry, immunofluorescence or flat-mount assays. In order to analyze the autophagy pathway, some mice received an intraperitoneal (i.p.) injection of 60 mg/kg chloroquine (CQ, Sigma-Aldrich, St. Louis, MO, United States) diluted in sterile phosphate buffered saline (PBS) 4 h before sacrifice. At least four mice per group were used for each condition depending on the experiment. Experimental procedures were designed and approved by the Institutional Animal Care and Use Committee (CICUAL) of the Faculty of Chemical Sciences, National University of Córdoba (Res. HCD 1199/17). All efforts were made to reduce the number of animals used.

Blood Glucose Measurements

Plasma glucose levels were determined in tail vein blood samples, using the Free Style Optium blood glucose meter (Abbot

Laboratories Argentina) in fasted (overnight, $n = 4$) or non-fasted mice ($n = 8$). The measurements were performed at the same time of day in each experimental condition.

Intraperitoneal Glucose Tolerance Test

The i.p. glucose tolerance test (IPGTT) was performed at 4 months of feeding. Animals were fasted overnight before the experiments. For the IPGTT, mice received an i.p. 1 g/kg (body weight) of glucose injection. Blood samples for plasma glucose measurement were collected from the tail vein at time 0 (before glucose injection) and 30, 60, and 120 min after glucose administration ($n = 4$). The area under the curve (AUC) was calculated using the trapezoidal rule estimation by GraphPad Prism 7.0 software.

Lipid Profile and Insulin Levels

At the end of the experimental period and prior euthanasia, triglycerides, high-density lipoprotein (HDL) cholesterol, low-density lipoprotein (LDL) cholesterol, total cholesterol and insulin were measured after overnight fasting, in heparinized blood samples collected from cardiac puncture in anesthetized animals via i.p. with ketamine (35 mg/kg)/xylazine (3.5 mg/kg). Different plasmatic cholesterol forms and triglyceride concentrations were determined using automatized commercial kits by enzymatic colorimetric methods (Roche, Buenos Aires, Argentina, $n = 6 - 8$). Insulin was measured by ELISA (Crystal Chem, United States, $n = 4$).

Electroretinography (ERG)

Electroretinographic activity was recorded after 2, 4, and 6 months of feeding according to previously described procedures (Ridano et al., 2017; Lorenc et al., 2018; Subirada et al., 2019). Briefly, after overnight dark adaptation and under dim red illumination, mice were anesthetized with ketamine/xylazine (i.p.), the pupils were dilated with 1% tropicamide (Midryl, Alcon, Buenos Aires, Argentina) and the cornea was lubricated with gel drops of 0.4% polyethylene glycol 400 and 0.3% propylene glycol (Systane, Alcon, Buenos Aires, Argentina) to prevent damage. After body temperature stabilization on a 37°C warming pad for 10 min, mice were exposed to a light stimulus at a distance of 20 cm. A reference electrode was inserted on the back between the ears, a grounding electrode was attached to the tail, and a gold electrode was placed in contact with the central cornea. Electroretinograms (ERG) were simultaneously recorded from both eyes and ten responses to not dimmed flashes of white led light (5 cd.s/m2, 0.2 Hz) from a photic stimulator (light-emitting diodes) set at maximum brightness were amplified, filtered (1.5-Hz low-pass filter, 1000 high-pass filter, notch activated) and averaged (Akonic BIO-PC, Argentina).

The a-wave was measured as the difference in amplitude between the recording at onset and trough of the negative deflection, and the b-wave amplitude was measured from the trough of the a-wave to the peak of the b-wave. The latencies of the a- and b-waves were measured from the time of flash presentation to the trough of the a-wave or the peak of the

b-wave, respectively. Responses were averaged across the two eyes for each mouse ($n = 6 - 12$).

Oscillatory potentials (OPs) were assessed as previously described (Moreno et al., 2005). Briefly, the same photic stimulator with a 0.2 Hz frequency and filters of high (300 Hz) or low (100 Hz) frequency were used. The OPs amplitude was estimated by measuring the heights from the baseline drawn between the troughs of successive wavelets to their peaks. The sum of three central peaks of OPs was used for statistical analysis. Responses were averaged across the two eyes for each mouse ($n = 6 - 12$).

Vascular Permeability

Vascular permeability was analyzed by measuring albumin–Evans blue complex leakage from retinal vessels as previously described (Ma et al., 1997; Barcelona et al., 2016). Briefly, mice ($n = 3$) were injected intravenous (i.v.) through the vein of the tail with a solution of Evans blue (2% w/v dissolved in PBS). Immediately after injection, animals turned visibly blue, confirming the dye uptake and distribution. After 48 h, mice were transcardially perfused with saline solution and flat-mounted retinas were obtained. Microphotographs were taken using identical exposure time, brightness, and contrast settings (Fernandez et al., 2011).

Labeling of Flat-Mount Retinas

Mice were euthanized at 4 months of diet and eyes were enucleated and fixed with freshly prepared 4% paraformaldehyde (PFA) for 2 h at room temperature. Corneas were removed with scissors along the limbus and the whole retinas were dissected. Then, they were blocked and permeabilized in Tris-buffered saline (TBS) containing 5% Bovine Serum Albumin (BSA, Sigma-Aldrich, United States) and 0.1% Triton-X-100 during 6 h at 4°C. After that, retinas were incubated overnight with Isolectin IB4 Alexa fluor-488 conjugated (GSA-IB4) from Molecular Probes, Inc. (1/100; Eugene, OR, United States) in combination with rabbit polyclonal Anti-Glial Fibrillary Acidic Protein (GFAP) antibody from Dako (1/200; Carpinteria, CA, United States) or mouse polyclonal alpha Smooth Muscle Actin (α-SMA) antibody from Dako (1/100; Carpinteria, CA, United States). Then, retinas were washed with TBS 0.1% Triton-X-100 and incubated with secondary antibodies including goat against rabbit or mouse IgG conjugated with Alexa Fluor 488 and 594 (1/250; Molecular Probes, Eugene, OR, United States) during 1 h at room temperature. Retinas were then washed with TBS containing 0.1% Triton-X-100, stored in PBS at 4°C and examined by confocal laser-scanning microscopy (Olympus FluoView FV1200; Olympus Corp., New York, NY, United States). Each image is the flatten result of 10 photos (10 μm) taken at plane z. Vascular density, vascular diameter and branching of the vasculature of the different experimental groups were quantified from GSA-IB4 immunostained flats, three different flats of each experimental group were average ($n = 3$). The vascular density was quantified as fluorescence intensity labeling (% area), using a square of 200 mm^2 (see scheme of quantification in **Figure 3B**) which was positioned in nine different places in each microphotograph, using Image J Fiji software (National Institutes of Health, Bethesda, MD, United States). The vascular diameter was quantified as the average (pixels) of three measurements in different places of three big arterioles in each microphotograph. Three areas of quantification were defined by using concentric circles around the optic nerve separated by 200 μm (see scheme of quantification in **Figure 3B**). Representative image and quantification at only one height is shown as no significant difference was observed at any height measured. The branching was quantified counting the primary branches from a big arteriole, since the optic nerve to the periphery. α-SMA immunostaining was quantified as fluorescence intensity labeling (% area) from four different flat-mounts of each experimental group ($n = 4$) using Image J Fiji software (National Institutes of Health, Bethesda, MD, United States).

Retinal Cryosection, Protein Extract and RNA Sample Preparation

For cryosection, eyes after 4 months of feeding were enucleated, fixed during 2 h with 4% PFA at room temperature, and incubated overnight in 10, 20, and 30% of sucrose in PBS at 4°C. Then, they were embedded in optimum cutting temperature (OCT, Tissue-TEK, Sakura) compound, and 10-μm-thick radial sections were obtained by using a cryostat, according to general methods (Subirada et al., 2019). Retinal cryosections were then stored at −20°C under dry conditions until immunohistochemical analysis. Neural retinas were dissected from Retinal Pigmentary Epithelium/choroid layers for Western blot and qRT-PCR analysis (Ridano et al., 2017; Lorenc et al., 2018). Protein extracts were obtained from retinas after homogenization with a lysis buffer containing 20 mM Tris-HCl pH 7.5, 137 mM NaCl, 2 mM EDTA pH 8, 1% Nonidet P40, 1 mM phenylmethylsulfonyl fluoride (PMSF), 2 mM sodium ortovanadate and protease inhibitor cocktail (Sigma Aldrich, St. Louis, MO, United States), and were sonicated during 20 s at 40% amplitude. In addition, some neural retinas were disrupted in 500 μL Trizol (Invitrogen) and were stored at −80°C until RNA extraction.

Immunofluorescence

Immunostaining was performed as described previously (Ridano et al., 2017; Lorenc et al., 2018; Subirada et al., 2019). Briefly, mouse cryosections were washed in PBS, blocked with 2% of BSA in PBS containing 0.1% Tween 20, for 1 h and then incubated overnight at 4°C with the following primary antibodies: rabbit polyclonal Anti-GFAP antibody from Dako (1/100; Carpinteria, CA, United States), rabbit polyclonal anti-LC3B (1/100; L7543, Sigma Aldrich) and mouse monoclonal anti-p62 (1/100; ab56416, Abcam). Then, sections were washed with 0.1% Tween 20 in PBS and incubated with secondary antibodies including goat against rabbit or mouse IgG conjugated with Alexa Fluor 488 or 594 (1/250; Molecular Probes, Eugene, OR, USA) during 1 h at room temperature. The sections were also counterstained with Hoechst 33258 (1:3000; Molecular Probes) for 7 min. After a thorough rinse, the sections were mounted with Fluor Save (Calbiochem, La Jolla, CA, United States) and cover slipped. The labeling was visualized using a confocal laser-scanning microscope (Olympus Fluo View FV300 or FV1200; Olympus

Corp., New York, NY, United States). Finally, images from three different retinas from each experimental group ($n = 3$), were processed with Image J software (National Institutes of Health, Bethesda, MD, United States). Negative controls without incubation with primary antibody were carried out to detect unspecific staining (data not shown). Negative controls without incubation with primary antibody were carried out to detect unspecific staining (data not shown). Vesicle quantification: in each cryosection, two images were acquired at the central area, next to the optic nerve head. Images were taken with oil 40X objective in the best confocal resolution condition. A total of 10 consecutive images were acquired in z plane, with a step size of 1 μm. The quantification of the number of LC3B positive vesicles was carried out in deconvolved images with ImageJ FIJI software, analyze particles plugin. The measurement of the number of puncta was done in a standard ROI (20 μm × 20 μm) area and further correlated to the number of nuclei present in the ROI. At least 5 ROIs were quantified from each layer of the retina in each slide for every condition.

Western Blot

Protein concentration of retinal extracts were determined by a Bicinchoninic Acid Protein Assay Kit (Pierce BCA, Thermo Scientific, United States) and 10 – 20 μg of proteins were electrophoresed in 10 or 15% sodium dodecyl sulphate polyacrylamide gel electrophoresis (SDS-PAGE). After electrophoresis, proteins were transferred to nitrocellulose membranes (Amersham Hybond ECL; GE Healthcare Bio-Sciences AB, Uppsala, Sweden). To prevent non-specific binding, membranes were blocked with 5% BSA in TBS containing 0.1% Tween-20 (TBST) during at least 1 h at room temperature. Then, blots were incubated with primary antibodies diluted in TBST or 1% BSA in TBST for 1 h at room temperature or overnight at 4°C, according to the antibody. The following primary antibodies were used: rabbit polyclonal anti-GFAP (1/1000; Dako, Carpinteria, CA, United States, $n = 4$), mouse monoclonal anti- glutamine synthetase (GS) (1/500; Millipore Corporation, MA, United States, $n = 5$), goat polyclonal anti-serum albumin (1/5000; Abcam, Argentina, n = 3), rabbit anti-LC3B (1/1000; Sigma-Aldrich, United States, $n = 3$), mouse monoclonal anti SQSTM1/p62 (1/1000; Abcam, $n = 3$) and loading proteins such as, mouse monoclonal anti-β actin (1/2000; Sigma-Aldrich, United States) or mouse monoclonal anti-α tubulin (1/2000; Sigma-Aldrich). Blots were incubated with IRDye 800 CW or IRDye 695 CW donkey anti-rabbit IgG, IRDye 800 CW or IRDye 695 CW donkey anti-mouse IgG or IRDye 695 CW donkey anti-goat IgG antibodies (1/15000 in TBS with 1% BSA) for 1 h, protected from light. After washing with TBST, membranes were visualized and quantified using the Odyssey Infrared Imaging System (LI-COR, Inc., Lincoln, NE, United States). All the assays were performed in triplicate and results are representative of at least three independent experiments ($n = 3 – 5$).

qRT-PCR

Total RNA was extracted from neural retinas using Trizol (Invitrogen), according to the manufacturer's instructions and was processed as previously reported (Ridano et al., 2017;

Subirada et al., 2019). Briefly, 1 μg of total RNA was reverse-transcribed in a total volume of 20 μL using random primers (Invitrogen, Buenos Aires, Argentina) and 50 U of M-MLV reverse transcriptase (Promega Corp.). For qPCR, cDNA was mixed with 1x SYBR Green PCR Master Mix (Applied Biosystems) and the forward and reverse primers (LC3B forward: CGC TTG CAG CTC AAT GCT AAC/LC3B reverse: CTC GTA CAC TTC GGA GAT GGG, Hypoxia-inducible factor-1α (HIF-1α) forward: CACCGATTCGCCATGGA/HIF-1α reverse: TTCGACGTTCAGAACTCATCTTTT, Vascular endothelial growth factor (VEGF) forward: AGAGCAGAAGTCCCATGAAGTGA/VEGF reverse: TCAATCGGACGGCAGTAGCT, Tumoral necrosis factor-α (TNF-α) forward: AGCCGATG GGTTGTACCTTGTCTA/, TNF-α reverse: TGAGAT AGCAAATCGGCTGACGGT and Interleukin-6 (IL-6) forward: ATCCAGTTGCCTTCTTGGGACTGA/IL-6 reverse: TAAGCCTCCGACTTGTGAAGTGGT), were carried out on an Applied Biosystems 7500 Real- Time PCR System with Sequence Detection Software v1.4. The cycling conditions included a hot start at 95°C for 10 min, followed by 40 cycles at 95°C for 15 s and 60°C for 1 min. Specificity was verified by melting curve analysis. Results were normalized to β-actin forward: GGCTGTATTCCCCTCCATCG/β-actin reverse: CCAGTTGGTAACAATGCCATGT. Relative gene expression was calculated according to the $2-\Delta\Delta Ct$ method. Each sample was analyzed in triplicate. No amplification was observed using as template water or RNA samples incubated without reverse transcriptase during the cDNA synthesis (data not shown). All the assays were performed in triplicate and results are representative of at least three independent experiments ($n = 3 - 4$).

TUNEL Assay

Cell death was examined by terminal deoxynucleotidyltransferase biotin dUTP nick end labeling (TUNEL) assay (Roche, Mannheim, Germany) following the manufacturer's instructions. The peroxidase label was detected with diaminobenzidine hydrochloride (Sigma-Aldrich, United States). Slides were counterstained with methyl green to visualize retinal layers and then mounted with DPX Mounting Media (Sigma-Aldrich, United States). Negative controls without enzyme were processed in order to avoid false positive results (data not shown). For each section, TUNEL-positive nuclei staining brown were counted (nucleus/mm) from three randomly selected fields on either side of the optic nerve and the average values from three slices/eye were combined to produce a mean value of each mouse ($n = 3$). Images were obtained under a light microscope (Nikon Eclipse TE2000-E, Japan).

Statistical Analysis

Statistical analysis was performed using the GraphPad Prism 7.0 software. A p-value < 0.05 was considered statistically significant. Parametric or non-parametric tests were used according to variance homogeneity evaluated by F or Barlett's tests. Kruskal–Wallis followed by Dunn's multiple comparisons post-test or two-way ANOVA followed by Bonferroni multiple comparisons

post-test. Data represent the mean ± standard error of the mean (SEM) or the median with the interquartile range depending on parametric or non-parametric test.

RESULTS

Fructose Diet Triggered MetS in ApoE-KO Mice

Representative biochemical parameters of plasma lipid profile were quantified in WT mice and ApoE-KO mice fed with ND or FD at 2, 4, and 6 months. Triglyceride levels were similar in all experimental groups at 2 months of diet (**Figure 1A**). However, at 4 months significant differences were observed in WT mice fed with FD ($p < 0.001$) and ApoE-KO mice with either ND ($p < 0.001$) or FD ($p < 0.0001$) compared with WT ND group (**Figure 1A**). Interestingly, at 6 months of diet, an additional increase was observed for triglycerides in ApoE-KO FD ($p < 0.05$) compared with ApoE-KO ND group, whereas in WT mice fed with FD group it returned to baseline levels (**Figure 1A**). Regarding the total cholesterol levels, a clearly significant difference was observed between ApoE-KO and WT mice, independently of the diet, at every evaluated time point (**Figure 1B**, $p < 0.0001$). Notably, total cholesterol in the ApoE-KO FD group was significantly higher than ApoE-KO ND group (**Figure 1B**, $p < 0.0001$). Plasma HDL cholesterol significantly increased in hypercholesterolemic mice ($p < 0.001$) compared to WT mice at 2 and 4 months regardless of the diet, and they began to decline at 6 months in ApoE-KO FD group (**Figure 1C**). In addition, a significant increase in the LDL cholesterol level was observed throughout the period evaluated in ApoE-KO mice ($p < 0.0001$) compared to WT mice, and this rise was higher in ApoE-KO FD group ($p < 0.0001$) compared with ApoE-KO ND group (**Figure 1D**).

In a previous study, we reported an increased concentration of plasma glucose in ApoE-KO mice fed with FD at 2 months of diet (Cannizzo et al., 2012), which was confirmed in this study under fasting and non-fasting conditions. A significant increase in the fasting glucose levels was observed in ApoE-KO FD group as compared with WT ND group (**Figure 1E**, $p < 0.05$), whereas in non-fasting conditions, it was shown an additional significant difference between ApoE-KO groups (**Figure 1F**, $p < 0.001$). Fasted insulin was higher in ApoE-KO FD group ($p < 0.01$) compared with WT ND mice at 2 months of diet. At 4 months, insulinemia was higher in ApoE-KO ND group ($p < 0.01$) and also in ApoE-KO FD group ($p < 0.0001$), showing an additional rise in ApoE-KO FD group ($p < 0.0001$) compared with ApoE-KO ND group (**Figure 1G**). Finally, in order to evaluate the ability of the mice to metabolize glucose, the IPGTT was performed in all groups of animals at 4 months of diet. Glucose levels assessed before and 30, 60, and 120 min after an i.p. administration of 1 g/kg of glucose, showed a significant increase in ApoE-KO FD group compared with ApoE-KO ND mice after 30 min of glucose injection (**Figure 1H**, $p < 0.01$). The average of AUC is showed in **Figure 1I**. Higher values of AUC were observed for the ApoE-KO FD group ($p < 0.0001$) when compared with ApoE-KO ND group

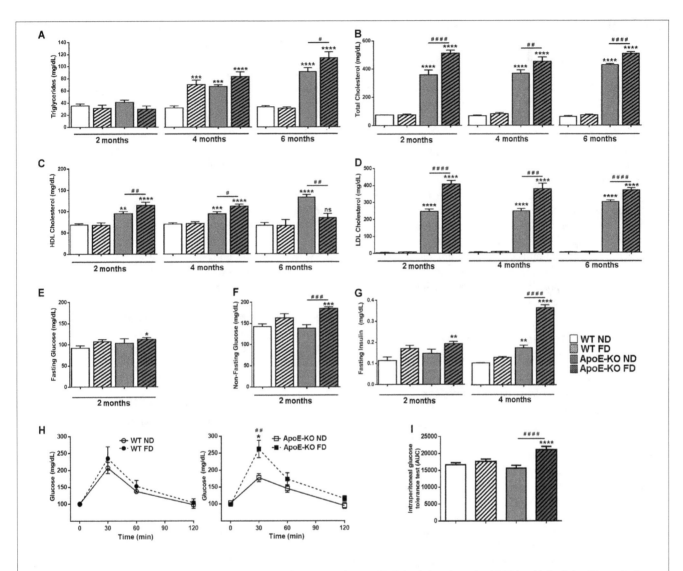

FIGURE 1 | Metabolic profile of peripheral blood in WT and ApoE-KO mice fed with ND or FD during 2, 4, or 6 months. **(A)** Triglyceride levels (mg/dl), $n = 6 - 8$. **(B)** Total cholesterol levels (mg/dl), $n = 6 - 8$. **(C)** HDL-cholesterol levels (mg/dl), $n = 6 - 8$. **(D)** LDL-cholesterol levels (mg/dl), $n = 6 - 8$. **(E)** Glycemic levels (mg/dl) in fasted mice ($n = 4$). **(F)** Glycemic levels (mg/dl) in non-fasted mice ($n = 8$). **(G)** Insulin levels (mg/dl) in fasted mice ($n = 4$). **(H)** Glycemic levels (mg/dl) before (time 0) and 30, 60, and 120 min after glucose injection (1 g/Kg, i.p.) of the different experimental groups at 4 months of diet (all experimental groups were statistically analyzed together but were shown in two graphs for better visualization, $n = 4$) **(I)** IPGTT, bars show the AUC quantification of glycemic levels of graph **(H)**. Data correspond to mean ± SEM. Two-way ANOVA followed by Bonferroni *post hoc* test. Not significant (ns), *$p < 0.05$, **$p < 0.01$, ***$p < 0.001$, and ****$p < 0.0001$ vs. WT ND; #$p < 0.05$, ##$p < 0.01$, ###$p < 0.001$, and ####$p < 0.0001$ ApoE-KO FD vs. ApoE-KO ND.

whereas no differences were observed between WT ND and FD groups (**Figure 1I**).

Taken together, these results demonstrated that 2 months of fructose intake triggered metabolic derangements in spontaneously hypercholesterolemic ApoE-KO mice, which mimics human MetS characterized by dyslipidemia, high insulin levels and hyperglycemia.

Fructose Diet Promoted Neuronal Impairment in the Inner Nuclear Layer of ApoE-KO Mice Retinas

Next, we analyzed the functional status of the retinas by scotopic ERG at 2, 4, and 6 months of diet. The a-wave amplitude was

lower, although not statistically significant, in both ApoE-KO (ND, $p < 0.9999$ and FD, $p = 0.9865$) groups at 2 months of diet respect to WT ND group, differing significantly at 4 months even for the WT DF group ($p < 0.05$) (**Figure 2A**). These ERG changes were maintained at 6 months of diet. Regarding the a-wave implicit time, no changes were observed among the experimental groups at every evaluated time points (**Figure 2A**). At 2 months of diet, the b-wave amplitude and -implicit time values showed a similar profile as the a-wave, excepting that both ApoE-KO (ND and FD) groups evidenced an early reduction in b-wave amplitude ($p < 0.05$) (**Figure 2B**). This effect was maintained at 4 and 6 months of diet in WT FD mice as well as in both ApoE-KO mice groups whereas the b-implicit time did not show changes.

Regarding the sum of OPs amplitude, a progressive decrease in the ApoE-KO groups (ND and FD) as well as in WT FD respect to WT ND group was observed at 4 months of diet. This reduction was more pronounced in the ApoE-KO mice at 6 months of FD ($p < 0.0001$) (**Figure 2C**). Representative scotopic ERG traces at 4 months of diet are also shown in **Figure 2**. In line with these results, TUNEL- positive cell nuclei were detected in retinas of ApoE-KO mice in either ND or FD at 4 months of diet (**Figure 2D**). Quantitative analysis showed a significant increase in the number of TUNEL positive cells in ganglion cell layer (GCL) in both ApoE-KO groups ($p < 0.01$) while an additional increase in the inner nuclear layer (INL; mainly neurons such as bipolar and amacrine cells), was observed in the ApoE-KO FD group ($p < 0.001$) (**Figure 2E**). The number of TUNEL positive cells showed no significant difference in INL and GCL between ApoE-KO groups at 6 months of FD (data not shown). Overall, these results reflected an early deterioration in retinal function and cell viability in ApoE-KO mice, which was intensified with the progressive fructose intake.

Fructose Diet Induced Vascular Permeability and Astrocyte Impairment in ApoE-KO Mice

Examination of GSA-IB4-labeled blood vessels in flat-mounted whole retinas was carried out at 4 months of FD. It showed a clear demarcation into large retinal vessels (arteries and veins) and retinal capillaries (**Figure 3A**). Quantitative measurements of major arteriolar blood vessel diameter showed a similar mean value for all experimental groups. In addition, the closely meshed microvasculature did not show any differences in density among groups. Similarly, blood vessels showed a regular branching aspect (**Figure 3B**). Next, we stained retinal flat-mounts with an antibody against α-SMA to analyze coverage of retinal blood vessels with smooth muscle cells. Interestingly, a loss of α-SMA positive cells was mainly observed in retinas of ApoE-KO mice after 4 months of FD (**Figure 3C**, $p = 0,075$). Then, we tested VEGF gene expression and its upstream factor, HIF-1α, as markers of the pro-angiogenic response in retinal extracts. Whereas HIF-1α mRNA levels did not differ among groups (**Figure 3D**), a slight but significant increase in VEGF mRNA level was observed in WT FD mice in comparison with retinas from the WT ND group ($p < 0.05$) (**Figure 3D**). Nevertheless, neither HIF-1α nor VEGF mRNA levels were modified in ApoE-KO (ND and FD) groups.

Next, we evaluated the Blood-Retinal Barrier (BRB) permeability in flat-mounted retinas by the albumin–Evans blue-complex leakage technique. In WT and ApoE-KO ND groups, the dye was exclusively observed within the vessel lumen of the retinal vasculature, with very low background fluorescence levels. However, focal sites of leakage were observed in WT and ApoE-KO mice fed with FD, with the dye diffusely distributed through the retinal parenchyma (**Figure 3E**). A common approach to quantify alterations in retinal vascular permeability is to determine retinal serum albumin as an endogenous marker for vascular leakage (Vinores et al., 1989; Vinores et al., 1990). We found increased levels of albumin in retinal extracts of WT

($p < 0.01$) and ApoE-KO ($p < 0.001$) mice fed 4 months with FD by Western blot assay (**Figure 3F**).

Considering these results, then we investigated astrocyte integrity by analyzing GFAP immunoreactivity in flat-mounted retinas at 4 month of FD. As shown in **Figure 3G**, in WT ND and FD as well as in ApoE-KO ND retinas, an intense GFAP immunoreactivity was observed in star-shaped astrocytes adjacent to the inner limiting membrane (**Figure 3G**). Western blot analysis confirmed the results seen by immunofluorescence and the quantification revealed a significant decrease of the GFAP protein expression in the ApoE-KO FD group ($p < 0.01$). Levels of GS, a glutamate detoxification enzyme, showed no changes among groups (**Figure 3H**). Moreover, it was demonstrated by GFAP staining on retinal cryosections that Müller glial cells (MGCs) remained not activated among groups (**Figure 3I**). In line with this result, no changes were seen in mRNA expression of IL-6 and TNF-α in retinal extracts, neither in WT and ApoE-KO FD mice nor in ApoE-KO ND group compared with WT ND group, after 4 months of diet (data not shown). Together, these results demonstrated that FD induced vascular permeability and astrocyte impairment without disclosing an outstanding participation of pro-angiogenic and pro- inflammatory pathways in ApoE-KO mice.

Fructose Diet Induced Autophagy Deficient Activation in Retinas of ApoE-KO Mice

Recently, autophagy has demonstrated an important role in the eye diseases such as retinopathies as either a pro-survival or pro-death mechanism (Arroba et al., 2016; Boya et al., 2016; Cammalleri et al., 2016; Lopes de Faria et al., 2016; Dehdashtian et al., 2018; Subirada et al., 2019). In this sense, changes in the autophagy flux have been described in conditions of hyperglycemia and hyperlipidemia (Meng et al., 2017). On that basis, our aim was to determine if this catabolic process was modified early in retinas of ApoE-KO FD mice. For this purpose, samples were obtained at 4 months of diet, period at which changes in the retinal function were detected by ERG assay. Increased levels of LC3B mRNA in retinal extracts of WT FD ($p < 0.05$) and ApoE-KO ND ($p < 0.01$) mice respect to WT ND group were demonstrated by qRT-PCR assay. In ApoE-KO FD the levels of LC3B mRNA were similar to WT ND group (**Figure 4A**), suggesting a minor synthesis of proteins involved in the maintenance of the normal autophagy mechanism. Thus, the autophagy pathway was evaluated. For these experiments, we used an i.p. injection of CQ to monitor autophagosome accumulation by lysosomal blockade. Western blot assays showed that while p62/SQSTM1, a selective substrate of autophagy, did not change in ApoE-KO FD mice, an upregulation was observed in WT FD ($p < 0.01$) and ApoE-KO ND mice ($p < 0.01$). A similar trend was seen for protein levels of LC3BII, where this difference did not reach statistical significance (**Figure 4B**), correlating with the qRT-PCR data. Then, we focused on analysis of the number of autophagosomes located in GCL and INL where we had previously detected TUNEL positive cells and related ERG abnormalities. Quantitative analysis showed an increase in LC3B

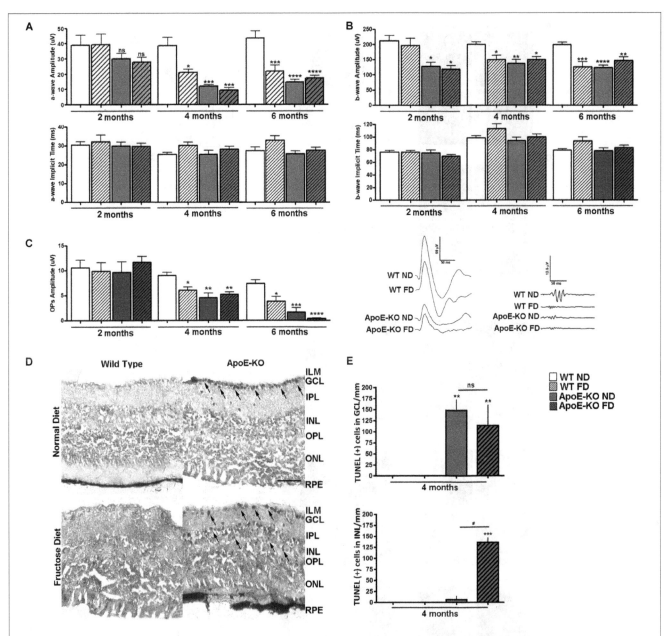

FIGURE 2 | Scotopic ERG after white led flash (5 cd.s/m2, 0.2 Hz) in WT and ApoE-KO mice fed with ND or FD during 2, 4, or 6 months (*n* = 6 – 12). **(A)** Bars represent the average of the amplitude (top panel) and implicit time (bottom panel) of a wave (ms) of the different experimental groups. **(B)** Bars represent the average of the amplitude (top panel) and implicit time (bottom panel) of b wave (ms) of the different experimental groups. **(C)** Bars represent the average of the OPs amplitudes, obtained by sum of OPs 2, OPs 3, and OPs 4, of the different experimental groups. The panel show representative registers of mixed response (scale 50 uV/50 ms) and OPs (scale 12.5 uV/50 ms) at 4 months of diet. **(D)** Representative photomicrographs of cell death analysis by TUNEL/DAB and methyl green counterstaining, in retinal cryosections (10 μm) of the different experimental groups at 4 months of diet (*n* = 3). Cell death was observed as TUNEL positive cells (arrows) in GCL of ApoE-KO (ND and FD) mice and in INL of ApoE-KO FD mice, scale bar: 50 μm, 400x magnification. **(E)** Bars represent the average number of TUNEL positive cells/mm in GCL and INL of retinas of the different experimental groups at 4 months of diet. Data correspond to mean ± SEM (*n* = 4 – 14, depending on the experiment). Two-way ANOVA followed by Bonferroni *post hoc* test or Kruskal–Wallis followed by Dunn's *post hoc* test. Not significant (ns), *$p < 0.05$, **$p < 0.01$, ***$p < 0.001$, and ****$p < 0.0001$ vs. WT ND; ns, #$p < 0.05$ ApoE-KO FD vs. ApoE-KO ND. ILM, inner limiting membrane; GCL, ganglion cell layer; IPL, inner plexiform layer; INL, inner nuclear layer; OPL, outer plexiform layer; ONL, outer nuclear layer; RPE, retinal pigmentary epithelium.

puncta in the GCL in WT FD ($p < 0.0001$) and a trend in ApoE-KO ND ($p = 0.0597$) while the ApoE-KO FD mice group showed an statistically reduction in LC3B puncta compared with WT ND ($p < 0.05$) or ApoE-KO ND mice ($p < 0.0001$) (**Figure 4C**).

Regarding the INL, a similar increase was observed in WT FD ($p < 0.0001$) and ApoE-KO ND ($p < 0.0001$) groups whereas no changes were observed in ApoE-KO at 4 months of FD respect to WT ND group (**Figure 4C**).

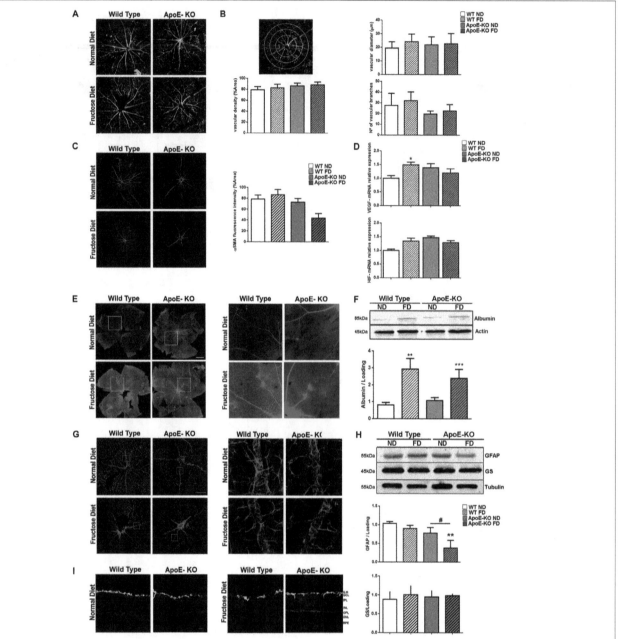

FIGURE 3 | Vascular analysis. **(A)** Representative photomicrographs (scale of 100 μm, 100x magnification) of GSA-IB4 labeled (green) blood vessels in flat-mounts of the central area of whole retinas in the different experimental groups at 4 months of diet (n = 3). **(B)** Scheme of quantification (top left panel), bars represent the average vascular density (% area, bottom left panel), the average vascular diameter (μm, top right panel) and the average vascular branching (bottom right panel) of flat-mounted whole retinas of mice from the different experimental groups at 4 months of diet. **(C)** representative photomicrographs (scale 100 μm, 50x magnification) of α-SMA labeled (red) blood vessels in flat-mounts of the central area of whole retinas of mice from the different experimental groups at 4 months of diet (n = 4). Bars represent the average vascular density (% area). **(D)** Bars represent the average VEGF (top panel) and HIF-1α (bottom panel) mRNA levels relative to actin in mouse retinal extracts of the different experimental groups at 4 months of diet (n = 4). **(E)** Representative photomicrographs (scale 500 μm, 100x magnification) of albumin–Evans blue-complex leakage (red) in flat-mounts of the whole retinas in mice from the different experimental groups at 4 months of diet (n = 3). Square indicate the place of 1000x magnification, scale 250 μm. **(F)** Bars represent albumin protein relative to actin levels in retinal extracts of mice from the different experimental groups at 4 months of diet (bottom panel, n = 3). Representative blot is showed (top panel). **(G)** representative photomicrographs (scale of 100 μm, 50x magnification) of GFAP labeled (red) in flat-mounted central area of the whole retinas of mice from the different experimental groups at 4 months of diet (n = 3). Squares indicate the place of 500x magnification, scale 500 μm. **(H)** Bars represent average protein expression of GFAP (n = 4) and GS (n = 5) relative to tubulin in retinal extracts of mice from the different experimental groups at 4 months of diet (bottom panel). Representative blot is showed (top panel).
(I) Representative photomicrographs (scale 25 μm, 200x magnification) of GFAP label (green) in retinal criosections (10 μm) of mice from the different experimental groups at 4 months of diet (n = 3). Data correspond to mean ± SEM. Two-way ANOVA followed by Bonferroni *post hoc* test or Kruskal–Wallis followed by Dunn's *post hoc* test. *p < 0.05, **p < 0.01, and ***p < 0.001 vs. WT ND, #p < 0.05 ApoE-KO FD vs. ApoE-KO ND. GCL, ganglion cell layer; IPL, inner plexiform layer; INL, inner nuclear layer; OPL, outer plexiform layer; ONL, outer nuclear layer.

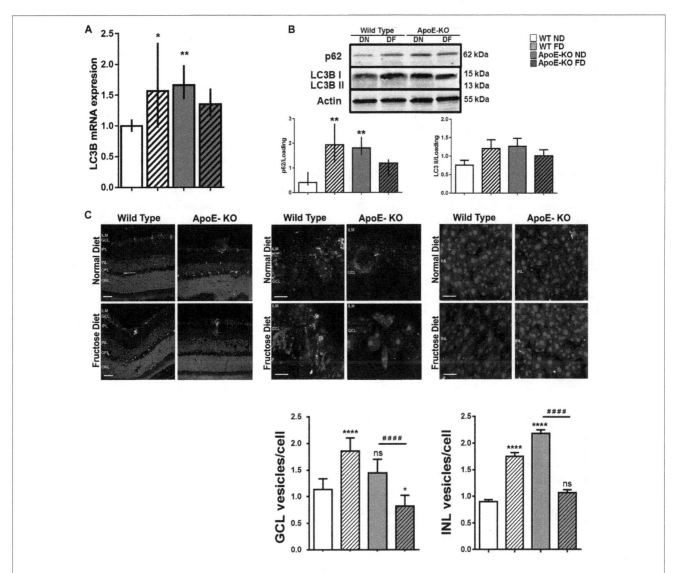

FIGURE 4 | Autophagy pathway evaluation. **(A)** Bars represent the average LC3B mRNA levels relative to actin in mice retinal extracts from the different experimental groups at 4 months of diet. **(B)** Bars represent average protein expression of LC3B I (15 kDa), LC3B II (13 kDa) and p62 relative to actin, in retinal extracts of mice from the different experimental groups at 4 months of diet and 4 h after an i.p. CQ injection (bottom panel). Representative protein blot is showed (top panel). **(C)** Representative photomicrographs (scale 25 μm, 200x magnification) of LC3B label (red) and p62 label (green) in retinal cryosections (10 μm) of mice of the different experimental groups at 4 months of diet, 4 h after an i.p. CQ injection (top left panel). Squares indicate the place of 2000x magnification of the GCL (top central panel) and INL (top right panel); scale 250 μm. Bars represent the quantification of the average of LC3B positive vesicles/cell in GCL (bottom left panel) and in INL (bottom right panel). Data correspond to mean ± SEM (n = 3). Two-way ANOVA followed by Bonferroni *post hoc* test or Kruskal–Wallis followed by Dunn's *post hoc* test. Not significant (ns), *$p < 0.05$, **$p < 0.01$, and ***$p < 0.0001$ vs. WT ND; ####$p < 0.0001$ ApoE-KO FD vs. ApoE-KO ND. ILM, inner limiting membrane; GCL, ganglion cell layer; IPL, inner plexiform layer; INL, inner nuclear layer; OPL, outer plexiform layer; ONL, outer nuclear layer; RPE, retinal pigmentary epithelium.

These findings clearly showed defective autophagy pathway activation in retinas from ApoE-KO mice fed with FD, correlating with retinal dysfunction observed at 4 months of diet.

DISCUSSION

In this study, WT and ApoE-KO mice were used to investigate the effect of metabolic alterations on retinal tissue induced by fructose feeding. These studies included functional retinal analysis over time as well as vascular, glial and neuronal response. Our results showed that WT mice fed with FD as well as ApoE-KO ND mice evidenced some metabolic alterations that were correlated with a mild retinal damage. However, only ApoE-KO mice fed with fructose exhibited hallmark features of MetS, associated with neuronal impairment and mild vascular alterations in the retina.

ApoE plays a critical role in lipoprotein metabolism contributing to the removal of chylomicrons, VLDL and IDL remnants by its interaction with the specific high affinity hepatic

ApoE receptor as well as with the hepatic LDL receptor (Plump et al., 1992). Thus, ApoE deficiency causes the inability to eliminate these lipoprotein remnants and consequently increases total cholesterol and triglycerides in circulation. Our findings indicated that 2 months of fructose intake, triggered metabolic derangements in spontaneously hypercholesterolemic ApoE-KO mice, mimicking MetS characterized by dyslipidemia, high insulin levels and hyperglycemia. Total cholesterol levels showed a significant increase at 2 months of FD in ApoE-KO mice differentiating from both WT groups and even from ApoE-KO ND group, which was maintained throughout the evaluated time points. A similar profile was obtained with LDL cholesterol whereas the HDL cholesterol level in ApoE-KO FD group was similar to WT ND at 6 months of FD. Therefore, a decrease in the HDL/LDL cholesterol ratio was observed in ApoE-KO FD mice. Regarding the triglycerides levels, an increase was observed in both ApoE-KO mice groups since 4 months of diet becoming remarkably different with the fructose ingestion at 6 months respect to ApoE-KO ND. It is of interest to note that plasmatic levels of triglycerides increased in WT mice at 4 months of FD. Observations from numerous mechanistic studies in cells, animals, healthy volunteers, and patients clearly demonstrated that fructose has lipogenic potential. Hepatic fructose metabolism rapidly produces gluconeogenesis and precursors for lipogenesis, while intermediary fructose metabolites also act as nutritional regulators of the major transcription factors that control these pathways. Accordingly, fructose ingestion increases plasma triglyceride levels (Chong et al., 2007; Parks et al., 2008; Teff et al., 2009). However, decreased levels of triglycerides observed in WT FD mice at 6 months suggested a hepatic homeostatic compensation.

The combination of genetic condition and carbohydrate-rich diet mimicked metabolic alterations experienced by individuals before the onset of frank diabetes such as fasting and non-fasting hyperglycemia, which were accompanied by hyperinsulinemia and glucose intolerance (Nathan et al., 2007; Mbata et al., 2017). These metabolic features compatible with MetS in humans were accurately reproduced in ApoE-KO FD, but not in the other experimental groups. Thus, altered lipid and carbohydrate profile associated with hyperinsulinemia clearly highlights to ApoE-KO FD mice as a novel animal model with characteristics of human MetS.

It is known that abnormal visual and retinal function usually precedes morphological alterations that characterize retinopathies in humans (Juen and Kieselbach, 1990; Gardner et al., 1997; Verma et al., 2009). The function of the neural components of the INL and the outer nuclear layer (ONL), assessed by ERG, is usually altered prior to the development of fundoscopically evident retinopathy changes. The most common ERG abnormality observed in these patients is a reduction in the amplitude and/or an increase in implicit time of OPs (Holopigian et al., 1992; Wachtmeister, 1998; Harrison et al., 2011; Bronson-Castain et al., 2012). Concerning the ERG results, most of the functional changes observed at 2 and 4 months of diet mainly correlated with ApoE-KO phenotype rather than any extra effect of diet. However, at 6 months, abolished OPs amplitude was observed in ApoE KO FD respect to WT ND, which represents

the functional response of neuronal cells located in the INL, the most affected retinal layer by the fructose intake. These changes may be attributed to synaptic contacts loss and even neuronal death, correlating with TUNEL assay.

Regarding the microvascular alterations, ApoE-KO mice showed vascular leakage, changes in the astrocyte integrity and reduced retinal label for α-SMA accompanied by plasmatic protein extravasation at 4 months of FD. α-SMA is restricted to vascular smooth muscle cells that surround larger vessels in the normal retina (Trost et al., 2013) whereas astrocytes help to maintain vessel integrity (Zhang and Stone, 1997) and keep the barrier properties of the retinal vascular endothelium (Barber et al., 2000; Fernandez et al., 2011). Impairment of astrocytes has been reported to play a pivotal role in inner BRB breakdown, resulting in the production of vasogenic edema (Chan-Ling and Stone, 1992; Gardner et al., 1997; Rungger-Brandle et al., 2000). In the same way, an enhanced production of VEGF also underlies an increased permeability of the BRB (Kaur et al., 2008). Here, results showed Evans blue complex leakage and increased level of albumin in retinal homogenates in both WT and ApoE-KO mice fed with fructose, which suggests reduced ability to maintain BRB properties. However, despite the fact that WT and ApoE-KO FD mice showed similar vascular permeability alterations in retina the mechanisms involved in both mice groups seem to be different. Whereas in WT FD mice an increased in VEGF mRNA expression seems to be the responsible, in ApoE-KO FD mice it could be attributed to astrocyte abnormalities evidenced by reduced GFAP immunoreactivity.

Müller glial cells are the main glial cells of the retina. These cells are involved in control of angiogenesis, neurotrophic support and through their activation allow the reduction of neurotoxicity by removing metabolic waste products (Bringmann et al., 2006; Subirada et al., 2018). Despite gliosis is a feature of retinal pathology (Mizutani et al., 1998; Gardner et al., 2002), our results showed absence of GFAP reactivity in MGCs in ApoE-KO FD mice retinas at 4 months. These findings were correlated with low levels of pro-inflammatory markers such as IL-6 and TNF-α (data not shown) in whole retinal extracts indicating early stages of retinopathy.

Autophagy is a highly sensitive cellular process induced in response to a wide range of stressful conditions and its deregulation has been implicated in retinal pathologies (Boya et al., 2016; Chai et al., 2016; Amato et al., 2018). In this sense, changes in mRNA and protein levels of autophagy markers have been described in conditions of hyperglycemia and hyperlipidemia (Fu et al., 2016; Meng et al., 2017). Here, we showed that ApoE-KO FD mice retinas, in response to severe metabolic stress, were unable to increase LC3B mRNA and protein level. Confirmation of these results was obtained by immunohistochemical analysis that revealed an increased number of autophagosomes (punctate LC3B staining), mainly in the INL, in WT FD and ApoE-KO ND mice, after the CQ injection. Because of its constant recycling, LC3B transcription is not frequently increased under soft transient autophagy activation. However, when this increase persist along the time, newly synthetized protein will be necessary to support the autophagosomes formation as part of LC3BII is degraded together with the cargo. This is the effect observed in WT FD and APOE-KO ND mice, where a minimal chronic increase in LC3BII protein may require a rise in the level of transcription. All cell types rely on one or more aspects of autophagy to maintain structure and/or function in the retina (Frost et al., 2014). However, the ability to respond will depend on the status of the cell as well as the intensity and duration of the stimuli (Boya et al., 2016; Fu et al., 2016). Here, we demonstrated that retinas from WT FD mice and ApoE-KO ND mice, experienced autophagy activation and cell survival, while in mice under more severe metabolic stress as ApoE-KO FD the altered retinal function and neuronal cell death correlated with a deficient autophagy pathway activation.

Probably, the autophagy variations in ApoE-KO FD is not the mechanism underlying cell death, but the lack of activation of this pathway would be able to shift the balance to cell death in stressed cells. In this sense, it has been described several crosstalk between autophagy and apoptosis or pyroptosis, then changes in one pathway can directly or indirectly modify the cell fate (D'Arcy, 2019; Liu, 2019). Our results encourage us to keep on working in this model to unravel cellular alterations in early stages of retinopathy. Despite the small differences observed among conditions, this research showed that mice with MetS have defective autophagy activation, therefore a potential treatment could contemplate this deficit and should differ from the treatment used in hypercholesterolemic patients.

Recently, it has been shown that in rats fed with a high fructose (60%) plus high fat (9% saturated) diet, the deregulation in glucose metabolism would be the key event in the onset of weak retinal abnormalities (Vidal et al., 2019). Herein, our results clearly demonstrated that both lipid and carbohydrate derangements contributed to the early and progressive retinal impairment. In this sense, 10% of fructose in drinking water was sufficient to induce MetS as was previously reported (Wong et al., 2016). It has been reported that early visual changes caused by type 2 diabetes include color vision losses and abnormal full-field ERG (Lecleire-Collet et al., 2011; Gualtieri et al., 2013). Whereas Vidal et al. (2019) reported not changes in latencies and amplitudes of both a- and b-waves at any time, we found significant changes in the ERG response highlights a progressive reduction mainly in the OPs amplitude which strength these findings.

Taken together, our results demonstrated that ApoE-KO mice, from 2 months of FD began to present biochemical alterations representative of MetS, with deleterious consequences on retinal function, BRB permeability, as well as on intracellular recycling

mechanisms. It is likely that the progression of chronic effects alter several intracellular metabolic pathways leading to complete retinal dysfunction. Therefore, these results validate ApoE-KO mice fed with FD as a suitable model of human MetS exhibiting changes associated with early signs of retinopathy, which allows to analyze the pathophysiological mechanisms involved in the progression of retinal disease as well as to develop possible therapeutic strategies in the future.

ETHICS STATEMENT

All mice were handled according to guidelines of the ARVO Statement for the Use of Animals in Ophthalmic and Vision Research. Experimental procedures were designed and approved by the Institutional Animal Care and Use Committee (CICUAL) of the School of Chemical Sciences, National University of Córdoba (Res. HCD 1199/17). All efforts were made to reduce the number of animals used.

AUTHOR CONTRIBUTIONS

MP, PB, and MS conceived and planned the experiments. MP, PB, PS, and MR carried out the experiments. MP, PB, GC, and MS interpreted the data. GC and CC contributed to the new reagents and analytic tools, analyzed, discussed the data, and reviewed critically the manuscript. MP and MS drafted, wrote, edited, and reviewed critically the manuscript. All authors had final approval of the submitted and published versions.

ACKNOWLEDGMENTS

We thank Gabriel Forzinetti and Natalia Baez for technical assistance in the biochemical determinations, José Luna-Pinto for advice and contributions from the clinical experience in ophthalmology, and Victoria Vaglienti for careful reading the manuscript. We also thank Carlos Mas, María Pilar Crespo, Cecilia Sampedro, and Gonzalo Quassollo of CEMINCO (Centro de Micro y Nanoscopía Córdoba, CONICET-UNC, Córdoba, Argentina) for assistance in confocal microscopy, to Soledad Miró and Victoria Blanco for dedicated animal care and Laura Gatica for histological assistance. MP and MR were postdoctoral fellow of CONICET, PS is posdoctoral fellow of CONICET, and PB, GC, CC, and MS are members of the Research Career of CONICET.

REFERENCES

Amato, R., Catalani, E., Dal Monte, M., Cammalleri, M., Di Renzo, I., and Perrotta, C. (2018). Autophagy-mediated neuroprotection induced by octreotide in an ex vivo model of early diabetic retinopathy. *Pharmacol. Res.* 128, 167–178. doi: 10.1016/j.phrs.2017.09.022

Arroba, A. I., Rodriguez-de la Rosa, L., Murillo-Cuesta, S., Vaquero-Villanueva, L., Hurle, J. M., and Varela-Nieto, I. (2016). Autophagy resolves early retinal inflammation in Igf1-deficient mice. *Dis. Model Mech.* 9, 965–974. doi: 10.1242/dmm.026344

Barber, A. J., Antonetti, D. A., and Gardner, T. W. (2000). Altered expression of retinal occludin and glial fibrillary acidic protein in experimental diabetes. The Penn State Retina Research Group. *Invest. Ophthalmol. Vis. Sci.* 41, 3561–3568.

Barcelona, P. F., Sitaras, N., Galan, A., Esquiva, G., Jmaeff, S., and Jian, Y. (2016). p75NTR and its ligand ProNGF activate paracrine mechanisms etiological to the vascular, inflammatory, and neurodegenerative pathologies of diabetic retinopathy. *J. Neurosci.* 36, 8826–8841. doi: 10.1523/JNEUROSCI.4278-15.2016

Boya, P., Esteban-Martinez, L., Serrano-Puebla, A., Gomez-Sintes, R., and Villarejo-Zori, B. (2016). Autophagy in the eye: development, degeneration, and aging. *Prog. Retin. Eye Res.* 55, 206–245. doi: 10.1016/j.preteyeres.2016.08.001

Bringmann, A., Pannicke, T., Grosche, J., Francke, M., Wiedemann, P., and Skatchkov, S. N. (2006). Muller cells in the healthy and diseased retina. *Prog. Retin. Eye Res.* 25, 397–424. doi: 10.1016/j.preteyeres.2006.05.003

Bronson-Castain, K. W., Bearse, M. A. Jr., Neuville, J., Jonasdottir, S., King-Hooper, B., and Barez, S. (2012). Early neural and vascular changes in the adolescent type 1 and type 2 diabetic retina. *Retina* 32, 92–102. doi: 10.1097/IAE.0b013e318219deac

Cammalleri, M., Dal Monte, M., Locri, F., Lista, L., Aronsson, M., and Kvanta, A. (2016). The urokinase receptor-derived peptide UPARANT mitigates angiogenesis in a mouse model of laser-induced choroidal neovascularization. *Invest. Ophthalmol. Vis. Sci.* 57, 2600–2611. doi: 10.1167/iovs.15-18758

Cannizzo, B., Lujan, A., Estrella, N., Lembo, C., Cruzado, M., and Castro, C. (2012). Insulin resistance promotes early atherosclerosis via increased proinflammatory proteins and oxidative stress in fructose-fed ApoE-KO mice. *Exp. Diabetes Res.* 2012:941304. doi: 10.1155/2012/941304

Chai, P., Ni, H., Zhang, H., and Fan, X. (2016). The evolving functions of autophagy in ocular health: a double-edged sword. *Int. J. Biol. Sci.* 12, 1332–1340. doi: 10.7150/ijbs.16245

Chan-Ling, T., and Stone, J. (1992). Degeneration of astrocytes in feline retinopathy of prematurity causes failure of the blood-retinal barrier. *Invest. Ophthalmol. Vis. Sci.* 33, 2148–2159.

Chong, M. F., Fielding, B. A., and Frayn, K. N. (2007). Mechanisms for the acute effect of fructose on postprandial lipemia. *Am. J. Clin. Nutr.* 85, 1511–1520. doi: 10.1093/ajcn/85.6.1511

D'Arcy, M. S. (2019). Cell death: a review of the major forms of apoptosis, necrosis and autophagy. *Cell Biol. Int.* 43, 582–592. doi: 10.1002/cbin.11137

Dehdashtian, E., Mehrzadi, S., Yousefi, B., Hosseinzadeh, A., Reiter, R. J., and Safa, M. (2018). Diabetic retinopathy pathogenesis and the ameliorating effects of melatonin; involvement of autophagy, inflammation and oxidative stress. *Life Sci.* 193, 20–33. doi: 10.1016/j.lfs.2017.12.001

Dorrell, M. I., Aguilar, E., Jacobson, R., Trauger, S. A., Friedlander, J., and Siuzdak, G. (2010). Maintaining retinal astrocytes normalizes revascularization and prevents vascular pathology associated with oxygen-induced retinopathy. *Glia* 58, 43–54. doi: 10.1002/glia.20900

Fernandez, D. C., Sande, P. H., Chianelli, M. S., Aldana Marcos, H. J., and Rosenstein, R. E. (2011). Induction of ischemic tolerance protects the retina from diabetic retinopathy. *Am. J. Pathol.* 178, 2264–2274. doi: 10.1016/j.ajpath.2011.01.040

Forouhi, N. G., Luan, J., Hennings, S., and Wareham, N. J. (2007). Incidence of Type 2 diabetes in England and its association with baseline impaired fasting glucose: the Ely study 1990-2000. *Diabet Med.* 24, 200–207. doi: 10.1111/j.1464-5491.2007.02068.x

Frost, L. S., Mitchell, C. H., and Boesze-Battaglia, K. (2014). Autophagy in the eye: implications for ocular cell health. *Exp. Eye Res.* 124, 56–66. doi: 10.1016/j.exer.2014.04.010

Fu, D., Yu, J. Y., Yang, S., Wu, M., Hammad, S. M., and Connell, A. R. (2016). Survival or death: a dual role for autophagy in stress-induced pericyte loss in diabetic retinopathy. *Diabetologia* 59, 2251–2261. doi: 10.1007/s00125-016-4058-5

Fu, Z., Nian, S., Li, S. Y., Wong, D., Chung, S. K., and Lo, A. C. (2015). Deficiency of aldose reductase attenuates inner retinal neuronal changes in a mouse model of retinopathy of prematurity. *Graefes Arch. Clin. Exp. Ophthalmol.* 253, 1503–1513. doi: 10.1007/s00417-015-3024-0

Gardner, T. W., Antonetti, D. A., Barber, A. J., LaNoue, K. F., and Levison, S. W. (2002). Diabetic retinopathy: more than meets the eye. *Surv. Ophthalmol.* 47(Suppl. 2), S253–S262. doi: 10.1016/s0039-6257(02)00387-9

Gardner, T. W., Lieth, E., Khin, S. A., Barber, A. J., Bonsall, D. J., and Lesher, T. (1997). Astrocytes increase barrier properties and ZO-1 expression in retinal vascular endothelial cells. *Invest. Ophthalmol. Vis. Sci.* 38, 2423–2427.

Gualtieri, M., Feitosa-Santana, C., Lago, M., Nishi, M., and Fix Ventura, D. (2013). Early visual changes in diabetic patients with no retinopathy measured by color discrimination and electroretinography. *Psychol. Neurosci.* 6, 227–234. doi: 10.3922/j.psns.2013.2.11

Harrison, W. W., Bearse, M. A. Jr., Ng, J. S., Jewell, N. P., Barez, S., and Burger, D. (2011). Multifocal electroretinograms predict onset of diabetic retinopathy in adult patients with diabetes. *Invest. Ophthalmol. Vis. Sci.* 52, 772–777. doi: 10.1167/iovs.10-5931

Holopigian, K., Seiple, W., Lorenzo, M., and Carr, R. (1992). A comparison of photopic and scotopic electroretinographic changes in early diabetic retinopathy. *Invest. Ophthalmol. Vis. Sci.* 33, 2773–2780.

Ibrahim, M. S., Pang, D., Randhawa, G., and Pappas, Y. (2019). Risk models and scores for metabolic syndrome: systematic review protocol. *BMJ Open* 9:e027326. doi: 10.1136/bmjopen-2018-027326

Juen, S., and Kieselbach, G. F. (1990). Electrophysiological changes in juvenile diabetics without retinopathy. *Arch. Ophthalmol.* 108, 372–375. doi: 10.1001/archopht.1990.01070050070033

Kaur, C., Foulds, W. S., and Ling, E. A. (2008). Blood-retinal barrier in hypoxic ischaemic conditions: basic concepts, clinical features and management. *Prog. Retin. Eye Res.* 27, 622–647. doi: 10.1016/j.preteyeres.2008.09.003

Keenan, J. D., Fan, A. Z., and Klein, R. (2009). Retinopathy in nondiabetic persons with the metabolic syndrome: findings from the Third national health and nutrition examination survey. *Am. J. Ophthalmol.* 147, 934.e2–944.e2. doi: 10.1016/j.ajo.2008.12.009

Kim, S. H., Munemasa, Y., Kwong, J. M., Ahn, J. H., Mareninov, S., and Gordon, L. K. (2008). Activation of autophagy in retinal ganglion cells. *J. Neurosci. Res.* 86, 2943–2951. doi: 10.1002/jnr.21738

Lecleire-Collet, A., Audo, I., Aout, M., Girmens, J. F., Sofroni, R., and Erginay, A. (2011). Evaluation of retinal function and flicker light-induced retinal vascular response in normotensive patients with diabetes without retinopathy. *Invest. Ophthalmol. Vis. Sci.* 52, 2861–2867. doi: 10.1167/iovs.10-5960

Liu, L., Yue, S., Wu, J., Zhang, J., Lian, J., and Teng, W. (2015). Prevalence and risk factors of retinopathy in patients with or without metabolic syndrome: a population-based study in Shenyang. *BMJ Open* 5:e008855. doi: 10.1136/bmjopen-2015-008855

Liu, T. (2019). Regulation of inflammasome by autophagy. *Adv. Exp. Med. Biol.* 1209, 109–123. doi: 10.1007/978-981-15-0606-2_7

Liu, X., Wang, D., Liu, Y., Luo, Y., Ma, W., and Xiao, W. (2010). Neuronal-driven angiogenesis: role of NGF in retinal neovascularization in an oxygen-induced retinopathy model. *Invest. Ophthalmol. Vis. Sci.* 51, 3749–3757. doi: 10.1167/iovs.09-4226

Lopes de Faria, J. M., Duarte, D. A., Montemurro, C., Papadimitriou, A., Consonni, S. R., Lopes, et al. (2016). Defective autophagy in diabetic retinopathy. *Invest. Ophthalmol. Vis. Sci.* 57, 4356–4366. doi: 10.1167/iovs.16-19197

Lorenc, V. E., Subirada Caldarone, P. V., Paz, M. C., Ferrer, D. G., Luna, J. D., and Chiabrando, G. A. (2018). IGF-1R regulates the extracellular level of active MMP-2, pathological neovascularization, and functionality in retinas of OIR mouse model. *Mol. Neurobiol.* 55, 1123–1135. doi: 10.1007/s12035-017-0386-9

Ma, N., Madigan, M. C., Chan-Ling, T., and Hunt, N. H. (1997). Compromised blood-nerve barrier, astrogliosis, and myelin disruption in optic nerves during fatal murine cerebral malaria. *Glia* 19, 135–151.

Mbata, O., Abo El-Magd, N. F., and El-Remessy, A. B. (2017). Obesity, metabolic syndrome and diabetic retinopathy: beyond hyperglycemia. *World J. Diabetes* 8, 317–329. doi: 10.4239/wjd.v8.i7.317

Meng, X. H., Chen, B., and Zhang, J. P. (2017). Intracellular Insulin and Impaired Autophagy in a Zebrafish model and a Cell Model of Type 2 diabetes. *Int. J. Biol. Sci.* 13, 985–995. doi: 10.7150/ijbs.19249

Mizutani, M., Gerhardinger, C., and Lorenzi, M. (1998). Muller cell changes in human diabetic retinopathy. *Diabetes* 47, 445–449. doi: 10.2337/diabetes.47.3.445

Moreno, M. C., Marcos, H. J., Oscar Croxatto, J., Sande, P. H., Campanelli, J., and Jaliffa, C. O. (2005). A new experimental model of glaucoma in rats through intracameral injections of hyaluronic acid. *Exp. Eye Res.* 81, 71–80. doi: 10.1016/j.exer.2005.01.008

Nathan, D. M., Davidson, M. B., DeFronzo, R. A., Heine, R. J., Henry, R. R., and Pratley, R. (2007). Impaired fasting glucose and impaired glucose tolerance: implications for care. *Diabetes Care* 30, 753–759. doi: 10.2337/dc07-9920

Parks, E. J., Skokan, L. E., Timlin, M. T., and Dingfelder, C. S. (2008). Dietary sugars stimulate fatty acid synthesis in adults. *J. Nutr.* 138, 1039–1046. doi: 10.1093/jn/138.6.1039

Peng, X. Y., Wang, F. H., Liang, Y. B., Wang, J. J., Sun, L. P., and Peng, Y. (2010). Retinopathy in persons without diabetes: the Handan Eye Study. *Ophthalmology* 117, 531–537, 537.e2–e2. doi: 10.1016/j.ophtha.2009.07.045

Plump, A. S., Smith, J. D., Hayek, T., Aalto-Setala, K., Walsh, A., and Verstuyft, J. G. (1992). Severe hypercholesterolemia and atherosclerosis in apolipoprotein E-deficient mice created by homologous recombination in ES cells. *Cell* 71, 343–353. doi: 10.1016/0092-8674(92)90362-g

Ridano, M. E., Subirada, P. V., Paz, M. C., Lorenc, V. E., Stupirski, J. C., and Gramajo, A. L. (2017). Galectin-1 expression imprints a neurovascular phenotype in proliferative retinopathies and delineates responses to anti-VEGF. *Oncotarget* 8, 32505–32522. doi: 10.18632/oncotarget.17129

Rodriguez-Muela, N., Germain, F., Marino, G., Fitze, P. S., and Boya, P. (2012). Autophagy promotes survival of retinal ganglion cells after optic nerve axotomy in mice. *Cell Death Differ.* 19, 162–169. doi: 10.1038/cdd.2011.88

Rungger-Brandle, E., Dosso, A. A., and Leuenberger, P. M. (2000). Glial reactivity, an early feature of diabetic retinopathy. *Invest. Ophthalmol. Vis. Sci.* 41, 1971–1980.

Schwartz, E. A., and Reaven, P. D. (2006). Molecular and signaling mechanisms of atherosclerosis in insulin resistance. *Endocrinol. Metab. Clin. North Am.* 35, 525–549, viii. doi: 10.1016/j.ecl.2006.06.005

Sherling, D. H., Perumareddi, P., and Hennekens, C. H. (2017). Metabolic syndrome. *J. Cardiovasc. Pharmacol. Ther.* 22, 365–367. doi: 10.1177/1074248416686187

Subirada, P. V., Paz, M. C., Ridano, M. E., Lorenc, V. E., Fader, C. M., and Chiabrando, G. A. (2019). Effect of autophagy modulators on vascular, glial, and neuronal alterations in the oxygen-induced retinopathy mouse model. *Front. Cell Neurosci.* 13:279. doi: 10.3389/fncel.2019.00279

Subirada, P. V., Paz, M. C., Ridano, M. E., Lorenc, V. E., Vaglienti, M. V., and Barcelona, P. F. (2018). A journey into the retina: muller glia commanding survival and death. *Eur. J. Neurosci.* 47, 1429–1443. doi: 10.1111/ejn.13965

Tappy, L., and Rosset, R. (2019). Health outcomes of a high fructose intake: the importance of physical activity. *J. Physiol.* 597, 3561–3571. doi: 10.1113/JP278246

Teff, K. L., Grudziak, J., Townsend, R. R., Dunn, T. N., Grant, R. W., and Adams, S. H. (2009). Endocrine and metabolic effects of consuming fructose- and glucose-sweetened beverages with meals in obese men and women: influence of insulin resistance on plasma triglyceride responses. *J. Clin. Endocrinol. Metab.* 94, 1562–1569. doi: 10.1210/jc.2008-2192

Thierry, M., Pasquis, B., Buteau, B., Fourgeux, C., Dembele, D., and Leclere, L. (2015). Early adaptive response of the retina to a pro-diabetogenic diet: impairment of cone response and gene expression changes in high-fructose fed rats. *Exp. Eye Res.* 135, 37–46. doi: 10.1016/j.exer.2015.04.012

Trost, A., Schroedl, F., Lange, S., Rivera, F. J., Tempfer, H., and Korntner, S. (2013). Neural crest origin of retinal and choroidal pericytes. *Invest. Ophthalmol. Vis. Sci.* 54, 7910–7921. doi: 10.1167/iovs.13-12946

Verma, A., Rani, P. K., Raman, R., Pal, S. S., Laxmi, G., and Gupta, M. (2009). Is neuronal dysfunction an early sign of diabetic retinopathy? Microperimetry and spectral domain optical coherence tomography (SD-OCT) study in individuals with diabetes, but no diabetic retinopathy. *Eye* 23, 1824–1830. doi: 10.1038/eye.2009.184

Vidal, E., Lalarme, E., Maire, M. A., Febvret, V., Gregoire, S., and Gambert, S. (2019). Early impairments in the retina of rats fed with high fructose/high fat diet are associated with glucose metabolism deregulation but not dyslipidaemia. *Sci. Rep.* 9:5997. doi: 10.1038/s41598-019-42528-9

Vinores, S. A., Gadegbeku, C., Campochiaro, P. A., and Green, W. R. (1989). Immunohistochemical localization of blood-retinal barrier breakdown in human diabetics. *Am. J. Pathol.* 134, 231–235.

Vinores, S. A., McGehee, R., Lee, A., Gadegbeku, C., and Campochiaro, P. A. (1990). Ultrastructural localization of blood-retinal barrier breakdown in diabetic and galactosemic rats. *J. Histochem. Cytochem.* 38, 1341–1352. doi: 10.1177/38.9.2117624

Wachtmeister, L. (1998). Oscillatory potentials in the retina: what do they reveal. *Prog. Retin. Eye Res.* 17, 485–521.

Wen, Y. T., Zhang, J. R., Kapupara, K., and Tsai, R. K. (2019). mTORC2 activation protects retinal ganglion cells via Akt signaling after autophagy induction in traumatic optic nerve injury. *Exp. Mol. Med.* 51, 1–11. doi: 10.1038/s12276-019-0298-z

Wild, S., Roglic, G., Green, A., Sicree, R., and King, H. (2004). Global prevalence of diabetes: estimates for the year 2000 and projections for 2030. *Diabetes Care* 27, 1047–1053. doi: 10.2337/diacare.27.5.1047

Wong, S. K., Chin, K. Y., Suhaimi, F. H., Fairus, A., and Ima-Nirwana, S. (2016). Animal models of metabolic syndrome: a review. *Nutr. Metab.* 13, 1–12. doi: 10.1186/s12986-016-0123-9

Wong, T. Y., Duncan, B. B., Golden, S. H., Klein, R., Couper, D. J., Klein, B. E., et al. (2004). Associations between the metabolic syndrome and retinal microvascular signs: the atherosclerosis risk in communities study. *Invest. Ophthalmol. Vis. Sci.* 45, 2949–2954. doi: 10.1167/iovs.04-0069

Zarei, R., Anvari, P., Eslami, Y., Fakhraie, G., Mohammadi, M., and Jamali, A. (2017). Retinal nerve fibre layer thickness is reduced in metabolic syndrome. *Diabet Med.* 34, 1061–1066. doi: 10.1111/dme.13369

Zhang, Y., and Stone, J. (1997). Role of astrocytes in the control of developing retinal vessels. *Invest. Ophthalmol. Vis. Sci.* 38, 1653–1666.

9

The Role of the Interplay Between Autophagy and NLRP3 Inflammasome in Metabolic Disorders

Shuangyu Lv, Honggang Wang* and Xiaotian Li

Institute of Biomedical Informatics, Bioinformatics Center, School of Basic Medical Sciences, Henan University, Kaifeng, China

Correspondence:
Honggang Wang
whg197167@vip.henu.edu.cn;
whg1975316@sina.com

Autophagy is an important and conserved cellular pathway in which cells transmit cytoplasmic contents to lysosomes for degradation. It plays an important role in maintaining the balance of cell composition synthesis, decomposition and reuse, and participates in a variety of physiological and pathological processes. The nucleotide-binding oligomerization domain-like receptor family, pyrin domain-containing 3 (NLRP3) inflammasome can induce the maturation and secretion of Interleukin-1 beta (IL-1β) and IL-18 by activating caspase-1. It is involved in many diseases. In recent years, the interplay between autophagy and NLRP3 inflammasome has been reported to contribute to many diseases including metabolic disorders related diseases. In this review, we summarized the recent studies on the interplay between autophagy and NLRP3 inflammasome in metabolic disorders to provide ideas for the relevant basic research in the future.

Keywords: autophagy, NLRP3 inflammasome, glucose metabolic disorders, uric acid metabolic disorders, inflammation-related metabolic disorders

INTRODUCTION

Autophagy is a closely coordinated process that isolates proteins and damaged or aged organelles in double membrane vesicles called autophagosomes which eventually fuse with lysosomes, leading to the degradation of isolated components (Behrends et al., 2010). It plays an important role in maintaining the balance of cell synthesis, decomposition and reuse (Wei et al., 2016). Abnormal autophagy is involved in the development of the pathological processes such as cardiomyopathy (Mclendon et al., 2014), neurodegenerative diseases (Mclendon et al., 2014), type II diabetes (Sarparanta et al., 2017), and cancer (Amaravadi et al., 2011). The nucleotide-binding oligomerization domain-like receptor family, pyrin domain-containing 3 (NLRP3) inflammasome can induce the maturation and secretion of interleukin-1 beta (IL-1β) and IL-18 by activating caspase-1 (Schroder and Tschopp, 2010; Strowig et al., 2012). Studies have shown that the abnormal activation of NLRP3 inflammasome contributes to many diseases including type 2 diabetes, atherosclerosis, and steatohepatitis (Mridha et al., 2017; Van Der Heijden et al., 2017; Zhai et al., 2018). Recently, more and more studies have shown that there is an interplay between autophagy and NLRP3 inflammasome in macrophage and the interplay plays an important role in many diseases including metabolic diseases, the mechanism of which remains to be elucidated (Biasizzo and Kopitar-Jerala, 2020). In this review, the interplay between autophagy and the NLRP3 inflammasome and its mechanism are explored in metabolic disorders to provide ideas for the relevant basic research in the future.

OVERVIEW OF AUTOPHAGY

Autophagy is a conserved process of self-sustaining internal environment stability, in which abnormal proteins and organelles are encapsulated by the bilayer membranes and transported to lysosomes for subsequent degradation (Sir et al., 2010; Qiu et al., 2014). Autophagy can be categorized as microautophagy, macroautophagy and chaperone-mediated autophagy according to the inducing signal, action time, target type, and transport pathway into lysosomes (Feng et al., 2014; Gomes et al., 2017). Macroautophagy, the most studied autophagy, is mainly responsible for the degradation of organelles and microorganisms. In this process, the degraded substance is encapsulated by a double membrane vesicle to form autophagosome, which then fuses with lysosome for degradation (Cheon et al., 2019). Microautophagy, without forming autophagosome, mainly degrades cell components by directly engulfing the cytoplasm at the lysosomal membrane through invagination and or septation (Oku and Sakai, 2018). Chaperone-mediated autophagy is a selective autophagy process in which intracellular proteins are transported to lysosomal chambers after binding with chaperones, then digested by lysosomal enzymes (Kaushik and Cuervo, 2012; **Figure 1**). Moreover, mitochondrial autophagy, also called mitophagy, is a special kind of autophagy, which selectively degrades organelle mitochondria and is largely responsible for mitochondrial quality control (Ashrafi and Schwarz, 2013; Ney, 2015). There are many factors affecting autophagy, such as Ca^{2+} concentration, immune or inflammatory stimulation, endoplasmic reticulum stress, nutritional deficiency, and accumulation of damaged cells or organelles (Tooze and Yoshimori, 2010; Mizushima et al., 2011). Under physiological conditions, autophagy often occurs at the basic maintenance level. When the body is in a pathological state, significantly enhanced autophagy can clear the abnormal proteins in cells, which is conducive to cell survival (Glick et al., 2010). The effect of autophagy on cells is a "double-edged sword," because if autophagy is maintained at a high level, autophagy will lead to cell death (Liu and Levine, 2015; Garcia-Huerta et al., 2016). Autophagy plays a key role in many basic physiological processes, including development, protein quality control, innate immunity and cell survival. It is well known that abnormal autophagy contributes to the occurrence of many diseases, including cancer, liver diseases, neurodegenerative diseases, type-II diabetes, and inflammation (Debnath, 2011; Murrow and Debnath, 2013). So far, the mechanism of autophagy in diseases is not fully clear.

OVERVIEW OF NLRP3 INFLAMMASOME

Inflammasome, a complex composed of many proteins, is an important part of the innate immune system and used to detect the presence of the infection, the pathogens and the metabolic alarms in cells (Elliott and Sutterwala, 2015; Jo et al., 2016). Five major inflammasomes have been identified: NLRP1, NLRC4, RIG-I, AIM2 and NLRP3. These inflammasomes consist of inflammasome adaptor protein, an active NLRP receptor, caspase-1, and apoptosis-associated speck-like protein containing CARD (ASC) (Barbe et al., 2014). NLRP3 inflammasome is the most thoroughly studied inflammasome which is mainly expressed in myeloid cells such as macrophages (O'connor et al., 2003). When the host is stimulated by the exogenous or endogenous stimuli, NLRP3 is activated to lead to the recruitment of pro-caspase-1 and ASC in macrophages. Stimulated NLRP3 interacts with pro-caspase-1 and ASC to form a large cytoplasmic complex, thus activating caspase-1. Actived caspase-1 cleaves pro-IL-1β and pro-IL-18 into IL-1β and IL-18, which induces inflammation by promoting the production of chemokines, proinflammatory cytokines and growth factors (Prochnicki et al., 2016; **Figure 2**). NLRP3 inflammasome was activated in two steps. The first signals (signal 1) indicating infection or tissue damage, including toll like receptor 4, a pattern recognition receptor capable of recognizing lipopolysaccharide (LPS) and a series of endogenous risk signals, activate the inflammatory transcription factor NF-κβ and increase the expression of NLRP3, pro-IL-1β, and pro-IL-18. Then, the second activation signal (signal 2) indicating cell damage, including extracellular adenosine triphosphate (ATP), urate and cholesterol crystal, induces the assembly of inflammasome and the autolysis of procaspase-1, activates caspase-1, and cleaves pro-IL-1β and pro-IL-18 into their active forms (Sokolova et al., 2019). Abnormal activation of NLRP3 inflammasome can lead to a variety of diseases including metabolic diseases (Meyers and Zhu, 2020).

THE INTERPLAY BETWEEN AUTOPHAGY AND NLRP3 INFLAMMASOME IN GLUCOSE AND LIPID METABOLIC DISORDERS

The Interplay Between Autophagy and NLRP3 Inflammasome in Impaired Wound Healing

In recent years, the prevalence of diabetes has increased significantly and become an important public health problem in the world (Balakumar et al., 2016). An important characteristic of diabetes is impaired wound healing (Falanga, 2005). It has been reported that NLRP3 inflammasome-mediated inflammatory response in macrophage is one of the key factors of impaired wound healing in diabetic mice (Bitto et al., 2014). Dai et al. (2017) found that high glucose (HG) activated NLRP3 inflammasome, increased the level of IL-1β and ROS production, and suppressed autophagy by decreasing the protein expression

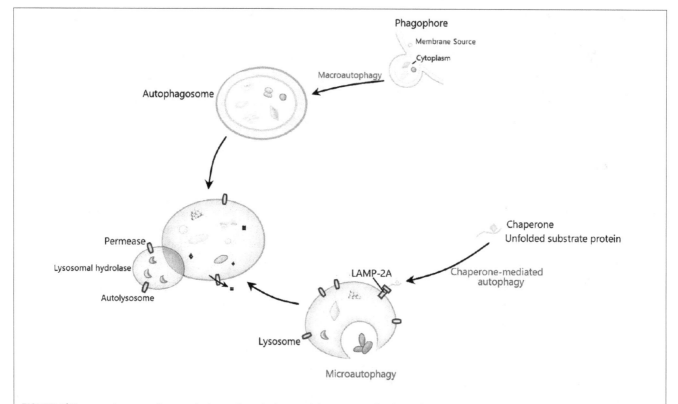

FIGURE 1 | The general process of macroautophagy, microautophagy, and chaperone-mediated autophagy. Macroautophagy mainly degrades organelles and microorganisms. The degraded substances are first encapsulated by double membrane vesicles to form autophagosomes, and then fuse with lysosomes for degradation. Microautophagy does not form autophagosomes, but mainly degrades cell components by directly engulfing the cytoplasm at the lysosomal membrane through invagination and or septation. Chaperone-mediated autophagy is a selective autophagy process in which degraded proteins are transported to lysosomal chambers after binding with chaperones, and then digested by lysosomal enzymes.

of LC3-II and increasing the protein expression of p62 in macrophages from human diabetic wound. Pre-treatment with resveratrol (an autophagy agonist) counteracted the effects of HG, suggesting that autophagy mediated the HG-induced NLRP3 inflammasome and the ROS production was involved in autophagy-associated NLRP3 inflammasome activation. Moreover, the application of ROS scavenger NAC notably inhibited HG-induced NLRP3 inflammasome, indicating that enhancing autophagy supressed HG-induced NLRP3 inflammasome through reducing ROS production. Autophagy can selectively remove the damaged mitochondria from which ROS mainly comes (Ding et al., 2014; Yang et al., 2014), therefore, it can be inferred that autophagy can inhibit ROS-mediated NLRP3 inflammasome activation through clearing damaged mitochondria, which suggests a new treatment strategy for diabetic wound healing. The relationship among autophagy, ROS and NLRP3 inflammasome needs further study.

The Interplay Between Autophagy and NLRP3 Inflammasome in Diabetic Nephropathy

Consistent with the above, ROS-mediated NLRP3 inflammasome activation is also involved in diabetic nephropathy (DN). DN is one of the major microvascular complications of diabetes,

and has become a common cause of end-stage renal disease (Gao et al., 2016). Many studies have shown that autophagy and inflammation play a key role in the pathological process of DN (Kitada et al., 2011; Feng et al., 2016). Gao et al. (2019) found that in glomerular mesangial cells stimulated by HG, the levels of NLRP3 inflammasome, IL-1β and ROS were increased, indicating that ROS-mediated NLRP3 inflammasome was activated to promote the development of DN. HG promoted autophagy in a short period (<12 h), but inhibited autophagy in a long period (72 h). Meanwhile, HG increased the level of ROS, NLRP3 inflammasome and IL-1β in a time-dependent manner, moreover, treatment cells with rapamycin (a specific activator of autophagy) for 72 h decreased the levels of NLRP3 inflammasome, IL-1β and ROS, suggesting that HG-regulated autophagy negatively regulated ROS-mediated NLRP3 inflammasome. In summary, in a short period of treatment, HG-induced autophagy inhibits ROS-mediated NLRP3 inflammasome and improve DN, while a long period of treatment, HG inhibits autophagy to activates ROS-mediated NLRP3 inflammasom to aggravate DN. The reason may be that HG causes mitochondrial damage, which induces autophagy to clear the damaged mitochondria-derived ROS. In a short period of time, the inhibition of HG on autophagy was less than the induction of ROS on autophagy, so the level of autophagy increased. With the extension

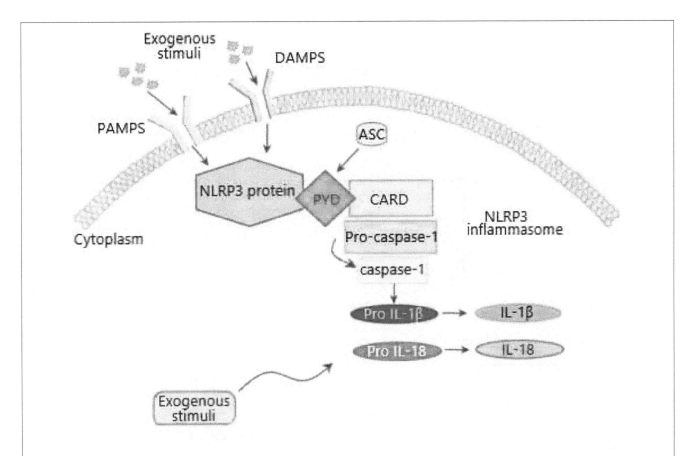

FIGURE 2 | Overview of NLRP3 inflammasome activation process. NLRP3 inflammasome is composed of sensor NLRP3 protein, adapter apoptosis related spot like protein (ASC) containing N-terminal PYRIN-PAAD-DAPIN domain (PYD), C-terminal caspase recruitment domain (CARD), and effector pro-caspase-1. When cells are stimulated by pathogen related molecular patterns (PAMPS) and damage related molecular patterns (DAMPS), NLRP3 inflammasome is activated. Activated NLRP3 interacts with ASC through PYD domain, and pro-caspase-1 binds to ASC through CARD to form a large cytoplasmic complex, thus activating caspase-1. Active caspase-1 cleaves proinflammatory cytokines interleukin-1 β (IL-1β), and IL-18 from their precursors into bioactive forms that induce inflammation.

of time, the induction of autophagy weakens, while high glucose inhibits autophagy to activate ROS-mediated NLRP3 inflammasome.

In addition to the above glomerular mesangial cell inflammation, NLRP3 inflammasome-mediated inflammation of tubulointerstitial also contributes to the development of DN (Chen et al., 2013; Hwang et al., 2017). Optineurin (OPTN), initially considered to be a regulator of NF-κβ signaling, is an important regulator of mitophagy in patients with DN, and reducing OPTN expression leads to premature senescence of renal tubular cells to promote DN (Slowicka et al., 2016; Chen et al., 2018). The results of Chen et al. (2019) showed that the expression of optineurin (OPTN) was reduced and correlated negatively with NLRP3 inflammasome activation in patients with DN. In primary mouse renal tubular epithelial cells (RTECs) treated with HG, the expression level of OPTN significantly decreased, the level of NLRP3 expression, cleaved caspase-1, and IL-1β, and the release of IL-1β increased. Moreover, the expression of mitochondrial fission protein Drp1 increased, and the expression of mitochondrial fusion protein Mitofusin 2 and mitochondrial membrane potential decreased, indicating that HG inhibited OPTN, activated NLRP3 inflammasome-mediated

inflammation and promoted mitochondrial dysfunction. While overexpression of OPTN in RTECs counteracted the HG effects on OPTN and NLRP3 inflammasome-mediated inflammation, and silencing of OPTN had the opposite result, suggesting that OPTN inhibited HG-induced activation of NLRP3 inflammasome. HG impaired mitophagy by decreasing the level of LC3II in RTECs. The mitophagy-specific inhibitor (Mdivi-1) could activate NLRP3 inflammasome in the presence of HG, while the autophagy agonist (Torin) had the opposite effect, indicating that mitophagy supressed NLRP3 inflammasome activation induced by HG. In addition, overexpression of OPTN notably increased mitophagy and silencing of OPTN induces mtROS production and activation of NLRP3 inflammasome. Collectively, it can be inferred that OPTN inhibited HG-induced NLRP3 inflammasome by enhancing mitophagy-mediated clearance of ROS. The mechanism of OPTN regulating mitophagy, especially the signal pathway, needs to be further elucidated.

On the contrary to autophagy-mediated regulation of the NLRP3 inflammasome, NLRP3 inflammasome also can regulate autophagy. In podocytes of DN mice induced by high-fat diet/streptozotocin (HFD/STZ), the number of autophagosomes decreased and the level of NLRP3 inflammasome expression and renal proinflammatory cytokines such as IL-1β increased, meanwhile, the similar results were obtained in human DN biopsies, suggesting that podocyte autophagy was inhibited and NLRP3 inflammasome was activated. In podocyte, with the activation of NLRP3 inflammasome by LPS plus ATP, the ratio of LC3II/I, the expression level of beclin 1 and nephrin (which meant podocyte injury), and the formation of autophagosomes decreased, indicating that podocyte autophagy is inhibited by the activation of NLRP3 inflammasome to aggravate the damage of podocyte. While silencing NLRP3 by siRNA had the opposite results. Therefore, appropriate changes of autophagy and inflammasome may potentially improve DN (Hou et al., 2020). The specific mechanism of NLRP3 negatively regulating autophagy needs to be further explored.

The Interplay Between Autophagy and NLRP3 Inflammasome in Diabetic Cardiomyopathy

Diabetic cardiomyopathy (DCM) is an important complication of diabetes and associated with inflammation, oxidative stress, impaired calcium homeostasis and mitochondrial damage (Huynh et al., 2014; Kobayashi and Liang, 2015). Autophagy and NLRP3 inflammasome have been reported to be involved in the pathological process of DCM (Xie et al., 2011; Luo et al., 2014). Visceral adipose tissue derived serine protease inhibitor (vaspin), firstly discovered in 2005, is an adipokine, which has significant anti-inflammatory effect (Li et al., 2008). In STZ-induced diabetes rat model, Vaspin improved cardiac function, cardiomyocyte apoptosis, myocardial tissue morphology and mitochondrial morphology to alleviate DCM. Mechanistic studies of the above effects revealed that LC3II/I ratio decreased and p62 expression increased in diabetic hearts, while Vaspin treatment abrogated the change to promote autophagy. Moreover, Vaspin also suppressed NLRP3 inflammasome through reducing the expression level of NLRP3 inflammasome and IL-1β. In HG-induced H9C2 cells, treatment with the autophagy inhibitor (3-MA) abolished the inhibitory effects of Vaspin on NLRP3 inflammasome, indicating that Vaspin alleviated STZ-induced myocardial injury by suppressing NLRP3 inflammasome activation via promoting autophagy. In addition, Vaspin inhibits ROS production and mitochondrial membrane depolarization in HG-induced H9C2 cells (Li et al., 2019). It can be inferred that there may be two mechanisms of myocardial protection in the above process: one is that Vaspin-induced autophagy can clear the damaged mitochondria to reduce the production of ROS to inhibit NLRP3 inflammasome; another is Vaspin improve damaged mitochondria to reduce the production of ROS to inhibit NLRP3 inflammasome.

The Interplay Between Autophagy and NLRP3 Inflammasome in Obesity-Induced Insulin Resistance

Obesity causes chronic low-grade inflammation, leading to insulin resistance, which is characteristic of type 2 diabetes mellitus (Xu et al., 2003; Arkan et al., 2005; Shoelson et al., 2007).

It has been reported that NLRP3 inflammasome perceives obesity related risk signals and participate in inflammation and insulin resistance caused by obesity (Vandanmagsar et al., 2011). Berberine (BBR) is a natural plant product and beneficial to diabetes and dyslipidemia (Kong et al., 2004; Turner et al., 2008). Zhou et al. (2017) found that BBR could significantly inhibit the activation of NLRP3 inflammasome and the release of IL-1β induced by saturated fatty acid palmitate (PA) in bone marrow-derived macrophages (BMDMs). Moreover, it also significantly increased the autophagy level and decreased mitochondrial ROS production in LPS plus PA-treated macrophages, while Beclin1 (an autophagy marker gene) knockout and 3-MA reversed the inhibitory effect of BBR on NLRP3 inflammasome and mitochondrial ROS production, indicating that BBR suppressed NLRP3 inflammasome-mediated inflammation and mitochondrial ROS production through enhancing autophagy. In addition, BBR could increase phosphorylation of AMPK (adenosine activated protein kinase) and caused a decrease of mammalian target of rapamycin (mTOR) in LPS plus PA-treated BMDMs, AMPK inhibitor, Ara-A, blocked most of the effects of BBR, suggesting that AMPK signal may be involved in BBR-induced autophagy. The similar effects of BBR were obtained in a HFD induced insulin resistance model. In conclusion, BBR inhibit obesity-induced inflammation and insulin resistance by activating AMPK dependent autophagy through suppressing mitochondrial ROS production in adipose tissue macrophages, which needs to be further studied. Targeting the effect of autophagy on NLRP3 with oral small molecule compound BBR might improve insulin resistance. Similar to the above results, our previous studies have shown that enhancing autophagy by hydrogen sulfide (H₂S) suppresses NLRP3 inflammasome through AMPK-mTOR pathway in L02 cells induced by oleic acid (Wang et al., 2019). AMPK-mTOR pathway is an important signaling pathway for the interaction between autophagy and NLRP3 inflammasome.

The Interplay Between Autophagy and NLRP3 Inflammasome in High Fat and High Sugar Diets-Induced Heart Damage

High energy diets rich in fat and *high sugar* leads to low-grade systemic inflammatory response and increases the risk of cardiovascular disease (CVD) (Minihane et al., 2015). NLRP3 inflammasome-mediated inflammation plays an important role in the cardiomyopathy of rats treated with HFD and STZ (Luo et al., 2014). Genetic ablation of NLRP3 or inhibition of NLRP3 by MCC950 could relieve high-sugar diet (HSD), HFD or high sugar/fat diet induced obesity, cardiomyocyte apoptosis and inflammation, and improve the antioxidant capacity to ameliorate cardiac injury. Mechanistic studies revealed that genetic ablation of NLRP3 or inhibition of NLRP3 by MCC950 could induce autophagy by increasing LC3-II level and decreasing p62 level (Pavillard et al., 2017). HFD-induced obesity can impair autophagy in cardiomyocytes (He et al., 2012), while the inhibition of NLRP3-inflammasome and promotion of autophagy can improve HFD-induced cardiac injury (Abderrazak et al., 2015). Collectively, it can be inferred that inhibition of NLRP3-inflammasome improve HSD, HFD, or high sugar/fat diet induced heart damage through promoting autophagy, which needs to be further explored. It is predicted that therapeutic targetting of autophagy/NLRP3 inflammasomes can improve obesogenic diet-induced heart injury.

THE INTERPLAY BETWEEN AUTOPHAGY AND NLRP3 INFLAMMASOME IN URIC ACID METABOLISM DISORDERS

Uric acid nephropathy (UAN) is one of the most common metabolic diseases, which leads to kidney damage (Wu et al., 2012; Hou et al., 2014). Urate can activate NLRP3 inflammasome and NLRP3 inflammasome-mediated inflammation is involved in kidney injury (Wang et al., 2012). Hu et al. (2018) found that uric acid activated NLRP3 inflammasome, promoted caspase-1 activation, and induced renal inflammation, leading to the generation and development of UAN. Weicao, a traditional Chinese medicine preparation, could reduce uric acid, improve proteinuria and renal insufficiency and reduce renal tissue crystals to avoid renal interstitial fibrosis. It also reduced the levels of NLRP3 inflammasome, IL-18 and IIL-1β, and significantly increased the levels of beclin-1, LC3-II, and LC3-II/LC3-I ratio, suggesting that Weicao inhibited NLRP3 inflammasome-mediated inflammation and promoted autophagy to improve UAN. In addition, autophagy inhibitor 3-MA abolished the effects of Weicao on NLRP3 inflammasome, suggesting autophagy mediated the inhibitory effect of Weicao on NLRP3 inflammasome activation. NLRP3 inflammasome activator, ATP, blocked the effects of Weicao capsule on autophagy, indicating that NLRP3 inflammasome participated in Weicao induction of autophagy. The similar results were obtained in vitro. Collectively, Weicao could ameliorate renal injury of UAV rats through inhibiting NLRP3 inflammasome and inducing autophagy. It is predicted that therapeutic targetting of autophagy/NLRP3 inflammasomes can ameliorate UAN. The relationship between autophagy and NLRP3 inflammasome is very complex, which needs to be further studied.

THE INTERPLAY BETWEEN AUTOPHAGY AND NLRP3 INFLAMMASOME IN OTHER TYPES OF METABOLIC DISORDERS

The Interplay Between Autophagy and Nlrp3 Inflammasome in Aging Related Metabolic Disorders

Endothelial cell senescence is an important factor in the pathogenesis of senile vascular diseases, which has been observed in diabetic CVDs (Yokoi et al., 2006). Studies have shown that autophagy is closely related to the accelerated aging of vascular endothelial cells, and enhanced autophagy may have a strong anti-aging effect (Wohlgemuth et al., 2014; Lee et al., 2015). Purple sweet potato pigment (PSPC), a flavonoid compound isolated from purple sweet potato, can inhibit the aging of endothelial cells of diabetic patients (Sun et al., 2015). Sun et al. (2019) found that PSPC promoted autophagy by increasing LC3 II and decreasing p62 level and suppressed the premature senescence of endothelial cells induced by HG. The similar results were obtained in diabetic mice in vivo. Rapamycin, an autophagy promotor, inhibited HG-induced endothelial cell senescence, while 3-MA accelerated endothelial cell senescence, indicating that autophagy mediated PSPC suppression of endothelial cell senescence. Moreover, PSPC and Rapamycin suppressed HG-induced NLRP3 inflammasome, and 3-MA abolished the inhibitory effect of PSPC on NLRP3 inflammasome, suggesting that PSPC suppressed NLRP3 inflammasome by promoting autophagy. P62, an autophagic receptor, acts as a molecular bridge to deliver substrates to autophagosomes (Seibenhener et al., 2004). P62 binded to NLRP3 inflammasome and transported it to lysosome for degradation. In the senescent endothelium of diabetic mice, HG impaired autophagy to inhibit P62-NLRP3 inflammasome degradation in lysosome, while PSPC had the opposite effects, which was the mechanism that PSPC inhibits NLRP3 inflammasome by promoting autophagy (Sun et al., 2019).

Nucleotide-binding oligomerization domain-like receptor family, pyrin domain-containing 3 inflammasome-mediated inflammation disorder is closely related to aging-related metabolic disorders (Finkel, 2015; Cordero et al., 2018). Marin-Aguilar et al. (2020) found that MCC950, a specific NLRP3 inhibitor, could reduce body weight, increase insulin sensitivity, improve hepatic metabolic dysfunction by reducing hepatic transaminases, lactate dehydrogenase, and creatine phosphokinase and alleviate steatosis and fibrosis in aged mice. Mechanistic studies revealed that MCC950 inhibited PI3K/Akt/mTOR pathway and enhanced autophagy by increasing LC3-II level and decreasing p62 level to improve the metabolism and liver dysfunction of old mice in vivo and in vitro. It can be inferred that NLRP3 inflammasome inhibition with MCC950 improves metabolism disorder via promoting autophagy through inhibiting PI3K/Akt/mTOR pathway in aged mice, which needs to be further studied by using autophagy inhibitors and the activator of PI3K/Akt/mTOR pathway.

The Interplay Between Autophagy and NLRP3 Inflammasome in Inflammation-Related Metabolic Disorders

Evidence indicates that mild chronic inflammation, including adipose tissue inflammation, contributes to metabolic disorders and is associated with many metabolic diseases, such as type 2 diabetes mellitus, insulin resistance and

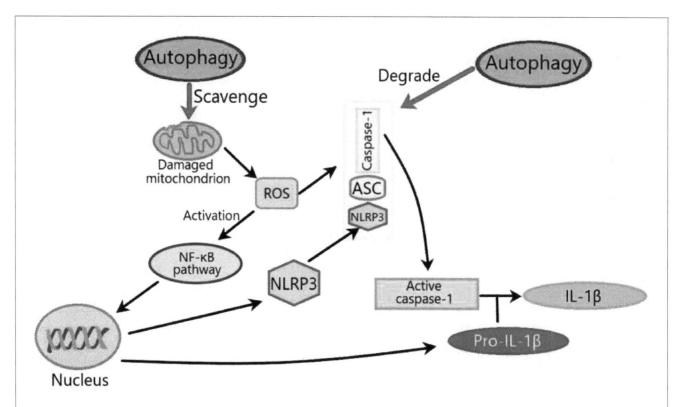

FIGURE 3 | Two mechanisms of the effects of autophagy on NLRP3 inflammasome in metabolic disorders. There are two mechanisms of the effects of autophagy on NLRP3 inflammasome: one is that autophagy inhibits NLRP3 inflammasome by scavenging ROS from damaged mitochondria. Mitochondria-derived ROS can activate NF-κβ pathway to promote the transcription of NLRP3 and pro-IL-1β, thus activating NLRP3 inflammasome. The other is that autophagy inhibits NLRP3 inflammasome through degrading inflammasome components such as pro-IL-1β, NLRP3, caspase-1, or ASC. ROS, Reactive oxygen species; NF-κβ, nuclear factor kappa-B; ASC, apoptosis-associated speck-like protein.

obesity (Weisberg et al., 2003; Lumeng and Saltiel, 2011; Harte et al., 2013). IL-1β activated by NLRP3 inflammasome can worse insulin resistance in human adipocytes (Gao et al., 2014), moreover, inhibition of IL-1β can reduce hyperglycemia in obese/diabetic rats (Ehses et al., 2009). So, inhibition of NLRP3 inflammasome-mediated production of IL-1β can improve the metabolic disorder associated with adipose tissue inflammation. AEDC is a cycloartane triterpenoid isolated from the whole plant of *Amanita vaginata* (Fang et al., 2019). Zhang et al. (2020) found that AEDC suppressed LPS plus ATP-induced NLRP3 inflammasome activation and IL-1β secretion in THP-1 macrophages. Moreover, LPS plus ATP notably decreased the protein levels of Atg5, Atg7, beclin 1 and the ratio of LC3-II/LC3-I and increased the level of p62, while AEDC had opposite effects, indicating that AEDC restored autophagy impaired by LPS plus ATP. 3-MA abolished the AEDC suppression of NLRP3 inflammasome activation induced by LPS plus ATP, suggesting that AEDC inhibited LPS plus ATP-induced NLRP3 inflammasome activation by promoting autophagy. Mechanistic studies showed that AEDC increased the expression level of NAD$^+$-dependent deacetylase sirtuin-3 (SIRT3) deacetylase and enhanced its deacetylation activity to restore mitochondrial dysfunction induced by LPS plus ATP. 3-TYP, a selective SIRT3 inhibitor, reversed AEDC effect on autophagy, indicating that AEDC

inhibited NLRP3 inflammasome activation to ameliorate inflammation-related metabolic disorders by promoting autophagy via SIRT3. Here, autophagy still suppresses NLRP3 inflammasome by clearing damaging mitochondria derived ROS.

CONCLUSION

The interplay between autophagy and NLRP3 inflammasome plays an important role in metabolic disorders. In this review, there are two mechanisms of the effects of autophagy on NLRP3 inflammasome in metabolic disorders: One is that autophagy suppresses NLRP3 inflammasome by inhibiting ROS production through scavenging damaged mitochondria. ROS released from mitochondria can activate the NF-κβ pathway to promote the transcription of NLRP3 and pro-IL-1β, thus activating NLRP3 inflammasome. The other is that autophagy can isolate and promote the degradation of inflammasome components such as pro-IL-1β, NLRP3, caspase-1, and ASC (**Figure 3**). Generally speaking, in addition to the above two ways, autophagy also inhibits NLRP3 inflammasome by phosphorylating NLRP3 (Cao et al., 2019). Whether autophagy can influence NLRP3 inflammasome by phosphorylating NLRP3 in metabolic disorders remains to be clarified.

Although the interplay between autophagy and NLRP3 inflammasome has potential therapeutic value in metabolic disorders, its mechanism has not been fully explained. For example, in metabolic disorders, does autophagy promote the activation of the NLRP3 inflammasome? What is the mechanism of NLRP3 inflammasome acting on autophagy? And are there any side effects of targeting autophagy/NLRP3 inflammasome to improve metabolic disorder? With the deepening of the research, targeting autophagy/NLRP3 inflammasome will provide a new method for the treatment of metabolic disorders related diseases.

AUTHOR CONTRIBUTIONS

HW devised, wrote, and funded the review. SL wrote and funded the review. XL drew the pictures of the review.

REFERENCES

Abderrazak, A., Couchie, D., Mahmood, D. F. D., Elhage, R., Vindis, C., Laffargue, M., et al. (2015). Anti-inflammatory and antiatherogenic effects of the NLRP3 inflammasome inhibitor arglabin in ApoE(2).Ki mice fed a high-fat diet. *Circulation* 131, 1061–1070. doi: 10.1161/circulationaha.114.013730

Amaravadi, R. K., Lippincott-Schwartz, J., Yin, X. M., Weiss, W. A., Takebe, N., Timmer, W., et al. (2011). Principles and current strategies for targeting autophagy for cancer treatment. *Clin. Cancer Res.* 17, 654–666. doi: 10.1158/1078-0432.ccr-10-2634

Arkan, M. C., Hevener, A. L., Greten, F. R., Maeda, S., Li, Z. W., Long, J. M., et al. (2005). IKK-beta links inflammation to obesity-induced insulin resistance. *Nat. Med.* 11, 191–198. doi: 10.1038/nm1185

Ashrafi, G., and Schwarz, T. L. (2013). The pathways of mitophagy for quality control and clearance of mitochondria. *Cell Death Differ.* 20, 31–42. doi: 10.1038/cdd.2012.81

Balakumar, P., Maung-U, K., and Jagadeesh, G. (2016). Prevalence and prevention of cardiovascular disease and diabetes mellitus. *Pharmacol. Res.* 113, 600–609. doi: 10.1016/j.phrs.2016.09.040

Barbe, F., Douglas, T., and Saleh, M. (2014). Advances in Nod-like receptors (NLR) biology. *Cytokine Growth Factor Rev.* 25, 681–697. doi: 10.1016/j.cytogfr.2014.07.001

Behrends, C., Sowa, M. E., Gygi, S. P., and Harper, J. W. (2010). Network organization of the human autophagy system. *Nature* 466, 68–76. doi: 10.1038/nature09204

Biasizzo, M., and Kopitar-Jerala, N. (2020). Interplay between NLRP3 inflammasome and autophagy. *Front. Immunol.* 11:591803. doi: 10.3389/fimmu.2020.591803

Bitto, A., Altavilla, D., Pizzino, G., Irrera, N., Pallio, G., Colonna, M. R., et al. (2014). Inhibition of inflammasome activation improves the impaired pattern of healing in genetically diabetic mice. *Br. J. Pharmacol.* 171, 2300–2307. doi: 10.1111/bph.12557

Cao, Z., Wang, Y., Long, Z., and He, G. (2019). Interaction between autophagy and the NLRP3 inflammasome. *Acta Biochim. Biophys. Sin. (Shanghai)* 51, 1087–1095. doi: 10.1093/abbs/gmz098

Chen, K., Dai, H., Yuan, J., Chen, J., Lin, L., Zhang, W., et al. (2018). Optineurin-mediated mitophagy protects renal tubular epithelial cells against accelerated senescence in diabetic nephropathy. *Cell Death Dis.* 9:105.

Chen, K., Feng, L., Hu, W., Chen, J., Wang, X., Wang, L., et al. (2019). Optineurin inhibits NLRP3 inflammasome activation by enhancing mitophagy of renal tubular cells in diabetic nephropathy. *FASEB J.* 33, 4571–4585. doi: 10.1096/fj.201801749rrr

Chen, K., Zhang, J., Zhang, W., Zhang, J., Yang, J., Li, K., et al. (2013). ATP-P2X4 signaling mediates NLRP3 inflammasome activation: a novel pathway of diabetic nephropathy. *Int. J. Biochem. Cell Biol.* 45, 932–943. doi: 10.1016/j.biocel.2013.02.009

Cheon, S. Y., Kim, H., Rubinsztein, D. C., and Lee, J. E. (2019). Autophagy, cellular aging and age-related human diseases. *Exp. Neurobiol.* 28, 643–657. doi: 10.5607/en.2019.28.6.643

Cordero, M. D., Williams, M. R., and Ryffel, B. (2018). AMP-activated protein kinase regulation of the NLRP3 inflammasome during aging. *Trends Endocrinol. Metab.* 29, 8–17. doi: 10.1016/j.tem.2017.10.009

Dai, J., Zhang, X., Li, L., Chen, H., and Chai, Y. (2017). Autophagy inhibition contributes to ROS-producing NLRP3-dependent inflammasome activation and cytokine secretion in high glucose-induced macrophages. *Cell. Physiol. Biochem.* 43, 247–256. doi: 10.1159/000480367

Debnath, J. (2011). The multifaceted roles of autophagy in tumors-implications for breast cancer. *J. Mammary Gland Biol. Neoplasia* 16, 173–187. doi: 10.1007/s10911-011-9223-3

Ding, Z., Liu, S., Wang, X., Dai, Y., Khaidakov, M., Deng, X., et al. (2014). LOX-1, mtDNA damage, and NLRP3 inflammasome activation in macrophages: implications in atherogenesis. *Cardiovasc. Res.* 103, 619–628. doi: 10.1093/cvr/cvu114

Ehses, J. A., Lacraz, G., Giroix, M. H., Schmidlin, F., Coulaud, J., Kassis, N., et al. (2009). IL-1 antagonism reduces hyperglycemia and tissue inflammation in the type 2 diabetic GK rat. *Proc. Natl. Acad. Sci. U.S.A.* 106, 13998–14003. doi: 10.1073/pnas.0810087106

Elliott, E. I., and Sutterwala, F. S. (2015). Initiation and perpetuation of NLRP3 inflammasome activation and assembly. *Immunol. Rev.* 265, 35–52. doi: 10.1111/imr.12286

Falanga, V. (2005). Wound healing and its impairment in the diabetic foot. *Lancet* 366, 1736–1743. doi: 10.1016/s0140-6736(05)67700-8

Fang, Z. J., Zhang, T., Chen, S. X., Wang, Y. L., Zhou, C. X., Mo, J. X., et al. (2019). Cycloartane triterpenoids from *Actaea vaginata* with anti-inflammatory effects in LPS-stimulated RAW264.7 macrophages. *Phytochemistry* 160, 1–10. doi: 10.1016/j.phytochem.2019.01.003

Feng, H., Gu, J., Gou, F., Huang, W., Gao, C., Chen, G., et al. (2016). High glucose and lipopolysaccharide prime NLRP3 inflammasome via ROS/TXNIP pathway in mesangial cells. *J. Diabetes Res.* 2016:6973175.

Feng, Y., He, D., Yao, Z., and Klionsky, D. J. (2014). The machinery of macroautophagy. *Cell Res.* 24, 24–41. doi: 10.1038/cr.2013.168

Finkel, T. (2015). The metabolic regulation of aging. *Nat. Med.* 21, 1416–1423.

Gao, C., Chen, J., Fan, F., Long, Y., Tang, S., Jiang, C., et al. (2019). RIPK2-mediated autophagy and negatively regulated ROS-NLRP3 inflammasome signaling in GMCs stimulated with high glucose. *Mediators Inflamm.* 2019:6207563.

Gao, D., Madi, M., Ding, C., Fok, M., Steele, T., Ford, C., et al. (2014). Interleukin-1 beta mediates macrophage-induced impairment of insulin signaling in human primary adipocytes. *Am. J. Physiol. Endocrinol. Metab.* 307, E289–E304.

Gao, H. X., Regier, E. E., and Close, K. L. (2016). International diabetes federation world diabetes congress 2015. *J. Diabetes* 8, 300–304.

Garcia-Huerta, P., Troncoso-Escudero, P., Jerez, C., Hetz, C., and Vidal, R. L. (2016). The intersection between growth factors, autophagy and ER stress: a new target to treat neurodegenerative diseases? *Brain Res.* 1649, 173–180. doi: 10.1016/j.brainres.2016.02.052

Glick, D., Barth, S., and Macleod, K. F. (2010). Autophagy: cellular and molecular mechanisms. *J. Pathol.* 221, 3–12. doi: 10.1002/path.2697

Gomes, L. R., Menck, C. F. M., and Cuervo, A. M. (2017). Chaperone-mediated autophagy prevents cellular transformation by regulating MYC proteasomal degradation. *Autophagy* 13, 928–940. doi: 10.1080/15548627.2017.1293767

Harte, A. L., Tripathi, G., Piya, M. K., Barber, T. M., Clapham, J. C., Al-Daghri, N., et al. (2013). NF kappa B as a potent regulator of inflammation in human adipose tissue, Influenced by depot, adiposity, T2DM status, and TNF alpha. *Obesity* 21, 2322–2330. doi: 10.1002/oby.20336

He, C., Bassik, M. C., Moresi, V., Sun, K., Wei, Y., Zou, Z., et al. (2012). Exercise-induced BCL2-regulated autophagy is required for muscle glucose homeostasis. *Nature* 481, 511–515. doi: 10.1038/nature10758

Hou, S. X., Zhu, W. J., Pang, M. Q., Jeffry, J., and Zhou, L. L. (2014). Protective effect of iridoid glycosides from *Paederia* scandens (LOUR.) MERRILL (Rubiaceae) on uric acid nephropathy rats induced by yeast and potassium oxonate. *Food Chem. Toxicol.* 64, 57–64. doi: 10.1016/j.fct.2013.11.022

Hou, Y., Lin, S., Qiu, J., Sun, W., Dong, M., Xiang, Y., et al. (2020). NLRP3 inflammasome negatively regulates podocyte autophagy in diabetic nephropathy. *Biochem. Biophys. Res. Commun.* 521, 791–798. doi: 10.1016/j.bbrc.2019.10.194

Hu, J., Wu, H., Wang, D., Yang, Z., Zhuang, L., Yang, N., et al. (2018). Weicao capsule ameliorates renal injury through increasing autophagy and NLRP3 degradation in UAN rats. *Int. J. Biochem. Cell Biol.* 96, 1–8. doi: 10.1016/j.biocel.2018.01.001

Huynh, K., Bernardo, B. C., Mcmullen, J. R., and Ritchie, R. H. (2014). Diabetic cardiomyopathy: mechanisms and new treatment strategies targeting antioxidant signaling pathways. *Pharmacol. Ther.* 142, 375–415. doi: 10.1016/j.pharmthera.2014.01.003

Hwang, S., Park, J., Kim, J., Jang, H. R., Kwon, G. Y., Huh, W., et al. (2017). Tissue expression of tubular injury markers is associated with renal function decline in diabetic nephropathy. *J. Diabetes Complications* 31, 1704–1709. doi: 10.1016/j.jdiacomp.2017.08.009

Jo, E. K., Kim, J. K., Shin, D. M., and Sasakawa, C. (2016). Molecular mechanisms regulating NLRP3 inflammasome activation. *Cell. Mol. Immunol.* 13, 148–159. doi: 10.1038/cmi.2015.95

Kaushik, S., and Cuervo, A. M. (2012). Chaperone-mediated autophagy: a unique way to enter the lysosome world. *Trends Cell Biol.* 22, 407–417. doi: 10.1016/j.tcb.2012.05.006

Kitada, M., Takeda, A., Nagai, T., Ito, H., Kanasaki, K., and Koya, D. (2011). Dietary restriction ameliorates diabetic nephropathy through anti-inflammatory effects and regulation of the autophagy via restoration of Sirt1 in diabetic wistar fatty (fa/fa) rats: a model of type 2 diabetes. *Exp. Diabetes Res.* 2011:908185.

Kobayashi, S., and Liang, Q. (2015). Autophagy and mitophagy in diabetic cardiomyopathy. *Biochim. Biophys. Acta Mol. Basis Dis.* 1852, 252–261. doi: 10.1016/j.bbadis.2014.05.020

Kong, W. J., Wei, J., Abidi, P., Lin, M. H., Inaba, S., Li, C., et al. (2004). Berberine is a novel cholesterol-lowering drug working through a unique mechanism distinct from statins. *Nat. Med.* 10, 1344–1351. doi: 10.1038/nm1135

Lee, M. J., Kim, E. H., Lee, S. A., Kang, Y. M., Jung, C. H., Yoon, H. K., et al. (2015). Dehydroepiandrosterone prevents linoleic acid-induced endothelial cell senescence by increasing autophagy. *Metab. Clin. Exp.* 64, 1134–1145. doi: 10.1016/j.metabol.2015.05.006

Li, Q., Chen, R., Moriya, J., Yamakawa, J., Sumino, H., Kanda, T., et al. (2008). A novel adipocytokine, visceral adipose tissue-derived serine protease inhibitor (vaspin), and obesity. *J. Int. Med. Res.* 36, 625–629. doi: 10.1177/147323000803600402

Li, X., Ke, X., Li, Z., and Li, B. (2019). Vaspin prevents myocardial injury in rats model of diabetic cardiomyopathy by enhancing autophagy and inhibiting inflammation. *Biochem. Biophys. Res. Commun.* 514, 1–8. doi: 10.1016/j.bbrc.2019.04.110

Liu, Y., and Levine, B. (2015). Autosis and autophagic cell death: the dark side of autophagy. *Cell Death Differ.* 22, 367–376. doi: 10.1038/cdd.2014.143

Lumeng, C. N., and Saltiel, A. R. (2011). Inflammatory links between obesity and metabolic disease. *J. Clin. Invest.* 121, 2111–2117. doi: 10.1172/jci57132

Luo, B., Li, B., Wang, W., Liu, X., Xia, Y., Zhang, C., et al. (2014). NLRP3 gene silencing ameliorates diabetic cardiomyopathy in a type 2 diabetes rat model. *PLoS One* 9:e104771. doi: 10.1371/journal.pone.0104771

Marin-Aguilar, F., Castejon-Vega, B., Alcocer-Gomez, E., Lendines-Cordero, D., Cooper, M. A., De La Cruz, P., et al. (2020). NLRP3 inflammasome inhibition by MCC950 in aged mice improves health via enhanced autophagy and PPAR alpha activity. *J. Gerontol. A Biol. Sci. Med. Sci.* 75, 1457–1464. doi: 10.1093/gerona/glz239

Mclendon, P. M., Ferguson, B. S., Osinska, H., Bhuiyan, M. S., James, J., Mckinsey, T. A., et al. (2014). Tubulin hyperacetylation is adaptive in cardiac proteotoxicity by promoting autophagy. *Proc. Natl. Acad. Sci. U.S.A.* 111, E5178–E5186.

Meyers, A. K., and Zhu, X. (2020). The NLRP3 inflammasome: metabolic regulation and contribution to inflammaging. *Cells* 9:1808. doi: 10.3390/cells9081808

Minihane, A. M., Vinoy, S., Russell, W. R., Baka, A., Roche, H. M., Tuohy, K. M., et al. (2015). Low-grade inflammation, diet composition and health: current research evidence and its translation. *Br. J. Nutr.* 114, 999–1012. doi: 10.1017/s0007114515002093

Mizushima, N., Yoshimori, T., and Ohsumi, Y. (2011). "The role of Atg proteins in autophagosome formation," in *Annual Review Of Cell And Developmental Biology*, Vol. 27, eds R. Schekman, L. Goldstein, and R. Lehmann, (Palo Alto, CA: Annual reviews), 107–132. doi: 10.1146/annurev-cellbio-092910-154005

Mridha, A. R., Wree, A., Robertson, A. A. B., Yeh, M. M., Johnson, C. D., Van Rooyen, D. M., et al. (2017). NLRP3 inflammasome blockade reduces liver inflammation and fibrosis in experimental NASH in mice. *J. Hepatol.* 66, 1037–1046. doi: 10.1016/j.jhep.2017.01.022

Murrow, L., and Debnath, J. (2013). Autophagy as a stress-response and quality-control mechanism: implications for cell injury and human disease. *Ann. Rev. Pathol.* 8, 105–137. doi: 10.1146/annurev-pathol-020712-163918

Ney, P. A. (2015). Mitochondrial autophagy: origins, significance, and role of BNIP3 and NIX. *Biochim. Biophys. Acta Mol. Cell Res.* 1853, 2775–2783. doi: 10.1016/j.bbamcr.2015.02.022

O'connor, W., Harton, J. A., Zhu, X. S., Linhoff, M. W., and Ting, J. P. Y. (2003). Cutting edge: CIAS1/cryopyrin/PYPAF1/NALP3/CATERPILLER 1.1 is an inducible inflammatory mediator with NF-kappa B suppressive properties. *J. Immunol.* 171, 6329–6333. doi: 10.4049/jimmunol.171.12.6329

Oku, M., and Sakai, Y. (2018). Three distinct types of microautophagy based on membrane dynamics and molecular machineries. *Bioessays* 40:e1800008.

Pavillard, L. E., Canadas-Lozano, D., Alcocer-Gomez, E., Marin-Aguilar, F., Pereira, S., Robertson, A. A. B., et al. (2017). NLRP3-inflammasome inhibition prevents high fat and high sugar diets-induced heart damage through autophagy induction. *Oncotarget* 8, 99740–99756. doi: 10.18632/oncotarget.20763

Prochnicki, T., Mangan, M. S., and Latz, E. (2016). Recent insights into the molecular mechanisms of the NLRP3 inflammasome activation. *F1000Research* 5, F1000FacultyRev-1469.

Qiu, D. M., Wang, G. L., Chen, L., Xu, Y. Y., He, S., Cao, X. L., et al. (2014). The expression of beclin-1, an autophagic gene, in hepatocellular carcinoma associated with clinical pathological and prognostic significance. *BMC Cancer* 14:327. doi: 10.1186/1471-2407-14-327

Sarparanta, J., Garcia-Macia, M., and Singh, R. (2017). Autophagy and mitochondria in obesity and type 2 diabetes. *Curr. Diabetes Rev.* 13, 352–369.

Schroder, K., and Tschopp, J. (2010). The inflammasomes. *Cell* 140, 821–832.

Seibenhener, M. L., Babu, J. R., Geetha, T., Wong, H. C., Krishna, N. R., and Wooten, M. W. (2004). Sequestosome 1/p62 is a polyubiquitin chain binding protein involved in ubiquitin proteasome degradation. *Mol. Cell. Biol.* 24, 8055–8068. doi: 10.1128/mcb.24.18.8055-8068.2004

Shoelson, S. E., Herrero, L., and Naaz, A. (2007). Obesity, inflammation, and insulin resistance. *Gastroenterology* 132, 2169–2180.

Sir, D., Tian, Y., Chen, W. L., Ann, D. K., Yen, T. S. B., and Ou, J. H. J. (2010). The early autophagic pathway is activated by hepatitis B virus and required for viral DNA replication. *Proc. Natl. Acad. Sci. U.S.A.* 107, 4383–4388. doi: 10.1073/pnas.0911373107

Slowicka, K., Vereecke, L., and Van Loo, G. (2016). Cellular functions of optineurin in health and disease. *Trends Immunol.* 37, 621–633. doi: 10.1016/j.it.2016.07.002

Sokolova, M., Ranheim, T., Louwe, M. C., Halvorsen, B., Yndestad, A., and Aukrust, P. (2019). NLRP3 inflammasome: a novel player in metabolically induced inflammation-potential influence on the myocardium. *J. Cardiovasc. Pharmacol.* 74, 276–284. doi: 10.1097/fjc.0000000000000704

Strowig, T., Henao-Mejia, J., Elinav, E., and Flavell, R. (2012). Inflammasomes in health and disease. *Nature* 481, 278–286. doi: 10.1038/nature10759

Sun, C., Diao, Q., Lu, J., Zhang, Z., Wu, D., Wang, X., et al. (2019). Purple sweet potato color attenuated NLRP3 inflammasome by inducing autophagy to delay endothelial senescence. *J. Cell. Physiol.* 234, 5926–5939. doi: 10.1002/jcp.28003

Sun, C., Fan, S., Wang, X., Lu, J., Zhang, Z., Wu, D., et al. (2015). Purple sweet potato color inhibits endothelial premature senescence by blocking the NLRP3 inflammasome. *J. Nutr. Biochem.* 26, 1029–1040. doi: 10.1016/j.jnutbio.2015. 04.012

Tooze, S. A., and Yoshimori, T. (2010). The origin of the autophagosomal membrane. *Nat. Cell Biol.* 12, 831–835. doi: 10.1038/ncb091 0-831

Turner, N., Li, J. Y., Gosby, A., To, S. W. C., Cheng, Z., Miyoshi, H., et al. (2008). Berberine and its more biologically available derivative, dihydroberberine, inhibit mitochondrial respiratory complex I: a mechanism for the action of berberine to activate AMP-activated protein kinase and improve insulin action. *Diabetes* 57, 1414–1418. doi: 10.2337/db07-1552

Van Der Heijden, T., Kritikou, E., Venema, W., Van Duijn, J., Van Santbrink, P. J., Slutter, B., et al. (2017). NLRP3 inflammasome inhibition by MCC950 reduces atherosclerotic lesion development in apolipoprotein E-deficient mice-brief report. *Arterioscler. Thromb. Vasc. Biol.* 37, 1457–1461. doi: 10.1161/atvbaha.117.309575

Vandanmagsar, B., Youm, Y. H., Ravussin, A., Galgani, J. E., Stadler, K., Mynatt, R. L., et al. (2011). The NLRP3 inflammasome instigates obesity-induced inflammation and insulin resistance. *Nat. Med.* 17, 179–188. doi: 10.1038/nm. 2279

Wang, C., Pan, Y., Zhang, Q. Y., Wang, F. M., and Kong, L. D. (2012). Quercetin and allopurinol ameliorate kidney injury in STZ-treated rats with regulation of renal NLRP3 inflammasome activation and lipid accumulation. *PLoS One* 7:e38285. doi: 10.1371/journal.pone.0038285

Wang, H., Zhong, P., and Sun, L. (2019). Exogenous hydrogen sulfide mitigates NLRP3 inflammasome-mediated inflammation through promoting autophagy via the AMPK-mTOR pathway. *Biol. Open* 8:bio043653. doi: 10.1242/bio. 043653

Wei, C., Gao, J., Li, M., Li, H., Wang, Y., Li, H., et al. (2016). Dopamine D2 receptors contribute to cardioprotection of ischemic post-conditioning via activating autophagy in isolated rat hearts. *Int. J. Cardiol.* 203, 837–839.

Weisberg, S. P., Mccann, D., Desai, M., Rosenbaum, M., Leibel, R. L., and Ferrante, A. W. (2003). Obesity is associated with macrophage accumulation in adipose tissue. *J. Clin. Invest.* 112, 1796–1808.

Wohlgemuth, S. E., Calvani, R., and Marzetti, E. (2014). The interplay between autophagy and mitochondrial dysfunction in oxidative stress-induced cardiac aging and pathology. *J. Mol. Cell. Cardiol.* 71, 62–70.

Wu, X., Liu, L., Xie, H., Liao, J., Zhou, X., Wan, J., et al. (2012). Tanshinone IIA prevents uric acid nephropathy in rats through NF-kappa B inhibition. *Planta Med.* 78, 866–873.

Xie, Z., Lau, K., Eby, B., Lozano, P., He, C., Pennington, B., et al. (2011). Improvement of cardiac functions by chronic metformin treatment is associated with enhanced cardiac autophagy in diabetic OVE26 mice. *Diabetes* 60, 1770–1778.

Xu, H. Y., Barnes, G. T., Yang, Q., Tan, Q., Yang, D. S., Chou, C. J., et al. (2003). Chronic inflammation in fat plays a crucial role in the development of obesity-related insulin resistance. *J. Clin. Invest.* 112, 1821–1830.

Yang, S., Xia, C., Li, S., Du, L., Zhang, L., and Zhou, R. (2014). Defective mitophagy driven by dysregulation of rheb and KIF5B contributes to mitochondrial reactive oxygen species (ROS)-induced nod-like receptor 3 (NLRP3) dependent proinflammatory response and aggravates lipotoxicity. *Redox Biol.* 3, 63–71.

Yokoi, T., Fukuo, K., Yasuda, O., Hotta, M., Miyazaki, J., Takemura, Y., et al. (2006). Apoptosis signal-regulating kinase 1 mediates cellular senescence induced by high glucose in endothelial cells. *Diabetes* 55, 1660–1665.

Zhai, Y., Meng, X., Ye, T., Xie, W., Sun, G., and Sun, X. (2018). Inhibiting the NLRP3 inflammasome activation with MCC950 ameliorates diabetic encephalopathy in db/db mice. *Molecules* 23:522.

Zhang, T., Fang, Z., Linghu, K. G., Liu, J., Gan, L., and Lin, L. (2020). Small molecule-driven SIRT3-autophagy-mediated NLRP3 inflammasome inhibition ameliorates inflammatory crosstalk between macrophages and adipocytes. *Br. J. Pharmacol.* 177, 4645–4665.

Zhou, H., Feng, L., Xu, F., Sun, Y., Ma, Y., Zhang, X., et al. (2017). Berberine inhibits palmitate-induced NLRP3 inflammasome activation by triggering autophagy in macrophages: a new mechanism linking berberine to insulin resistance improvement. *Biomed. Pharmacother.* 89, 864–874.

10

SESTRINs: Emerging Dynamic Stress-Sensors in Metabolic and Environmental Health

Seung-Hyun Ro[1]*, Julianne Fay[1], Cesar I. Cyuzuzo[1], Yura Jang[1,2], Naeun Lee[3], Hyun-Seob Song[3,4] and Edward N. Harris[1]

[1] Department of Biochemistry, University of Nebraska-Lincoln, Lincoln, NE, United States, [2] Department of Neurology, Institute for Cell Engineering, Johns Hopkins University School of Medicine, Baltimore, MD, United States, [3] Department of Biological Systems Engineering, University of Nebraska-Lincoln, Lincoln, NE, United States, [4] Department of Food Science and Technology, Nebraska Food for Health Center, University of Nebraska-Lincoln, Lincoln, NE, United States

*Correspondence:
Seung-Hyun Ro
shro@unl.edu;
shro1129@gmail.com

Proper timely management of various external and internal stresses is critical for metabolic and redox homeostasis in mammals. In particular, dysregulation of mechanistic target of rapamycin complex (mTORC) triggered from metabolic stress and accumulation of reactive oxygen species (ROS) generated from environmental and genotoxic stress are well-known culprits leading to chronic metabolic disease conditions in humans. Sestrins are one of the metabolic and environmental stress-responsive groups of proteins, which solely have the ability to regulate both mTORC activity and ROS levels in cells, tissues and organs. While Sestrins are originally reported as one of several p53 target genes, recent studies have further delineated the roles of this group of stress-sensing proteins in the regulation of insulin sensitivity, glucose and fat metabolism, and redox-function in metabolic disease and aging. In this review, we discuss recent studies that investigated and manipulated Sestrins-mediated stress signaling pathways in metabolic and environmental health. Sestrins as an emerging dynamic group of stress-sensor proteins are drawing a spotlight as a preventive or therapeutic mechanism in both metabolic stress-associated pathologies and aging processes at the same time.

Keywords: Sestrins, environmental stress, aging, metabolic disease, obesity/inflammation, mTORC, ROS, cancer

INTRODUCTION OF SESTRINs

SESTRINs (Sestrin1, 2, and 3, gene name: *Sesn*) are a classical family of stress-inducible proteins that regulate metabolism through sensing nutrient level and redox status in cells, tissues and organs. *Sesn1* (aka *PA26*) was originally identified as one of the p53 tumor suppressor target genes in a tetracycline-dependent manner (Buckbinder et al., 1994) and located in chromosome 6q21 (Velasco-Miguel et al., 1999). *Sesn1* is also largely expressed ubiquitously in almost all tissues including the pancreas, kidney, skeletal muscle, lung, and brain (Budanov et al., 2002) and activated in a p53-dependent manner under oxidative and irradiation stresses (Sablina et al., 2005; Budanov and Karin, 2008). *Sesn2* (aka *Hi95*) was identified by microarray in Hif1-independent hypoxia condition of glioblastoma A172 cells and located in chromosome 1p35.3 (Budanov et al., 2002). *Sesn2* is activated by DNA damaging oxidative stress and overnutrition stress in the lung, liver, adipose, kidney and pancreas (Budanov et al., 2002; Lee et al., 2012). *Sesn3* was originally identified by *in silico* data base search and located in chromosome 11q21 (Budanov et al., 2002; Peeters et al., 2003). *Sesn3* is activated by FoxO1 and 3 (Nogueira et al., 2008; Chen et al., 2010; Hagenbuchner et al., 2012) and overexpressed in skeletal muscle, intestine, liver, adipose, kidney, colon and brain (Peeters et al., 2003). However, *Sesn3* is somewhat redundant to *Sesn2* in metabolic function and autophagy induction in liver and colon tissues (Lee et al., 2012; Ro et al., 2016). Although ectopically expressed Sestrin2 protein is mostly found in cytoplasm (Parmigiani et al., 2014), recent studies suggest that Sestrin2 is associated with mitochondria (Kim H. et al., 2020; Kovaleva et al., 2020), nucleus (Tu et al., 2018; Wang L.X. et al., 2020), and endoplasmic reticulum (ER) (Wang L.X. et al., 2020) depending on intra- or extra- cellular stress conditions. Those three Sestrin paralogues have a common antioxidant function that suppresses reactive oxygen species (ROS) (Lee et al., 2013; Wang et al., 2017). Another shared function is that Sestrins activate AMP-activated protein kinase (AMPK), inhibiting the mechanistic target of rapamycin complex 1 (mTORC1) (Parmigiani and Budanov, 2016). Upregulation of mTORC1 has been shown to lead to the accelerated development of several obesity-induced and age-related pathologies, such as lipid accumulation, inflammation, glucose tolerance, insulin resistance, ER stress, mitochondrial dysfunction, protein aggregate formation, cardiac arrhythmia and muscle degeneration (Um et al., 2006; Zoncu et al., 2011). Sestrins are considered to improve obesity-induced and age-related pathologies by inhibiting mTORC1. Protein kinase B (AKT) activation through mTORC2 activation by Sestrins leads to improved insulin sensitivity in obesity and diabetes (Dong, 2015; Kazyken et al., 2019; Knudsen et al., 2020). These pathologies were remedied by inhibition of mTORC1, activation of mTORC2/AKT and the use of antioxidants, which shows that the mTORC- and ROS-controlling functions of Sestrins are indeed important for metabolism and cellular homeostasis (**Figure 1A**).

By sensing nutrient and redox-activity levels, Sestrins can integrate cellular signal transduction through their conserved residues and translational and transcriptional modifications (**Figure 1B**). Recent studies of the X-ray crystal structure of Sestrin2 show that it belongs to the family of globin-like α-helix-fold proteins, consisting of 23 helices and no β-sheets, structured by well-conserved Sesn-A [AA 66–239, *N*-terminal structuring domain (NTD)], Sesn-B [AA 254–294, loop linker domain] and Sesn-C [AA308-480, *C*-terminal domain (CTD)] domains among species. Sesn-A and Sesn-C structure are very similar but they have distinctive functions. Sesn-A and Sesn-C are connected by flexible loop linker domain Sesn-B whose functions are not yet known (Kim H. et al., 2015; Ho et al., 2016; Saxton et al., 2016b). Sesn-A has an evolutionarily conserved Cys125 residue with a thiol side chain that has antioxidant function through reducing ROS accumulation (Budanov et al., 2004; Ro et al., 2014a; Kim H. et al., 2015). Knowing the unique structural features of human Sestrin2, several genetic variations and protein modification studies reported the dynamic roles of *Sesn2* in nutrient-sensing, redox-active function, and signal transduction in relation to disease status. K13 and K48 of Sesn-A are ubiquitinated by E3 ligase ring finger protein 186 (RNF186)

and ring-box protein 1 (RBX-1) respectively, causing Sestrin2's degradation in the proteasome (Kumar and Shaha, 2018a; Lear et al., 2019). Using a high-throughput whole-genome single-cell sequencing, Hou et al. (2012) reported that P87S missense mutation of *Sesn2* was found in patients with a certain type of blood cancer, myeloproliferative neoplasms (MPNs), causing aggressive progression of neoplasms. Interestingly, several phosphorylation sites are identified and regulated by unc-51 like autophagy activating kinase 1 (ULK1). ULK1 phosphorylates T232/S249/S279 residues of Sestrin2 which inhibits Sestrin2's binding with leucine in high nutrient condition (Kimball et al., 2016). Exercise increases the same phosphorylation profile of Sestrin2 and improves skeletal muscle metabolism (Zeng et al., 2017, 2018b). ULK1 also phosphorylates S73 and S254 to activate the autophagic clearance of mitochondria in response to copper-induced oxidative stress (Kim H. et al., 2020). L261 and E451 are identified as essential residues for leucine binding in HEK293 cells (Lee et al., 2016; Saxton et al., 2016a,b; Wolfson et al., 2016). DD406/7 are identified as key residues for GTPase-activating protein (GAP) activity toward recombination activating genes (RAGs) (GATOR) 2 binding so that Sestrin2 can inhibit mTORC1 association with lysosome for its activation (Kim H. et al., 2015; Ho et al., 2016). LSD1, upon deacetylation by histone deacetylase 1 (HDAC1), reduced the methylations of H3K4me2 in the promoter region of *Sesn2*, thereby suppressed the gene expression of *Sesn2* in chronic renal failure (CRF) (Zhou et al., 2020). Jumonji domain-containing protein D3 (JMJD3), a histone demethylase, inhibited the transcription of *Sesn2* by reducing the methylations of H3K27me3 in the promoter region of *Sesn2* in cardiomyopathy (Wang P. et al., 2020). Although dense methylation of CpG islands of *Sesn3* was identified in 20% of endometrial cancers (Zighelboim et al., 2007), the transcriptional regulation (e.g., methylation and demethylation) of *Sesn* genes needs further investigation (Ambrosio et al., 2019). Knowing that Sestrin2 stability, redox-active function, nutrient sensing, and interaction with other proteins can be regulated through those identified residues (**Figure 1B**), the development of methodology measuring the activity of specific Sestrin2 functional residues would be a promising venue combating against stress-induced pathologies.

Metabolic dysregulation induces Sestrins as a defense mechanism against obesity and metabolic diseases (Lee et al., 2012; Parmigiani and Budanov, 2016; Dalina et al., 2018). Important key features of cellular function are the regulation of insulin sensitivity, lipid/fatty acid (FA) metabolism, ER stress, and autophagy (Lee et al., 2012, 2020; Park et al., 2014). Glucose starvation, ER stress, amino acid deprivation and mitochondrial dysfunction induces Sestrins as a protective mechanism (Park et al., 2014; Ro et al., 2015; Ye et al., 2015; Ding et al., 2016; Garaeva et al., 2016; Saveljeva et al., 2016). Sestrins are central nutrient status sensors and regulates AMPK, mTORC and subsequent downstream metabolic pathways. Sestrin2 improves insulin sensitivity, prevents excessive lipid accumulation and alleviates ER stress by inhibiting mTORC1 through AMPK activation (Budanov and Karin, 2008) and GATOR binding (Chantranupong et al., 2014; Parmigiani et al., 2014; Kim J.S. et al., 2015) (**Figure 1A**).

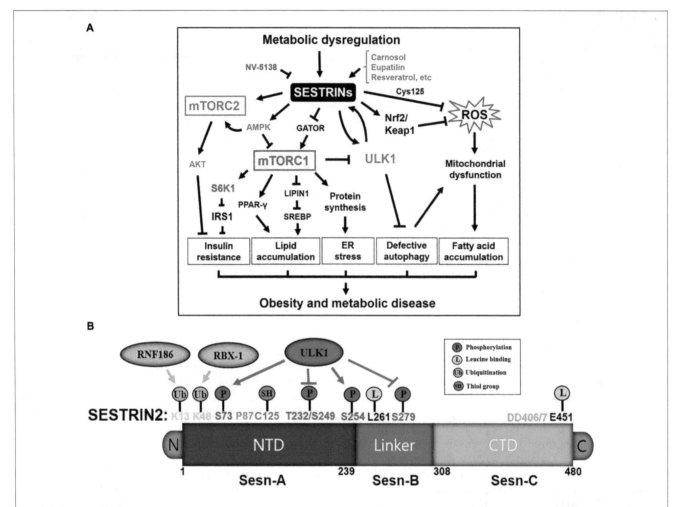

FIGURE 1 | Diagrams depicting the Sestrins-mediated stress signaling pathways and functional domains of Sestrin2 in the regulation of metabolism and disease. **(A)** Schematic diagram of Sestrins/mTORC/ROS pathways in obesity and metabolic diseases induced by metabolic dysregulation stress. Sestrins improve insulin sensitivity by blocking mTORC1/ribosomal protein S6 kinase 1(S6K1) and activating AMPK and mTORC1/AKT pathway. Sestrins also inhibit lipid accumulation and ER stress via mTORC1 inhibition through activating AMPK and binding GATOR2. Sestrins activate autophagy and mitophagy through mTORC1 inhibition and ULK1 activation, which contributes to reducing ROS and removing dysfunctional mitochondria. ULK1 phosphorylates Sestrin2 to induce mitophagy, and phosphorylated Sestrin2 activates ULK1 to further induce autophagy as positive feedback mechanism. Sestrins protect cells, tissues and organs by alleviating stresses and pathologies associated with obesity and metabolic dysfunctions. **(B)** Sestrin2 functional domains (Sesn-A, Sesn-B, and Sesn-C domains) and residues for: (i) protein stability and turnover through ubiquitinations by RNF186 and RBX-1; (ii) redox homeostasis through ROS regulation (Cys125); and (iii) nutrient sensing and regulation through leucine binding, ULK1 activation, and autophagy induction.

Tao et al. (2015) reported that Sestrin3 prevents insulin resistance by activating mTORC2/AKT pathways in the liver. Sestrin2 also activates AKT through mTORC2 and GATOR2 (MIOS/WDR24/SEH1L/WDR59/SEC13) bindings (Kowalsky et al., 2020). Sestrins can eliminate ROS by inducing antioxidants enzymes by activating nuclear factor erythroid 2-related factor 2 (Nrf2) through p62 (gene name: SQSTM1)-dependent degradation of Kelch-like ECH-associated protein 1 (Keap1) pathways, which can reduce the damaged mitochondria, improve fat metabolism, and maintain mitochondrial function in mammalian cells (Bae et al., 2013). Knockdown of Sestrin2 aggravates the atherosclerotic process in human umbilical vein endothelial and THP-1 cell lines and C57BL/6 mice by increasing pro-inflammatory response (Hwang et al., 2017). Sestrin2 suppresses sepsis by inhibiting prolonged nod-like receptor (NLR) family pyrin domain containing 3 (NLRP3)-inflammasome activation (Kim et al., 2016) and protects macrophage by inhibiting TLR-induced pro-inflammatory signaling (Yang et al., 2015). Lysine-specific demethylase 1 (LSD1) suppresses oxidized low-density lipoprotein (Ox-LDL)-induced inflammation by promoting Sestrin2-mediated PI3K/AKT/mTOR pathway activation (Zhuo et al., 2019). Recently, Navitor Pharmaceuticals developed Sestrin2-specific inhibitor, a leucine analog NV-5138, and try to treat the major depressive disorder (MDD) by activating mTORC1 in the brain (Hasegawa et al., 2019; Kato et al., 2019; Sengupta et al., 2019). However, one of the main causes of obesity, inflammation and metabolic disease is the hyperactivation of mTORC1, so the development of Sestrin2-specific activator compound or drug would be a potential therapeutic (Dong, 2015). Indeed, several recent studies suggest that synthetic chemicals or naturally occurring compounds induces Sestrins gene expression as adaptive defense mechanisms upon various cellular damaging stresses (Sanchez-Alvarez et al., 2019). In the examples of *Sesn2* induction, synthetic drugs such as eupatilin (Jegal et al., 2016), topotecan (TPT) (Chen et al., 2015), tanshinone IIA (TIIA) (Yen et al., 2018), and cheliensisin A (ChlA)-F (Hua et al., 2018) induce autophagy by increasing *Sesn2* expression as cellular defense upon oxidative stress and DNA damage. The naturally occurring resveratrol inhibits hepatic lipogenesis through *Sesn2* induction (Jin et al., 2013), thus keeping fatty liver in check. Nelfinavir/bortezomib (Bruning et al., 2013) and protopanaxadiol (PPD) (Jin et al., 2019) are known to induce *Sesn2* through protein kinase R (PKR)-like endoplasmic reticulum kinase (PERK)/ cyclic AMP-dependent transcriptional factor (ATF) 4 activation upon ER stress. Albeit the increasing therapeutic potential of allosteric modulation of Sestrin2 is promising, the unexpected side effects should be thoroughly examined by animal studies and human clinical trials.

SESTRINs IN NUTRIENT STRESS-SENSING AND METABOLIC DYSFUNCTION

In modern westernized society, excessive consumption of fat and sugar combined with sedentary life style causes an exponential increase in the number of patients with obesity and metabolic diseases such as diabetes, cardiovascular disease, and cancer (Bidwell, 2017; Pallazola et al., 2019; Leisegang et al., 2020). Hyperactivation of mTORC1 is one of the underlying mechanisms causing insulin resistance, lipid accumulation, ER stress, defective autophagy function and mitochondrial dysfunction (Um et al., 2006; Zoncu et al., 2011; Tao and Xu, 2020). Here, we reviewed Sestrins, potent inhibitors of mTORC1, and its mechanism for preventing nutrient-associated stress and metabolic dysfunctions.

After *Sesn1* was originally identified as one of the p53 target genes in the late 90's (Velasco-Miguel et al., 1999), *Sesn2* was also identified under the control of p53 to induce autophagy under DNA damage and oxidative stress (Maiuri et al., 2009). When S18 of p53, a phosphorylated target of ataxia-telangiectasia mutated (ATM) kinase, was mutated to Ala in p53 ^{S18A} knock-in mice, these mice developed a diabetic phenotype with abnormal glucose homeostasis and insulin resistance within 6 months of age. This phenotype was alleviated with ectopically overexpressed Sestrin2, suggesting that Sestrin2 has an anti-diabetic effect (Armata et al., 2010). Indeed, Sestrin2 and 3 have a protective effect against obesity-induced metabolic dysfunction and insulin resistance, which is revealed by investigating the liver and adipose tissues of *Sesn2/3* double knockout (DKO) mice (Lee et al., 2012). *Sesn2* ablation exacerbates obesity-induced mTORC1-S6K activation, and moreover, the concomitant ablation of *Sesn2* and *Sesn3* provokes hepatic mTORC1-S6K activation and insulin resistance even in the absence of nutritional overload and obesity (Lee et al., 2012). Although *Sesn2* is suggested to be dominant over *Sesn3* in the previous adipose and liver metabolism studies, each Sestrin

have unique stress-specific regulatory functions. Sestrin2-AMPK axis alleviates hyperglycemia-induced glomerular injury caused by high glucose, high level of ROS and decreased level of nitric oxide (Eid et al., 2013). Sestrin3 reduces lipid accumulation of chronic alcohol-induced liver injury (Kang et al., 2014). And this demonstrates an important homeostatic function for the stress-inducible Sestrin protein family in the control of mammalian lipid and glucose metabolism. It is shown that *Sesn3* liver-specific knockout (KO) mice exhibit insulin resistance and glucose intolerance, and *Sesn3* transgenic mice were protected against insulin resistance induced by a high fat diet (HFD). Also, it has been demonstrated that the *Sesn3* insulin-sensitizing effect is largely independent of AMPK, and *Sesn3* can activate AKT via mTORC2 to regulate hepatic insulin sensitivity and glucose metabolism (Tao et al., 2014). However, the study using adipose-specific Sestrin2 overexpressing mice (PG-*Sesn2*) suggests that Sestrin2 interferes with brown adipose tissue (BAT)-specific expression of uncoupling protein 1 (UCP1) through suppression of ROS-mediated p38 MAPK activation, and resulted in the undesirable accumulation of lipids in BAT (Ro et al., 2014a). These results indicate that maintaining the physiological level and activity of Sestrins in each tissues are critical for metabolic homeostasis and may provide a new therapeutic approach for the prevention of obesity, insulin resistance and diabetes.

Regular physical exercises benefit human health by protecting humans against obesity and metabolic dysfunctions including insulin resistance, glucose intolerance and galactose malabsorption. However, the mechanism of how Sestrins are induced by exercise and their beneficial effects on human health are not completely understood (Nascimento et al., 2013). AMPK and TORC1 are cellular energy sensors that respond in a reciprocal manner to environmental conditions such as nutrient supply or cellular stress to control metabolism and growth in insulin-sensitive tissues like skeletal muscle. A recent study suggests that exercise induces direct interaction between Sestrin2 and AMPK and improves insulin sensitivity through autophagy induction (Li et al., 2017). The expression levels of both Sestrin2 and 3 along with autophagy activity were increased in skeletal muscle of HFD-fed mice after long-term physical exercises (Liu et al., 2015). Both Sestrin2 and 3 directly bind with AMPK and promotes glucose uptake in skeletal muscle in wild type (C57BL/6) and but not in *AMPKα2$^{-/-}$* mice (Morrison et al., 2015; Wang et al., 2018). Sestrins were directly induced by exercise and its phosphorylation by ULK1 kinase was observed along with autophagy induction which improved metabolic parameters, prevented atrophy and maintained mitochondrial mass in muscle (Li et al., 2019; Xu et al., 2019; Kim M. et al., 2020; Segales et al., 2020). Acute exercise increased Sestrin1 whereas chronic exercise up to 4 weeks increased both Sestrin1 and 2 in mice suggesting that Sestrins have distinct functions on the intensity and duration of the exercise (Crisol et al., 2018). In these studies, Sestrins were suggested as plausible cellular mechanism by which exercise protects against metabolic diseases.

Chronic hyperactivation of mTORC1 is one of the hallmarks of tumor proliferation and growth as cancer cells rapidly synthesize proteins, lipids and cellular components in response to metabolic dysregulation, hypoxic environment and genetic mutation stresses (Guertin and Sabatini, 2007; Jones and Thompson, 2009). mTORC1-specific inhibitors such as rapamycin, metformin and aspirin suppresses intestinal and breast cancer initiation and growth (Faller et al., 2015; Pulito et al., 2017). mTORC1/2 inhibitor torin suppresses hepatocellular carcinoma (HCC) cell growth (Wang et al., 2015). Although mTOR inhibitors were widely used previously, efficacy and safety on cancer patients are controversial due to their side effects (Kalender et al., 2010; Blagosklonny, 2011; Din et al., 2012). Knowing that Sestrins are specific mTORC1 inhibitors through AMPK activation and GATOR binding, Sestrin-based therapeutics are emerging as a novel anti-cancer and tumor treatment with less off-target effects. Here, we have reviewed how Sestrins act on tumor suppression and progression in two different aspects. Recent studies identified that Sestrin2 is down-regulated in colorectal cancer and overexpression of Sestrin2 inhibited colon carcinogenesis through mTORC1 inhibition (Wei J.L. et al., 2015; Wei et al., 2017; Ro et al., 2016). Loss of heterozygosity in *Sesn1* (6q21) and *Sesn2* (1p35) is frequently detected in human solid tumors (Ragnarsson et al., 1999; Velasco-Miguel et al., 1999). Sestrins are targets of p53 which, under normal conditions, prevents the outgrowth of cancer cells. There is evidence in the literature which shows that chronic stress-induced inactivation of the p53 target, Sestrin family, promotes the outgrowth of cancer cells. For some examples, inactivation of p53 and repression of *Sesn1/3* contribute to Ras oncogene-induced ROS accumulation and genetic instability in immortalized embryonic fibroblasts (Kopnin et al., 2007). *Sesn2*-deficient mouse embryonic fibroblast (MEF) cells were significantly more susceptible to oncogenic stresses (Budanov and Karin, 2008). *Sesn2* inhibition promotes A549, human a non-small cell lung carcinoma, cell growth (Sablina et al., 2005), and its expression level is negatively correlated with the lung cancer survival rate (Chae et al., 2020). *Sesn3* induces apoptosis of human non-small cell lung cancer (NSCLC) cells in dietary compound cucurbitacin B treatment (Khan et al., 2017). *Sesn3*-deficiency developed severe HCC via hedgehog pathway activation in *Sesn3* KO mice (Liu et al., 2019). In the recent study, knockdown of *Sesn2* promoted the cell growth, migration, and oxidative stress of HEC-1A and ishikawa endometrial cancer cells through mTOC1 hyperactivation (Shin et al., 2020). These findings suggested that Sestrins have a tumor suppressive function through downstream activation by p53.

On the contrary to Sestrins' tumor suppressive role, other studies suggest that Sestrins would promote cancer cell proliferation and growth in nutrient-deficient or oxygen-limited (hypoxic) conditions because Sestrins can activate autophagy and reduces ROS in the hypoxic cancer microenvironment (Maiuri et al., 2009). *Sesn2* promotes tumorigenesis and chemo-resistance under Ultraviolet B (UVB) stress and chemo-therapeutics by activating AKT in human squamous cell carcinomas (SCCs) and melanoma cells (Zhao et al., 2014). Both UVB and UVA induce *Sesn2* upregulation in melanocytes and melanoma cells suggesting the oncogenic role of *Sesn2* in melanoma skin cancer (Zhao et al., 2017). The gene expression of *Sesn2* upregulated by miR182-5p suppression in arsenic treatment functions as an antioxidant in Uppsala 87 malignant glioma (U87MG), human

lung adenocarcinoma H1299, and A549 cell lines (Lin et al., 2018). *Sesn2* would promote colorectal cancer cell growth in the iron-rich environment by suppressing ROS (Kim et al., 2019). Sestrins promote anchorage-independent (anoikis resistance) growth of human endometrial cancer cells (Kozak et al., 2019). Despite Sestrins' contribution on early tumor growth, Sestrins suppress late stages of carcinogenesis in a mouse lung cancer model and A549 cells (Ding et al., 2019). Carnosol, a dietary diterpene from rosemary, induces Sestrins as antioxidants in apoptotic death of HepG2 human hepatoma and HCT116 and SW480 human colorectal carcinoma cells (Tong et al., 2017; Yan et al., 2018). Sestrins promote cell death of breast cancer cells upon irradiation and DNA-damaging drug treatment through mTORC1 inhibition (Sanli et al., 2012). On the other hand, Sestrins may block oxidative damage-associated chemotherapy by reducing ROS (Budanov and Karin, 2008; Hagenbuchner et al., 2012). Sestrins were upregulated upon drug treatments in various type of pre- and mature-tumors as cell survival mechanism: head and neck cancers (Won et al., 2019), non-alcoholic steatohepatitis (Huang et al., 2020), HCC (Dai et al., 2018), osteosarcoma (Yen et al., 2018), acute pancreatitis (Norberg et al., 2018), colitis (Ro et al., 2016), bladder cancer (Hua et al., 2018), and prostate cancer (Fu et al., 2018; Shan et al., 2019). The distinctive roles of Sestrins as tumor suppressor or oncogene in the early or late stages of cancers need further investigation (Sanchez-Alvarez et al., 2019). These results might lead to a novel anti-tumor therapy through the cancer type- and cancer stage-dependent administration or induction of Sestrins.

SESTRINs IN ENVIRONMENTAL STRESS AND AGING

Aging or shortening of lifespan is closely connected with the exposure to oxidative stress, DNA damaging agents, losing immunity, and metabolic dysregulation (Lee et al., 2013; Wei Y. et al., 2015; Srivastava, 2017; Dalina et al., 2018; Fan et al., 2020; Sun et al., 2020). As human life expectancy has extended, the importance of healthy aging or elderly health is increasing and drawing significant attention among the general public. Since Sestrins are known to have anti-aging effect by removing oxidative stress, improving cellular metabolism and immunity, their therapeutic role in healthy aging and elderly health has been emerging subject of scientific studies (Budanov et al., 2010; Lee et al., 2010a; Budanov, 2011; Martyn and Kaneki, 2020). In this section, we have reviewed the essential function of Sestrins as a barometer of stress and indicator of human health at the molecular level focusing on the recent reports.

Sestrins possess two important functions that contribute to protecting cells, tissues and organs against environmental stress and aging (**Figure 2A**). First, Sestrins function as antioxidants, promoting regeneration of peroxiredoxins (Prxs), one of the major ROS scavengers in cells (Budanov et al., 2004; Ro et al., 2014a, 2015). Initially, mammalian Sestrins shows very low similarity to any proteins performed by the basic local alignment search tool (BLAST) search and position-specific scoring matrix (PSSM) analysis (Budanov et al., 2004, 2010).

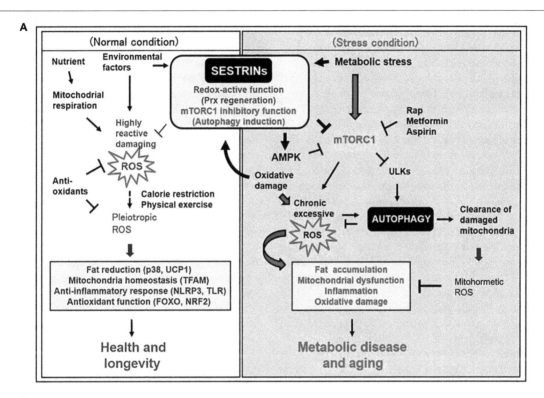

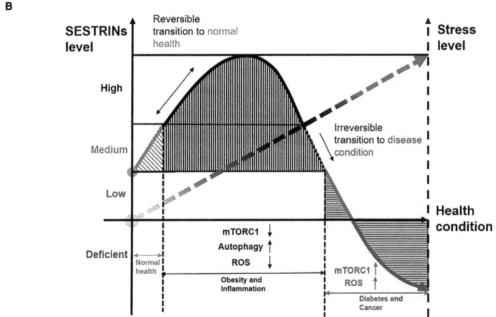

FIGURE 2 | Diagrams depicting the roles of Sestrins in managing stress levels and health conditions. **(A)** Diagram depicting the possible roles of Sestrins in the regulation of ROS and autophagy in mammalian cells. (*Normal condition*) Redox-active function of Sestrins may suppress highly reactive damaging ROS and maintain pleiotropic ROS level such as mitohormesis in mammalian cells under normal nutrient and environmental factors. (*Stress condition*) Sestrins are induced by metabolic or genotoxic stresses such as overnutrition and oxidative damage. Chronic activation of mTORC1 may induce chronic excessive ROS, which results in aging-associated phenotypes such as fat accumulation, mitochondrial dysfunction, inflammation, and oxidative damage in mammalian cells. However, Sestrins inhibit mTORC1 activity and subsequently induce or regulate autophagy activity in the cells and tissues. Activated autophagy removes oxidized proteins and also clear damaged mitochondria which are producing excessive harmful ROS. Overall, Sestrins-mediated autophagy regulates the ROS level to trigger redox adaptations under stress conditions. The underlying mechanism of how pleiotropic level of ROS is maintained by Sestrins-mediated autophagy signaling pathway needs further investigation. **(B)** Graphic diagram explaining the correlation between Sestrins and stress levels in health and disease conditions.

However, residues 100–175 AA shared sequence and structure homology with alkyl hydroperoxidase D (AhpD) which is a *Mycobacterium tuberculosis* hydrogen peroxide reductase and regenerating oxidized bacterial Prxs AhpC by ROS or reactive nitrogen species (RNS). AhpD is a disulfide reductase but Sestrin2 might be a cysteine sulfinyl reductase regenerating oxidized Prxs (Budanov et al., 2004) although it remains controversial (Woo et al., 2009). Further investigation on the role of Sestrins in anti-oxidant defense related to Prxs which confer thiol oxidation of a majority of cytosolic proteins including aurora kinase A (Perkins et al., 2015; Stocker et al., 2018; Byrne et al., 2020) and promote longevity by regulating nutrient signaling protein kinase A (Bodvard et al., 2017; Roger et al., 2020) is warranted to resolve this controversy. Sestrin2 reduces alkylhydroperoxide radicals and ROS accumulation through Cys125 (Ro et al., 2014a; Kim H. et al., 2015). Second, Sestrins stimulate autophagy by inhibiting rapamycin-sensitive mTORC1 comprising of mTOR and Raptor (Kim et al., 2002), through activating AMPK or through binding with GATOR2 (Kim H. et al., 2015; Kim J.S. et al., 2015). Inducing autophagy also contributes to the suppression of ROS, because it eliminates dysfunctional mitochondria that produce the pathogenic level of ROS (Salminen et al., 2012; Ashrafi and Schwarz, 2013). Sestrins also induce the gene expression of antioxidant enzymes via Nrf2 activation through autophagy-mediated degradation of Keap1 (Bae et al., 2013). Sestrin2 associates with autophagy kinase ULK1 and binds with autophagy adaptor protein p62 to activate autophagy (Ro et al., 2014b; Lim et al., 2015). This autophagy activity was significantly blocked when *Sesn2* KO MEF cells were treated with rapamycin as an autophagy inducer (Lee et al., 2012). Recent studies indicate that Sestrin2 activates the autophagic clearance of damaged mitochondria through Parkin-ULK1-Beclin1 activation (Kumar and Shaha, 2018b) and also induces mitophagy in macrophages and renal tubular cells (Ishihara et al., 2013; Kim et al., 2016). ULK1 phosphorylates Sestrin2 at S73 and S254 to induce mitophagy upon copper-catalyzed oxidative stress (Kim H. et al., 2020). Although recent study suggests that Sestrin2 is colocalized with mitochondria and regulates some mitochondrial functions (Kovaleva et al., 2020), its direct translocation into mitochondria and involvement in maintaining mitochondrial

antioxidant enzymes function and ROS level remain unknown.

Given the existence of three distinct paralogues in mammalian Sestrins (Sestrin1/2/3), *Drosophila melanogaster* (*D. melanogaster*) and *Caenorhabditis elegans* (*C. elegans*) have single Sestrin in their genomes, namely *dSesn* and *cSesn*, respectively. Like mammalian Sestrins, *dSesn* is highly expressed in cardiac and skeletal muscle tissues and fat body (Lee et al., 2010b). *dSesn*-null mutant *D. melanogaster* significantly exhibited multiple age-associated degenerative pathologies, including mitochondrial dysfunction, lipid accumulation, cardiac dysfunction, and muscle degeneration. Among these pathologies, mitochondria dysfunction and accompanying fat accumulation was well pronounced (Lee et al., 2010b), which is well correlated with the muscle- and fat body-specific expression patterns of *dSesn*. These pathologies were ameliorated by administering antioxidants and/or autophagy inducers such

as metformin and rapamycin (Lee et al., 2010b). Other genetic results also suggest that the ROS- and autophagy-regulating functions of Sestrins are important for muscle and fat body homeostasis in *D. melanogaster* (Lee et al., 2010a,b). Considering that Sestrins are potent inducers of autophagy (Maiuri et al., 2009) and that *dSesn*-deficient flies and *Sesn2/3*-deficient mice are defective in autophagy function (Lee et al., 2010b, 2012; Bae et al., 2013), it is highly speculated that Sestrins-regulated autophagy is beneficial for metabolic tissue homeostasis and protective against metabolic dysfunctions. *dSesn* reduces oxidative stress from chromium [Cr(IV)]-induced neuronal cell death (Singh and Chowdhuri, 2018). Recent studies also reported that *C. elegans*, lack sulfiredoxin (Srx) but encode *cSesn* (*Sesn1* orthologue), remove oxidative stress and increase longevity (Thamsen et al., 2011; Yang et al., 2013). Since both ROS accumulation and autophagy inhibition are among the common molecular pathologies underlying human metabolic dysfunctions and aging, Sestrins may also have tissue-specific protective roles distinctively from conserved functions in most metabolic tissues (e.g., adipose, brain, colon, liver, cardiac muscle, and skeletal muscle) which are very sensitive to redox regulation and aging (Liu et al., 2015; Li et al., 2017).

Recent studies suggest that Sestrins improve longevity and elderly health by suppressing ROS, regulating autophagy activity and protecting metabolic dysfunction in muscle, heart and brain (Rai et al., 2018; Chen et al., 2019; Cordani et al., 2019; Fan et al., 2020; Liu et al., 2020; Segales et al., 2020; Sun et al., 2020). The level of Sestrins expression is downregulated in aged men although it has no clear correlation with autophagy activity, mTORC1 activity and antioxidant regulation (Zeng et al., 2018a). Both *Sesn1* and *2* levels are significantly decreased in patients with sarcopenic muscle disease (Rajan et al., 2020). Resistant exercise but not dietary protein increased the *Sesn2* level and its phosphorylation in the skeletal muscle of elderly humans (Zeng et al., 2018b) and aged mice (Lenhare et al., 2017). The following are examples in the way Sestrins are involved with symptoms of aging. *Sesn2* is induced in patients with hypertension (Fang et al., 2020) and overexpressed *Sesn2* was protective against cardiomyopathy (Li et al., 2019; Wang P. et al., 2019) and cardiac dysfunction via extracellular signal-regulated protein kinases (ERK)1/2 inhibition (Dong B. et al., 2017) and liver kinase B (LKB)1-mediated AMPK activation (Morrison et al., 2015). *Sesn2* also prevents age-related intolerance to myocardial infarction via AMPK/peroxisome proliferator-activated receptor gamma coactivator 1-alpha (PGC-1α) pathway (Quan et al., 2018), ischemia and reperfusion injury (Quan et al., 2017), atrial fibrillation (Dong Z. et al., 2017), radiation-induced myocardium damage (Zeng et al., 2016) in human and rodent models. These studies indicate that maintaining the homeostatic level of *Sesn2* is protective against cardiovascular aging (Liu et al., 2020; Sun et al., 2020). *Sesn2* promoted autophagy in the brain and prevented neurodegenerative diseases by alleviating oxidative stress (Chen et al., 2019; Luo et al., 2020). *Sesn2* protects neuronal cells from cerebral ischemia-reperfusion injury by increasing Nrf2, Srx1, and thioredoxin (Trx) 1 (Zhang and Zhang, 2018).

Sesn3 positively regulates a pro-convulsant gene network in the human epileptic hippocampus (Johnson et al., 2015). As a non-canonical function of the Sestrin family, Sestrins improve life-long immunity and extend longevity through enhancing natural killer cell function (Pereira et al., 2020) and vaccine responsiveness (Lanna et al., 2017). *Sesn3* promotes the generation of macrophage-mediated helper T cells in colitis (Ge et al., 2020). Taken together, Sestrins' canonical and non-canonical functions contribute to the protection against the aging process and extend healthy lifespan.

PERSPECTIVE ON SESTRINs AS STRESS SENSING-PROTEINS IN METABOLIC DISEASE AND AGING

During the most recent decade, the research on Sestrin2 was increased exponentially according to PubMed and google scholar analysis data (Wang L.X. et al., 2019). Unlike other kinases or transcription factors, a group of Sestrins protein family confers unique dual functions: sensing nutrient stress and reducing oxidative stress. These unique features of stress-inducible protein Sestrins are becoming an intriguing theme among research groups around the world. It is still debatable that maintaining low level of ROS or RNS is actually beneficial to the human body similar to vaccination rather than completely removing all (Kenny et al., 2019; Klaus and Ost, 2020). For example, mitohormesis refers to maintain physiological levels of ROS or RNS which would benefit but could harm tissues and organs at an excessive level (Yun and Finkel, 2014; Barcena et al., 2018; Palmeira et al., 2019). In the current literature, ROS is emerging as a pleiotropic physiological signaling agent in addition to their characteristics as highly reactive damaging species (Holmstrom and Finkel, 2014; Sies and Jones, 2020). For instance, metformin, a well-known anti-diabetic drug, extends the life-span of worms through the production of low levels of mitochondrial ROS and Prxs PRDX-2 (De Haes et al., 2014). Low levels of H_2O_2 extends the life-span of yeast in a Prx-dependent manner (Goulev et al., 2017) and an endogenous

amino-acid metabolite, namely N-acetyl-L-tyrosine (NAT), was recently shown to reduce tumor growth in mice via mitohormesis (Matsumura et al., 2020). Sestrins could be functionally similar to Prx by fine-tuning a pleitropic level of ROS, which might be beneficial for human health, but the underlying mechanism needs further interrogation. Another intriguing speculation is that Sestrins can be induced by various stress conditions in the earlier inflammation and metabolic dysfunction stage, then they act as a cellular defense mechanism by suppressing mTORC1, inducing autophagy and removing ROS. When the stress level goes over the threshold which indicates the metabolic diseases and aging conditions, the Sestrins level goes down in tissues and organs and human can suffer from the irrevocable conditions confronting pain and death (**Figure 2B**). Initially, the upregulation of Sestrins is observed as a defense mechanism in the tissues under metabolic stress and inflammation or during predisposition stage of metabolic syndrome (Lee et al., 2012; Ro et al., 2016), as chronic stress conditions sustain, the level of Sestrins is dramatically suppressed in the etiology of disease conditions such as type 2 diabetes, dyslipidemia, colon cancer development and muscle aging progression (Wei J.L. et al., 2015; Ro et al., 2016; Kim M. et al., 2020; Segales et al., 2020; Sundararajan et al., 2020). In recent human studies, secreted Sestrin2 level in the serum of obese children, diabetic nephropathy patients, and elderly sarcopenia adults is significantly lower and associated with metabolic dysfunction (Nourbakhsh et al., 2017; Mohany and Al Rugaie, 2020; Rajan et al., 2020), suggesting that the expression or the secretion of Sestrin2 is somehow blocked in the disease state. Measuring tissue- or individual patient-specific Sestrins level could be used as a direct health or stress sensors, and proper timely administration of active Sestrins would be emerging preventive or therapeutic methods for those who are suffering from metabolic diseases and aging-associated pathologies.

AUTHOR CONTRIBUTIONS

All authors contributed to the article and approved the submitted version.

REFERENCES

Ambrosio, S., Ballabio, A., and Majello, B. (2019). Histone methyl-transferases and demethylases in the autophagy regulatory network: the emerging role of KDM1A/LSD1 demethylase. *Autophagy* 15, 187–196. doi: 10.1080/15548627.2018.1520546

Armata, H. L., Golebiowski, D., Jung, D. Y., Ko, H. J., Kim, J. K., and Sluss, H. K. (2010). Requirement of the ATM/p53 tumor suppressor pathway for glucose homeostasis. *Mol. Cell. Biol.* 30, 5787–5794.

Ashrafi, G., and Schwarz, T. L. (2013). The pathways of mitophagy for quality control and clearance of mitochondria. *Cell Death Differ.* 20, 31–42. doi: 10.1038/cdd.2012.81

Bae, S. H., Sung, S. H., Oh, S. Y., Lim, J. M., Lee, S. K., Park, Y. N., et al. (2013). Sestrins activate Nrf2 by promoting p62-dependent autophagic degradation of Keap1 and prevent oxidative liver damage. *Cell Metab.* 17, 73–84. doi: 10.1016/j.cmet.2012.12.002

Barcena, C., Mayoral, P., and Quiros, P. M. (2018). Mitohormesis, an antiaging paradigm. *Int. Rev. Cell Mol. Biol.* 340, 35–77. doi: 10.1016/bs.ircmb.2018.05.002

Bidwell, A. J. (2017). Chronic fructose ingestion as a major health concern: Is a sedentary lifestyle making it worse? A review. *Nutrients* 9:549. doi: 10.3390/nu9060549

Blagosklonny, M. V. (2011). Rapamycin-induced glucose intolerance: hunger or starvation diabetes. *Cell Cycle* 10, 4217–4224.

Bodvard, K., Peeters, K., Roger, F., Romanov, N., Igbaria, A., Welkenhuysen, N., et al. (2017). Light-sensing via hydrogen peroxide and a peroxiredoxin. *Nat. Commun.* 8:14791. doi: 10.1038/ncomms14791

Bruning, A., Rahmeh, M., and Friese, K. (2013). Nelfinavir and bortezomib inhibit mTOR activity via ATF4-mediated sestrin-2 regulation. *Mol. Oncol.* 7, 1012–1018. doi: 10.1016/j.molonc.2013.07.010

Buckbinder, L., Talbott, R., Seizinger, B. R., and Kley, N. (1994). Gene regulation by temperature-sensitive p53 mutants: identification of p53 response genes. *Proc. Natl. Acad. Sci. U.S.A.* 91, 10640–10644. doi: 10.1073/pnas.91.22.10640

Budanov, A. V. (2011). Stress-responsive sestrins link p53 with redox regulation and mammalian target of rapamycin signaling. *Antioxid. Redox Signal.* 15, 1679–1690. doi: 10.1089/ars.2010.3530

Budanov, A. V., and Karin, M. (2008). p53 target genes sestrin1 and sestrin2 connect genotoxic stress and mTOR signaling. *Cell* 134, 451–460. doi: 10.1016/j.cell.2008.06.028

Budanov, A. V., Lee, J. H., and Karin, M. (2010). Stressin' Sestrins take an aging fight. *EMBO Mol. Med.* 2, 388–400. doi: 10.1002/emmm.201000097

Budanov, A. V., Sablina, A. A., Feinstein, E., Koonin, E. V., and Chumakov, P. M. (2004). Regeneration of peroxiredoxins by p53-regulated sestrins, homologs of bacterial AhpD. *Science* 304, 596–600. doi: 10.1126/science.1095569

Budanov, A. V., Shoshani, T., Faerman, A., Zelin, E., Kamer, I., Kalinski, H., et al. (2002). Identification of a novel stress-responsive gene Hi95 involved in regulation of cell viability. *Oncogene* 21, 6017–6031. doi: 10.1038/sj.onc.1205877

Byrne, D. P., Shrestha, S., Galler, M., Cao, M., Daly, L. A., Campbell, A. E., et al. (2020). Aurora A regulation by reversible cysteine oxidation reveals evolutionarily conserved redox control of Ser/Thr protein kinase activity. *Sci. Signal.* 13:eaax2713. doi: 10.1126/scisignal.aax2713

Chae, H. S., Gil, M., Saha, S. K., Kwak, H. J., Park, H. W., Vellingiri, B., et al. (2020). Sestrin2 expression has regulatory properties and prognostic value in lung cancer. *J. Pers. Med.* 10:109. doi: 10.3390/jpm10030109

Chantranupong, L., Wolfson, R. L., Orozco, J. M., Saxton, R. A., Scaria, S. M., Bar-Peled, L., et al. (2014). The Sestrins interact with GATOR2 to negatively regulate the amino-acid-sensing pathway upstream of mTORC1. *Cell Rep.* 9, 1–8. doi: 10.1016/j.celrep.2014.09.014

Chen, C. C., Jeon, S. M., Bhaskar, P. T., Nogueira, V., Sundararajan, D., Tonic, I., et al. (2010). FoxOs inhibit mTORC1 and activate Akt by inducing the expression of Sestrin3 and Rictor. *Dev. Cell* 18, 592–604. doi: 10.1016/j.devcel.2010.03.008

Chen, J. H., Zhang, P., Chen, W. D., Li, D. D., Wu, X. Q., Deng, R., et al. (2015). ATM-mediated PTEN phosphorylation promotes PTEN nuclear translocation and autophagy in response to DNA-damaging agents in cancer cells. *Autophagy* 11, 239–252. doi: 10.1080/15548627.2015.1009767

Chen, S. D., Yang, J. L., Lin, T. K., and Yang, D. I. (2019). Emerging roles of sestrins in neurodegenerative diseases: counteracting oxidative stress and beyond. *J. Clin. Med.* 8:1001. doi: 10.3390/jcm8071001

Cordani, M., Sanchez-Alvarez, M., Strippoli, R., Bazhin, A. V., and Donadelli, M. (2019). Sestrins at the interface of ROS control and autophagy regulation in health and disease. *Oxid. Med. Cell. Longev.* 2019:1283075. doi: 10.1155/2019/1283075

Crisol, B. M., Lenhare, L., Gaspar, R. S., Gaspar, R. C., Munoz, V. R., da Silva, A. S. R., et al. (2018). The role of physical exercise on Sestrin1 and 2 accumulations in the skeletal muscle of mice. *Life Sci.* 194, 98–103. doi: 10.1016/j.lfs.2017.12.023

Dai, J., Huang, Q., Niu, K., Wang, B., Li, Y., Dai, C., et al. (2018). Sestrin 2 confers primary resistance to sorafenib by simultaneously activating AKT and AMPK in hepatocellular carcinoma. *Cancer Med.* 7, 5691–5703. doi: 10.1002/cam4.1826

Dalina, A. A., Kovaleva, I. E., and Budanov, A. V. (2018). [Sestrins are Gatekeepers in the Way from Stress to Aging and Disease]. *Mol. Biol.* 52, 948–962. doi: 10.1134/S0026898418060046

De Haes, W., Frooninckx, L., Van Assche, R., Smolders, A., Depuydt, G., Billen, J., et al. (2014). Metformin promotes lifespan through mitohormesis via the

peroxiredoxin PRDX-2. *Proc. Natl. Acad. Sci. U.S.A.* 111, E2501–E2509. doi: 10.1073/pnas.1321776111

Din, F. V., Valanciute, A., Houde, V. P., Zibrova, D., Green, K. A., Sakamoto, K., et al. (2012). Aspirin inhibits mTOR signaling, activates AMP-activated protein kinase, and induces autophagy in colorectal cancer cells. *Gastroenterology* 142, 1504–1515.e3. doi: 10.1053/j.gastro.2012.02.050

Ding, B., Haidurov, A., Chawla, A., Parmigiani, A., van de Kamp, G., Dalina, A., et al. (2019). p53-inducible SESTRINs might play opposite roles in the regulation of early and late stages of lung carcinogenesis. *Oncotarget* 10, 6997–7009. doi: 10.18632/oncotarget.27367

Ding, B., Parmigiani, A., Divakaruni, A. S., Archer, K., Murphy, A. N., and Budanov, A. V. (2016). Sestrin2 is induced by glucose starvation via the unfolded protein response and protects cells from non-canonical necroptotic cell death. *Sci. Rep.* 6:22538. doi: 10.1038/srep22538

Dong, B., Xue, R., Sun, Y., Dong, Y., and Liu, C. (2017). Sestrin 2 attenuates neonatal rat cardiomyocyte hypertrophy induced by phenylephrine via inhibiting ERK1/2. *Mol. Cell. Biochem.* 433, 113–123.

Dong, X. C. (2015). The potential of sestrins as therapeutic targets for diabetes. *Expert Opin. Ther. Targets* 19, 1011–1015. doi: 10.1517/14728222.2015.1044976

Dong, Z., Lin, C., Liu, Y., Jin, H., Wu, H., Li, Z., et al. (2017). Upregulation of sestrins protect atriums against oxidative damage and fibrosis in human and experimental atrial fibrillation. *Sci. Rep.* 7:46307. doi: 10.1038/srep46307

Eid, A. A., Lee, D. Y., Roman, L. J., Khazim, K., and Gorin, Y. (2013). Sestrin 2 and AMPK connect hyperglycemia to Nox4-dependent endothelial nitric oxide synthase uncoupling and matrix protein expression. *Mol. Cell. Biol.* 33, 3439–3460.

Faller, W. J., Jackson, T. J., Knight, J. R., Ridgway, R. A., Jamieson, T., Karim, S. A., et al. (2015). mTORC1-mediated translational elongation limits intestinal tumour initiation and growth. *Nature* 517, 497–500. doi: 10.1038/nature13896

Fan, X., Zeng, Y., Song, W., Li, J., Ai, S., Yang, D., et al. (2020). The role of Sestrins in the regulation of the aging process. *Mech. Ageing Dev.* 188, 111251. doi: 10.1016/j.mad.2020.111251

Fang, C., Yang, Z., Shi, L., Zeng, T., Shi, Y., Liu, L., et al. (2020). Circulating sestrin levels are increased in hypertension patients. *Dis. Markers* 2020:3787295. doi: 10.1155/2020/3787295

Fu, H., Song, W., Wang, Y., Deng, W., Tang, T., Fan, W., et al. (2018). Radiosensitizing effects of Sestrin2 in PC3 prostate cancer cells. *Iran. J. Basic Med. Sci.* 21, 621–624. doi: 10.22038/IJBMS.2018.18283.4923

Garaeva, A. A., Kovaleva, I. E., Chumakov, P. M., and Evstafieva, A. G. (2016). Mitochondrial dysfunction induces SESN2 gene expression through Activating Transcription Factor 4. *Cell Cycle* 15, 64–71. doi: 10.1080/15384101.2015.1120929

Ge, L., Xu, M., Brant, S. R., Liu, S., Zhu, C., Shang, J., et al. (2020). Sestrin3 enhances macrophage-mediated generation of T helper 1 and T helper 17 cells in a mouse colitis model. *Int. Immunol.* 32, 421–432. doi: 10.1093/intimm/dxaa016

Goulev, Y., Morlot, S., Matifas, A., Huang, B., Molin, M., Toledano, M. B., et al. (2017). Nonlinear feedback drives homeostatic plasticity in H2O2 stress response. *eLife* 6:e23971. doi: 10.7554/eLife.23971

Guertin, D. A., and Sabatini, D. M. (2007). Defining the role of mTOR in cancer. *Cancer Cell* 12, 9–22. doi: 10.1016/j.ccr.2007.05.008

Hagenbuchner, J., Kuznetsov, A., Hermann, M., Hausott, B., Obexer, P., and Ausserlechner, M. J. (2012). FOXO3-induced reactive oxygen species are regulated by BCL2L11 (Bim) and SESN3. *J. Cell Sci.* 125(Pt 5), 1191–1203. doi: 10.1242/jcs.092098

Hasegawa, Y., Zhu, X., and Kamiya, A. (2019). NV-5138 as a fast-acting antidepressant via direct activation of mTORC1 signaling. *J. Clin. Invest.* 129, 2207–2209. doi: 10.1172/JCI129702

Ho, A., Cho, C. S., Namkoong, S., Cho, U. S., and Lee, J. H. (2016). Biochemical basis of sestrin physiological activities. *Trends Biochem. Sci.* 41, 621–632. doi: 10.1016/j.tibs.2016.04.005

Holmstrom, K. M., and Finkel, T. (2014). Cellular mechanisms and physiological consequences of redox-dependent signalling. *Nat. Rev. Mol. Cell Biol.* 15, 411–421. doi: 10.1038/nrm3801

Hou, Y., Song, L., Zhu, P., Zhang, B., Tao, Y., Xu, X., et al. (2012). Single-cell exome sequencing and monoclonal evolution of a JAK2-negative myeloproliferative neoplasm. *Cell* 148, 873–885. doi: 10.1016/j.cell.2012.02.028

Hua, X., Xu, J., Deng, X., Xu, J., Li, J., Zhu, D. Q., et al. (2018). New compound ChlA-F induces autophagy-dependent anti-cancer effect via upregulating

Sestrin-2 in human bladder cancer. *Cancer Lett.* 436, 38–51. doi: 10.1016/j.canlet.2018.08.013

Huang, M., Kim, H. G., Zhong, X., Dong, C., Zhang, B., Fang, Z., et al. (2020). Sestrin 3 protects against diet-induced nonalcoholic steatohepatitis in mice through suppression of transforming growth factor beta signal transduction. *Hepatology* 71, 76–92. doi: 10.1002/hep.30820

Hwang, H. J., Jung, T. W., Choi, J. H., Lee, H. J., Chung, H. S., Seo, J. A., et al. (2017). Knockdown of sestrin2 increases pro-inflammatory reactions and ER stress in the endothelium via an AMPK dependent mechanism. *Biochim. Biophys. Acta Mol. Basis Dis.* 1863, 1436–1444. doi: 10.1016/j.bbadis.2017.02.018

Ishihara, M., Urushido, M., Hamada, K., Matsumoto, T., Shimamura, Y., Ogata, K., et al. (2013). Sestrin-2 and BNIP3 regulate autophagy and mitophagy in renal tubular cells in acute kidney injury. *Am. J. Physiol. Renal Physiol.* 305, F495–F509. doi: 10.1152/ajprenal.00642.2012

Jegal, K. H., Ko, H. L., Park, S. M., Byun, S. H., Kang, K. W., Cho, I. J., et al. (2016). Eupatilin induces Sestrin2-dependent autophagy to prevent oxidative stress. *Apoptosis* 21, 642–656.

Jin, H. R., Du, C. H., Wang, C. Z., Yuan, C. S., and Du, W. (2019). Ginseng metabolite Protopanaxadiol induces Sestrin2 expression and AMPK activation through GCN2 and PERK. *Cell Death Dis.* 10:311.

Jin, S. H., Yang, J. H., Shin, B. Y., Seo, K., Shin, S. M., Cho, I. J., et al. (2013). Resveratrol inhibits LXRalpha-dependent hepatic lipogenesis through novel antioxidant Sestrin2 gene induction. *Toxicol. Appl. Pharmacol.* 271, 95–105. doi: 10.1016/j.taap.2013.04.023

Johnson, M. R., Behmoaras, J., Bottolo, L., Krishnan, M. L., Pernhorst, K., Santoscoy, P. L. M., et al. (2015). Systems genetics identifies Sestrin 3 as a regulator of a proconvulsant gene network in human epileptic hippocampus. *Nat. Commun.* 6:6031. doi: 10.1038/ncomms7031

Jones, R. G., and Thompson, C. B. (2009). Tumor suppressors and cell metabolism: a recipe for cancer growth. *Genes Dev.* 23, 537–548. doi: 10.1101/gad.1756509

Kalender, A., Selvaraj, A., Kim, S. Y., Gulati, P., Brule, S., Viollet, B., et al. (2010). Metformin, independent of AMPK, inhibits mTORC1 in a rag GTPase-dependent manner. *Cell Metab.* 11, 390–401. doi: 10.1016/j.cmet.2010.03.014

Kang, X., Petyaykina, K., Tao, R., Xiong, X., Dong, X. C., and Liangpunsakul, S. (2014). The inhibitory effect of ethanol on Sestrin3 in the pathogenesis of ethanol-induced liver injury. *Am. J. Physiol. Gastrointest. Liver Physiol.* 307, G58–G65. doi: 10.1152/ajpgi.00373.2013

Kato, T., Pothula, S., Liu, R. J., Duman, C. H., Terwilliger, R., Vlasuk, G. P., et al. (2019). Sestrin modulator NV-5138 produces rapid antidepressant effects via direct mTORC1 activation. *J. Clin. Invest.* 129, 2542–2554. doi: 10.1172/JCI126859

Kazyken, D., Magnuson, B., Bodur, C., Acosta-Jaquez, H. A., Zhang, D., Tong, X., et al. (2019). AMPK directly activates mTORC2 to promote cell survival during acute energetic stress. *Sci. Signal.* 12:eaav3249. doi: 10.1126/scisignal.aav3249

Kenny, T. C., Gomez, M. L., and Germain, D. (2019). Mitohormesis, UPR(mt), and the complexity of mitochondrial DNA landscapes in cancer. *Cancer Res.* 79, 6057–6066.

Khan, N., Jajeh, F., Khan, M. I., Mukhtar, E., Shabana, S. M., and Mukhtar, H. (2017). Sestrin-3 modulation is essential for therapeutic efficacy of cucurbitacin B in lung cancer cells. *Carcinogenesis* 38, 184–195. doi: 10.1093/carcin/bgw124

Kim, D. H., Sarbassov, D. D., Ali, S. M., King, J. E., Latek, R. R., Erdjument-Bromage, H., et al. (2002). mTOR interacts with raptor to form a nutrient-sensitive complex that signals to the cell growth machinery. *Cell* 110, 163–175.

Kim, H., An, S., Ro, S. H., Teixeira, F., Jin Park, G., Kim, C., et al. (2015). Janus-faced Sestrin2 controls ROS and mTOR signalling through two separate functional domains. *Nat. Commun.* 6:10025. doi: 10.1038/ncomms10025

Kim, H., Jeon, B. T., Kim, I. M., Bennett, S. J., Lorch, C. M., Viana, M. P., et al. (2020). Sestrin2 Phosphorylation by ULK1 induces autophagic degradation of mitochondria damaged by copper-induced oxidative stress. *Int. J. Mol. Sci.* 21:6130. doi: 10.3390/ijms21176130

Kim, J. S., Ro, S. H., Kim, M., Park, H. W., Semple, I. A., Park, H. L., et al. (2015). Sestrin2 regulates mTOR complex 1 (mTORC1) through modulation of GATOR complexes. *Sci. Rep.* 5:9502. doi: 10.1038/srep09502

Kim, M., Sujkowski, A., Namkoong, S., Gu, B., Cobb, T., Kim, B., et al. (2020). Sestrins are evolutionarily conserved mediators of exercise benefits. *Nat. Commun.* 11:190.

Kim, H., Yin, K., Falcon, D. M., and Xue, X. (2019). The interaction of Hemin and Sestrin2 modulates oxidative stress and colon tumor growth. *Toxicol. Appl. Pharmacol.* 374, 77–85. doi: 10.1016/j.taap.2019.04.025

Kim, M. J., Bae, S. H., Ryu, J. C., Kwon, Y., Oh, J. H., Kwon, J., et al. (2016). SESN2/sestrin2 suppresses sepsis by inducing mitophagy and inhibiting NLRP3 activation in macrophages. *Autophagy* 12, 1272–1291. doi: 10.1080/15548627.2016.1183081

Kimball, S. R., Gordon, B. S., Moyer, J. E., Dennis, M. D., and Jefferson, L. S. (2016). Leucine induced dephosphorylation of Sestrin2 promotes mTORC1 activation. *Cell. Signal.* 28, 896–906. doi: 10.1016/j.cellsig.2016.03.008

Klaus, S., and Ost, M. (2020). Mitochondrial uncoupling and longevity - A role for mitokines? *Exp. Gerontol.* 130, 110796. doi: 10.1016/j.exger.2019.110796

Knudsen, J. R., Fritzen, A. M., James, D. E., Jensen, T. E., Kleinert, M., and Richter, E. A. (2020). Growth factor-dependent and -independent activation of mTORC2. *Trends Endocrinol. Metab.* 31, 13–24. doi: 10.1016/j.tem.2019.09.005

Kopnin, P. B., Agapova, L. S., Kopnin, B. P., and Chumakov, P. M. (2007). Repression of sestrin family genes contributes to oncogenic Ras-induced reactive oxygen species up-regulation and genetic instability. *Cancer Res.* 67, 4671–4678.

Kovaleva, I. E., Tokarchuk, A. V., Zheltukhin, A. O., Dalina, A. A., Safronov, G. G., Evstafieva, A. G., et al. (2020). Mitochondrial localization of SESN2. *PLoS One* 15:e0226862. doi: 10.1371/journal.pone.0226862

Kowalsky, A. H., Namkoong, S., Mettetal, E., Park, H. W., Kazyken, D., Fingar, D. C., et al. (2020). The GATOR2-mTORC2 axis mediates Sestrin2-induced AKT Ser/Thr kinase activation. *J. Biol. Chem.* 295, 1769–1780. doi: 10.1074/jbc.RA119.010857

Kozak, J., Wdowiak, P., Maciejewski, R., and Torres, A. (2019). Interactions between microRNA-200 family and Sestrin proteins in endometrial cancer cell lines and their significance to anoikis. *Mol. Cell. Biochem.* 459, 21–34.

Kumar, A., and Shaha, C. (2018a). RBX1-mediated ubiquitination of SESN2 promotes cell death upon prolonged mitochondrial damage in SH-SY5Y neuroblastoma cells. *Mol. Cell. Biochem.* 446, 1–9.

Kumar, A., and Shaha, C. (2018b). SESN2 facilitates mitophagy by helping Parkin translocation through ULK1 mediated Beclin1 phosphorylation. *Sci. Rep.* 8:615.

Lanna, A., Gomes, D. C., Muller-Durovic, B., McDonnell, T., Escors, D., Gilroy, D. W., et al. (2017). A sestrin-dependent Erk-Jnk-p38 MAPK activation complex inhibits immunity during aging. *Nat. Immunol.* 18, 354–363. doi: 10.1038/ni.3665

Lear, T. B., Lockwood, K. C., Ouyang, Y., Evankovich, J. W., Larsen, M. B., Lin, B., et al. (2019). The RING-type E3 ligase RNF186 ubiquitinates Sestrin-2 and thereby controls nutrient sensing. *J. Biol. Chem.* 294, 16527–16534. doi: 10.1074/jbc.AC119.010671

Lee, J. H., Bodmer, R., Bier, E., and Karin, M. (2010a). Sestrins at the crossroad between stress and aging. *Aging* 2, 369–374. doi: 10.18632/aging.100157

Lee, J. H., Budanov, A. V., Park, E. J., Birse, R., Kim, T. E., Perkins, G. A., et al. (2010b). Sestrin as a feedback inhibitor of TOR that prevents age-related pathologies. *Science* 327, 1223–1228. doi: 10.1126/science.1182228

Lee, J. H., Budanov, A. V., and Karin, M. (2013). Sestrins orchestrate cellular metabolism to attenuate aging. *Cell Metab.* 18, 792–801. doi: 10.1016/j.cmet.2013.08.018

Lee, J. H., Budanov, A. V., Talukdar, S., Park, E. J., Park, H., Park, H.-W., et al. (2012). Maintenance of metabolic homeostasis by Sestrin2 and Sestrin3. *Cell Metab.* 16, 311–321.

Lee, J. H., Cho, U. S., and Karin, M. (2016). Sestrin regulation of TORC1: Is Sestrin a leucine sensor? *Sci. Signal.* 9:re5. doi: 10.1126/scisignal.aaf2885

Lee, S., Shin, J., Hong, Y., Shin, S. M., Shin, H. W., Shin, J., et al. (2020). Sestrin2 alleviates palmitate-induced endoplasmic reticulum stress, apoptosis, and defective invasion of human trophoblast cells. *Am. J. Reprod. Immunol.* 83:e13222. doi: 10.1111/aji.13222

Leisegang, K., Sengupta, P., Agarwal, A., and Henkel, R. (2020). Obesity and male infertility: mechanisms and management. *Andrologia*. doi: 10.1111/and.13617 [Epub ahead of print].

Lenhare, L., Crisol, B. M., Silva, V. R. R., Katashima, C. K., Cordeiro, A. V., Pereira, K. D., et al. (2017). Physical exercise increases Sestrin 2 protein levels and induces autophagy in the skeletal muscle of old mice. *Exp. Gerontol.* 97, 17–21. doi: 10.1016/j.exger.2017.07.009

Li, H., Liu, S., Yuan, H., Niu, Y., and Fu, L. (2017). Sestrin 2 induces autophagy and attenuates insulin resistance by regulating AMPK signaling in C2C12 myotubes. *Exp. Cell Res.* 354, 18–24. doi: 10.1016/j.yexcr.2017.03.023

Li, R., Huang, Y., Semple, I., Kim, M., Zhang, Z., and Lee, J. H. (2019). Cardioprotective roles of sestrin 1 and sestrin 2 against doxorubicin cardiotoxicity. *Am. J. Physiol. Heart Circ. Physiol.* 317, H39–H48. doi: 10.1152/ajpheart.00008.2019

Lim, J., Lachenmayer, M. L., Wu, S., Liu, W., Kundu, M., Wang, R., et al. (2015). Proteotoxic stress induces phosphorylation of p62/SQSTM1 by ULK1 to regulate selective autophagic clearance of protein aggregates. *PLoS Genet.* 11:e1004987. doi: 10.1371/journal.pgen.1004987

Lin, L. T., Liu, S. Y., Leu, J. D., Chang, C. Y., Chiou, S. H., Lee, T. C., et al. (2018). Arsenic trioxide-mediated suppression of miR-182-5p is associated with potent anti-oxidant effects through up-regulation of SESN2. *Oncotarget* 9, 16028–16042. doi: 10.18632/oncotarget.24678

Liu, X., Niu, Y., Yuan, H., Huang, J., and Fu, L. (2015). AMPK binds to Sestrins and mediates the effect of exercise to increase insulin-sensitivity through autophagy. *Metabolism* 64, 658–665. doi: 10.1016/j.metabol.2015.01.015

Liu, Y., Du, X., Huang, Z., Zheng, Y., and Quan, N. (2020). Sestrin 2 controls the cardiovascular aging process via an integrated network of signaling pathways. *Ageing Res. Rev.* 62:101096. doi: 10.1016/j.arr.2020.101096

Liu, Y., Kim, H. G., Dong, E., Dong, C., Huang, M., Liu, Y., et al. (2019). Sesn3 deficiency promotes carcinogen-induced hepatocellular carcinoma via regulation of the hedgehog pathway. *Biochim. Biophys. Acta Mol. Basis Dis.* 1865, 2685–2693. doi: 10.1016/j.bbadis.2019.07.011

Luo, L., Wu, J., Qiao, L., Lu, G., Li, J., and Li, D. (2020). Sestrin 2 attenuates sepsis-associated encephalopathy through the promotion of autophagy in hippocampal neurons. *J. Cell. Mol. Med.* 24, 6634–6643. doi: 10.1111/jcmm.15313

Maiuri, M. C., Malik, S. A., Morselli, E., Kepp, O., Criollo, A., Mouchel, P. L., et al. (2009). Stimulation of autophagy by the p53 target gene Sestrin2. *Cell Cycle* 8, 1571–1576.

Martyn, J. A. J., and Kaneki, M. (2020). Muscle atrophy and the sestrins. *N. Engl. J. Med.* 383, 1279–1282. doi: 10.1056/NEJMcibr2003528

Matsumura, T., Uryu, O., Matsuhisa, F., Tajiri, K., Matsumoto, H., and Hayakawa, Y. (2020). N-acetyl-l-tyrosine is an intrinsic triggering factor of mitohormesis in stressed animals. *EMBO Rep.* 21:e49211. doi: 10.15252/embr.201949211

Mohany, K. M., and Al Rugaie, O. (2020). Association of serum sestrin 2 and betatrophin with serum neutrophil gelatinase associated lipocalin levels in type 2 diabetic patients with diabetic nephropathy. *J. Diabetes Metab. Disord.* 19, 249–256.

Morrison, A., Chen, L., Wang, J., Zhang, M., Yang, H., Ma, Y., et al. (2015). Sestrin2 promotes LKB1-mediated AMPK activation in the ischemic heart. *FASEB J.* 29, 408–417.

Nascimento, E. B., Osler, M. E., and Zierath, J. R. (2013). Sestrin 3 regulation in type 2 diabetic patients and its influence on metabolism and differentiation in skeletal muscle. *Am. J. Physiol. Endocrinol. Metab.* 305, E1408–E1414. doi: 10.1152/ajpendo.00212.2013

Nogueira, V., Park, Y., Chen, C. C., Xu, P. Z., Chen, M. L., Tonic, I., et al. (2008). Akt determines replicative senescence and oxidative or oncogenic premature senescence and sensitizes cells to oxidative apoptosis. *Cancer Cell* 14, 458–470. doi: 10.1016/j.ccr.2008.11.003

Norberg, K. J., Nania, S., Li, X., Gao, H., Szatmary, P., Segersvard, R., et al. (2018). RCAN1 is a marker of oxidative stress, induced in acute pancreatitis. *Pancreatology* 18, 734–741. doi: 10.1016/j.pan.2018.08.005

Nourbakhsh, M., Sharifi, R., Ghorbanhosseini, S. S., Javad, A., Ahmadpour, F., Razzaghy Azar, M., et al. (2017). Evaluation of plasma TRB3 and Sestrin 2 levels in obese and normal-weight children. *Child. Obes.* 13, 409–414. doi: 10.1089/chi.2017.0082

Pallazola, V. A., Davis, D. M., Whelton, S. P., Cardoso, R., Latina, J. M., Michos, E. D., et al. (2019). A Clinician's guide to healthy eating for cardiovascular disease prevention. *Mayo Clin. Proc. Innov. Qual. Outcomes* 3, 251–267. doi: 10.1016/j.mayocpiqo.2019.05.001

Palmeira, C. M., Teodoro, J. S., Amorim, J. A., Steegborn, C., Sinclair, D. A., and Rolo, A. P. (2019). Mitohormesis and metabolic health: the interplay between ROS, cAMP and sirtuins. *Free Radic. Biol. Med.* 141, 483–491. doi: 10.1016/j.freeradbiomed.2019.07.017

Park, H. W., Park, H., Ro, S. H., Jang, I., Semple, I. A., Kim, D. N., et al. (2014). Hepatoprotective role of Sestrin2 against chronic ER stress. *Nat. Commun.* 5:4233.

Parmigiani, A., and Budanov, A. V. (2016). Sensing the environment through sestrins: implications for cellular metabolism. *Int. Rev. Cell Mol. Biol.* 327, 1–42. doi: 10.1016/bs.ircmb.2016.05.003

Parmigiani, A., Nourbakhsh, A., Ding, B., Wang, W., Kim, Y. C., Akopiants, K., et al. (2014). Sestrins inhibit mTORC1 kinase activation through the GATOR complex. *Cell Rep.* 9, 1281–1291. doi: 10.1016/j.celrep.2014.10.019

Peeters, H., Debeer, P., Bairoch, A., Wilquet, V., Huysmans, C., Parthoens, E., et al. (2003). PA26 is a candidate gene for heterotaxia in humans: identification of a novel PA26-related gene family in human and mouse. *Hum. Genet.* 112, 573–580.

Pereira, B. I., De Maeyer, R. P. H., Covre, L. P., Nehar-Belaid, D., Lanna, A., Ward, S., et al. (2020). Sestrins induce natural killer function in senescent-like CD8(+) T cells. *Nat. Immunol.* 21, 684–694.

Perkins, A., Nelson, K. J., Parsonage, D., Poole, L. B., and Karplus, P. A. (2015). Peroxiredoxins: guardians against oxidative stress and modulators of peroxide signaling. *Trends Biochem. Sci.* 40, 435–445. doi: 10.1016/j.tibs.2015.05.001

Pulito, C., Mori, F., Sacconi, A., Goeman, F., Ferraiuolo, M., Pasanisi, P., et al. (2017). Metformin-induced ablation of microRNA 21-5p releases Sestrin-1 and CAB39L antitumoral activities. *Cell Discov.* 3:17022. doi: 10.1038/celldisc.2017.22

Quan, N., Sun, W., Wang, L., Chen, X., Bogan, J. S., Zhou, X., et al. (2017). Sestrin2 prevents age-related intolerance to ischemia and reperfusion injury by modulating substrate metabolism. *FASEB J.* 31, 4153–4167. doi: 10.1096/fj.201700063R

Quan, N., Wang, L., Chen, X., Luckett, C., Cates, C., Rousselle, T., et al. (2018). Sestrin2 prevents age-related intolerance to post myocardial infarction via AMPK/PGC-1alpha pathway. *J. Mol. Cell. Cardiol.* 115, 170–178. doi: 10.1016/j.yjmcc.2018.01.005

Ragnarsson, G., Eiriksdottir, G., Johannsdottir, J. T., Jonasson, J. G., Egilsson, V., and Ingvarsson, S. (1999). Loss of heterozygosity at chromosome 1p in different solid human tumours: association with survival. *Br. J. Cancer* 79, 1468–1474. doi: 10.1038/sj.bjc.6690234

Rai, N., Venugopalan, G., Pradhan, R., Ambastha, A., Upadhyay, A. D., Dwivedi, S., et al. (2018). Exploration of novel anti-oxidant protein sestrin in frailty syndrome in elderly. *Aging Dis.* 9, 220–227. doi: 10.14336/AD.2017.0423

Rajan, S. P., Anwar, M., Jain, B., Khan, M. A., Dey, S., and Dey, A. B. (2020). Serum sestrins: potential predictive molecule in human sarcopenia. *Aging Clin. Exp. Res.* doi: 10.1007/s40520-020-01642-9 [Epub ahead of print].

Ro, S. H., Nam, M., Jang, I., Park, H. W., Park, H., Semple, I. A., et al. (2014a). Sestrin2 inhibits uncoupling protein 1 expression through suppressing reactive oxygen species. *Proc. Natl. Acad. Sci. U.S.A.* 111, 7849–7854. doi: 10.1073/pnas.1401787111

Ro, S. H., Semple, I. A., Park, H., Park, H., Park, H. W., Kim, M., et al. (2014b). Sestrin2 Promotes Unc-51-like Kinase 1 (ULK1)-Mediated Phosphorylation of p62/sequestosome-1. *FEBS J.* 281, 3816–3827.

Ro, S. H., Semple, I., Ho, A., Park, H. W., and Lee, J. H. (2015). Sestrin2, a Regulator of Thermogenesis and Mitohormesis in Brown Adipose Tissue. *Front. Endocrinol.* 6:114. doi: 10.3389/fendo.2015.00114

Ro, S.-H., Xue, X., Ramakrishnan, S. K., Cho, C.-S., Namkoong, S., Jang, I., et al. (2016). Tumor suppressive role of Sestrin2 during colitis and colon carcinogenesis. *eLife* 5:e12204. doi: 10.7554/eLife.12204

Roger, F., Picazo, C., Reiter, W., Libiad, M., Asami, C., Hanzen, S., et al. (2020). Peroxiredoxin promotes longevity and H2O2-resistance in yeast through redox-modulation of protein kinase A. *eLife* 9:e60346. doi: 10.7554/eLife.60346

Sablina, A. A., Budanov, A. V., Ilyinskaya, G. V., Agapova, L. S., Kravchenko, J. E., and Chumakov, P. M. (2005). The antioxidant function of the p53 tumor suppressor. *Nat. Med.* 11, 1306–1313. doi: 10.1038/nm1320

Salminen, A., Ojala, J., Kaarniranta, K., and Kauppinen, A. (2012). Mitochondrial dysfunction and oxidative stress activate inflammasomes: impact on the aging process and age-related diseases. *Cell. Mol. Life Sci.* 69, 2999–3013.

Sanchez-Alvarez, M., Strippoli, R., Donadelli, M., Bazhin, A. V., and Cordani, M. (2019). Sestrins as a therapeutic bridge between ROS and autophagy in cancer. *Cancers* 11:1415. doi: 10.3390/cancers11101415

Sanli, T., Linher-Melville, K., Tsakiridis, T., and Singh, G. (2012). Sestrin2 modulates AMPK subunit expression and its response to ionizing radiation in breast cancer cells. PLoS One 7:e32035. doi: 10.1371/journal.pone.0032035

Saveljeva, S., Cleary, P., Mnich, K., Ayo, A., Pakos-Zebrucka, K., Patterson, J. B., et al. (2016). Endoplasmic reticulum stress-mediated induction of SESTRIN 2 potentiates cell survival. Oncotarget 7, 12254–12266. doi: 10.18632/oncotarget.7601

Saxton, R. A., Knockenhauer, K. E., Schwartz, T. U., and Sabatini, D. M. (2016a). The apo-structure of the leucine sensor Sestrin2 is still elusive. Sci. Signal. 9:ra92. doi: 10.1126/scisignal.aah4497

Saxton, R. A., Knockenhauer, K. E., Wolfson, R. L., Chantranupong, L., Pacold, M. E., Wang, T., et al. (2016b). Structural basis for leucine sensing by the Sestrin2-mTORC1 pathway. Science 351, 53–58. doi: 10.1126/science.aad2087

Segales, J., Perdiguero, E., Serrano, A. L., Sousa-Victor, P., Ortet, L., Jardi, M., et al. (2020). Sestrin prevents atrophy of disused and aging muscles by integrating anabolic and catabolic signals. Nat. Commun. 11:189.

Sengupta, S., Giaime, E., Narayan, S., Hahm, S., Howell, J., O'Neill, D., et al. (2019). Discovery of NV-5138, the first selective Brain mTORC1 activator. Sci. Rep. 9:4107.

Shan, J., Al-Muftah, M. A., Al-Kowari, M. K., Abuaqel, S. W. J., Al-Rumaihi, K., Al-Bozom, I., et al. (2019). Targeting Wnt/EZH2/microRNA-708 signaling pathway inhibits neuroendocrine differentiation in prostate cancer. Cell Death Discov. 5:139. doi: 10.1038/s41420-019-0218-y

Shin, J., Bae, J., Park, S., Kang, H. G., Shin, S. M., Won, G., et al. (2020). mTOR-dependent role of sestrin2 in regulating tumor progression of human endometrial cancer. Cancers 12:2515. doi: 10.3390/cancers12092515

Sies, H., and Jones, D. P. (2020). Reactive oxygen species (ROS) as pleiotropic physiological signalling agents. Nat. Rev. Mol. Cell Biol. 21, 363–383.

Singh, P., and Chowdhuri, D. K. (2018). Modulation of sestrin confers protection to Cr(VI) induced neuronal cell death in Drosophila melanogaster. Chemosphere 191, 302–314. doi: 10.1016/j.chemosphere.2017.10.037

Srivastava, S. (2017). The mitochondrial basis of aging and age-related disorders. Genes 8:398. doi: 10.3390/genes8120398

Stocker, S., Maurer, M., Ruppert, T., and Dick, T. P. (2018). A role for 2-Cys peroxiredoxins in facilitating cytosolic protein thiol oxidation. Nat. Chem. Biol. 14, 148–155. doi: 10.1038/nchembio.2536

Sun, W., Wang, Y., Zheng, Y., and Quan, N. (2020). The emerging role of sestrin2 in cell metabolism, and cardiovascular and age-related diseases. Aging Dis. 11, 154–163. doi: 10.14336/AD.2019.0320

Sundararajan, S., Jayachandran, I., Subramanian, S. C., Anjana, R. M., Balasubramanyam, M., Mohan, V., et al. (2020). Decreased Sestrin levels in patients with type 2 diabetes and dyslipidemia and their association with the severity of atherogenic index. J. Endocrinol. Invest. doi: 10.1007/s40618-020-01429-9 [Epub ahead of print].

Tao, R., Xiong, X., Liangpunsakul, S., and Dong, X. C. (2014). Sestrin 3 protein enhances hepatic insulin sensitivity by direct activation of the mTORC2-Akt signaling. Diabetes 64, 1211–1223. doi: 10.2337/db14-0539

Tao, R., Xiong, X., Liangpunsakul, S., and Dong, X. C. (2015). Sestrin 3 protein enhances hepatic insulin sensitivity by direct activation of the mTORC2-Akt signaling. Diabetes 64, 1211–1223.

Tao, T., and Xu, H. (2020). Autophagy and obesity and diabetes. Adv. Exp. Med. Biol. 1207, 445–461. doi: 10.1007/978-981-15-4272-5_32

Thamsen, M., Kumsta, C., Li, F., and Jakob, U. (2011). Is overoxidation of peroxiredoxin physiologically significant? Antioxid. Redox Signal. 14, 725–730. doi: 10.1089/ars.2010.3717

Tong, X. P., Ma, Y. X., Quan, D. N., Zhang, L., Yan, M., and Fan, X. R. (2017). Rosemary Extracts Upregulate Nrf2, Sestrin2, and MRP2 Protein Level in Human Hepatoma HepG2 Cells. Evid. Based Complement. Alternat. Med. 2017:7359806. doi: 10.1155/2017/7359806

Tu, J., Li, W., Li, S., Liu, W., Zhang, Y., Wu, X., et al. (2018). Sestrin-mediated inhibition of stress-induced intervertebral disc degradation through the enhancement of autophagy. Cell. Physiol. Biochem. 45, 1940–1954. doi: 10.1159/000487970

Um, S. H., D'Alessio, D., and Thomas, G. (2006). Nutrient overload, insulin resistance, and ribosomal protein S6 kinase 1, S6K1. Cell Metab. 3, 393–402. doi: 10.1016/j.cmet.2006.05.003

Velasco-Miguel, S., Buckbinder, L., Jean, P., Gelbert, L., Talbott, R., Laidlaw, J., et al. (1999). PA26, a novel target of the p53 tumor suppressor and member of the GADD family of DNA damage and growth arrest inducible genes. Oncogene 18, 127–137. doi: 10.1038/sj.onc.1202274

Wang, C., Wang, X., Su, Z., Fei, H., Liu, X., and Pan, Q. (2015). The novel mTOR inhibitor Torin-2 induces autophagy and downregulates the expression of UHRF1 to suppress hepatocarcinoma cell growth. Oncol. Rep. 34, 1708–1716. doi: 10.3892/or.2015.4146

Wang, L. X., Zhu, X. M., Luo, Y. N., Wu, Y., Dong, N., Tong, Y. L., et al. (2020). Sestrin2 protects dendritic cells against endoplasmic reticulum stress-related apoptosis induced by high mobility group box-1 protein. Cell Death Dis. 11:125.

Wang, L. X., Zhu, X. M., and Yao, Y. M. (2019). Sestrin2: its potential role and regulatory mechanism in host immune response in diseases. Front. Immunol. 10:2797. doi: 10.3389/fimmu.2019.02797

Wang, P., Lan, R., Guo, Z., Cai, S., Wang, J., Wang, Q., et al. (2020). Histone Demethylase JMJD3 mediated doxorubicin-induced cardiomyopathy by suppressing SESN2 expression. Front. Cell Dev. Biol. 8:548605. doi: 10.3389/fcell.2020.548605

Wang, P., Wang, L., Lu, J., Hu, Y., Wang, Q., Li, Z., et al. (2019). SESN2 protects against doxorubicin-induced cardiomyopathy via rescuing mitophagy and improving mitochondrial function. J. Mol. Cell. Cardiol. 133, 125–137. doi: 10.1016/j.yjmcc.2019.06.005

Wang, M., Xu, Y., Liu, J., Ye, J., Yuan, W., Jiang, H., et al. (2017). Recent insights into the biological functions of sestrins in health and disease. Cell. Physiol. Biochem. 43, 1731–1741. doi: 10.1159/000484060

Wang, T., Niu, Y., Liu, S., Yuan, H., Liu, X., and Fu, L. (2018). Exercise improves glucose uptake in murine myotubes through the AMPKalpha2-mediated induction of Sestrins. Biochim. Biophys. Acta Mol. Basis Dis. 1864, 3368–3377. doi: 10.1016/j.bbadis.2018.07.023

Wei, J. L., Fang, M., Fu, Z. X., Zhang, S. R., Guo, J. B., Wang, R., et al. (2017). Sestrin 2 suppresses cells proliferation through AMPK/mTORC1 pathway activation in colorectal cancer. Oncotarget 8, 49318–49328. doi: 10.18632/oncotarget.17595

Wei, J. L., Fu, Z. X., Fang, M., Guo, J. B., Zhao, Q. N., Lu, W. D., et al. (2015). Decreased expression of sestrin 2 predicts unfavorable outcome in colorectal cancer. Oncol. Rep. 33, 1349–1357. doi: 10.3892/or.2014.3701

Wei, Y., Zhang, Y. J., Cai, Y., and Xu, M. H. (2015). The role of mitochondria in mTOR-regulated longevity. Biol. Rev. Camb. Philos. Soc. 90, 167–181. doi: 10.1111/brv.12103

Wolfson, R. L., Chantranupong, L., Saxton, R. A., Shen, K., Scaria, S. M., Cantor, J. R., et al. (2016). Sestrin2 is a leucine sensor for the mTORC1 pathway. Science 351, 43–48. doi: 10.1126/science.aab2674

Won, D. H., Chung, S. H., Shin, J. A., Hong, K. O., Yang, I. H., Yun, J. W., et al. (2019). Induction of sestrin 2 is associated with fisetin-mediated apoptosis in human head and neck cancer cell lines. J. Clin. Biochem. Nutr. 64, 97–105.

Woo, H. A., Bae, S. H., Park, S., and Rhee, S. G. (2009). Sestrin 2 is not a reductase for cysteine sulfinic acid of peroxiredoxins. Antioxid. Redox Signal. 11, 739–745. doi: 10.1089/ARS.2008.2360

Xu, D., Shimkus, K. L., Lacko, H. A., Kutzler, L., Jefferson, L. S., and Kimball, S. R. (2019). Evidence for a role for Sestrin1 in mediating leucine-induced activation of mTORC1 in skeletal muscle. Am. J. Physiol. Endocrinol. Metab. 316, E817–E828. doi: 10.1152/ajpendo.00522.2018

Yan, M., Vemu, B., Veenstra, J., Petiwala, S. M., and Johnson, J. J. (2018). Carnosol, a dietary diterpene from rosemary (Rosmarinus officinalis) activates Nrf2 leading to sestrin 2 induction in colon cells. Integr. Mol. Med. 5:10.15761/IMM.1000335. doi: 10.15761/IMM.1000335

Yang, J. H., Kim, K. M., Kim, M. G., Seo, K. H., Han, J. Y., Ka, S. O., et al. (2015). Role of sestrin2 in the regulation of proinflammatory signaling in macrophages. Free Radic. Biol. Med. 78, 156–167. doi: 10.1016/j.freeradbiomed.2014.11.002

Yang, Y. L., Loh, K. S., Liou, B. Y., Chu, I. H., Kuo, C. J., Chen, H. D., et al. (2013). SESN-1 is a positive regulator of lifespan in Caenorhabditis elegans. Exp. Gerontol. 48, 371–379. doi: 10.1016/j.exger.2012.12.011

Ye, J., Palm, W., Peng, M., King, B., Lindsten, T., Li, M. O., et al. (2015). GCN2 sustains mTORC1 suppression upon amino acid deprivation by inducing Sestrin2. Genes Dev. 29, 2331–2336. doi: 10.1101/gad.269324.115

Yen, J. H., Huang, S. T., Huang, H. S., Fong, Y. C., Wu, Y. Y., Chiang, J. H., et al. (2018). HGK-sestrin 2 signaling-mediated autophagy contributes to antitumor efficacy of Tanshinone IIA in human osteosarcoma cells. Cell Death Dis. 9:1003.

Yun, J., and Finkel, T. (2014). Mitohormesis. *Cell Metab.* 19, 757–766. doi: 10.1016/j.cmet.2014.01.011

Zeng, N., D'Souza, R. F., Figueiredo, V. C., Markworth, J. F., Roberts, L. A., Peake, J. M., et al. (2017). Acute resistance exercise induces Sestrin2 phosphorylation and p62 dephosphorylation in human skeletal muscle. *Physiol. Rep.* 5:e13526. doi: 10.14814/phy2.13526

Zeng, N., D'Souza, R. F., Mitchell, C. J., and Cameron-Smith, D. (2018a). Sestrins are differentially expressed with age in the skeletal muscle of men: A cross-sectional analysis. *Exp. Gerontol.* 110, 23–34. doi: 10.1016/j.exger.2018.05.006

Zeng, N., D'Souza, R. F., Sorrenson, B., Merry, T. L., Barnett, M. P. G., Mitchell, C. J., et al. (2018b). The putative leucine sensor Sestrin2 is hyperphosphorylated by acute resistance exercise but not protein ingestion in human skeletal muscle. *Eur. J. Appl. Physiol.* 118, 1241–1253.

Zeng, Y. C., Chi, F., Xing, R., Zeng, J., Gao, S., Chen, J. J., et al. (2016). Sestrin2 protects the myocardium against radiation-induced damage. *Radiat. Environ. Biophys.* 55, 195–202.

Zhang, L. L., and Zhang, Z. J. (2018). Sestrin2 aggravates oxidative stress of neurons by decreasing the expression of Nrf2. *Eur. Rev. Med. Pharmacol. Sci.* 22, 3493–3501. doi: 10.26355/eurrev_201806_15176

Zhao, B., Shah, P., Budanov, A. V., Qiang, L., Ming, M., Aplin, A., et al. (2014). Sestrin2 protein positively regulates AKT enzyme signaling and survival in human squamous cell carcinoma and melanoma cells. *J. Biol. Chem.* 289, 35806–35814. doi: 10.1074/jbc.M114.595397

Zhao, B., Shah, P., Qiang, L., He, T. C., Budanov, A., and He, Y. Y. (2017). Distinct Role of Sesn2 in Response to UVB-Induced DNA Damage and UVA-Induced Oxidative Stress in Melanocytes. *Photochem. Photobiol.* 93, 375–381. doi: 10.1111/php.12624

Zhou, J., Zhou, H., Liu, C., Huang, L., Lu, D., and Gao, C. (2020). HDAC1-mediated deacetylation of LSD1 regulates vascular calcification by promoting autophagy in chronic renal failure. *J. Cell. Mol. Med.* 24, 8636–8649. doi: 10.1111/jcmm.15494

Zhuo, X., Wu, Y., Yang, Y., Gao, L., Qiao, X., and Chen, T. (2019). Knockdown of LSD1 meliorates Ox-LDL-stimulated NLRP3 activation and inflammation by promoting autophagy via SESN2-mesiated PI3K/Akt/mTOR signaling pathway. *Life Sci.* 233:116696. doi: 10.1016/j.lfs.2019.116696

Zighelboim, I., Goodfellow, P. J., Schmidt, A. P., Walls, K. C., Mallon, M. A., Mutch, D. G., et al. (2007). Differential methylation hybridization array of endometrial cancers reveals two novel cancer-specific methylation markers. *Clin. Cancer Res.* 13, 2882–2889.

Zoncu, R., Efeyan, A., and Sabatini, D. M. (2011). mTOR: from growth signal integration to cancer, diabetes and ageing. *Nat. Rev. Mol. Cell Biol.* 12, 21–35. doi: 10.1038/nrm3025

11

Metabolic Syndrome and Autophagy: Focus on HMGB1 Protein

Vincenza Frisardi[1]*, Carmela Matrone[2] and Maria Elisabeth Street[3]

[1] Clinical and Nutritional Laboratory, Department of Geriatric and NeuroRehabilitation, Arcispedale Santa Maria Nuova
(AUSL-IRCCS), Reggio Emilia, Italy, [2] Division of Pharmacology, Department of Neuroscience, School of Medicine, University
of Naples Federico II, Naples, Italy, [3] Division of Paediatric Endocrinology and Diabetology, Paediatrics, Department
of Mother and Child, Arcispedale Santa Maria Nuova (AUSL-IRCCS), Reggio Emilia, Italy

*Correspondence:
Vincenza Frisardi
vincenza.frisardi@ausl.re.it

Metabolic syndrome (MetS) affects the population worldwide and results from several factors such as genetic background, environment and lifestyle. In recent years, an interplay among autophagy, metabolism, and metabolic disorders has become apparent. Defects in the autophagy machinery are associated with the dysfunction of many tissues/organs regulating metabolism. Metabolic hormones and nutrients regulate, in turn, the autophagy mechanism. Autophagy is a housekeeping stress-induced degradation process that ensures cellular homeostasis. High mobility group box 1 (HMGB1) is a highly conserved nuclear protein with a nuclear and extracellular role that functions as an extracellular signaling molecule under specific conditions. Several studies have shown that HMGB1 is a critical regulator of autophagy. This mini-review focuses on the involvement of HMGB1 protein in the interplay between autophagy and MetS, emphasizing its potential role as a promising biomarker candidate for the early stage of MetS or disease's therapeutic target.

Keywords: metabolic syndrome, autophagy, HMBG1, cellular homeostasis, insulin resistance, oxidative stress

INTRODUCTION

Metabolic syndrome (MetS) increases significantly morbidity and all-cause mortality worldwide (Cornier et al., 2008; Alamdari et al., 2020; Watanabe and Kotani, 2020). MetS is linked to cognitive decline and Alzheimer's disease (AD), and this has suggested the term "metabolic-cognitive syndrome" (Frisardi et al., 2010). Over the past few decades, the prevalence of MetS, cardiovascular disease, and dementia has risen rapidly. The increasing worldwide prevalence of childhood obesity and diabetes in the young (DeBoer, 2019; Weihe and Weihrauch-Blûher, 2019) has promoted the search for biochemical markers of MetS to identify its prodromal phase or to predict the evolutionary risk. Autophagy is a degradation process facilitating homeostasis and intracellular energy balance. Emerging discoveries showed the complex and reciprocal interplay between autophagy and metabolism (Martinez-Lopez et al., 2017; Raj et al., 2020). Obesity, fatty liver disease and diabetes, the principal components of MetS, show dysregulated hepatic autophagy (Zhang et al., 2018; Allaire et al., 2019). Vice versa, glycolysis alters the autophagy self-fueling derangements in other metabolic pathways (Kiffin et al., 2006). A ubiquitous small chromatin-linked non-histone peptide, High Mobility Group Box-1 (HMGB1), has gained attention lately as a critical promoter of autophagy processes (Huebener et al., 2014). HMGB1 levels are related to inflammation (Cal et al., 2015), insulin resistance (IR), hyperglycemia (Migazzi et al., 2021), and MetS (Jialal et al., 2014; Chen et al., 2020a). Understanding the molecular bases for these processes is essential for developing new diagnostic biomarkers and identifying new therapeutic target and subpopulations at risk. Not all obese subjects have Mets, while lean subjects could develop MetS-linked cardiovascular complications.

METABOLIC SYNDROME (MetS): DYSFUNCTIONAL ADIPOSITY AND IR

Metabolic and vascular factors, especially visceral obesity and IR, characterize MetS (Cornier et al., 2008). Measuring IR is demanding, and the lack of assay standardization makes new syndrome markers necessary. Chronic pro-inflammatory and pro-thrombotic states, non-alcoholic fatty liver disease (NAFLD) (Lonardo et al., 2020), and sleep apnea (Castaneda et al., 2018) contribute to the MetS entity (Jabalie et al., 2019). MetS represents a clinical spectrum where a lag time exists between a single risk factor, the syndrome's definition and clinical consequences. Receiving a diagnosis of MetS is already too late (Reaven, 2006) compared to the possibility of having molecular markers of disease's evolving risk. Adipose tissue (AT) is metabolically active (Kershaw and Flier, 2004; Iozzo and Guzzardi, 2016). Chronic nutrient surplus and hyperinsulinemia increase adipocytes metabolic glucose flux and lead to cell hypertrophy. As adipocytes reach the critical size, precursor cells differentiate (Longo et al., 2019). In this context, lipogenic and antilipolytic control is impaired with reduced insulin sensitivity and ectopic fat accumulation. Therefore, the inability to buffer excess metabolic substrates from nutritional overload exposes other tissues to lipotoxicity (Cornier et al., 2011). There are functional differences between healthy (insulin sensitive) and unhealthy (IR) obesity. Inflammation can induce DNA damage, such as DNA double-strand breaks (DSBs), which increase inflammation. Obesity also modifies the immune cells (Olefsky and Glass, 2010; Trim et al., 2018). Explicitly, in the AT of obese subjects, monocytes polarize to M1 macrophages and display several cytokines (including TNF-α, IL-6, HMGB1) (Zhang et al., 2017). This molecular shift aggravates the chronic inflammatory state and IR. Furthermore, an increased formation of advanced glycation products (AGE) and their signaling via specific receptors (RAGE), including redox mechanisms, mediate vascular dysfunction and end-organ failure in MetS (Fournet et al., 2018).

OVERVIEW ON AUTOPHAGY

Although firstly described in 1963, only in the 1990s autophagy mechanisms were elucidated with identifying autophagy-related genes (ATG) in yeast (Takeshige et al., 1992; Klionsky, 2007; Mizushima, 2018). In eukaryotic, energy deprivation and/or intense physical activity trigger the cellular self-digestion processes to secure sufficient nutrient supply (Klionsky, 2007; Maiuri et al., 2007; Mizushima et al., 2008; Levine et al., 2011; Rubinsztein et al., 2011). Besides its role in preserving normal cellular functions, autophagy participates in several diseases (Jiang and Mizushima, 2014). Many stress conditions lead to a progressive accumulation of toxic molecular components and activate autophagic processes (Leidal et al., 2018) that rely upon three primary types: microautophagy, macroautophagy, and chaperone-mediated autophagy (CMA). Macroautophagy differs from the others because the waste of damaged organelles, unneeded cellular materials, and pathogenic agents are first sequestered and encapsulated in double-membrane vesicles (autophagosomes). Then, by trafficking from the cytoplasm to the lysosomes, autophagosomes fuse with lysosomes, and their contents can be either recycled or degraded (Mehrpour et al., 2010; Lamb et al., 2013; **Figure 1**). Six main steps (initiation, nucleation, elongation closure, maturation, and degradation or extrusion) characterize autophagy; each of these is highly regulated (**Figure 1**). Beclin 1 (BCN1) belongs to the autophagy machinery, and it plays its effects by the activation of specific (BCN1)-binding proteins, autophagic inducers and autophagic inhibitors in a cell- or tissue-dependent fashion (Cuomo et al., 2019). Autophagy induction might counteract SARS-CoV-2 infection (Carmona-Gutierrez et al., 2020). Although it is far beyond the goal of this review, the speculation of autophagy as a possible druggable target in SARS-CoV-2 is undeniably and surely deserves further investigations, also regarding the hypothesized link among obesity, IR and COVID-19 (Frisardi, 2020; Street, 2020).

AUTOPHAGY AND MetS: THE VICIOUS CIRCLE

Various metabolic disorders showed functional defects in autophagy (Ichimura and Komatsu, 2011; Ueno and Komatsu, 2017; Barbosa et al., 2018; Ren et al., 2018; Zhang et al., 2018). Over the last years, the use of mice models, yeast screen and genome-wide analysis has considerably amplified our knowledge about this topic (Li et al., 2016; Kuma et al., 2017). Silencing of ATG promotes obesity and triggers metabolic complications. Consistently, ATG overexpression improves the metabolic profile in aged mice (Pyo et al., 2013). Since fasting activates autophagy, dietary interventions promoting autophagy has been explored (Martinez-Lopez et al., 2017). Different metabolic phenotypes have been described in various tissues, suggesting that autophagy genes are differentially expressed and activated in a tissue- and stage-specific manner during the development. However, it is worth to note that deficits in the autophagy genes, at systemic rather than tissue-specific level, affect cell adaptation to metabolic stress more and facilitates the progression from a risk factor (ex. obesity) to full-blown diseases (Lim et al., 2014; Ren et al., 2018). Nutrient limitation and multiple stress conditions upregulate autophagy because this latter serves cytoprotective functions and, reducing cellular death, limits the following inflammatory state. Indeed, autophagy could represent a protective mechanism following myocardial infarction (Czaja, 2010). Autophagy regulates adipocyte differentiation, lipid metabolism, endothelial activity, pancreatic β-cell maturation, molecular processes related to inflammation/immune responses (Ryter et al., 2014) and storing of lipids. Whenever autophagy is inhibited, lipids accumulate, and many processes' dysregulation

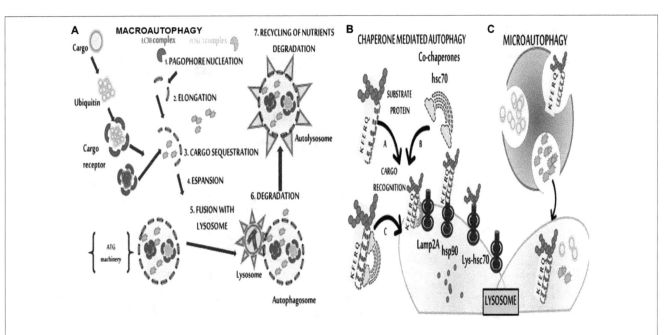

FIGURE 1 | Schematic representation of macroautophagy, chaperone-mediated autophagy (CMA), and microautophagy. **(A)** In macroautophagy, cargos are sequestered by phagophores, which elongate and form a double membranous structure, the autophagosome. Autophagosomes then fuse with the lysosome to form autolysosomes. (1) Nucleation consists of the formation of the phagophore. A class III of phosphoinositide 3-kinases (PI3K) complex consisting of beclin 1 (BCN1), Phosphatidylinositol 3-kinase catalytic subunit type 3 (PIK3C3), Phosphoinositide 3-kinase regulatory subunit 4 (PIK3R4), UV radiation resistance-associated gene protein (UVRAG), and Autophagy And Beclin 1 Regulator 1 (AMBRA1) is required for phagophore formation. (2) Microtubule-associated proteins 1A/1B light chain 3B (MAP1LC3) complex anchors to the membrane via a phosphoethanolamine (PE) anchor (LC3-II) and triggers the elongation. (3) The phagophore sequesters cytosolic cargo and forms a double-membranous vesicle, the autophagosome. (4) Maturation, the completed autophagosome undergoes multiple maturation steps. (5) Docking and fusion, the autophagosome is released into the lysosome/autolysosome to be degraded by lysosomal hydrolases or to become available for re-usage (6). **(B)** In CMA **(left)**, substrate proteins that can be damaged by various factors, such as reactive oxygen species (ROS), bind the Lysosomial-Heat shock cognate 71 kDa protein (Lys-Hsc70) chaperone through a specific amino acid sequence (the KFERQ motif) and are transported across the lysosomal membrane for degradation via interaction with lysosomal-associated membrane protein 2A (Lamp2A) proteins. **(C)** Microautophagy **(right)** involves the direct engulfment of portions of the cytoplasm into lysosomes.

occurs (Czaja, 2010). Briefly, cell-intrinsic effects (e.g., nutrient metabolism, mitochondria, and lipid droplet homeostasis), cell-extrinsic effects (e.g., the release of pro-inflammatory cytokines), and potentially lack of feedback inhibition of insulin and mTOR-C1 (mammalian target of rapamycin-complex 1) signaling pathways interfere with autophagy mechanisms. As in a vicious circle, defects in autophagy accelerates lifestyle-induced obesity that, in turn, inhibits autophagy in the liver, muscle and AT, worsening symptomatic features of MetS (**Figure 2**; Yang et al., 2010; Ruderman et al., 2013; Kaur and Debnath, 2015; Ren and Xu, 2015; Che et al., 2018; Zhang et al., 2018; Menikdiwela et al., 2020). In obesity, autophagy is suppressed via an increase in mTOR activity, which is involved in different cardiovascular pathophysiology (Wang et al., 2007; Che et al., 2018; Samidurai et al., 2018). Chronic obesity related-stress with a dysregulation of insulin/mTOR signaling (Wang et al., 2007; Sohrabi et al., 2019; Menikdiwela et al., 2020) lead to autophagy machinery disruption (**Figure 2**). During fasting, neuroendocrine signals [e.g., insulin and Insulin Growth Factor 1 decrease vs. glucagon, fibroblast growth factor 21 (FGF21) increase] regulate autophagy tightly. Commonly, these neurohormonal signals are altered in obesity (Levine and Kroemer, 2019). Mesenchymal stem cells from patients with diabetes and MetS show changes in oxidative stress and autophagy (Kornicka et al., 2018). Both

lipogenesis and adipogenesis are redox-sensitive; healthy obesity is consistent with the lack of the redox stress signature (Jankovic et al., 2015; Bañuls et al., 2017; Böhm et al., 2020). On the contrary, constant nutritional overload and oxidative pressure may compromise autophagy machinery ability to counteract metabolic derangement. As oxidative injuries accumulate, irreversible damage appears with signaling pathways disruption. Consistently, data suggest that oxidative injury may precede adipocyte dysfunction and other metabolic disorders even in yet metabolically healthy obese subjects (Jankovic et al., 2015). Evidence support an association between mitochondrial dysfunction and MetS in prediabetic and diabetic states (Bugger and Abel, 2008; Montgomery, 2019; Böhm et al., 2020). Mitophagy (selective autophagy in mitochondria) is a vital mechanism to keep stable the metabolic homeostasis (Xu et al., 2020). Therefore, enhancement of autophagy activity might be a novel therapeutic approach against organ failure's evolving metabolic disorders.

HMGB1: A MULTIFACETED PROTEIN

High mobility group box 1 (HMGB1) is an evolutionarily highly conserved small chromatin-linked non-histone peptide, first

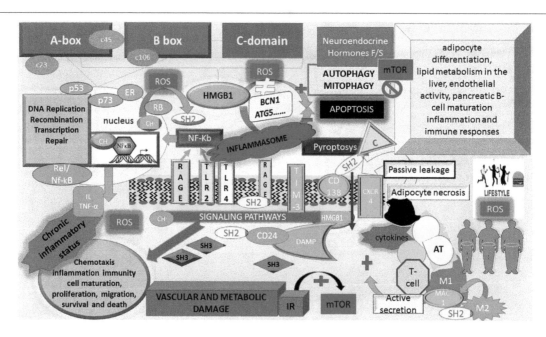

FIGURE 2 | The schematic interplay among HMBG1, autophagy, and Metabolic Syndrome. HMGB1, High mobility group box 1; c23, c46, c106, cysteine at 23, 46, 106 position; ROS, reactive oxygen species; BCN1, Beclin-1; ATG, autophagy-related genes; Neuroendocrine hormones F/S, fasting/starvation; mTOR, mammalian target of rapamycin; NF-кb, nuclear factor kappa-light-chain-enhancer of activated B cells; IL, interleukines; TNF-α, tumor necrosis factor-alpha; p53, protein 53; p73, protein 73; RB, retinoblastoma protein; Rel/Nf-кB, member of Rel/Nf-кB family; ER, estrogen receptor; C, caspases, non-canonical inflammasome; RAGE, advanced glycosylation end product-specific receptor; TLR2 and TLR4, Toll-like Receptor 2 and 4; TIM-3, T-cell immunoglobulin mucin-3; CXCR4, chemokine C-X-C motif receptor 4; Mac-1, macrophage-1 antigen; CD138, syndecan-1; CD24, cluster of differentiation 24; M, macrophages; IR, Insulin Resistance; AT, Adipose Tissue. HMGB1 functions as a Damage Associated Molecular Pattern (DAMP) protein in the extracellular space. A mixture of different HMBG1 isoforms (CH = reduced form; SH2: disulfide HMGB1, SH3 oxidized form) in the extracellular space activates different pathway signaling. As the disulfide HMGB1 is responsible for autophagy activation, which counteracts the metabolic consequences of MetS. During an overload of food nutrients, there is an increase in ROS. The oxidative environment modifies the Reduced/oxidized HMGB1 ratio, increasing the dysregulation in Insulin/mTOR signaling, which blocks the autophagy machinery. It follows an increased risk for the "unhealthy" obese to develop MetS complications due to an unbalance among the downstream IR pathway, chronic inflammatory pattern and inability to counteract metabolic derangements via autophagy machinery disruption. HMGB1 is an autophagic regulator that mediates stress response: in normal condition, cytosolic HMGB1 as BECN1-binding protein induces autophagy. Extracellular HMGB1 binds RAGE, which inhibits mTOR and promotes autophagy. In chronic obesity and switching from insulin-sensitive to IR state, change in oxidative environment modifies the HMBG1 activity altering its inducer role in autophagy. In the nucleus, HMBG1 interact with and enhances the activities of number of transcription factors, including p53, p73, RB, Rel/Nf-кB, and ER. Once released, HMBG1 binds to various receptors to activate DAMP signaling involved in multiple cellular processes. Inflammasomes are a cytosolic multiprotein complex formation that are recruited by external pathogen and/or internal stimuli. Chronic inflammasomes lead to chronic inflammatory status increasing the risk of clinical consequences of MetS. HMGB1 triggers C (Caspase-4/caspase-5) which are components of the "non-canonical inflammasome" with cytokines release and induction of pyroptosis (a kind of proinflammatory cell death combining features of both apoptosis and necrosis).

identified in the HMG family. HMGB1 (215 amino acids) is organized in three distinct regions: Box A and Box B and the C-terminal domain. While Box A and B are essential for the HMGB1 binding to DNA and thereby regulating transcription of target genes, the C-terminal domain contains the binding sites for RAGE and Toll-like receptor (TLR) (Livesey et al., 2012; Jiang et al., 2020). Each of these receptors mediates HMGB1 signals (Park et al., 2004), also activating the NF-κB proinflammatory pathway (nuclear factor kappa-light-chain-enhancer of activated B cells) (Jiang et al., 2020; **Figure 2**). NF-κB was also detected in the mitochondria, where it intervenes in mitochondrial dynamics, apoptosis, respiratory control, gene expression, and disease mechanisms (Albensi, 2019). HMGB1 is involved in maintaining genomic structure and function, and it is predominantly located in the nucleus in the reduced form Tang et al. (2010a). However, a small amount of HMBG1 is also present in the cytosol, which controls cell stress responses and inhibits apoptosis (Yang et al., 2013). During inflammation, HMGB1 promotes autophagy via binding to BCN1 and ATG5

and regulating mitochondrial morphology and function (Zhu et al., 2015; **Figure 2**).

HMBG1 can be released either passively from damaged cells or actively from immunologically activated immune cells under distress conditions. Extracellular HMGB1 acts as an alarmin and a Damage Associated Molecular Pattern (DAMP) protein (Raucci et al., 2019) by binding to several pathogen-associated molecular patterns (PAMPs) (Jiang et al., 2020) and activating downstream signals (**Figure 2**). An excessive accumulation of extracellular HMGB1 has been associated with the pathogenesis of many disorders, including diabetes (Wang et al., 2016; Zhang et al., 2020; Li and Lu, 2021). HMGB1 has several extracellular receptors (**Figure 2**). Actually, only RAGE and TLR4 are mainly studied and reported receptors (Andersson et al., 2018). HMGB1 serves as a redox sensor. In this regard, the three conserved redox-sensitive cysteine residues Cys23, Cys45, and Cys106 play a critical role (Li et al., 2003). Depending on the redox state, HMGB1 switches from the active to the inactive conformation. In particular, when Cys106 is oxidized, HMGB1 is inactive and likely promotes immune tolerance with the release of proinflammatory cytokines. Moreover, Cys106 oxidation induces the HMGB1 dimerization in cells exposed to oxidative stress. It follows that HMGB1 binds to DNA with a higher affinity than monomeric HMGB1, protects DNA from damage due to hydroxyl free radicals and prevents cell death (Kwak et al., 2021).

Conversely, the reduced HMGB1 form switches its activity into the proinflammatory state (Zhang et al., 2017). Although the oxidized HMGB1 is thought to be non-inflammatory, a role in promoting the intrinsic apoptotic pathway has been reported (Tang et al., 2010b). Moreover, a mixture of oxidized/reduced HMGB1 isoforms has been described in the extracellular compartments exerting different effects on cell defense mechanisms (Xue et al., 2020).

HMGB1, AUTOPHAGY AND MetS: A SUGGESTIVE TRIANGULATION

Accumulating evidence supports the relationship between autophagy and HMGB1. There is a mutual regulation where one's inhibition affects the release of the other (Zhang et al., 2017), while uncontrolled autophagy increases the HMGB1 release (Tang et al., 2010b; Kim et al., 2020). HMGB1 is crucial for normal autophagy functioning (Tang et al., 2010a; Foglio et al., 2019). As a transcriptional co-factor, HMGB1 regulates the expression of heat shock protein β-1 (Tang et al., 2011; Foglio et al., 2019), which sustains dynamic intracellular trafficking during autophagy. Cytosolic HMGB1 competes with Bcl-2 for interaction with BCN1 by intramolecular disulfide bridge of HMGB1 promoting BCN1-mediated autophagosomes (Kang et al., 2010; Tang et al., 2010a; Foglio et al., 2019). HMGB1 triggers autophagy through binding to RAGE (Tang et al., 2010a). This latter is a positive regulator of autophagy and a negative regulator of apoptosis during oxidative stress, DNA damage, and hypoxia (Kang et al., 2010). In *in vitro* and *in vivo* experiments, deletion, depletion or inhibition of HMGB1 reduces autophagy (Tang et al., 2010a,b). HMGB1-mediated autophagy prevents a worse evolution of several diseases (Kang et al., 2014). In contrast, conditional knockdown of HMGB1 in the liver or heart does not affect autophagy and mitochondrial quality (Huebener et al., 2014). These conflicting results could be imputable first to the difference in cellular line; second, we can hypothesize that as a DAMP, over secreted HMBG1 could play its role in a paracrine mode by linking RAGE in the target organ. In the Huebener et al. (2014) experiment, HMGB1 was deleted in hepatocytes but not in non-parenchymal liver cells. RAGE expression was only found on ductal cells and Kupffer's cells but not on hepatocytes and this could the explanation of why in the experiment performed by Huebener et al. (2014) deleted HMBG1 in hepatocytes does not alter mitophagy, autophagy, or gene expression.

Furthermore, in basal condition, maybe HMBG1 could be dispensable for autophagy. Nevertheless, under stress conditions, if we modify the cellular micro-macro environment, for example, by aging, cumulating oxidative damage or nutrients overload, HMBG1 could be essential (Ferrara et al., 2020). In atherosclerotic lesions in human carotid, BCN1 was found

to co-localize with HMGB1 and were both found in foamy macrophages suggesting an interplay between HMGB1 and autophagy in atherosclerosis (Umahara et al., 2020). Further studies are re required to investigate the HMGB1 contributes to autophagy in tissue-specific contexts and conditions.

Differently than in the inflammation (Cal et al., 2015; Yao et al., 2015; Biscetti et al., 2019) and autophagy, the role exerted by HMGB1 in MetS and its potential contribution to cardiovascular complications remains mostly unexplored despite the increasing number of evidence underlining this association (van Niekerk et al., 2019). A linear relationship has been consistently observed among HMGB1 levels and inflammation, IR, and hyperglycemia (Montanini et al., 2016; Cirillo et al., 2019, 2020). In particular, a study comparing control mice to MetS mice, fed with a high-fat diet, showed increased secretion of HMGB1 in the AT of the affected mice (Jialal et al., 2014). Increased circulating HMGB1 concentrations have been described in obese children with MetS compared to healthy controls (Arrigo et al., 2013).

Further, in adipocytes, HMGB1 secretion is regulated by c-Jun (Shimizu et al., 2016), a downstream mediator of the insulin receptor. HMGB1 is implicated in the development of non-alcoholic fatty liver Disease (NAFLD) by insulin receptor downstream effectors (Arrigo et al., 2013; Wang et al., 2015; Giacobbe et al., 2016). Obese pregnant women as children show high serum HMGB1 levels (Arrigo et al., 2013; Giacobbe et al., 2016), directly associated with body mass index. Circulating HMGB1 significantly increase in obese individuals and T2D patients (Wang et al., 2015). However, a larger sample size will be necessary to support the clinical relevance of HMGB1 as a potential and viable biomarker for the early diagnosis of obesity. As secreted by the macrophages within AT (Bonaldi et al., 2003), HMGB1 may promote inflammation by binding to receptors on effector cell membranes, leading to inflammatory mediators (IL-6 and TNF-α). In turn, the release of IL-6 and TNF-α leads to increased HMGB1 release, resulting in a cascade amplification of inflammation (Zhang et al., 2019).

High mobility group box 1-gene-deficient mice show several metabolic defects and die of hypoglycemia. Obese individuals are more prone to DNA damage than normal-weight adolescents (Azzarà et al., 2016; Rohde et al., 2020) but have improved the potential to repair occurred lesions. Different repair kinetics of DSBs in obese versus lean derived lymphocytes, along with differences in HMGB1 expression level, have been reported, and specifically, cytoplasmic HMGB1 is more abundant in VAT (visceral adipose tissue) of obese compared with lean subjects (Azzarà et al., 2016). To find early biomarkers of autophagy/apoptosis unbalance concerning MetS principally, HMGB1 could represent a seducing molecule (Foglio et al., 2019). Although most evidence came from studies on cancer cell lines, speculation could be made as the cancer cells are exposed to a metabolically demanding environment (Marijt et al., 2019). Conjectures concerning a pivotal role for HMBG1 could also derive from the observed increased risk among obese subjects in morbidity and mortality related to COVID-19 (Seidu et al., 2020). Shortly, HMGB1 is (1) related to an increased risk of thrombosis; (2) HMGB1 gene polymorphisms are associated with hypertension; (3) HMGB1 regulates ACE II receptors which act as a counterbalance to the Angiotensin-converting enzyme (ACE), the central component of the renin-angiotensin system (Chen et al., 2020b) essential for SARS-CoV-2 infection (Chen et al., 2020b; Street, 2020; **Figure 1B**). *In vitro* studies have shown that in bronchial epithelial cells, hyperglycemia increases HMGB1 while it is lowered by insulin (Montanini et al., 2016; Seidu et al., 2020), suggesting that this protein might be a vulnerability marker besides a therapeutic target.

CONCLUSION

This mini-review focused on the hypothetical involvement of HMGB1 in the current hot topic of autophagy and MetS to prompt debate and promote further experimental studies. Chronic nutrient overload impairs the autophagy mechanism's ability to counteract the lifestyle-induced metabolic processes,

and it appears that autophagy defects play a role in determining the cardiovascular complications of MetS. HMGB1, among many other functions, also regulates autophagy and therefore represents an attractive biomarker of disease evolution and a possible therapeutic target. Obese subjects have elevated serum levels of HMGB1. We underlined the possible importance of the reducing/oxidized HMGB1 ratio for predicting the risk of disease evolution in obese healthy subjects using a conceptual "autophagy bridge." Early diagnosis of a metabolic state that will progress to MetS complications is of crucial importance.

AUTHOR CONTRIBUTIONS

VF conceived of the presented idea and planned the manuscript. CM conceived **Figure 1** and VF conceived of **Figure 2**. All authors shared the leading role in writing the manuscript, read and agreed to the published version of the manuscript.

REFERENCES

Alamdari, N. M., Rahimi, F. S., Afaghi, S., Zarghi, A., Qaderi, S., Tarki, F. E., et al. (2020). The impact of metabolic syndrome on morbidity and mortality among intensive care unit admitted COVID-19 patients. *Diabetes Metab. Syndr.:Clin. Res. Rev.* 14, 1979–1986. doi: 10.1016/j.dsx.2020.10.012

Albensi, B. C. (2019). What Is Nuclear Factor Kappa B (NF-κB) Doing in and to the Mitochondrion? *Front. Cell Dev. Biol.* 2019:00154. doi: 10.3389/fcell.2019.00154

Allaire, M., Rautou, P. E., Codogno, P., and Lotersztajn, S. (2019). Autophagy in liver diseases: time for translation? *J. Hepatol.* 70, 985–998. doi: 10.1016/j.jhep.2019.01.026

Andersson, U., Yang, H., and Harris, H. (2018). High-mobility group box 1 protein (HMGB1) operates as an alarmin outside as well as inside cells. *Semin Immunol.* 38, 40–48. doi: 10.1016/j.smim.2018.02.011

Arrigo, T., Chirico, V., Salpietro, V., Munafò, C., Ferraù, V., Gitto, E., et al. (2013). High-mobility group protein B1: a new biomarker of metabolic syndrome in obese children. *Eur. J. Endocrinol.* 68, 631–638. doi: 10.1530/EJE-13-0037

Azzarà, A., Pirillo, C., Giovannini, C., Federico, G., and Scarpato, R. (2016). Different repair kinetic of DSBs induced by mitomycin C in peripheral lymphocytes of obese and normal weight adolescents. *Mutat Res.* 789, 9–14. doi: 10.1016/j.mrfmmm.2016.05.001

Bañuls, C., Rovira-Llopis, S., Lopez-Domenech, S., Diaz-Morales, N., Blas-Garcia, A., Veses, S., et al. (2017). Oxidative and endoplasmic reticulum stress is impaired in leukocytes from metabolically unhealthy vs healthy obese individuals. *Int. J. Obes.* 41, 1556–1563. doi: 10.1038/ijo.2017.147

Barbosa, M. C., Grosso, R. A., and Fader, C. M. (2018). Hallmarks of Aging: An Autophagic Perspective. *Front. Endocrinol.* 9:790. doi: 10.3389/fendo.2018.00790

Biscetti, F., Rando, M. M., Nardella, E., Cecchini, A. L., Pecorini, G., Landolfi, R., et al. (2019). High mobility group box-1 and diabetes mellitus complications: state of the art and future perspectives. *Int. J. Mol. Sci.* 20:E6258.

Böhm, A., Keuper, M., Meile, T., Zdichavsky, M., Fritsche, A., Häring, H. U., et al. (2020). Increased mitochondrial respiration of adipocytes from metabolically unhealthy obese compared to healthy obese individuals. *Sci. Rep.* 10:12407. doi: 10.1038/s41598-020-69016-9

Bonaldi, T., Talamo, F., Scaffidi, P., Ferrera, D., Porto, A., Bachi, A., et al. (2003). Monocytic cells hyperacetylate chromatin protein HMGB1 to redirect it towards secretion. *EMBO J.* 22, 5551–5560. doi: 10.1093/emboj/cdg516

Bugger, H., and Abel, E. D. (2008). Molecular mechanisms for myocardial mitochondrial dysfunction in the metabolic syndrome. *Clin. Sci.* 114, 195–210. doi: 10.1042/CS20070166

Cal, J., Yuan, H., Wang, Q., Yang, H., Al-Abed, Y., Hua, Z., et al. (2015). HMGB1-driven inflammation and intimal hyperplasia after arterial injury involves cell-specific actions mediated by TLR4. *Arterioscler. Thromb. Vasc. Biol.* 35, 2579–2593. doi: 10.1161/ATVBAHA.115.305789

Carmona-Gutierrez, D., Bauer, M. A., Zimmermann, A., Kainz, K., Hofer, S. J., Kroemer, G., et al. (2020). Digesting the crisis: autophagy and coronaviruses. *Microb. Cell* 7, 119–128. doi: 10.15698/mic2020.05.715

Castaneda, A., Jauregui-Maldonado, E., Ratnani, I., Varon, J., and Surani, S. (2018). Correlation between metabolic syndrome and sleep apnea. *World J. Diabetes* 9, 66–71. doi: 10.4239/wjd.v9.i4.66

Che, Y., Wang, Z., Yuan, Y., Zhang, N., Jin, Y., Wan, C., et al. (2018). Role of autophagy in a model of obesity: A long-term high fat diet induces cardiac dysfunction. *Mole. Med. Rep.* 18, 3251–3261. doi: 10.3892/mmr.2018.9301

Chen, L., Long, X., Xu, Q., Tan, J., Wang, G., Cao, Y., et al. (2020b). Elevated serum levels of S100A8/A9 and HMGB1 at hospital admission are correlated with inferior clinical outcomes in COVID-19 patients. *Cell Mol. Immunol.* 17, 992–994. doi: 10.1038/s41423-020-0492-x

Chen, L., Zhu, H., Su, S., Harshfield, G., Sullivan, J., Webb, C., et al. (2020a). High-Mobility Group Box-1 Is Associated With Obesity, Inflammation, and Subclinical Cardiovascular Risk Among Young Adults. *Arterioscler. Thromb. Vasc. Biol.* 2020:314599. doi: 10.1161/atvbaha.120.314599

Cirillo, F., Catellani, C., Lazzeroni, P., Sartori, C., Nicoli, A., Amarri, S., et al. (2019). MiRNAs Regulating Insulin Sensitivity Are Dysregulated in Polycystic Ovary Syndrome (PCOS) Ovaries and Are Associated With Markers of Inflammation and Insulin Sensitivity. *Front. Endocrinol.* 13:879. doi: 10.3389/fendo.2019.00879

Cirillo, F., Catellani, C., Lazzeroni, P., Sartori, C., Tridenti, G., Vezzani, C., et al. (2020). HMGB1 is increased in adolescents with polycystic ovary syndrome (PCOS) and decreases after treatment with myo-inositol (MYO) in combination with alpha-lipoic acid (ALA). *Gynecol. Endocrinol.* 36, 588–593. doi: 10.1080/09513590.2020.1725967

Cornier, M. A., Dabelea, D., Hernandez, T. L., Lindstrom, R. C., Steig, A. J., Stob, N. R., et al. (2008). The metabolic syndrome. *Endocr. Rev.* 29, 777–822. doi: 10.1210/er.2008-0024

Cornier, M. A., Després, J. P., Davis, N., Grossniklaus, D. A., Klein, S., Lamarche, B., et al. (2011). Assessing adiposity: A scientific statement from the American Heart Association. *Circulation* 124, 1996–2019. doi: 10.1161/CIR.0b013e318233bc6

Cuomo, F., Altucci, L., and Cobellis, G. (2019). Autophagy Function and Dysfunction: Potential Drugs as Anti-Cancer Therapy. *Cancers* 11:1465. doi: 10.3390/cancers11101465

Czaja, M. J. (2010). Autophagy in health and disease. 2. Regulation of lipid metabolism and storage by autophagy: pathophysiological implications. *Am. J. Physiol. Cell Physiol.* 298, C973–C978. doi: 10.1152/ajpcell.00527.2009

DeBoer, M. D. (2019). Assessing and Managing the Metabolic Syndrome in Children and Adolescents. *Nutrients* 11:1788. doi: 10.3390/nu11081788

Ferrara, M., Chialli, G., Ferreira, L. M., Ruggieri, E., Careccia, G., Preti, A., et al. (2020). Oxidation of HMGB1 Is a Dynamically Regulated Process in Physiological and Pathological Conditions. *Front. Immunol.* 11:1122. doi: 10.3389/fimmu.2020.01122

Foglio, E., Pellegrini, L., Germani, A., Russo, M. A., and Limana, F. (2019). HMGB1-mediated apoptosis and autophagy in ischemic heart diseases. *Vasc. Biol.* 1, H89–H96. doi: 10.1530/VB-19-0013

Fournet, M., Bonté, F., and Desmoulière, A. (2018). Glycation Damage: A Possible Hub for Major Pathophysiological Disorders and Aging. *Aging Dis.* 9, 880–900. doi: 10.14336/AD.2017.1121

Frisardi, V. (2020). Commentary: Coronavirus and Obesity: Could Insulin Resistance Mediate the Severity of Covid-19 Infection? *Front. Public Health* 8:351. doi: 10.3389/fpubh.2020.00351

Frisardi, V., Solfrizzi, V., Seripa, D., Capurso, C., Santamato, A., Sancarlo, D., et al. (2010). Metabolic-cognitive syndrome: a cross-talk between metabolic syndrome and Alzheimer's disease. *Ageing Res. Rev.* 9, 399–417. doi: 10.1016/j.arr.2010.04.007

Giacobbe, A., Granese, R., Grasso, R., Salpietro, V., Corrado, F., Giorgianni, G., et al. (2016). Association between maternal serum high mobility group box 1 levels and pregnancy complicated by gestational diabetes mellitus. *Nutr. Metab. Cardiovasc.* 26, 414–418. doi: 10.1016/j.numecd.2016.02.007

Huebener, P., Gwak, G. Y., Pradere, J. P., Quinzii, C. M., Friedman, R., Lin, C. S., et al. (2014). High Mobility Group Box 1 is Dispensable for Autophagy, Mitochondrial Quality Control and Organ Function in Vivo. *Cell Metab.* 19, 539–547. doi: 10.1016/j.cmet.2014.01.014

Ichimura, Y., and Komatsu, M. (2011). Pathophysiological role of autophagy: lesson from autophagy-deficient mouse models. *Exp. Anim.* 60, 329–345. doi: 10.1538/expanim.60.329

Iozzo, P., and Guzzardi, M. A. (2016). Cross-Talk Between Adipose Tissue Health, Myocardial Metabolism and Vascular Function: The Adipose-Myocardial and Adipose-Vascular Axes. *Curr. Pharm. Des.* 22, 59–67. doi: 10.2174/1381612822666151109111834

Jabalie, G., Ahmadi, M., Koushaeian, L., Eghbal-Fard, S., Mehdizadeh, A., Kamrani, A., et al. (2019). Metabolic syndrome mediates proinflammatory responses of inflammatory cells in preeclampsia. *Am. J. Reprod Immunol.* 81:e13086.

Jankovic, A., Korac, A., Buzadzic, B., Otasevic, V., Stancic, A., Daiber, A., et al. (2015). Redox implications in adipose tissue (dys)function–A new look at old acquaintances. *Redox Biol.* 6, 19–32. doi: 10.1016/j.redox.2015.06.018

Jialal, I., Rajamani, U., Adams-Huet, B., and Kaur, H. (2014). Circulating pathogen-associated molecular pattern - binding proteins and High Mobility Group Box protein 1 in nascent metabolic syndrome: implications for cellular Toll-like receptor activity. *Atherosclerosis* 236, 182–187. doi: 10.1016/j.atherosclerosis.2014.06.022

Jiang, L., Shao, Y., Tian, Y., Ouyang, C., and Wang, X. (2020). Nuclear Alarmin Cytokines in Inflammation. *J. Immunol. Res.* 4:7206451.

Jiang, P., and Mizushima, N. (2014). Autophagy and human diseases. *Cell Res.* 24, 69–79. doi: 10.1038/cr.2013.161

Kang, R., Chen, R., Zhang, Q., Hou, W., Wu, S., Cao, L., et al. (2014). HMGB1 in health and disease. (2014). *Mol. Aspects Med.* 40, 1–116. doi: 10.1016/j.mam.2014.05.001

Kang, R., Livesey, K. M., Zeh, H. J., Loze, M. T., and Tang, D. (2010). HMGB1: a novel Beclin 1-binding protein active in autophagy. *Autophagy* 6, 1209–1211. doi: 10.4161/auto.6.8.13651

Kaur, J., and Debnath, J. (2015). Autophagy at the crossroads of catabolism and anabolism. *Nat. Rev. Mol. Cell Biol.* 16, 461–472. doi: 10.1038/nrm4024

Kershaw, E. E., and Flier, J. S. (2004). Adipose tissue as an endocrine organ. *J. Clin. Endocrinol. Metab.* 89, 2548–2556. doi: 10.1210/jc.2004-0395

Kiffin, R., Bandyopadhyay, U., and Cuervo, A. M. (2006). Oxidative stress and autophagy. *Antioxid Redox Signal.* 8, 152–162. doi: 10.1089/ars.2006.8.152

Kim, Y. H., Kwak, M. S., Lee, B., Shin, J. M., Aum, S., Park, I. H., et al. (2020). Secretory autophagy machinery and vesicular trafficking are involved in HMGB1 secretion. *Autophagy* 2020:1826690. doi: 10.1080/15548627.2020.1826690

Klionsky, D. J. (2007). Autophagy: from phenomenology to molecular understanding in less than a decade. *Nat. Rev. Mole. Cell Biol.* 8, 931–937. doi: 10.1038/nrm2245

Kornicka, K., Houston, J., and Marycz, K. (2018). Dysfunction of Mesenchymal Stem Cells Isolated from Metabolic Syndrome and Type 2 Diabetic Patients as Result of Oxidative Stress and Autophagy may Limit Their Potential Therapeutic Use. *Stem Cell Rev. Rep.* 14, 337–345. doi: 10.1007/s12015-018-9809-x

Kuma, A., Komatsu, M., and Mizushima, N. (2017). Autophagy-monitoring and autophagy-deficient mice. *Autophagy* 13, 1619–1628. doi: 10.1080/15548627.2017.1343770

Kwak, M. S., Rhee, W. J., Lee, Y. J., Kim, H. S., Kim, Y. H., Kwon, M. K., et al. (2021). Reactive oxygen species induce Cys106-mediated anti-parallel HMGB1 dimerization that protects against DNA damage. *Redox Biol.* 40:101858. doi: 10.1016/j.redox.2021.101858

Lamb, C. A., Yoshimori, T., and Tooze, S. A. (2013). The autophagosome: origins unknown, biogenesis complex. *Nat. Rev. Mol. Cell Biol.* 14, 759–774. doi: 10.1038/nrm3696

Leidal, A. M., Levine, B., and Debnath, J. (2018). Autophagy and the cell biology of age-related disease. *Nat. Cell Biol.* 20, 1338–1348. doi: 10.1038/s41556-018-0235-8

Levine, B., and Kroemer, G. (2019). Biological Functions of Autophagy Genes: A Disease Perspective Cell. *Volume* 176, 11–42.

Levine, B., Mizushima, N., and Virgin, H. W. (2011). Autophagy in immunity and inflammation. *Nature* 469, 323–335. doi: 10.1038/nature09782

Li, J., Kokkola, R., Tabibzadeh, S., Yang, R., Ochani, M., Qiang, X., et al. (2003). Structural basis for the proinflammatory cytokine activity of high mobility group box 1. *Mol. Med.* 9, 37–45.

Li, L., and Lu, Y. Q. (2021). The Regulatory Role of High-Mobility Group Protein 1 in Sepsis-Related Immunity. *Front. Immunol.* 22:601815. doi: 10.3389/fimmu.2020

Li, W., Chen, M., Wang, E., Hu, L., Hawkesford, M. J., Zhong, L., et al. (2016). Genome-wide analysis of autophagy-associated genes in foxtail millet (Setaria italica L.) and characterization of the function of SiATG8a in conferring tolerance to nitrogen starvation in rice. *BMC Genomics.* 17:797. doi: 10.1186/s12864-016-3113-4

Lim, Y. M., Lim, H., Hur, K. Y., Quan, W., Lee, H. Y., Cheon, H., et al. (2014). Systemic autophagy insufficiency compromises adaptation to metabolic stress and facilitates progression from obesity to diabetes. *Nat. Commun.* 5:4934. doi: 10.1038/ncomms5934

Livesey, K. M., Kang, R., Vernon, P., Buchser, W., Loughran, P., Watkins, S. C., et al. (2012). p53/HMGB1 complexes regulate autophagy and apoptosis. *Cancer Res.* 72, 1996–2005. doi: 10.1158/0008-5472

Lonardo, A., Leoni, S., Alswat, K. A., and Fouad, Y. (2020). History of Nonalcoholic Fatty Liver Disease. *Int. J. Mol. Sci.* 21:5888. doi: 10.3390/ijms21165888

Longo, M., Zatterale, F., Naderi, J., Parrillo, L., Formisano, P., Raciti, G. A., et al. (2019). Adipose Tissue Dysfunction as Determinant of Obesity-Associated Metabolic Complications. *Int. J. Mol. Sci.* 20:2358. doi: 10.3390/ijms20092358

Maiuri, M. C., Zalckvar, E., Kimchi, A., and Kroemer, G. (2007). Self-eating and self-killing: crosstalk between autophagy and apoptosis. *Nat. Rev. Mol. Cell Biol.* 8, 741–752. doi: 10.1038/nrm2239

Marijt, K. A., Sluijter, M., Blijleven, L., Tolmeijer, S. H., Scheeren, F. A., van der Burg, S. H., et al. (2019). Metabolic stress in cancer cells induces immune escape through a PI3K-dependent blockade of IFNγ receptor signaling. *J. Immunother. Cancer* 7:152. doi: 10.1186/s40425-019-0627-8

Martinez-Lopez, N., Tarabra, E., Toledo, M., Schwartz, G. J., Kersten, S., and Singh, R. (2017). System-wide Benefits of Intermeal Fasting by Autophagy. *Cell Metab.* 26, 856.e–871.e. doi: 10.1016/j.cmet.2017.09.020

Mehrpour, M., Esclatine, A., Beau, I., and Codogno, P. (2010). Autophagy in health and disease. Regulation and significance of autophagy: an overview. *Am. J. Physiol. Cell Physiol.* 298, C776–C785. doi: 10.1152/ajpcell.00507.2009

Menikdiwela, K. R., Ramalingam, L., Rash, F., Wang, S., Dufour, J. M., Kalupahana, N. S., et al. (2020). Autophagy in metabolic syndrome: breaking the wheel by targeting the renin-angiotensin system. *Cell Death Dis.* 11:87. doi: 10.1038/s41419-020-2275-9

Migazzi, M., Dauriz, M., Cirillo, F., Catellani, C., Villani, M., Tosi, F., et al. (2021). Circulating HMGB1 Levels Are Associated With Glucose Clamp-Derived Measures of Insulin Resistance in Women With PCOS. *Accept. Endocr. Soc. Meeting** 2021.

Mizushima, N. (2018). A brief history of autophagy from cell biology to physiology and disease. *Nat. Cell Biol.* 20, 521–527. doi: 10.1038/s41556-018-0092-5

Mizushima, N., Levine, B., Cuervo, A. M., and Klionsky, D. J. (2008). Autophagy fights disease through cellular self-digestion. *Nature* 451, 1069–1075. doi: 10.1038/nature06639

Montanini, L., Cirillo, F., Smerieri, A., Pisi, G., Giardino, I., d'Apolito, M., et al. (2016). HMGB1 Is Increased by CFTR Loss of Function, Is Lowered by Insulin, and Increases In Vivo at Onset of CFRD. *J. Clin. Endocrinol. Metab.* 101, 1274–1281.

Montgomery, M. K. (2019). Mitochondrial Dysfunction and Diabetes: Is Mitochondrial Transfer a Friend or Foe? *Biology* 8:33. doi: 10.3390/biology8020033

Olefsky, J. M., and Glass, C. K. (2010). Macrophages, inflammation, and insulin resistance. *Annu. Rev. Physiol.* 72, 219–246. doi: 10.1146/annurev-physiol-021909-135846

Park, J. S., Svetkauskaite, D., He, Q., Kim, J. Y., Strassheim, D., Ishizaka, A., et al. (2004). Involvement of toll-like receptors 2 and 4 in cellular activation by high mobility group box 1 protein. *J. Biol. Chem.* 279, 7370–7377. doi: 10.1074/jbc.M306793200

Pyo, J. O., Yoo, S. M., Ahn, H. H., Nah, J., Hong, S. H., Kam, T. I., et al. (2013). Overexpression of Atg5 in mice activates autophagy and extends lifespan. *Nat. Commun.* 4:2300. doi: 10.1038/ncomms3300

Raj, S., Chandela, V., Kumar, A., Kesari, K. K., Asthana, S., Ruokolainen, J., et al. (2020). Molecular mechanisms of interplay between autophagy and metabolism in cancer. *Life Sci. Volume* 259, 118–184. doi: 10.1016/j.lfs.2020.118184

Raucci, A., Di Maggio, S., Scavello, F., D'Ambrosio, A., Bianchi, M. E., and Capogrossi, M. C. (2019). The Janus face of HMGB1 in heart disease: a necessary update. *Cell. Mole. Life Sci.* 76, 211–229. doi: 10.1007/s00018-018-2930-9

Reaven, G. M. (2006). The metabolic syndrome: is this diagnosis necessary? *Am. J. Clin. Nutr.* 83, 1237–1247. doi: 10.1093/ajcn/83.6.1237

Ren, J., Sowers, J. R., and Zhang, Y. (2018). Metabolic Stress, Autophagy, and Cardiovascular Aging: from Pathophysiology to Therapeutics. *Trends Endocrinol. Metab.* 29, 699–711. doi: 10.1016/j.tem.2018.08.001

Ren, S. Y., and Xu, X. (2015). Role of Autophagy in Metabolic Syndrome-Associated Heart Disease. *Biochim. Biophys. Acta* 1852, 225–231. doi: 10.1016/j.bbadis.2014.04.029

Rohde, K., Rønningen, T., La Cour Poulsen, L., Keller, M., and Blüher, M. (2020). Role of the DNA repair genes H2AX and HMGB1 in human fat distribution and lipid profiles. *BMJ Open Diab. Res. Care.* 8:e000831. doi: 10.1136/bmjdrc-2019-000831

Rubinsztein, D. C., Mariño, G., and Kroemer, G. (2011). Autophagy and aging. *Cell* 146, 682–695. doi: 10.1016/j.cell.2011.07.030

Ruderman, N. B., Carling, D., Prentki, M., and Cacicedo, J. M. (2013). AMPK, insulin resistance, and the metabolic syndrome. *J. Clin. Invest.* 123, 2764–2772. doi: 10.1172/JCI67227

Ryter, S. W., Koo, J. K., and Choi, A. M. (2014). Molecular regulation of autophagy and its implications for metabolic diseases. *Curr. Opin. Clin. Nutr. Metab. Care.* 7, 329–337. doi: 10.1097/MCO.0000000000000068

Samidurai, A., Kukreja, R. C., and Das, A. (2018). Emerging Role of mTOR Signaling-Related miRNAs in Cardiovascular Diseases. *Oxidat. Med. Cell. Long.* 2018:6141902. doi: 10.1155/2018/6141902

Seidu, S., Gillies, C., Zaccardi, F., Kunutsor, S. K., Hartmann-Boyce, J., Yates, T., et al. (2020). The impact of obesity on severe disease and mortality in people with SARS-CoV-2: A systematic review and meta-analysis. *Endocrinol. Diabetes Metab.* 14:e00176. doi: 10.1002/edm2.176

Shimizu, T., Yamakuchi, M., Biswas, K. K., Aryal, B., Yamada, S., Hashiguchi, T., et al. (2016). HMGB1 is secreted by 3T3-L1 adipocytes through JNK signaling and the secretion is partially inhibited by adiponectin. *Obesity* 24, 1913–1921. doi: 10.1002/oby.21549

Sohrabi, Y., Lagache, S. M. M., Schnack, L., Godfrey, R., Kahles, F., Bruemmer, D., et al. (2019). mTOR-Dependent Oxidative Stress Regulates oxLDL-Induced Trained Innate Immunity in Human Monocytes. *Front. Immunol.* 9:3155. doi: 10.3389/fimmu.2018.03155

Street, M. E. (2020). HMGB1: A possible crucial Therapeutic Target for Covid-19? *Horm. Res. Paediatr.* 2020:000508291. doi: 10.1159/000508291

Takeshige, K., Baba, M., Tsuboi, S., Noda, T., and Ohsumi, Y. (1992). Autophagy in yeast demonstrated with proteinase-deficient mutants and conditions for its induction. *J. Cell Biol.* 119, 301–311. doi: 10.1083/jcb.119.2.301

Tang, D., Kang, R., Cheh, C. W., Livesey, K. M., Liang, X., Schapiro, N. E., et al. (2010b). HMGB1 release and redox regulates autophagy and apoptosis in cancer cells. *Oncogene* 29, 5299–5310. doi: 10.1038/onc.2010.261

Tang, D., Kang, R., Livesey, K. M., Cheh, C. W., Farkas, A., Loughran, P., et al. (2010a). Endogenous HMGB1 regulates autophagy. *J. Cell Biol.* 190, 881–892. doi: 10.1083/jcb.200911078

Tang, D., Kang, R., Livesey, K. M., Kroemer, G., Billiar, T. R., Van Houten, B., et al. (2011). High-mobility group box 1 is essential for mitochondrial quality control. *Cell Metab.* 13, 701–711. doi: 10.1016/j.cmet.2011.04.008

Trim, W., Turner, J. E., and Thompson, D. (2018). Parallels in Immunometabolic Adipose Tissue Dysfunction with Ageing and Obesity. *Front. Immunol.* 9:169. doi: 10.3389/fimmu.2018.00169

Ueno, T., and Komatsu, M. (2017). Autophagy in the liver: functions in health and disease. *Nat. Rev. Gastroenterol. Hepatol* 14, 170–184. doi: 10.1038/nrgastro.2016

Umahara, T., Uchihara, T., Hirao, K., Shimizu, S., Hashimoto, T., Kohno, M., et al. (2020). Essential autophagic protein Beclin 1 localizes to atherosclerotic lesions of human carotid and major intracranial arteries. *J. Neurol. Sci.* 414:116836. doi: 10.1016/j.jns.2020.116836

van Niekerk, G., Davis, T., Patterton, H. G., and Engelbrecht, A. M. (2019). How Does Inflammation-Induced Hyperglycemia Cause Mitochondrial Dysfunction in Immune Cells? *Bioessays.* 41:e1800260. doi: 10.1002/bies.201800260

Wang, H., Qu, H., and Deng, H. (2015). Plasma HMGB-1 levels in subjects with obesity and type 2 diabetes: a cross-sectional study in China. *PLoS One* 10:e0136564. doi: 10.1371/journal.pone.0136564

Wang, L., Harris, T. E., Roth, R. A., and Lawrence, J. C. Jr. (2007). PRAS40 regulates mTORC1 kinase activity by functioning as a direct inhibitor of substrate binding. *J. Biol. Chem.* 282, 20036–20044. doi: 10.1074/jbc.M702376200

Wang, Y., Zhong, J., Zhang, X., Liu, Z., Yang, Y., Gong, Q., et al. (2016). The Role of HMGB1 in the Pathogenesis of Type 2 Diabetes. *J. Diabetes Res.* 2016:2543268. doi: 10.1155/2016/2543268

Watanabe, J., and Kotani, K. (2020). Metabolic Syndrome for Cardiovascular Disease Morbidity and Mortality Among General Japanese People: A Mini Review. *Vasc. Health Risk Manag.* 16, 149–155. doi: 10.2147/VHRM.S245829

Weihe, P., and Weihrauch-Blüher, S. (2019). Metabolic Syndrome in Children and Adolescents: Diagnostic criteria, therapeutic options and perspectives. *Curr. Obesity Rep.* 8, 472–479. doi: 10.1007/s13679-019-00357-x

Xu, Y., Shena, J., and Ran, Z. (2020). Emerging views of mitophagy in immunity and autoimmune diseases. *Autophagy* 16, 3–17. doi: 10.1080/15548627.2019.1603547

Xue, J., Suarez, J. S., Minaai, M., Li, S., Gaudino, G., Pass, H. I., et al. (2020). HMGB1 as a therapeutic target in disease. *J. Cell Physiol.* 26:30125. doi: 10.1002/jcp.30125

Yang, H., Antoine, D. J., Andersson, U., and Tracey, K. J. (2013). The many faces of HMGB1: molecular structure-functional activity in inflammation, apoptosis, and chemotaxis. *J. Leukocyte Biol.* 93, 865–873. doi: 10.1189/jlb.1212662

Yang, L., Li, P., Fu, S., Calay, E. S., and Hotamisligil, G. S. (2010). Defective Hepatic Autophagy in Obesity Promotes ER Stress and Causes Insulin Resistance. *Cell Metab.* 11, 467–478. doi: 10.1016/j.cmet.2010.04.005

Yao, Y., Guo, D., Yang, S., Lin, Y., He, L., Chen, J., et al. (2015). HMGB1 gene polymorphism is associated with hypertension in Han Chinese population. *Clin. Exp. Hypertens.* 37, 166.171. doi: 10.3109/10641963.2014.933963

Zhang, J., Chen, L., Wang, F., Zou, Y., Li, J., Luo, J., et al. (2020). Extracellular HMGB1 exacerbates autoimmune progression and recurrence of type 1 diabetes by impairing regulatory T cell stability. *Diabetologia* 63, 987–1001. doi: 10.1007/s00125-020-05105-8

Zhang, J., Zhang, L., Zhang, S., Yu, Q., Xiong, F., Huang, K., et al. (2017). HMGB1, an innate alarmin, plays a critical role in chronic inflammation of adipose tissue in obesity. *Mol. Cell Endocrinol.* 15, 103–111. doi: 10.1016/j.mce.2017.06.012

Zhang, Y., Sowers, J. R., and Ren, J. (2018). Targeting autophagy in obesity: from pathophysiology to management. *Nat. Rev. Endocrinol* 14, 356–376. doi: 10.1038/s41574-018-0009-1

Zhang, Y., Thery, F., Wu, N. C., Luhmann, E. K., Dussurget, O., Foecke, M., et al. (2019). The in vivo ISGylome links ISG15 to metabolic pathways and autophagy upon Listeria monocytogenes infection. *Nat. Commun.* 10. doi: 10.1038/s41467-019-13393-x

Zhu, X., Messer, J. S., Wang, Y., Lin, F., Cham, C. M., Chang, J., et al. (2015). Cytosolic HMGB1 controls the cellular autophagy/apoptosis checkpoint during inflammation. *J. Clin. Investig.* 125, 1098–1110. doi: 10.1172/JCI76344

12

Autophagy in Diabetes Pathophysiology: Oxidative Damage Screening as Potential for Therapeutic Management by Clinical Laboratory Methods

Ezekiel Uba Nwose [1,2]* and Phillip Taderera Bwititi [3]

[1] School of Community Health, Charles Sturt University, Orange, NSW, Australia, [2] Department of Public and Community Health, Novena University, Kwale, Nigeria, [3] School of Biomedical Sciences, Charles Sturt University, Wagga Wagga, NSW, Australia

Keywords: biomarkers, cause-and-effect, erythrocyte, laboratory tests, oxidative stress

*Correspondence:
Ezekiel Uba Nwose
enwose@csu.edu.au

INTRODUCTION—PHENOMENOLOGY

Autophagy or auto-phagocytosis is self-phagocytosis of tissues and cellular materials i.e., "self-maintenance." While phagocytosis normally refers to the innate immune process of white blood cells engulfing foreign bodies such as infectious materials, autophagy is a regulatory phenomenon of dysfunctional cellular components being removed (Kobayashi, 2015). Autophagy is inseparable from inflammation and oxidative stress phenomena (Turkmen, 2017); which are intricately involved in pathophysiology of diabetes mellitus (DM) (Muriach et al., 2014). The relationships between phenomena is shown in **Figure 1**.

Autophagy in association with oxidative stress is involved in pathophysiology. For instance, in the non-modifiable aging process, autophagy is involved in the associated oxidative stress and this can be assessed by glycation end-products as well as indices of lipid oxidation such as malondialdehyde (Moldogazieva et al., 2019). What is yet to be articulated for clinical translation in terms of laboratory assessment of autophagy is the concept of oxidative stress screening. A recent review highlights cell culture and electron microscopy methods (Yoshii and Mizushima, 2017) but not blood tests for oxidative stress indices. Thus, the gap between knowledge and practice are the apparent lack of acknowledgment of oxidative damage interplay between autophagy and metabolic diseases.

The objective of this paper is to bring to the fore the way in which clinical laboratory tests for oxidative stress panel can be used to assess autophagy in metabolic syndrome, especially the relevance of tests from different thematic sub-panels to establish cellular damage in metabolic syndrome. In this objective, cognizance is taken that metabolic syndrome is a constellation of diabetes and its cardiovascular complications including dyslipidaemia factor. For instance, abnormal cholesterol can exacerbate oxidative stress to increase autophagy in diabetes.

This opinion paper is organized in four sections. First three sections cover "causes, consequences, and therapeutic challenges" in terms of oxidative stress, effects on vascular physiology, and implications for management by laboratory methods, respectively. A brief fourth section is on availability of clinical laboratory tests for oxidative stress panel and how to interpret the results in terms of autophagy-inflammation interplay.

CAUSES OF AUTOPHAGY IN DIABETES—ERYTHROCYTE OXIDATIVE STRESS (EOS) PERSPECTIVE

Cellular oxidative stress can induce mitochondrial damage, which then requires autophagy to maintain homeostasis (Lee et al., 2012). Oxidative stress is a disturbance of the physiological control of oxidant/antioxidant (redox) balance, in which oxidants become dominant. It is a state in which a cell experiences alteration of cellular components, due to exposure to free radicals and other reactive oxygen species (ROS) beyond its antioxidant capacity (Sies, 1991). Redox reactions are essential for cellular functions such as the utilization of chemical energy from nutrients for the production of adenosine triphosphate. However, excessive oxidants expose cells including erythrocytes to oxidative stress (Kuhn et al., 2017).

EOS is a type of cellular oxidative stress, which arises from over-exposure of the cellular components of red blood cells to various ROS (Richards et al., 1998). It is a situation whereby the erythrocyte's functional mechanisms are impaired or overwhelmed by alteration in the normal metabolic and/or physiological activities that generate ROS (Taniyama and Griendling, 2003). Although the red cell has an efficient antioxidant system for the normal levels of oxidants generated in its membranes, the oxidant challenge can exceed the capacity of the antioxidant system (Fung and Zhang, 1990).

There is a tendency for imperfect reduction of oxygen in the mitochondrial electron transport systems e.g., the leak of superoxide radicals (Maxwell and Lip, 1997). The cascade reaction induced by the superoxide radicals involves antioxidant function of "reduced" glutathione (GSH) that leads to reduction in concentration and exacerbates EOS (McMullin, 1999; Boada et al., 2000; Ulusu et al., 2003). Thus, there are three possible sources of ROS that predispose the erythrocytes to oxidative stress:

- There exist special channels on the membrane by which superoxide radicals permeate the erythrocyte from the mitochondria of other cells (Richards et al., 1998). This is more so during hyperglycaemia or dyslipidaemia (Taniyama and Griendling, 2003). A discussed how EOS is strongly implicated in diabetes and its cardiovascular complications (Nwose et al., 2007a). Laboratory-based investigations have also reported on erythrocyte morphology or oxidative stress being associated with oxidative stress (Parthiban et al., 1995; Nwose et al., 2009; Gyawali et al., 2015). What is being advanced here is the EOS interplay with autophagy in metabolic syndrome (**Figure 1**).
- Secondly, the erythrocyte can paradoxically become oxidatively stressed from normal physiological processes (Kuhn et al., 2017). Due to the role of erythrocytes in oxygen transport and the presence of redox-active hemoglobin molecules, they generate pro-oxidant radicals by the Fenton reaction.

- Thirdly, there is hyperglycaemia-induced oxidative stress. Besides glycolysis being associated with oxidative stress in diabetic cardiovascular physiology (Zinman, 2003; Brownlee, 2005), there are points of pro-oxidant production when the erythrocyte is utilizing glucose to generate energy in the pentose phosphate pathway (Nwose et al., 2007a).
- Cellular oxidative stress can induce mitochondrial damage, which then requires autophagy to maintain homeostasis.

Therefore, point of emphasize is that fragments of damaged red blood cell materials are removed from the system by the phagocytosis function of the spleen—the basic cleaning function of the blood by spleen. In the context of splenectomy, red blood cells tend to acquire autophagic vacuoles (Holroyde and Gardner, 1970). Current research is yet to translate the basic science that EOS is followed by splenic autophagy of the damaged red blood cells. Therefore, what is being brought to the fore is a measurable perspective of autophagy in terms of EOS that is integral to diabetes and associated metabolic syndrome indices.

CONSEQUENCES—POTENTIAL IMPLICATIONS OF AUTOPHAGY-EOS INTERPLAY IN DIABETES

There can be autophagy of pancreatic beta-cells (Marasco and Linnemann, 2018), and this has implications, but is not the focus of this discussion. Mitochondrial oxidative stress and autophagy are implicated in diabetes (Muriach et al., 2014); and although red blood cells lack mitochondria, there are potential effects on glucose metabolic pathways. Whether in glycolysis or pentose phosphate pathway, the physiology to meet the cellular need of energy in the erythrocyte is associated with the propensity to deplete GSH content, which in turn leads to EOS. The aberrant state of EOS is of clinical importance in diabetes (Nwose et al., 2007a), especially because hyperglycaemia exacerbates oxidative stress (Yano et al., 2004).

In the diabetes pathophysiology, GSH level is depleted as it is converted to oxidized glutathione. This leads to reduced erythrocyte antioxidant capacity including impaired vitamin E regeneration system (Nwose et al., 2008a), which feedforward to constitutes a possible cause of EOS (Nwose et al., 2007a). Methaemoglobin reductase activity is the other pathway, which impairs GSH functions and potentially complicates the entire vitamin E recycling system (Nwose et al., 2008a).

Thus, diabetes is associated with a decrease of erythrocyte GSH level, which translates to antioxidant imbalance of the cell. Prolonged impairment of the vitamin E recycling in the red blood cell membrane amounts to EOS that damages the cell (Nwose et al., 2008a). What is being brought to the fore is that hyperglycaemia-induced EOS can cause autophagy and may complicate a cause-and-effect phenomenon in diabetes (**Figure 1**). Therefore, the laboratory perspective is to view autophagy and associated challenges as follows:

- Causes—oxidative stress
- Consequences—effects on cardiovascular physiology

Abbreviations: DM, diabetes mellitus; EOS, erythrocyte oxidative stress; GSH, reduced glutathione; MDA, Malondialdehyde; ROS, reactive oxygen species.

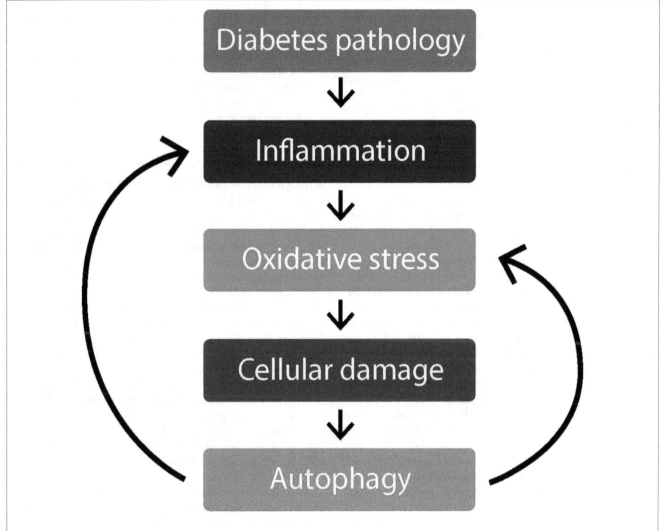

FIGURE 1 | Illustration* of relationship between autophagy and oxidative stress in diabetes mellitus. *This figure illustrates how autophagy is inseparable from inflammation and oxidative stress phenomena. Figure shows that autophagy is caused by (downward arrows), but it also exacerbates (backward arrows), inflammation, and oxidative stress in diabetes.

- Therapeutic challenges—implications for management by oxidative stress panel screening.

THERAPEUTIC CHALLENGES

Implications for Management by Laboratory Methods

For over two decades, research has demonstrated that changes in erythrocyte antioxidant and haem components in DM lead to complications such as cardiovascular diseases (Dominguez et al., 1998; Dumaswala et al., 2001; Memisogullari et al., 2003), but the question is how EOS is involved in macrovascular complications of DM. As illustrated (Nwose et al., 2007a), EOS may effect macrovascular events including increased blood viscosity, hypercoagulation, and endothelial dysfunction. It is noteworthy that these vascular events constitute Virchow's triad, which has been a subject of research (Makin et al., 2002; Lowe,

2003; Nwose et al., 2014); and shrouded in discussion (Bagot and Arya, 2008; Dickson, 2009; Malone and Agutter, 2009). There is also the effect of tissue hypoxia as discussed that can lead to high blood pressure hence exacerbate metabolic syndrome.

Endothelial Dysfunction Exacerbated by Metabolic Syndrome

There is knowledge of hyperglycaemia-induced endothelial dysfunction (De Vriese et al., 2000; Zinman, 2003); and that diabetic dyslipidaemia (component of metabolic syndrome) initiates a chronic inflammatory reaction that results in endothelial damage, which culminates in endothelial dysfunction such as atherosclerosis and coronary artery disease (Gonzalez and Selwyn, 2003). It is established that oxidative stress results in endothelial dysfunction, which has plasma homocysteine levels as clinical index (Dumaswala et al., 2001; Nwose et al., 2007a).

Blood Viscosity

This is an intrinsic resistance of blood flow in the vascular system (Lowe et al., 1997). Normally, erythrocyte membrane deformability is a physical property that enables cells to change shape and flow with little or no aggregation/friction. When EOS occurs through lipid peroxidation within the membrane, the cell membrane becomes more rigid and less adaptable (Suda et al., 1980). This makes the blood more viscous, which leads to the development of vascular abnormalities including atherothrombosis and endothelial dysfunction that are associated with coronary artery disease (Solans et al., 2000), as well as tissue hypoxia (El-Sayed et al., 2005). The implication in diabetes and dyslipidaemia has been highlighted (Nwose, 2010, 2013; Richards and Nwose, 2010; Nwose et al., 2014). The point advanced here is the potential, as part of oxidative damage indices for screening splenic autophagy of red blood cellular materials after EOS.

Imbalance of Coagulation and Fibrinolysis

There are several theories surrounding hypercoagulation in DM. For instance, hypo-fibrinolysis occurring as thrombomodulin-thrombin complex—which is formed on intact vascular endothelium—may activate thrombin-activatable fibrinolysis inhibitor (Yano, 2003). This suggestion is supported by the observation that hyperglycaemia and insulin enhance the synthesis and secretion of plasminogen activator inhibitor type 1 (Kohler and Grant, 2000). These findings imply that fibrinolysis and therefore the generation of D-dimer are reduced in DM. A seemingly opposing theory is that EOS leads to enhancement of events such as increased production of procoagulant tissue factors at the gene level (Brownlee, 2005), which imply that D-dimer changes in diabetes have not been adequately explained.

It has been reported that some coagulation markers such as D-dimer and fibrinogen are elevated in DM (Sommeijer et al., 2004). Preliminary reports have also shown increased D-dimer levels in DM (Nwose et al., 2007b). Therefore, it is advanced that D-dimer constitutes a potential option for oxidative damage screening (**Table 1**).

EOS-Induced Haemolytic Anemia Exacerbating High Blood Pressure

There is a likelihood that hyperglycaemia-depleted GSH occurs *via* either reduced regeneration due to deficient pentose phosphate pathway (McMullin, 1999), or enhanced hexosamine pathway flux (Brownlee, 2005). The effect is EOS, which leads to a sequence of membrane rigidity and lysis (Fung and Zhang, 1990). The impacts are both hyperviscosity and anemia, respectively. That is, disruption of the normal rheological properties (El-Sayed et al., 2005), which leads to a sequence of anemia, reduced blood/O_2 supply, ischaemia and subsequently angina, chronic ischaemic heart disease, myocardial infarction or sudden death (McCance et al., 2002). It is noteworthy that the homeostatic response to reduced blood/O_2 supply involves increase in cardiac output, which may lead to high blood pressure. Hence, evaluation of fluctuations in blood pressure can support oxidative stress panel.

Indeed, anemia is associated with an increased risk of diabetic macrovascular disease or metabolic syndrome *per se* (Thomas et al., 2006). Autophagy is implicated in anemia (Grosso et al., 2017), but what has not been given adequate attention is that:

- EOS compromises the free radical basis of anemia (Dumaswala et al., 2001)
- Anemia is an effect of autophagy-related EOS
- To date, there are no defined signs and symptoms of autophagy for clinical decision making.

Oxidative Stress Panel Indices for Autophagy—Screening Suggestion

There are limited laboratory methods for autophagy evaluation (Klionsky et al., 2016), especially in diabetes research and practice. Thus, the justification of this paper is to advance the role of oxidative stress panel indices for the screening of autophagy in people living with diabetes. For instance, this could be used to monitor therapeutic management of cardiovascular complications of diabetes.

Diagnostic laboratory markers include the traditional risk evaluation markers such as cholesterol and glucose profiles. Emerging biomarkers include C-reactive protein, D-dimer, and homocysteine (Tracy, 2003; Ridker et al., 2004), as well as oxidative stress indices that include GSH and MDA (Tsimikas, 2006; Gyawali et al., 2015; Nwose et al., 2018; Lubrano et al., 2019). Uric acid and albumin levels have been considered (Bwititi et al., 2012). Pending clear definition of the signs and symptoms of autophagy, it is recommendable that the common laboratory principle applies whereby more than three positive results from this suite of biomarkers may indicate high levels of autophagy, be adopted.

It is becoming more clear that pharmacological agents to promote autophagy work by mediating oxidative stress (Wu et al., 2020). This implies that autophagy status is associated with degree of oxidative stress. The contribution being made in this paper is that methods for clinical evaluation of oxidative stress used in research can be integrated into clinical practice.

Further, it has been established that oxidative damage must involve reduction in antioxidant status, increase in oxidant levels and evidence of cardiovascular effects such as hypercoagulation, endothelial dysfunction, and blood viscosity that could easily lead to diseases (Nwose et al., 2008b). Thus, laboratory screening of oxidative damage includes indices of oxidative stress indices and their effects (**Table 1**). Oxidative stress markers listed here are just examples of what is readily available. There are a whole lot of others (Keaney et al., 2003; Frijhoff et al., 2015).

Perhaps, it is pertinent to emphasize that although assessment of EOS and its role in autophagy would be a potential therapeutic screening method, what needs to be addressed is *"if it will be an effective indicator of overall metabolic dysregulation."* For this reason, it is pertinent to point out the concept of high cholesterol (indicated by lipid profile) being a factor that can exacerbate lipid peroxidation (i.e., oxidative stress) to increase autophagy in diabetes. Also, oxidative damage panel screening will show cardiovascular effect such as increased blood viscosity (Nwose, 2013). Thus, beyond e.g., blood glucose

Autophagy in Diabetes Pathophysiology: Oxidative Damage Screening as Potential for Therapeutic Management...

179

TABLE 1 | Oxidative damage panel useable in the laboratory as oxidative stress screening.

Theme	Biomarker	Expectation in oxidative stress	Sample type[a]
Oxidative stress	Glutathione (GSH)	Reduced antioxidant level	Heparin, citrate, EDTA blood (RBCs or plasma, serum)
	Malondialdehyde (MDA)[b]	Increased oxidant level	EDTA plasma, serum, saliva, urine, cell culture extracts, tissue extracts
	Isoprostane	Increased levels	Citrated or heparin plasma, urine
	Methaemoglobin (metHB)	Increased oxidant level	Citrate or heparin plasma, RBC hemolysate
Oxidative stress "cardiovascular" effect	Blood pressure	Increased	Auscultatory, oscillometry, ultrasound
	D-dimer	Increased hypercoagulability	Heparin, citrate plasma, whole blood
	Homocysteine	Increased endothelial dysfunction	Citrate, EDTA plasma, serum, urine
	Whole blood viscosity	Hyperviscosity/slowed blood flow	EDTA whole blood

[a]It is expected that lab protocol will establish separate reference range for every sample type used.
[b]Particularly to assess lipid peroxidation that is exacerbated in dyslipidaemia.

and cholesterol dysregulation, there are effects or subclinical pathophysiological indices.

This perspective recommendation advances the knowledge that oxidative stress induces autophagy (Hariharan et al., 2011; Turkmen, 2017; Gao, 2019; Moldogazieva et al., 2019). This therefore justifies carrying out laboratory tests for oxidative stress. The theme of this special issue, therapeutic challenges in the management of autophagy implies the need for monitoring of treatment using tests that assess therapeutic efficacy. It has recently been highlighted that targeting autophagy is a means to counteract oxidative stress in obesity (Pietrocola and Bravo-San Pedro, 2021). Another advantage is therefore identification of need for change in treatment regimen. For instance, there is indication of possible simultaneous induction of oxidative stress and autophagy in diabetes as well as obese patients (Klionsky et al., 2016). What this opinion paper contributes is the need to look at a panel of tests and the availability of the test methods.

CONCLUSION

Current considerations of autophagy acknowledge oxidative stress in the cause-and-effect physiology as well as therapeutic

modes of action. However, monitoring by laboratory methods is yet to integrate the available and validated oxidative stress parameters. What this opinion paper brings to fore is that tests for oxidative stress panel can be used to assess autophagy in metabolic syndrome, including diabetes and its cardiovascular complications, at no major cost.

AUTHOR CONTRIBUTIONS

EN and PB conceptualized the opinion. EN did the initial draft of main text. PB did the revision as well as the abstract and conclusion. Both authors contributed to the article and approved the submitted version.

ACKNOWLEDGMENTS

This opinion paper was predominantly based on, and represents a translational update of, several pieces of doctoral research work done more than 13 years ago. Kay Skinner from Charles Sturt University has kindly edited the manuscript to improve the English language and is hereby appreciated.

REFERENCES

Bagot, C. N., and Arya, R. (2008). Virchow's triad: a question of attribution. Br. J. Haematol. 143, 180–190. doi: 10.1111/j.1365-2141.2008.07323.x

Boada, J., Riog, T., Xavier, P., Gamez, A., Bartrons, R., Cascante, M., et al. (2000). Cells overexpressing fructose-2-6-bisphosphatase showed enhanced pentose phosphate pathway flux and resistance to oxidative stress. FEBS Lett. 480:261. doi: 10.1016/S0014-5793(00)01 950-5

Brownlee, M. (2005). The pathobiology of diabetic complications: a unifying mechanism. Diabetes 54, 1615–1625. doi: 10.2337/diabetes.54.6.1615

Bwititi, P., Nwose, U., Nielsen, S., Ruven, H., Kalle, W., Richards, R., et al. (2012). Serum uric acid and albumin levels and estimated glomerular filtration rate: oxidative stress considerations. Aust. J. Med. Sci. 33, 82–87.

De Vriese, A. S., Verbeuren, T. J., Van de Voorde, J., Lameire, N. H., and Vanhoutte, P. M. (2000). Endothelial dysfuntion in diabetes. *Br. J. Pharmacol.* 130, 963–974. doi: 10.1038/sj.bjp.0703393

Dickson, B. C. (2009). Virchow's triad. *Br. J. Haematol.* 145:433. doi: 10.1111/j.1365-2141.2009.07617.x

Dominguez, C., Ruiz, E., Gussinye, M., and Carrascosa, A. (1998). Oxidative stress at onset and in early stages of type I diabetes in children and adolescents. *Diabetes Care* 21, 1736–1742. doi: 10.2337/diacare.21.10.1736

Dumaswala, U. J., Zhuo, L., Mahajan, S., Nair, P. N. M., Shertzer, H. G., Dibello, P., et al. (2001). Glutathione protects chemokine-scavenging and antioxidative defense functions in human RBC. *Am. J. Physiol. Cell Physiol.* 280, C867–C873. doi: 10.1152/ajpcell.2001.280.4.C867

El-Sayed, M. S., Ali, N., and El-Sayed, A. Z. (2005). Haemorheology in exercise and training. *Sports Med.* 35, 649–670. doi: 10.2165/00007256-200535080-00001

Frijhoff, J., Winyard, P. G., Zarkovic, N., Davies, S. S., Stocker, R., Cheng, D., et al. (2015). Clinical relevance of biomarkers of oxidative stress. *Antioxid. Redox Signal.* 23, 1144–1170. doi: 10.1089/ars.2015.6317

Fung, L. W., and Zhang, Y. (1990). A method to evaluate the antioxidant system for radicals in erythrocyte membranes. *Free Radic. Biol. Med.* 9, 289–298. doi: 10.1016/0891-5849(90)90003-2

Gao, Q. (2019). Oxidative stress and autophagy. *Adv. Exp. Med. Biol.* 1206, 179–198. doi: 10.1007/978-981-15-0602-4_9

Gonzalez, M. A., and Selwyn, A. P. (2003). Endothelial dysfunction, inflammation, and prognosis in cardiovascular disease. *Am. J. Med.* 115, 99S–106S. doi: 10.1016/j.amjmed.2003.09.016

Grosso, R., Fader, C. M., and Colombo, M. I. (2017). Autophagy: a necessary event during erythropoiesis. *Blood Rev.* 31, 300–305. doi: 10.1016/j.blre.2017.04.001

Gyawali, P., Richards, R. S., Bwititi, P. T., and Nwose, E. U. (2015). Association of abnormal erythrocyte morphology with oxidative stress and inflammation in metabolic syndrome. *Blood Cells Mol. Dis.* 54, 360–363. doi: 10.1016/j.bcmd.2015.01.005

Hariharan, N., Zhai, P., and Sadoshima, J. (2011). Oxidative stress stimulates autophagic flux during ischemia/reperfusion. *Antioxid. Redox Signal.* 14, 2179–2190. doi: 10.1089/ars.2010.3488

Holroyde, C. P., and Gardner, F. H. (1970). Acquisition of autophagic vacuoles by human erythrocytes physiological role of the spleen. *Blood* 36, 566–575. doi: 10.1182/blood.V36.5.566.566

Keaney, J. F., Larson, M. G., Vasan, R. S., Wilson, P. W. F., Lipinska, I., Corey, D., et al. (2003). Obesity and systemic oxidative stress: clinical correlates of oxidative stress in the Framingham study. *Arterioscler. Thromb. Vasc. Biol.* 23, 434–439. doi: 10.1161/01.ATV.0000058402.34138.11

Klionsky, D. J., Abdelmohsen, K., Abe, A., Abedin, M. J., Abeliovich, H., Acevedo Arozena, A., et al. (2016). Guidelines for the use and interpretation of assays for monitoring autophagy (3rd edition). *Autophagy* 12, 1–222. doi: 10.1080/15548627.2015.1100356

Kobayashi, S. (2015). Choose delicately and reuse adequately: the newly revealed process of autophagy. *Biol. Pharm. Bull.* 38, 1098–1103. doi: 10.1248/bpb.b15-00096

Kohler, H. P., and Grant, P. J. (2000). Plasminogen-activator inhibitor type 1 and coronary artery disease. *New Engl. J. Med.* 342, 1792–1801. doi: 10.1056/NEJM200006153422406

Kuhn, V., Diederich, L., Keller, T. C. S., t, Kramer, C. M., Lückstädt, W., et al. (2017). Red blood cell function and dysfunction: redox regulation, nitric oxide metabolism, anemia. *Antioxid. Redox Signal.* 26, 718–742. doi: 10.1089/ars.2016.6954

Lee, J., Giordano, S., and Zhang, J. (2012). Autophagy, mitochondria, and oxidative stress: cross-talk and redox signalling. *Biochem. J.* 441, 523–540. doi: 10.1042/BJ20111451

Lowe, G. D. (2003). Virchow's triad revisited: abnormal flow. *Pathophysiol. Haemost. Thromb.* 33, 455–457. doi: 10.1159/000083845

Lowe, G. D., Lee, A. J., Rumley, A., Price, J. F., and Fowkes, F. G. (1997). Blood viscosity and risk of cardiovascular events: the Edinburgh artery study. *Br. J. Haematol.* 96, 168–173. doi: 10.1046/j.1365-2141.1997.8532481.x

Lubrano, V., Pingitore, A., Traghella, I., Storti, S., Parri, S., Berti, S., et al. (2019). Emerging biomarkers of oxidative stress in acute and stable coronary artery disease: levels and determinants. *Antioxidants (Basel)* 8:115. doi: 10.3390/antiox8050115

Makin, A., Silverman, S. H., and Lip, G. Y. H. (2002). Peripheral vascular disease and Virchow's triad for thrombogenesis. *QJM* 95, 199–210. doi: 10.1093/qjmed/95.4.199

Malone, P. C., and Agutter, P. S. (2009). Is 'Virchow's triad' useful? *Br. J. Haematol.* 145:839. doi: 10.1111/j.1365-2141.2009.07685.x

Marasco, M. R., and Linnemann, A. K. (2018). β-Cell autophagy in diabetes pathogenesis. *Endocrinology* 159, 2127–2141. doi: 10.1210/en.2017-03273

Maxwell, S. R. J., and Lip, G. Y. H. (1997). Free radicals and antioxidants in cardiovascular disease. *Br. J. Clin. Pharmacol.* 44, 307–317. doi: 10.1046/j.1365-2125.1997.t01-1-00594.x

McCance, K. L., Grey, T. C., and Huether, S. E. (2002). "Altered cellular and tissue biology," in *Pathophysiology: The Biologic Basis for Disease in Adults and Children, 4th Edn,* ed K. L. McCance (Maryland Heights, MO: Mosby), 48–51.

McMullin, M. F. (1999). The molecular basis of disorders of red cell enzymes. *J. Clin. Pathol.* 52, 241–244. doi: 10.1136/jcp.52.4.241

Memisogullari, R., Taysi, S., Bakan, E., and Capoglu, I. (2003). Antioxidant status and lipid peroxidation in type II diabetes mellitus. *Cell Biochem. Funct.* 21, 291–296. doi: 10.1002/cbf.1025

Moldogazieva, N. T., Mokhosoev, I. M., Mel'nikova, T. I., Porozov, Y. B., and Terentiev, A. A. (2019). Oxidative stress and advanced lipoxidation and glycation end products (ALEs and AGEs) in aging and age-related diseases. *Oxid. Med. Cell. Longev.* 2019:3085756. doi: 10.1155/2019/3085756

Muriach, M., Flores-Bellver, M., Romero, F. J., and Barcia, J. M. (2014). Diabetes and the brain: oxidative stress, inflammation, and autophagy. *Oxid. Med. Cell. Longev.* 2014:102158. doi: 10.1155/2014/102158

Nwose, E. U. (2010). Whole blood viscosity assessment issues V: prevalence in hypercreatinaemia, hyperglycaemia, and hyperlipidaemia. *North Am. J. Med. Sci.* 2, 403–408. doi: 10.4297/najms.2010.2408

Nwose, E. U. (2013). Blood viscosity, lipid profile, and lipid peroxidation in type-1 diabetic patients with good and poor glycemic control: the promise and reality. *North Am. J. Med. Sci.* 5, 567–568. doi: 10.4103/1947-2714.118926

Nwose, E. U., Bwititi, P. T., and Chalada, M. J. (2018). Influence of anticoagulants on determination of H2O2 levels in blood: comparison of citrate and EDTA. *Int. J. Pathol. Clin. Res.* 4:083. doi: 10.23937/2469-5807/1510083

Nwose, E. U., Jelinek, H. F., Richards, R. S., and Kerr, P. G. (2007a). Erythrocyte oxidative stress in clinical management of diabetes and its cardiovascular complication. *Br. J. Biomed. Sci.* 64, 35–43. doi: 10.1080/09674845.2007.11732754

Nwose, E. U., Jelinek, H. F., Richards, R. S., and Kerr, P. G. (2008a). The "vitamin E regeneration system" (VERS) and an algorithm to justify antioxidant supplementation in diabetes–a hypothesis. *Med. Hypotheses* 70, 1002–1008. doi: 10.1016/j.mehy.2007.07.048

Nwose, E. U., Jelinek, H. F., Richards, R. S., Tinley, P., and Kerr, P. G. (2009). Atherothrombosis and oxidative stress: the connection and correlation in diabetes. *Redox Rep.* 14, 55–60. doi: 10.1179/135100009X392458

Nwose, E. U., Richards, R. S., and Bwititi, P. T. (2014). Cardiovascular risks in prediabetes: preliminary data on "vasculopathy triad." *North Am. J. Med. Sci.* 6, 328–332. doi: 10.4103/1947-2714.136913

Nwose, E. U., Richards, R. S., Jelinek, H. F., and Kerr, P. G. (2007b). D-dimer identifies stages in the progression of diabetes mellitus from family history of diabetes to cardiovascular complications. *Pathology* 39, 252–257. doi: 10.1080/00313020701230658

Nwose, E. U., Richards, R. S., Kerr, P. G., Tinley, R., and Jelinek, H. F. (2008b). Oxidative damage indices for the assessment of subclinical diabetic macrovascular complications. *Br. J. Biomed. Sci.* 65, 136–141. doi: 10.1080/09674845.2008.11732817

Parthiban, A., Vijayalingam, S., Shanmugasundaram, K. R., and Mohan, R. (1995). Oxidative stress and the development of diabetic complications–antioxidants and lipid peroxidation in erythrocytes and cell membrane. *Cell Biol. Int.* 19, 987–993. doi: 10.1006/cbir.1995.1040

Pietrocola, F., and Bravo-San Pedro, J. M. (2021). Targeting autophagy to counteract obesity-associated oxidative stress. *Antioxidants (Basel)* 10:102. doi: 10.3390/antiox10010102

Richards, R. S., and Nwose, E. U. (2010). Blood viscosity at different stages of diabetes pathogenesis. *Br. J. Biomed. Sci.* 67, 67–70. doi: 10.1080/09674845.2010.11730293

Richards, R. S., Roberts, T. K., McGregor, N. R., Dunstan, R. H., and Butt, H. L. (1998). Erythrocyte antioxidant systems protect cultured endothelial cells against oxidant damage. *Biochem. Mol. Biol. Int.* 46, 857–865. doi: 10.1080/15216549800204402

Ridker, P. M., Brown, N. J., Vaughan, D. E., Harrison, D. G., and Mehta, J. L. (2004). Established and emerging plasma biomarkers in the prediction of first atherothrombotic events. *Circulation* 109(25 Suppl. 1), IV6–IV19. doi: 10.1161/01.CIR.0000133444.17 867.56

Sies, H. (1991). Oxidative stress: from basic research to clinical application. *Am. J. Med.* 91, S31–S38. doi: 10.1016/0002-9343(91)90281-2

Solans, R., Motta, C., Sol,á, R., La Ville, A. E., Lima, J., Simeón, P., et al. (2000). Abnormalities of erythrocyte membrane fluidity, lipid composition, and lipid peroxidation in systemic sclerosis: evidence of free radical-mediated injury. *Arthritis Rheum.* 43, 894–900. doi: 10.1002/1529-0131(200004)43:4<894::AID-ANR22>3.0.CO;2-4

Sommeijer, D. W., MacGillavry, M. R., Meijers, J. C. M., Zanten, A. P., Reitsma, P. H., and Ten Cate, H. (2004). Anti-inflammatory and anticoagulant effects of pravastatin in patients with type 2 diabetes. *Diabetes Care* 27, 468–474. doi: 10.2337/diacare.27.2.468

Suda, T., Maeda, N., and Shiga, T. (1980). Effect of cholesterol on human erythrocyte membrane. A spin label study. *J. Biochem. (Tokyo)* 87, 1703–1713. doi: 10.1093/oxfordjournals.jbchem.a132914

Taniyama, Y., and Griendling, K. K. (2003). Reactive oxygen species in the vasculature: molecular and cellular mechanisms. *Hypertension* 42, 1075–1081. doi: 10.1161/01.HYP.0000100443.09293.4F

Thomas, M. C., Cooper, M. E., Rossing, K., and Parving, H. H. (2006). Anaemia in diabetes: is there a rationale to TREAT? *Diabetologia* 49, 1151–1157. doi: 10.1007/s00125-006-0215-6

Tracy, R. P. (2003). Thrombin, inflammation, and cardiovascular disease: an epidemiologic perspective. *Chest* 124(3 Suppl.), 49S–57S. doi: 10.1378/chest.124.3_suppl.49S

Tsimikas, S. (2006). Measures of oxidative stress. *Clin. Lab. Med.* 26, 571–590. doi: 10.1016/j.cll.2006.06.004

Turkmen, K. (2017). Inflammation, oxidative stress, apoptosis, and autophagy in diabetes mellitus and diabetic kidney disease: the Four Horsemen of the Apocalypse. *Int. Urol. Nephrol.* 49, 837–844. doi: 10.1007/s11255-016-1488-4

Ulusu, N. N., Sahilli, M., Avci, A., Canbolat, O., Ozansoy, G., Ari, N., et al. (2003). Pentose phosphate pathway, glutathione-dependent enzymes, and antioxidant defense during oxidative stress in diabetic rodent brain and peripheral organs: effects of stobadine and vitamin E. *Neurochem. Res.* 28, 815–823. doi: 10.1023/A:1023202805255

Wu, D., Zhong, P., Wang, Y., Zhang, Q., Li, J., Liu, Z., et al. (2020). Hydrogen sulfide attenuates high-fat diet-induced non-alcoholic fatty liver disease by inhibiting apoptosis and promoting autophagy via reactive oxygen species/phosphatidylinositol 3-kinase/AKT/mammalian target of rapamycin signaling pathway. *Front. Pharmacol.* 11:585860. doi: 10.3389/fphar.2020.585860

Yano, M., Hasegawa, G., Ishii, M., Yamasaki, M., Fukuri, M., Nakamura, N., et al. (2004). Short-term exposure of high glucose concentration induces generation of reactive oxygen species in endothelial cells: implication for the oxidative stress associated with postprandial hyperglycaemia. *Redox Rep.* 9, 111–116. doi: 10.1179/135100004225004779

Yano, Y. (2003). "Diabetes pathogenesis: thrombin-activatable fibrinolysis inhibitor implicated in vascular damage," in *Diabetes Week* (Atlanta), 18.

Yoshii, S. R., and Mizushima, N. (2017). Monitoring and measuring autophagy. *Int. J. Mol. Sci.* 18:1865. doi: 10.3390/ijms1809 1865

Zinman, B. (2003). *Pathways Leading to Diabetic Microvascular Complications and the Latest Therapies CME.* Available online at: http://www.medscape.com/viewprogram/2636?src=search (accessed November 29, 2020).

13

Epigenetic Regulation of Adipogenesis in Development of Metabolic Syndrome

Richa Pant[1], Priyanka Firmal[1†], Vibhuti Kumar Shah[1†], Aftab Alam[2†] and Samit Chattopadhyay[1,3*]

[1] National Centre for Cell Science, SP Pune University Campus, Pune, India, [2] Roswell Park Comprehensive Cancer Center, Buffalo, NY, United States, [3] Department of Biological Sciences, BITS Pilani, Goa, India

*Correspondence:
Samit Chattopadhyay
samitc@goa.bits-pilani.ac.in;
samitchatterji@yahoo.com;
samit@iicb.res.in

† These authors have contributed
equally to this work

Obesity is one of the biggest public health concerns identified by an increase in adipose tissue mass as a result of adipocyte hypertrophy and hyperplasia. Pertaining to the importance of adipose tissue in various biological processes, any alteration in its function results in impaired metabolic health. In this review, we discuss how adipose tissue maintains the metabolic health through secretion of various adipokines and inflammatory mediators and how its dysfunction leads to the development of severe metabolic disorders and influences cancer progression. Impairment in the adipocyte function occurs due to individuals' genetics and/or environmental factor(s) that largely affect the epigenetic profile leading to altered gene expression and onset of obesity in adults. Moreover, several crucial aspects of adipose biology, including the regulation of different transcription factors, are controlled by epigenetic events. Therefore, understanding the intricacies of adipogenesis is crucial for recognizing its relevance in underlying disease conditions and identifying the therapeutic interventions for obesity and metabolic syndrome.

Keywords: obesity, adipogenesis, insulin resistance, metabolic syndrome, transgenerational inheritance

INTRODUCTION

Obesity is defined as excessive or abnormal fat accumulation in the body which may impair the health of an individual. Body mass index (BMI), which is considered the most simple and useful index of weight-for-height in the entire world, provides only a rough estimate to categorize people with obesity in adult population[1]. Therefore, the concept of metabolically healthy obesity and metabolically unhealthy obesity is gaining attention as in addition to gaining abdominal weight, hormonal and metabolic profile of an individual also counts (Naukkarinen et al., 2014). The increasing incidences of obesity ignited a huge interest in understanding the process promoting efficient energy storage and curtailing the adverse metabolic consequences of obesity such as diabetes, hypertension, dyslipidemia, atherosclerosis and fatty liver diseases. The ability of adipocytes to effectively store lipids prevents the toxic lipid accumulation in other organs. In fact, adipose tissue can expand in response to excess lipid accumulation to maintain the energy homeostasis (Wang et al., 2013) but the capacity of adipose tissue to store fat or to expand in response to fat storage is limited. Once exceeded, lipids might spill into other

---

[1] https://www.cancer.gov/about-cancer/causes-prevention/risk/obesity/obesity-fact-sheet

organs that are not suitable for fat storage resulting in insulin resistance (IR) and other metabolic complications (Tan and Vidal-Puig, 2008). Alteration in fat mass also results in alteration in adipokine profile of an individual. Obesity is linked with an increase in leptin concentration and a decrease in adiponectin levels (Matsubara et al., 2002). In addition to these two prototype adipokines, many other factors are known to get altered in obesity. Obese state is also identified by an increased macrophage infiltration in the adipose tissue. These macrophages and other immune cells infiltrated in the adipose tissue are a source of TNF-α, IL-6, and other cytokines that links obesity with inflammation and IR (Weisberg et al., 2003). Altered immune response and adipokine secretion are also known to increase the risks of certain cancers such as breast, ovarian, kidney, endometrial, colorectal, etc. (see text footnote 1). Past few decades have shown some great advancement in understanding transcriptional and epigenetic regulation of adipogenesis. Peroxisome-proliferator activator receptor γ (PPARγ) and CCAAT/enhancer binding protein α (C/EBPα) are the two key transcription factors which regulates the adipocyte formation. They work in co-ordination with transcriptional co-activators and epigenetic regulators modulating the gene expression profiles during adipocyte differentiation (Madsen et al., 2014). Advancement in molecular biology techniques unfolded the key mechanisms of epigenomic regulation during adipogenesis and revealed the significance of histone modification, DNA methylation, and chromatin remodeling in adipocytes differentiation (Lee et al., 2019). These epigenetic changes are influenced by certain environmental factors such as energy-rich foods, changes in sleep cycle, sedentary lifestyle, medicated drugs and environmental chemicals that have potential to reprogram the epigenetic patterns and induce adiposity (Gangwisch et al., 2005; McAllister et al., 2009). The environment-epigenetic interaction also results in transgenerational and lifestyle-induced obesity (Youngson and Morris, 2013). Moreover, exposure to high fat diet and environmental toxins *in utero* may affect the metabolic outcomes in future generations through epigenetic transgenerational inheritance of obesity (Vandegehuchte et al., 2010; Dunn and Bale, 2011).

This review focuses on the interplay between adipose tissue function, adipokines, systemic inflammatory profile and metabolic health. We have also discussed the transcriptional and epigenetic regulators involved in adipogenesis and their interaction with environment responsible for transgenerational inheritance of the disease. Understanding the molecular mechanism of adipogenesis and the complexities associated with it will help in finding the plausible therapeutic approaches for treatment of obesity.

ADIPOSE TISSUE: WHITE, BROWN AND MORE

Adipose tissue is a loose connective tissue which is critical in regulating energy metabolism, i.e., energy storage and expenditure. Adipocytes or the fat cells contribute around 35–70% of adipose tissue mass in an adult human. Besides

adipocytes, some other cell types like macrophages, blood cells, fibroblasts, endothelial cells, etc., are also present in the adipose tissue (Frühbeck, 2008). Morphologically, adipose tissue can be classified into three types: white, brown and beige. White adipose tissue (WAT) is mostly composed of unilocular adipocytes and its key function is to store surplus energy as triglycerides during excess nutrient condition. The stored triglycerides are utilized for energy generation under energy deficit conditions such as fasting, exercise or prolonged food deprivation (Li et al., 1993; Blüher, 2013). On the other hand, brown adipose tissue (BAT) consists of mitochondria-rich multilocular adipocytes. The main function of brown adipose tissue is to dissipate energy in the form of heat through mitochondrial uncoupling upon β-adrenergic stimulation (Foster and Frydman, 1979). BAT was formerly believed to have functional role in rodents, hibernating mammals, and partly in human infants but recently, adult humans have shown functional BAT upon mild cold exposure and activation of sympathetic nervous system (Cypess et al., 2013, 2015). β3-adrenergic receptor (β3-AR) agonist can stimulate human BAT thermogenesis and help in treatment of obesity and metabolic diseases (Cypess et al., 2015). A clinical trial of β3-AR agonist, mirabegron, stimulated BAT metabolic activity and increased WAT lipolysis in human subjects (Baskin et al., 2018). In addition to white and brown fat, there also exists a third type known as beige/brite fat. As the name implies, brite fat is the accumulation of brown adipocytes within the white fat depots. Beige cells have the unique ability to shift between energy storage and energy expenditure phenotype (Wu et al., 2012). A study by Zhang et al. demonstrated that embryo-derived white adipose stem cells (eWAsc) have excellent beige adipogenic potential. The study showed potential in widening the research on human adipocytes (Zhang et al., 2019). There also exists a functional relationship between angiogenesis and brite/beige adipocyte development. The pro-angiogenic conditions helps in proliferation of beige/brite adipocytes and transplantation of human brite adipocytes improves the systemic glucose homeostasis in diet induced obesity (DIO) mice model. Since brite adipocytes were found to enhance glucose homeostasis, they could be implied to have potential therapeutic benefits (Min et al., 2016).

Adipocytes have an astonishing plastic property, i.e., white adipocytes can trans-differentiate to brown adipocytes. In fact, during pregnancy and lactation, white adipocytes specific to mammary gland convert reversibly to milk producing epithelial cells (also called pink adipocytes because they appear pink at macroscopic level) and brown adipocytes trans-differentiate to myoepithelial cells (cells of alveolar glands) (**Figure 1**). Once the lactation period is over, pink adipocytes convert back to white and brown adipocytes (Morroni et al., 2004; Giordano et al., 2014).

The fat cells (adipocytes) develop from adipocyte precursor cells (pre-adipocytes) in a process called adipogenesis which occurs throughout the lifespan of an organism (Billon et al., 2007). The differentiation of pre-adipocytes to lipid-laden adipocytes is widely studied *in vitro*. Amongst all the studied cell lines, the most widely used ones which provide the important insights in regulating late steps of adipocyte development are 3T3-L1 and 3T3-F422A (Green and Meuth, 1974;

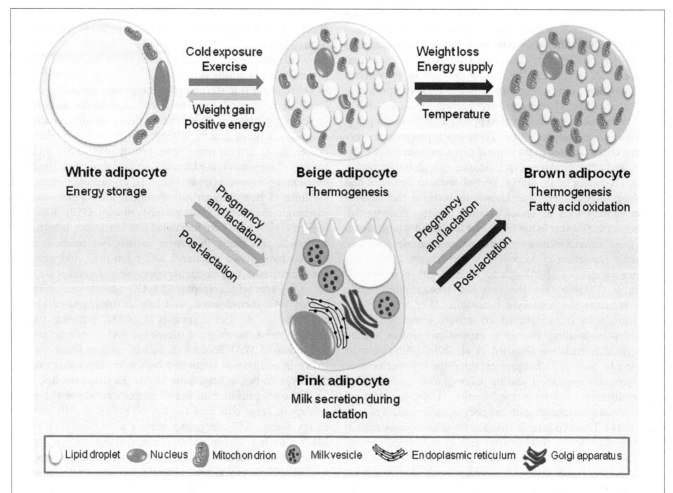

FIGURE 1 | Adipocytes have remarkable plastic properties. In usual scenario adipose tissue consists of white, brown and occasional beige adipocytes. The main function of white adipocytes is to store lipids to meet the metabolic requirements of the body while brown adipocytes are required for thermogenesis. Beige adipocytes have the ability to switch between energy storage and expenditure. However, during certain conditions like cold exposure or strenuous exercise, white adipocytes trans-differentiates to beige or brown adipocytes while during the state of positive energy when there is lack of lipid storage, brown/beige adipocytes can be converted back to white adipocytes to increase the energy stores. During pregnancy and lactation, subcutaneous white adipocytes of the breast tissue convert to pink adipocytes which are basically the milk secreting glands formed by lipid-rich elements and brown adipocytes trans-differentiate to myoepithelial cells of mammary glands. All these conversions are reversible, i.e., post-lactation, pink adipocytes convert back to white and brown adipocytes.

Green and Kehinde, 1975). Mouse embryonic stem cells (mESCs) also provide an alternate system for understanding early stages of adipogenesis (Billon et al., 2007). By using these biological tools, researchers have been able to recognize the key transcription factors involved in adipogenesis and many are still in the process of being identified.

ADIPOSE TISSUE DYSFUNCTION IN OBESITY AND METABOLIC DISEASES

Obesity is defined as excessive fat accumulation that may impair the health and wellbeing of an individual. Sedentary lifestyle, urbanization, easy affordability and accessibility to high calorie food may account for excess energy intake and weight gain within the population (Afshin et al., 2017). Apart from some parts of sub-Saharan Africa and Asia, the number of people with obesity surpasses the number of people who are underweight. Globally, this accounts for more deaths from obesity than malnutrition[2]. The development of obesity not only depends upon the balance between energy intake and expenditure but also on the balance between WAT and BAT. Unhealthy expansion of WAT is one of the major culprits contributing to obesity-associated metabolic complications.

White adipose tissue accounts for 5–50% of human body weight and has a central role in energy homeostasis (Kajimura, 2017). Anatomically, WAT can be categorized as visceral adipose tissue or VAT (intra-abdominal, surrounding the internal organs) and sub-cutaneous adipose tissue or SAT (under the skin). Amongst the two types, visceral fat is said to be strongly associated with increased metabolic risk than subcutaneous fat (Hayashi et al., 2008). Additionally, the associated risk factor

---

[2]https://www.who.int/news-room/fact-sheets/detail/obesity-and-overweight

is more pronounced in women than men (Fox et al., 2007). It has been observed that in 3D adipocyte-ECM culture, SAT ECM rescued the defects in glucose uptake and adipogenesis specific gene regulation in VAT adipocytes while VAT ECM impaired the adipocyte function in SAT adipocytes. This suggests the importance of extracellular matrix-adipocyte crosstalk in regulation of depot-specific adipocyte function in murine obesity and metabolic diseases (Strieder-Barboza et al., 2020).

In majority of lean and healthy individuals, WAT is mostly restricted to subcutaneous depots but in individuals with obese/overweight phenotype, WAT mass can expand ectopically in areas other than their specific depots as a result of lipodystrophy (Chait and den Hartigh, 2020). Lipodystrophy is a heterogenous group of disorder characterized by abnormal adipose tissue distribution. It can be congenital or acquired and is linked with the development of IR and related co-morbidities like type 2 diabetes (T2D), hyperglycemia, hyperlipidemia, non-alcoholic fatty liver disease (NAFLD), auto-immune hepatitis or viral hepatitis in case of human immunodeficiency virus (HIV)-associated lipodystrophy (Polyzos et al., 2019). There are essentially two mechanisms to explain the development of metabolic syndrome resulting from obesity: (a) accumulation of fat in liver and muscle or other cells of the body in addition to adipose tissue resulting in IR in these organs (Petersen and Shulman, 2006) and (b) release of adipokines and cytokines from the dysfunctional adipocytes (Saltiel, 2001; Scherer, 2006). In healthy states, these adipokines and cytokines maintain the metabolic homeostasis but in obesity, the hypertrophic adipocytes and the resident immune cells hasten the pro-inflammatory profile with altered secretion of these endocrine factors thereby contributing to metabolic diseases (Scheja and Heeren, 2019). However, not all individuals with obesity develop the associated metabolic problems. The sub-group of insulin-sensitive individuals with obesity showing normal hormonal and metabolic profiles despite of their BMIs in obese category (i.e., ≥ 30 kg/m^2) are classified as having "metabolically healthy obesity" (MHO) (Naukkarinen et al., 2014). These individuals are different from those having "metabolically unhealthy obesity" (MUHO) who are characterized by accumulation of intra-abdominal fat in visceral depots (central obesity), IR, pre-disposition to diabetes and other metabolic diseases (Karelis et al., 2005; Blüher, 2010). Individuals with MHO are defined as having abdominal obesity with waist circumference >88 cm in women and >102 cm in men. They might not develop any of the risk factors such as increased fasting plasma glucose, high triglycerides, low HDL cholesterol and high blood pressure, two or more of which are observed commonly in MUHO (Grundy et al., 2005; Janiszewski and Ross, 2010).

In mice and rat models, surgical removal of visceral fat pads using lipectomy improved the insulin sensitivity, longevity and decreased tumor proliferation (Gabriely et al., 2002; Lu et al., 2012). Not only in rodent models but adipose tissue removal from the mesentery of baboons (having insulin resistance and obese phenotype) also resulted in reversal of IR and significant weight loss (Andrew et al., 2018). These studies suggest the use of lipectomy as a potential clinical tool to ameliorate obesity associated co-morbidities. In summary, adipose tissue health is utmost important for maintaining the metabolic health of an individual. Any perturbance in adipose tissue function may result in long term health ailments.

ALTERED ADIPOKINE PRODUCTION AND THE RISK OF DEVELOPMENT OF METABOLIC DISORDERS

Adipose tissue is a metabolically active endocrine organ that secretes a range of adipokines and hormones which can have different functions in human body (Derosa et al., 2020). One of the first discoveries that recognized the role of adipose tissue as an endocrine organ was the positional cloning of obese (ob) gene and detection of its 16-KDa protein product leptin (Zhang et al., 1994). Subsequent studies revealed that daily administration of recombinant OB protein to ob/ob mice lowered their food intake, body fat percentage and serum concentration of glucose and insulin. Moreover, the energy expenditure and metabolic rate of these mice were also increased with this treatment, suggesting that OB protein stabilizes the metabolic status of ob/ob mice (Campfield et al., 1995; Halaas et al., 1995; Pelleymounter et al., 1995). Since then, leptin is known to regulate whole body metabolism through inhibiting food intake, restoring euglycemia and stimulating energy expenditure. In 2014, AstraZeneca's myalept/metreleptin (recombinant human leptin) was approved by the United States Food and Drug Administration to treat generalized lipodystrophy ([3]identifier: NCT00677313) (Ajluni et al., 2016). Recently, in a non-randomized crossover group study including patients with lipodystrophy, metreleptin was shown to improve insulin sensitivity and decrease circulating and hepatic triglycerides irrespective of their food intake (Brown et al., 2018). Another important protein, adiponectin, was originally described in 1995 as a 30 KDa secretory protein 'Acrp30' that was exclusively made in adipocytes (Scherer et al., 1995). Adiponectin functions to increase the insulin sensitivity, fatty acid oxidation and energy expenditure along with reduction in glucose production by liver (Galic et al., 2010). Adiponectin is also known to inhibit breast cancer growth by induction of cytotoxic autophagy in breast cancer cells through activation of AMPK-ULK1 axis (Chung et al., 2017). Altered adipokine production is usually associated with the risk of development of metabolic disorders. High levels of resistin and low levels of adiponectin could be predictive of future diabetic condition in people with obesity (Derosa et al., 2020). Apart from these two proteins, many different adipokines have been described in recent times that control the energy metabolism (Galic et al., 2010). An observational trial confirmed that people with obesity have higher levels of leptin, adipsin, retinol binding protein-4 (RBP-4), IL-6, high sensitivity-C reactive protein (Hs-CRP) and lower levels of adiponectin and visfatin as compared to lean people (Derosa et al., 2013). Recently, S100A4 was identified as a novel adipokine associated with IR and subcutaneous WAT inflammation/adipocytes hypertrophy irrespective of BMI although its significance as a circulating marker for dysfunctional

---

[3]https://clinicaltrials.gov/

WAT and IR is yet to be established (Arner et al., 2018). A newly discovered adipokine, asprosin, promoted the hepatic glucose release and inhibition of its activity could be used as an approach to counteract hyperinsulinism associated with metabolic disorders (Romere et al., 2016). Apelin is another adipokine which improves insulin sensitivity in humans and could be considered as a target for new therapeutic strategies to combat IR in patients with T2D (Gourdy et al., 2018). TGF-β2 is an exercise/lactate induced adipokine which improves the glucose tolerance and insulin sensitivity. HFD-fed mice treated with recombinant TGF-β2 showed reduced WAT inflammation and fat mass indicating the importance of exercise training on glucose and lipid metabolism (Takahashi et al., 2019).

Obesity related adipokines also play a role in etiology of different cancers. A decrease in adiponectin concentration and a corresponding increase in concentration of leptin, resistin, visfatin, IL-6, IL-8, and TNF-α are linked with progression of breast cancer (Gui et al., 2017). Moreover, decreased expression of adiponectin receptor is associated with the metastasis of human endometrioid adenocarcinoma (Yamauchi et al., 2012). Exposure of human breast cancer cell line MCF-7 to recombinant adiponectin resulted in AMPK activation and MAPK inactivation thereby inhibiting cell cycle progression. This indicates that adiponectin mediates anti-proliferative response in breast cancer cells (Dieudonne et al., 2006). Apart from adiponectin, nearly all the other adipokines exhibit pro-inflammatory and proliferative activities in cancer progression. For example resistin induces prostate cancer progression through activation of PI3K signaling pathway (Kim et al., 2011). Resistin also stimulates the expression of stromal cell-derived factor-1 (SDF-1) by activating p38 MAPK/NF-κB signaling pathway in human gastric carcinoma cells (Hsieh et al., 2014). A meta-analysis study revealed that serum leptin profile plays an important role in pathogenesis of breast cancer (Gu et al., 2019). Leptin crosstalks with various molecular mediators of the obesity such as VEGF, estrogen, IGF-1, insulin and inflammatory cytokines. Hyperactive leptin signaling potentiates these molecular mediators and leads to the activation of various oncogenic pathways resulting in enhanced proliferation and invasion of cancer cells (Saxena and Sharma, 2013). Accumulating evidences suggest that leptin induces EMT in cancer cells via different molecular pathways including JAK/STAT pathway, β-catenin activation via Akt/GSK3 and MTA/Wnt1 pathway, and activation of IL-8 via PI3K/Akt dependent pathway (Yan et al., 2012; Wang L. et al., 2015; Mullen and Gonzalez-Perez, 2016). Upregulation of pyruvate kinase muscle isozyme 2 (PKM2) along with activation of PI3K/AKT signaling can also be regarded as the potential candidate for breast cancer therapy (Wei et al., 2016). A recent research demonstrated that leptin results in the secretion of MMP2 and MMP9 in mammary epithelial cells via Src and FAK-dependent pathways (Olea-Flores et al., 2019). Leptin is also known to promote ovarian cancer invasion by inducing MMP7 expression through activation of ERK and JNK pathways (Ghasemi et al., 2018). The cell signaling events triggered by different adipokines are illustrated in **Figure 2**.

Leptin is often found to be associated with drug resistance. Tumor leptin expression in gastro-oesophageal adenocarcinomas

is associated with resistance to cytotoxic chemotherapy (Bain et al., 2014). Additionally, leptin receptor-positive glioblastoma cells were found to be temozolomide (TMZ)-resistant (Han et al., 2013). Also, the high circulating leptin concentration could counteract cisplatin-induced cytotoxicity in breast cancer cells (Nadal-Serrano et al., 2015). Therefore, the use of non-toxic leptin antagonists that interferes with leptin signaling could serve as a novel mechanism to target leptin-induced cancers (Candelaria et al., 2017).

In addition to WAT, recent studies also reported the contribution of BAT to release secretory molecules called 'batokines' which make BAT functionally similar to an endocrine organ. Fibroblast growth factor 21 (FGF21), IL-6, neuregulin-4 (NRG-4), and bone morphogenetic protein-8b (BMP8b) are amongst the first few batokines to be identified. The BAT-released endocrine factors can target peripheral tissues and affect systemic metabolism by interacting with central nervous system (Burýsek and Houstek, 1997; Hondares et al., 2011; Whittle et al., 2012; Wang et al., 2014). Peptidase M20 domain containing 1 (PM20D1) and Slit2 are two newly identified batokines that improves glucose homeostasis as well as regulate thermogenesis which might be used for the treatment of obesity and obesity associated metabolic disorders (Long et al., 2016; Svensson et al., 2016). In summary, adipokine/batokine-centered therapeutic strategies could pave the way for treatment of metabolic diseases and cancers.

INFLAMMATORY MEDIATORS IN OBESITY

Development of chronic low grade systemic inflammation is one of the primary consequences of obesity (Bekkering et al., 2020). High fat diet induces the expression of pro-inflammatory cytokines and inflammatory responsive proteins in the hypothalamus (an important part of brain responsible for controlling hunger and thermogenesis). Leptin and insulin provide signals to specific neurons in the hypothalamus to report about the energy stocks in response to high fat diet. This signaling is accompanied by an increased expression of c-Jun N-terminal kinase (JNK) and nuclear factor-κB (NF-κB) and thereby inducing IR in the hypothalamus (De Souza et al., 2005). Moreover, depletion of medio-basal hypothalamus (MBH) in mice resulted in enhanced leptin signaling and reduced food intake, signifying the importance of inflammation in hypothalamus-related weight gain (Valdearcos et al., 2014). In addition to this, consumption of HFD is accompanied by unfavorable changes in gut microbiota (a decrease in ratio of Firmicutes to Bacteroidetes), metabolic profile of feces and plasma proinflammatory factors (PGE_2 and TXB_2) which adversely affect the health of young adults (Wan et al., 2019).

In healthy and lean individuals, the resident immune cells of adipose tissue are indispensable for its function but in individuals with obesity, inflammation of adipose tissue is one of the major contributors to metabolic dysfunction including systemic IR and/or glucose intolerance. The resident cells of both innate and

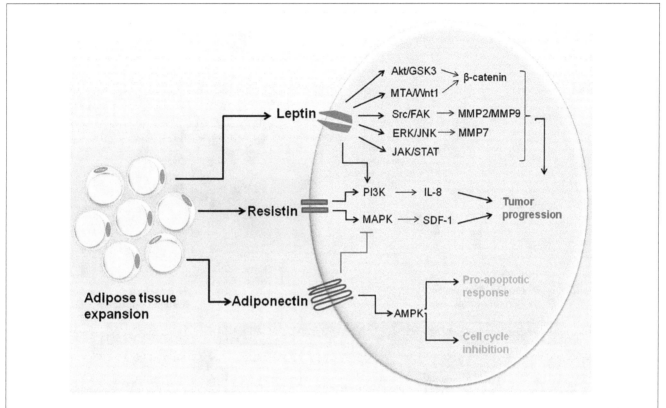

FIGURE 2 | Cell signaling events triggered by altered adipokine production during obesity. Expansion of adipose tissue in obese condition leads to altered adipokine production. High concentration of leptin and resistin results in the activation of different signaling pathways within the cell (Akt/GSK3, MTA/Wnt1, Src/FAK, ERK/JNK, JAK/STAT, PI3K, and MAPK). These signaling pathways ultimately lead to cancer cell invasion and metastasis. On the other hand, high adiponectin concentration leads to MAPK inhibition and AMPK inactivation which is responsible for its pro-apototic and anti-tumoral activities.

adaptive immune system in the adipose tissue take part in this process (**Figure 3**) and are described below.

Innate Immunity

Initial evidence to understand the connection between obesity and inflammation came from the finding that IR in the adipocytes is induced by macrophages (Pekala et al., 1983). Later, tumor necrosis factor-α (TNF-α) was identified as the molecule which mediated obesity-linked IR (Hotamisligil et al., 1993). Adipose tissue macrophages (ATMs) from lean mice show a different profile than ATMs of mice with obese phenotype. DIO shifts the activation state of ATMs from M2 anti-inflammatory state to M1 pro-inflammatory state exemplified by an increased expression of genes encoding TNF-α and NOS-2, which contribute to pathophysiological repercussions of obesity (Lumeng et al., 2007). Studies suggest that MCP-1/CCR2 axis is responsible for adipose tissue inflammation and development of obesity and IR (Kanda, 2006; Weisberg et al., 2006). Factors secreted from ATMs blocks the insulin action in adipocytes by down-regulating IRS-1 and GLUT4. Additionally, TNF-α neutralizing antibodies could partially reverse the IR induced by macrophage- conditioned media *in vitro* (Lumeng et al., 2007). ATMs isolated from mice and humans with obese phenotype have markers for increased *de novo* synthesis of phosphotidylcholine (PC) biosynthesis.

Deletion of phosphocholine cytidylyltransferase A (a rate-limiting enzyme in *de novo* PC synthesis) in a macrophage-specific manner improved adipose tissue inflammation and IR (Petkevicius et al., 2019). Additionally, Galectin-3 (Gal-3), a lectin secreted by macrophages, has been found to directly bind to insulin receptor and inhibit the downstream insulin signaling. Gal-3 could be used as an important target for treatment of IR as its inhibition in mice improved insulin sensitivity and glucose tolerance (Li P. et al., 2016). Latest studies have also started to identify epigenomic alterations in macrophages that determine their sensitivity upon metabolic stress induced by obesity. A co-repressor complex containing G protein pathway suppressor 2 (GPS2) was identified as one such epigenomic modifier whose function and expression in macrophages is dependent on the disease state (Fan et al., 2016). Moreover, activation of inflammasome (a protein complex facilitating maturation of pro-inflammatory cytokines IL-1β and 1L-18 by caspase-1 mediated cleavage) is crucial for impairment of insulin signaling in target tissues. It is observed that the presence of free fatty acids in HFD triggers the activation of NLRP3-ASC inflammasome in macrophages by AMPK autophagy-ROS signaling pathway resulting in impaired insulin signaling (Wen et al., 2011). The role of melatonin in alleviating inflammasome-induced pyroptosis by blocking NF-κB/gasdermin D (GSDMD) signal in adipose tissue of mice has also been observed (Liu et al., 2017). Receptor

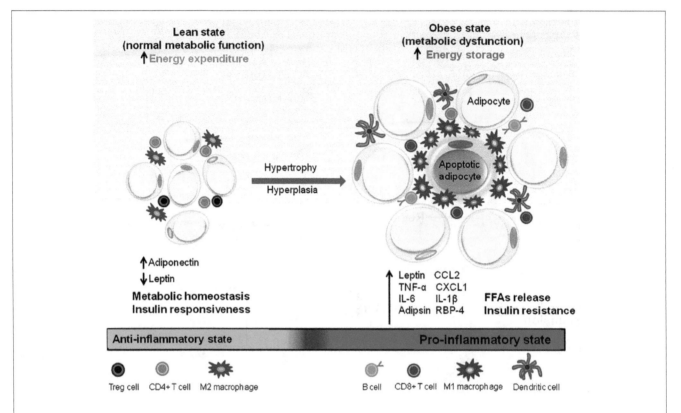

FIGURE 3 | Immune cell distribution in lean and obese state. In lean adipose tissue with normal metabolic function, M2 macrophages are uniformly distributed throughout the tissue. The lean AT milieu also consists of CD4+ T cells and Treg cells having anti-inflammatory properties. Adiponectin to leptin ratio is high which contributes to the insulin responsive state of the adipocytes. In obese state, macrophages switch to M1 type which forms a crown like structure (CLS) around the adipocytes. Adipocyte hypertrophy results in the rupture of adipocytes and releases FFAs. In addition to M1 macrophages, obese state is also associated with an increase in CD8+ T cells, dendritic cells and IgG antibody producing B cells responsible for pathogenic state of AT. Obesity is also associated with abnormal adipokine profile, i.e., increased release pro-inflammatory adipokines. Aberrant secretion of adipokines (leptin, IL-6, adipsin, RBP-4, and IL-1β), chemokines (CCL2 and CXCL1) and macrophage factors (TNF-α) causes metabolic dysfunction and insulin resistance.

for advanced glycation end products (RAGE), which is highly expressed in monocytes and macrophages and its ligand, high mobility group box 1 (HMGB1), are also found to be associated with development of obesity. Blockage of RAGE or neutralization of HMGB1 prevented HFD induced weight gain and improved glucose tolerance in mice model (Song et al., 2014; Montes et al., 2015). Also, the depletion of visceral adipose tissue macrophage from mice downregulated the genes involved in gluconeogenesis and lipogenesis which conferred protection from HFD induced obesity, IR and hepatic steatosis (Bu et al., 2013).

HFD is also reported to change the gut microbiome and cause dysbiosis which is considered one of the main factors contributing to colorectal cancer (CRC) susceptibility. Activation of MCP-1/CCR2 axis mediated by HFD-induced dysbiosis accelerated the incidences of advanced colorectal neoplasia (Liu et al., 2020). Specific gut bacteria also serve as a source of lipopolysaccharide (LPS) and increase the intestinal permeability along with the increase in systemic concentration of TNF-α and IL-6 in patients with T2D (Jayashree et al., 2014). A recent study demonstrated the role of TLR4 in LPS and saturated fatty acid mediated adipocytes dysfunction by stimulating inflammatory changes in adipocytes and macrophages (McKernan et al., 2020).

In addition to macrophages, other cells of innate immune system such as dendritic cells, mast cells, and neutrophils also contribute to development of obesity and IR. Accumulation of plasmacytoid DCs (pDCs) during obesity induces AT inflammation and T2D through their IFN-producing ability. IFNAR$^{-/-}$ mice and the mice lacking pDCs failed to develop obesity and other metabolic complication upon feeding with HFD (Hannibal et al., 2017). Recently, a gene ontology (GO) analysis identified the association of obesity with increased percentage and gene activation of neutrophils in young African-American male population (Xu et al., 2015). Additionally, genetic deficiency or pharmacological stabilization of mast cells was found to ameliorate glucose homeostasis as well as weight gain due to obesity (Liu et al., 2009). However, a novel study in human subjects identified the role of mast cells in cold-induced subcutaneous WAT beiging independent of BMI. This adipose beiging was attributed to release of histamine during mast cell degranulation (Finlin et al., 2019).

In total, macrophages along with other cells of innate immune system contribute in the development of obesity and insulin resistance.

Adaptive Immunity

While most of the studies on obesity, inflammation and IR are majorly directed toward the role of macrophages, recent investigations points to the significant participation of adaptive immune system in regulating obesity associated metabolic anomalies (Nishimura et al., 2009). A study reported that in obese state, CD8$^+$ T cells helped in macrophage recruitment and caused adipose tissue inflammation. Moreover, genetic or immunological depletion of CD8$^+$ T cells lowered the macrophage infiltration and adipose tissue inflammation, thereby ameliorated systemic IR. On the contrary, adoptive transfer of CD8$^+$ T cells to CD8-deficient mice exacerbated AT inflammation (Nishimura et al., 2009). Mice with obese phenotype and lacking αβ T cell (TCRb−/− mice) exhibited reduced inflammation of adipose tissue and skeletal muscle suggesting the important role of T_H1 cells in regulating inflammation and IR in obesity (Khan et al., 2014). Recently, a unique population of regulatory T cells, i.e., CD4$^+$Foxp3$^+$ T_{reg} cells, having anti-inflammatory properties were found to be highly enriched in visceral fat of mice with lean phenotype (Feuerer et al., 2009) and PPARγ was the central molecular initiator for accumulation and functioning of T_{reg} cells (Cipolletta et al., 2012). In addition to T cells, B cells also promote IR through activation of proinflammatory macrophages, T cells and production of pathogenic IgG antibodies. Depletion of B cells using anti-CD20 mAb in early stage of the disease can have therapeutic benefits in managing IR and associated co-morbidities (Winer et al., 2011). Also, B-cell null mice were found to be protected from obesity and systemic inflammation and had an increased ratio of anti-inflammatory regulatory T cells (DeFuria et al., 2013).

Altogether, these studies highlight the importance of both arms of immune system in adipose tissue inflammation and systemic IR in obese condition. Understanding the relationship between adipose tissue and immune cells could provide therapeutic targets for treating obesity and IR in future.

TRANSCRIPTIONAL REGULATION OF ADIPOCYTE DIFFERENTIATION

Multistage differentiation of pre-adipocytes or mesenchymal stem cells to adipocytes involves numerous transcription factors. The expression of these wide ranges of transcription factors regulates the differentiation process either positively or negatively. The core factors, PPARγ and C/EBP-α, along with several other proteins regulate the expansion of pre-adipocytes and thereby formation of lipid droplets in mature adipocytes (**Figure 4**; Herrera et al., 1989; Wu et al., 1999; Birsoy et al., 2008).

Positive Regulators of Adipogenesis
PPARγ and C/EBPs

PPARγ and C/EBPα are considered as the key regulators of adipogenesis that are vital for adipocyte differentiation both *in vitro* and *in vivo* (Rosen et al., 1999; Linhart et al., 2001). The initial stages of adipocyte differentiation require C/EBPβ and C/EBPδ that triggers the mitotic cell division and

clonal expansion (Tang et al., 2003). During the cell cycle progression from G1 to S phase, C/EBPβ is hyper-phosphorylated which leads to the activation GSK-3β and MAPK followed by mitotic division (Tang et al., 2005). Activation of GSK-3β and MAPK induces the transcription of PPARγ and C/EBPα for terminal differentiation of adipocytes. Although C/EBPα is an essential factor for adipocyte differentiation but it requires the presence of PPARγ to establish the adipogenic phenotype. In PPARγ$^{−/−}$ fibroblasts, C/EBPα was unable to induce any lipid accumulation whereas PPARγ could induce adipogenesis in C/EBPα$^{−/−}$ fibroblasts (Rosen et al., 2002). However, the complexity of adipogenesis *in vivo* is quite different and is temporally regulated. While C/EBPα is important for all white adipogenic requirement of an adult, the terminal adipogenesis in an embryo is completely independent of C/EBPα but requires PPARγ (Wang Q.A. et al., 2015). Although important, the presence of C/EBPα is not essential for adipocytes survival in adult stage (Wang Q.A. et al., 2015). The significance of PPARγ was also observed in *Pparg* null mice wherein these mice eventually developed diabetic nephropathy (Toffoli et al., 2017). The loss-of-function mutations in human *PPARG* results in the development of familial partial lipodystrophy type 3 (FPLD3) and other serious metabolic anomalies. Recently, a study reported that patients with FPLD3, harboring Arg308Pro (R308P) and Ala261Glu (A261E) PPARγ variants responded satisfactorily to synthetic PPARγ agonists (Agostini et al., 2018). Additionally, the systemic deletion of PPARγ in mice caused total lipoatrophy accompanied by organomegaly and hypermetabolism. *Pparg$^{Δ/Δ}$* mice also developed severe T2D and showed metabolic inflexibility (Gilardi et al., 2019). Altogether, the experimental data from different studies suggest that PPARγ is the master regulator of adipogenesis and the main role of C/EBPα is to maintain the expression of PPARγ.

Zinc Finger Proteins (ZFPs)

The family of ZFPs is known to regulate various biological functions and some of the ZFPs that play significant role in adipocyte differentiation are also well elucidated. Adipogenic stimulus results in increased expression of ZFP423 at both transcript and protein level in 3T3-L1 cells. Over expression of ZFP423 in non adipogenic cell line (NIH-3T3) resulted in their adipogenic differentiation via robust activation of PPARγ (Gupta et al., 2010). Furthermore, the overexpression of ZFP423 in low adipogenic cells resulted in increased competence of the cells to differentiate into mature adipocytes. However, the knockdown of ZFP423 in high adipogenic cells prevented their adipogenic differentiation. This differential regulation of ZFP423 in low and high adipogenic cells was found to be associated with DNA methylation of its promoter (Huang et al., 2012). Moreover, the recruitment of ZFP30 and its co-activator KRAB-associated protein 1 (KAP1) on PPARγ2 enhancer activates its expression and thus promotes adipogenesis (Chen et al., 2019).

Many other transcription factors like Sterol regulatory element-binding protein 1 (SREBP1), Cyclic AMP Response Element-Binding Protein (CREBP) and several proteins from Kruppel-like factor family (KLFs) like KLF4, KLF5, KLF9,

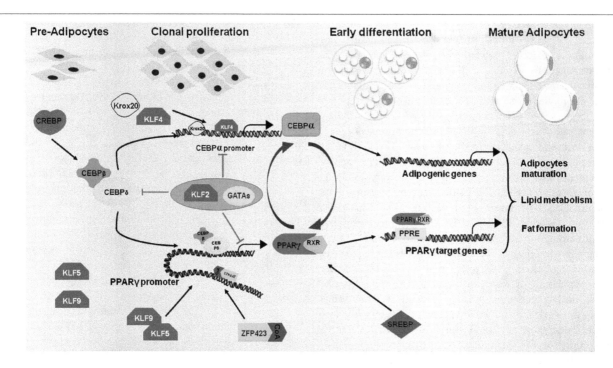

FIGURE 4 | Cascade of transcription factors in adipocyte differentiation. Many transcription factors act as positive regulators that express at different stages of adipocyte differentiation (pre-adipocytes to mature adipocytes). The differentiation process initiates upon induction of cells with adipogenic cocktail which helps in activation of certain transcription factors like CREBP, KLF4, 5, and 9, and CEBPβ/δ. CEBPβ and CEBPδ triggers the second wave of adipogenesis by activating PPARγ, CEBPα and SREBP. The PPAR proteins dimerizes with retinoic X receptor (RXR) for interaction with target promoters containing PPAR-response elements. PPARγ and CEBPα are the key proteins that targets the essential genes required for adipogenesis. To regulate the process of adipogenesis, some transcription factors like KLF2 and GATA2/3 act as negative regulators and inhibits the expression of CEBPα and PPARγ by direct or indirect repression of the transcription cascade.

KLF15 positively regulate the adipocyte differentiation at various stages by binding to the promoter of either PPARγ or C/EBPs (Tontonoz et al., 1993; Zhang et al., 2004; Oishi et al., 2005; Birsoy et al., 2008). For example, overexpression of SREBP1 in adipocytes as well as in HepG2 cells can induce PPARγ transcript expression suggesting that SREBP1 enhances PPARγ expression (Fajas et al., 1999). Likewise, CREBP positively regulate the expression of C/EBPβ by interacting with its promoter (Zhang et al., 2004). While KLF5 and KLF9 are known to bind to PPARγ2 promoter, KLF4 binds to C/EBPβ promoter along with Krox20, thereby regulating its expression in early phase of adipogenesis (Oishi et al., 2005; Pei et al., 2011).

Negative Regulators of Adipogenesis

Various signaling pathways and transcription factors help in maintaining the expression of positive regulators. The intricate balance between the positive and negative regulators is required for the efficient and regulated conversion of pre-adipocytes to lipid loaded mature adipocytes. The absence of negative regulators or increased expression of positive regulators may result in obesity and related disorders. These transcription factors are potential targets to control obesity and metabolic disorders.

GATA-Binding Factors

These zinc finger proteins bind to various promoters to regulate the cellular development and differentiation. GATA2 and GATA3

are abundantly expressed in pre-adipocytes and their expression decreases during adipocyte differentiation (Tong et al., 2000). Constitutive expression of GATA2 and GATA3 results in their interaction with either C/EBPα or C/EBPβ thereby inhibiting their activity (Tong et al., 2005). In general, GATAs subdues the adipogenesis process by two pathways, i.e., by interaction with PPARγ promoter and by protein-protein interaction which hinders the expression of C/EBP protein (Tong et al., 2000, 2005). GATA protein works along with cofactor Friend of GATA (FOG) and C-terminal binding proteins (CTBPs). FOG and CTBP protein interact with GATA2 in pre-adipocytes and inhibits the terminal differentiation of adipocytes (Jack and Crossley, 2010). Downregulation of GATA2 led to the pathogenesis of diseases like aplastic anemia, which was reported to have elevated expression of PPARγ (Xu et al., 2009). A recent study described GATA3 as a target gene of KLF-7 which inhibits chicken adipogenesis (Sun et al., 2020). Altogether, the interaction of GATAs with numerous proteins at different stages of adipogenesis keeps the positive adipogenic regulators in check and maintains the metabolic homeostasis.

In addition to GATA- binding factors, several other proteins like Pref-1, SIRT1, HDAC9 and transcriptional modulator TAZ also negatively regulate the differentiation of adipocytes by inhibiting the positive regulators at different stages of adipogenesis (Moon et al., 2002; Kurtev et al., 2004; Hong et al., 2005; Chatterjee et al., 2011). In contrast to other KLFs, KLF-2 inhibits the differentiation of adipocytes by interaction with a consensus motif 5′-CNCCC-3′ present in PPARγ2 promoter, thus limiting its expression (Sen Banerjee et al., 2003).

EPIGENETIC REGULATION OF ADIPOGENESIS

There are numerous epigenetic events involved at specific stages of adipocyte differentiation that eventually decide the fate of adipogenesis. Post Translational Modifications (PTMs) of histones such as Histone acetyltransferases (HATs), Histone deacetylases (HDACs), Histone methyltransferases (HMTs), and Histone demethylases (HDMs) have been reported to be crucial in shaping the adipogenesis process (Lizcano et al., 2011; Okuno et al., 2013). Along with histone PTMs, DNA methylation, chromatin remodeling and several microRNAs (miRNAs) also guide the adipogenesis program (**Figure 5**; Salma et al., 2004; Sakamoto et al., 2008; Peng et al., 2013). This part of the review focuses on the role of epigenetic regulation that ultimately dictates the adipocyte differentiation in normal scenarios and during metabolic disorders.

Histone Modifications

The constantly varying histone modifications are responsible for controlling the expression of various regulators of adipogenesis process namely Pref-1, C/EBP(α/β), PPARγ2 and aP2 (Zhang et al., 2012). MLL3/MLL4 are the most important H3K4 methyltransferases that are known to prime the enhancer before their activation thereby determining the ultimate cell fate (Wang et al., 2016). MLL3/MLL4 and CBP/p300 are also known as the super enhancer epigenomic regulators and activators that control the chromatin landscaping during adipocyte differentiation (Lai et al., 2017). Additionally, the mutations associated with MLL2 are responsible for lowering glucose tolerance in mice that could result in T2D (Goldsworthy et al., 2013). Similarly, cases of congenital hyperinsulinemia were observed in human infants having mutated *MLL2* gene (Yap et al., 2019). A genome wide histone modification examination uncovered the histone modification pattern of H3 that is frequently associated with obesity and diabetes (Jufvas et al., 2013). A study conducted on hyperphagic (ob/ob) mice and in mice with DIO has shown an increase in the acetylation level of lysine (K9, K18) on histone H3 at the gene promoter of TNF α and CCL2 in the liver tissue (Mikula et al., 2014). Moreover, a decreased methylation pattern of histone H3 (H3K4me3) was observed under high Isocitrate Dehydrogenase 1– α-Ketoglutarate (IDH1–α-KG) conditions, thus regulating the brown adipocyte differentiation in mice (Kang et al., 2020). This could be used as a therapeutic target for various metabolic syndromes. In a recent experiment conducted on human VAT, enhanced H3K4me3 marks were observed on the promoter region of various genes that are involved in adipogenesis, lipid metabolism and inflammatory pathways (Castellano-Castillo et al., 2019a). There are various protein arginine methyltransferases (Prmts) that are involved in regulating the expression of numerous regulators of adipogenesis. Studies revealed that overexpression of Prmt5 eventually

promotes adipocyte differentiation by upregulating PPARγ2 gene expression via forming an immature Promoter-enhancer looping (LeBlanc et al., 2012; Leblanc et al., 2016). Whereas, Prmt6 acts as a negative regulator of adipogenesis and is known to repress the activity of PPARγ (Hwang et al., 2019). Unlike Prmt5 and Prmt6, knockdown and overexpression of Pmrt7 did not affect the adipocyte differentiation; hence not all Prmts are important for regulating adipogenesis (Imbalzano et al., 2013).

Differential expression of HDACs is known to be associated with various metabolic conditions. For example, a case control experiment conducted on women with normal weight and women with obesity, showed a differential expression of HDAC2/4/5/6 that could be associated with obesity and inflammatory reactions related to obesity (Shanaki et al., 2020). Also, mice lacking *Hdac9* or *Hdac11* gene were found to have an increased whole-body energy consumption which protected them against DIO (Chatterjee et al., 2014; Sun et al., 2018). Moreover, the alteration in class I HDAC activity has been shown to shift the white adipocytes phenotype toward brown-like phenotype by modifying the histone marks (Ferrari et al., 2020). In addition to other HDACs, Class III HDACs (Sirtuins) are also known to regulate the adipocyte differentiation. Studies involving HFD-fed, *Sirt1* knockout mice model showed an increase in adipose tissue mass by promoting PPARγ activity, indicating a negative correlation between Sirt1 and adipogenesis (Mayoral et al., 2015). Complete *Sirt7* knockout in mice resulted in reduction of white adipose tissue which indicates that Sirt7 is a positive regulator of adipocyte differentiation (Fang et al., 2017). Additionally, mutation in Sirt6 has been found to disturb the adipogenesis phenomenon, as Sirt6 is essential for regulating the mitotic clonal expansion in cells via suppressing the expression of Kinesis heavy chain isoform 5C (Chen et al., 2017). A study in human SAT and VAT has shown that reduced Sirt1 and Sirt2 expression was associated with increased visceral adipose stem cells differentiation ability (Perrini et al., 2020). Similarly, knockdown of Jumonji domain containing protein 6 (JMJD6), a histone arginine demethylase, results in reduced expression of PPARγ2 and C/EBPα both at transcript as well as post transcription level, thereby inhibiting adipocyte differentiation (Hu et al., 2015). Later, studies revealed that the positive regulation of adipogenesis by JMJD6 is independent of its catalytic domain and requires its AT-hook like domain to interact with other important adipogenesis regulators by acting as a scaffold protein for them (Reyes-Gutierrez et al., 2019).

Statins are DNA methylation inhibitors and are known to regulate blood cholesterol but recently they are also found to be associated with a high risk of causing T2D. Statin treatment tends to reduce the methylation pattern on HDAC9 promoter that results in a reduced expression of key regulators of adipogenesis (Khamis et al., 2020). Keeping in consideration all the information obtained from various studies, modification of histone marks appears to be a potential therapeutic target for addressing numerous metabolic disorders.

DNA Methylation

The DNA methyltransferase (DNMT) family comprises of five main enzymes which regulate the *de novo* DNA methylation

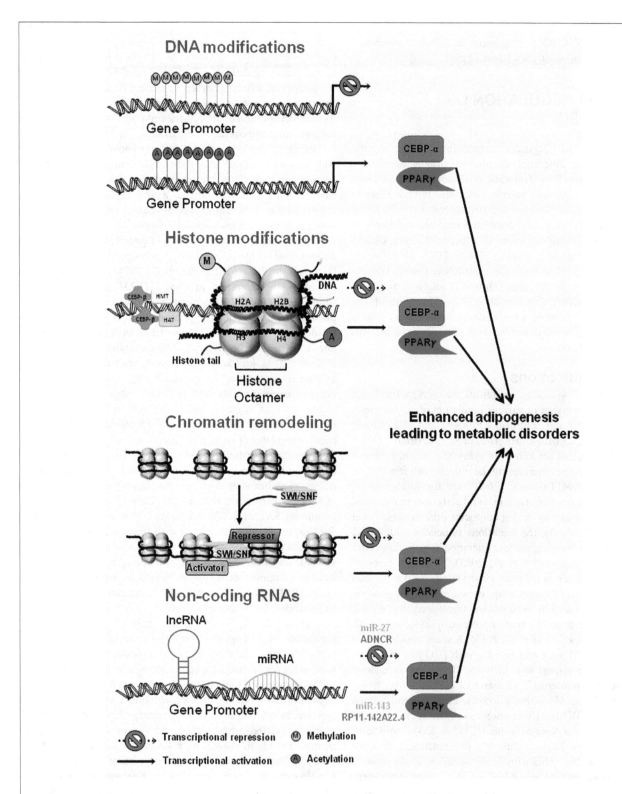

FIGURE 5 | Epigenetic modification of genes involved in adipogenesis. Methylation of gene promoters, that are necessary for adipogenesis, results in inactivation of the genes leading to reduced adipogenesis, whereas acetylation of promoter region brings about active adipocyte differentiation. Histone modification through HATs or HMTs that are recruited at the gene promoter by CEBPβ results in either activation or repression of the genes that are essential for adipogenesis. Chromatin remodeling complexes, such as SWI/SNF, tends to change the chromatin structure, thereby making the DNA either accessible or inaccessible for the transcription of adipogenesis specific genes to happen. Non-coding RNAs also govern the transcription of master regulators of adipogenesis by activating (miR-143, RP11-142A22.4) or repressing (miR-27, ADNCR) the transcription of key genes required for adipogenesis. Uncontrolled expression of genes involved in adipogenesis could ultimately lead to metabolic disorders.

(DNMT3A/3B) and adds methylation marks during replication (DNMT1) (Weber et al., 2007; Lyko, 2018). Earlier it was reported that reduced expression of DNMT1 by a novel miRNA (ACL-miR-148a) in 3T3-L1 cell line resulted in the promotion of adipogenesis by decreasing the DNA methylation marks on *PPARγ* (Londono Gentile et al., 2013). Later, it was revealed that DNA methylation has a biphasic effect on adipogenesis process where in the early stage, inhibition of methylation by 5-aza-dC promoted the adipocyte differentiation, while in late stage it inhibited the adipogenesis (Yang et al., 2016). Additionally, an altered global DNA methylation pattern during metabolic disorders has been observed on various genes involved in adipocyte differentiation, lipid metabolism, and inflammation (Castellano-Castillo et al., 2019b). A novel methylase enzyme, METTL4, responsible for the methylation of N^6- methyladenine (6ma) was found to promote adipogenesis in 3T3-L1 cells (Zhang Z. et al., 2020).

Modified cytosine(C) residue, 5-methylcytosine (5mC), established by DNMTs could easily be reverted to unmodified C by ten eleven translocation (TET) enzymes (Wu and Zhang, 2017). The mouse model having TET1/2 double knockout was found to have developmental abnormalities along with adipocyte differentiation defects because of the associated epigenetic instabilities (Wiehle et al., 2016). Recently global levels of 5mC were examined in the genome of 3T3-L1 cells. Among all the DNA demethylases, TET2 exhibited the major effect on adipocyte differentiation studies. Knockdown of *Tet2* resulted in enhanced adipogenesis and hence it is considered as an anti-adipogenic demethylase (Hou et al., 2020). Still a detailed gene knockout study in mice model is needed to further determine the involvement of TET1/2 in regulating adipogenesis.

Chromatin Dynamics and Remodeling

A dynamic chromatin is indispensable for an effective replication and transcription process to take place. Various ATP-dependent remodeling factors are required to carry out the chromatin remodeling. The SWItch/Sucrose Non Fermentable (SWI/SNF) is one such ATP-dependent family of chromatin remodeling complex which by utilizing brahma (BRM) or brahma-related bromodomain protein (BRG) makes the chromatin access easy through the rearrangement of nucleosomes (Kadoch and Crabtree, 2015). A study showed that involvement of C/EBP is essential in recruiting the SWI/SNF enzymes on PPARγ2 promoter in order to proceed with the adipogenesis process (Salma et al., 2004). Another study demonstrated that C/EBPα transactivation element III (TE-III) interacts with SWI/SNF chromatin remodeling complex to collaborate with TBP/TFIIB for adipocyte differentiation (Pedersen et al., 2001). Knockdown of Prmt5 has been found to decrease the binding of BRG1, a SWI/SNF ATPase that is required for activating PPARγ2. It eventually resulted in reduced adipogenesis because BRG1 failed to interact effectively with the PPARγ2 chromatin locus in the absence of Prmt5 (Leblanc et al., 2016). Although, the role of SWI/SNF for the activation of enhancers during cancer development has been widely studied (Nakayama et al., 2017), but its involvement in activating

adipogenesis related enhancers for effective gene expression is yet to be explored.

Non-coding RNAs

There are several non-coding (nc) RNAs, small nuclear RNAs (snRNAs), microRNAs (miRNAs), and long nc RNAs (lncRNAs) that are extensively involved in regulating various essential genes or transcription factors involved in numerous biological processes (Mercer et al., 2009; O'Brien et al., 2018). Many of these miRNAs and lncRNAs are also known to control the adipogenesis process by regulating the expression transcription factors involved in adipocyte differentiation during normal and diseased conditions (Hilton et al., 2013; Arner and Kulyté, 2015; Chen et al., 2018).

Initial miRNA microarray studies highlighted the increased expression of miR-143 in preadipocytes where it promoted the adipocyte differentiation via controlling the levels of ERK5 protein (Esau et al., 2004). An intronic miRNA, miR-33, which is present within the SREBP-2 gene has come up as an essential non coding RNA which transcriptionally controls the cholesterol homeostasis by inhibiting the adenosine triphosphate–binding cassette (ABC) transporter (Najafi-Shoushtari et al., 2010; Rayner et al., 2010). Further study conducted on miR-33 knockout mice has revealed an enhanced expression of SREBP-1 in these mice which leads to obesity and various hepatic complications (Horie et al., 2013). Additionally, miR-27 as well as miR-130 gene family were found to inhibit the master regulators (PPARγ, C/EBPα) of adipocyte differentiation and therefore considered negative regulators of adipogenesis (Lin et al., 2009; Lee et al., 2011). A microarray study has shown the presence of PPARγ regulated differential miRNA expression profile in human subcutaneous and visceral fat tissues. An increase in the expression of miR-378 has been observed upon pioglitazone (PPARγ agonist) treatment, where it was found to enhance the adipocyte differentiation in the subcutaneous tissue but no effect was seen on visceral tissue (Yu et al., 2014). miR-146 and miR-93 were found to inhibit the expression of Sirtuins (Sirt1, Sirt7, respectively) in order to regulate adipogenesis (Ahn et al., 2013; Cioffi et al., 2015). Another mi-RNA that came up as a positive regulator of adipocyte differentiation is miR-125-5p. It has been found to suppress the genes involved in cell cycle progression (G1/S) and results in enhanced expression of key adipogenesis associated genes (Ouyang et al., 2015). Recent transcriptome analysis performed on human mesenchymal stem cells focused upon those miRNAs that are somehow involved in the lipid droplet formation during adipogenesis and could be used as disease biomarkers for various metabolic disorders (Yi et al., 2020). A miRNA originated from hepatic exosome, miR-130a-3p, was found responsible for mediating a tissue cross-talk in order to regulate the glucose intolerance by inhibiting the PH domain leucine -rich repeat protein phosphatase 2 (PHLPP2) during adipocyte differentiation (Wu et al., 2020). Also, the novel role of miR-196b-5p in promoting adipogenesis by inhibiting the expression of tuberous sclerosis 1 (Tsc1) and transforming growth factor-β receptor 1 (TGFBR1) was established (Shi et al., 2020).

A few circulating lncRNAs, despite having no functional outcome, have also been found to be differentially expressed among lean people and in people with obesity. A transcriptome study carried out in bovine preadipocytes found a lncRNA, adipocyte differentiation-associated long non-coding RNA (ADNCR), that suppressed adipogenesis by inhibiting miR-204 which is a known repressor of Sirt1 (Li M. et al., 2016). Also, silencing of lncRNA H19 in BAT reduced adipocyte differentiation, whereas its absence enhanced adipogenesis in WAT (Schmidt et al., 2018). A global expression pattern study resulted in the identification of RP11-142A22.4, expression of which was found to be highly increased during adipocyte differentiation and hence it could be used as a therapeutic target for obesity (Zhang T. et al., 2020). Despite of all the available literature, a lot is yet to be explored in order to implement the findings for the treatment of metabolic disorders.

ENVIRONMENT-EPIGENETIC INTERACTION

The prevalence of obesity in modern environment can be understood with regard to evolution (Lev-Ran, 2001). Our primeval ancestors favored "thrifty" genotype that enabled them to efficiently store fat during a period of famine. The hunter gatherers had the cycles of feast and famine interspersed with cycles of physical activity and rest. Their ability to conserve energy by storing fat provided them with genetic advantage for selecting this genotype for unfavorable conditions (food scarcity). Therefore, these individuals were more likely to survive the periods of famine than lean individuals who were more prone to infectious diseases (Eaton et al., 1988; Chakravarthy and Booth, 2004). We, the modern day humans, have the continuous supply of food and are relatively physically inactive which abrogates the evolutionary programmed feast-famine and physical activity-rest cycles. So, carrying the thrifty genotype, turned out to be a risk factor for developing obesity and metabolic diseases (Chakravarthy and Booth, 2004).

The pathophysiology of obesity is highly complex and involves the interplay of environmental factors, lifestyle changes (nourishment, exercise, exposure to noxious substances) and gene expression factors. Additionally, the gene expression changes are believed to have associated epigenetic changes that link epigenetics with obesity (**Figure 6**; Youngson and Morris, 2013; Albuquerque et al., 2017). Several medications and environmental toxins are known to induce adiposity. For example administration of valproic acid (VPA; a histone deacetylase) in children for treatment of epilepsy lead to an increased risk of developing metabolic and endocrine disorders (Carmona-Vazquez et al., 2015). Sodium VPA is also linked with an increase in BMI, increased leptin levels, IR and hyperinsulinemia in these children (Rehman et al., 2017).

Nutrition and the type of diet directly influence epigenetic marking and have a role to play in obesity and related metabolic disorders. DNA and histone methyltransferases uses S-adenosyl-methionine (SAM) as methyl donors, availability of which is directly influenced by diet (Zeisel, 2009). SAM is formed by the diet supplemented with folate, Vitamin B6, B12, choline, and methionine and is critical for fetal development where it help in DNA methylation and proper brain development of the child. Deficiency of methyl donors might result in lifelong changes in gene expression and results in several health problems like IR and fatty liver (Sinclair et al., 2007). Moreover, supplementation of methyl donors can improve NAFLD in rats fed on obesogenic diet pointing to the fact that methyl supplementation might prove to be protective against obesity (Cordero et al., 2013). Some food components such as polyphenols and organosulfur compounds have also shown positive results in lowering obesity, inflammation, oxidative stress and cancers (Milagro et al., 2013). One such organosulfur compound is sulforaphane which is naturally present in cruciferous vegetables. Sulforaphane administered as broccoli extract reduced the fasting blood glucose and glycated hemoglobin (HbA1c) in patients with obesity and T2D (Axelsson et al., 2017).

Chemicals present in our environment, termed as obesogens, can also affect a person's susceptibility to obesity by helping in adipocyte differentiation *in vitro* and storage of fat *in vivo* (Gru et al., 2006). One of the ubiquitous obesogen is organotin, like tributyltin (TBT) which is widely used in industries and agriculture. Human exposure to organotin is possible through consumption of seafood contaminated with TBT used in marine shipping applications (Mattos et al., 2017). TBT activates all three RXR–PPAR-α, -γ, -δ heterodimers, mainly through its interaction with RXR and thereby promotes adipogenesis and lipid accumulation (le Maire et al., 2009). Other obesogens include phthalates, persistent organic pollutants, components of plastics and epoxy resins. In addition to acting through nuclear receptors, these obesogens can also induce epigenetic changes and alters the chromatin accessibility or architecture in adipose tissue (Chamorro-Garcia et al., 2017). RXR activation also alters the expression of enhancer of zeste homolog 2 (EZH2) which results in genome-wide reduction and redistribution of histone 3 lysine 27 trimethylation (H3K27me^3) repressive marks and promote adipose-lineage commitment (Shoucri et al., 2017).

Apart from the above listed factors, there are numerous other societal factors such as sleep patterns, sleep deprivation, chronic shift working which alter the circadian clock genes and disrupt metabolic integrity. Even a single night of sleeplessness can alter the transcriptional and epigenetic profile of circadian clock genes consequently resulting in reduced glucose tolerance and increased insulin sensitivity (Donga et al., 2010; Cedernaes et al., 2015; Morris et al., 2016).

TRANSGENERATIONAL INHERITANCE OF OBESITY

Environmental stress/exposure can reprogram the epigenetic patterns of germ cells (egg and sperm) which associate with the development of altered phenotypes in future generations through epigenetic transgenerational inheritance (Anway et al., 2005; Skinner et al., 2013). As a result of early life developmental plasticity, the risk of obesity begins *in utero*. This idea is in accordance with the Developmental Origins of Health

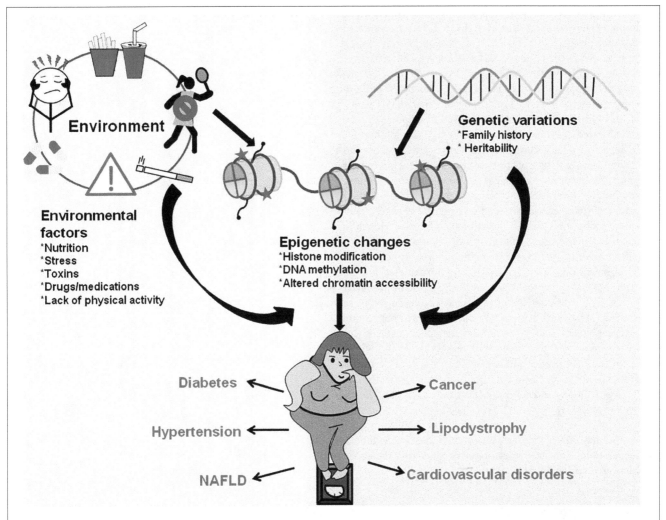

FIGURE 6 | Interaction between environment/genetic factors and epigenetic changes in establishment of obesity and obesity-associated metabolic disorders. Environmental factors like exposure to drugs/toxic chemicals, lack of physical activity, sedentary lifestyle, poor and unhealthy diet, stress/anxiety, smoking/alcohol abuse along with genetic makeup of an organism can have direct influence on epigenetic marks and result in increased adiposity. The changes in epigenetic landscape through various histone modifications, changes in chromatin accessibility and DNA methylation results in obesity and other metabolic disorders like diabetes, hypertension, lipodystrophy, cardiovascular diseases, NAFLD, cancer, etc.

and Diseases (DOHaD) hypothesis which seeks to understand the relationship between perinatal environmental conditions and disease manifestation in adulthood (Barker et al., 1989; Ravelli et al., 1999). Adipose tissue is regarded as the main target of developmental programming in a sex- and depot-specific manner. Despite of the difference in developmental time windows, similar mechanisms of adipose tissue programming exist across species. Nutritional status of mother largely affects the reprogramming of offspring's adipose tissue resulting in increased adipogenesis and lipogenesis, increased inflammation and impaired sympathetic activity thereby rendering them to disproportionate fat accumulation (Lecoutre et al., 2018). The excessive fat accumulation results in leptin and insulin resistance in these individuals predisposing them to metabolic syndrome (Muhlhausler and Smith, 2009). Maternal obesity in mice reduces the DNA methylation on Zfp423 promoter (i.e., reduced histone

modification H3K27me3), which is correlated with enhanced Zfp423 expression and adipogenesis in fetal progenitor cells which thereby predisposes the offspring to obesity and metabolic dysfunction later in life (Yang et al., 2013). Gestational obesity (OB) in rats is responsible for broad changes in lipogenic and adipogenic genes in the WAT of offspring. OB-dam offsprings shows an increased mRNA expression of SREBP-1, GLUT4 and a greater AKT phosphorylation. They also exhibit increased expression of adipogenic regulators like PPARγ, C/EBP-α and C/EBP-β associated with differentiation of WAT stromal-vascular cells. These transcriptional changes are also associated with certain epigenetic changes like alteration in DNA methylation of CpG sites and CpG island (CGI) shores proximal to developmentally important factors including Zfp234 and C/EBP-β (Borengasser et al., 2013). Evidence suggests that the ratio of omega-6 (n-6) relative to omega-3 (n-3) polyunsaturated fatty acids (PUFA) is essential in regulating perinatal adipogenesis (Rudolph et al., 2018). A diet rich in n-3 PUFA decreased adipose tissue mass and prevented the development of obesity in rodents (Madsen et al., 2005). Moreover, offsprings of transgenic mothers with low n-6/n-3 PUFA ratio in plasma during gestation and lactation had smaller adipocytes, reduced gene expression of certain pro-adipogenic markers (Pparg2, Fabp4, and Plin1), elevated circulating levels of adiponectin and hypermethylated proximal promoter of Pparg2 (Rudolph et al., 2018). Exposure to HFD during pregnancy may affect glucose and lipid metabolism of female offsprings through epigenetic changes in *Leptin* (methylation of H4K20) and *Adiponectin* (decrease in acetyl H3K9 levels and increase in dimethyl H3K9 levels) genes for multiple generations. These epigenetic changes result in metabolic abnormalities like weight gain, glucose and insulin intolerance, hypertension, abnormal adipocytokine levels, etc. The effects are much stronger if the HFD *in utero* continues for multiple generations. However, a switch to normal diet *in utero* may prevent the epigenetic changes caused by HFD and eliminate the metabolic effects after the normal diet is restored for three generations (Masuyama et al., 2015). Not only maternal obesity but paternal obesity also contributes to metabolic disturbances in future generations. Diet induced paternal obesity modulates the sperm miRNA profile and methylation status of germ cell which initiate the transmission of obesity and metabolic diseases to future generations and adversely affect the health of offspring (Fullston et al., 2013).

Apart from the dietary factors, several other environmental insults that have been identified in recent times which induce transgenerational inheritance of obesity and related metabolic disorders are listed in **Table 1**.

THERAPEUTIC STRATEGIES FOR OBESITY TREATMENT

Several clinical and epidemiological studies identify behavioral patterns including dietary habits as well as individual genetics to have direct correlation with metabolic syndrome and obesity. Apart from this, gut microbiome and environmental conditions also play a vital role in onset of obesity (Sonnenburg and Bäckhed, 2016). Additionally, if the calorie uptake is lowered, then the metabolic flux shifts toward catabolism of adipose tissues and glycogenolysis resulting in weight loss (Anton et al., 2018). Most of the strategies to control or treat obesity rely on calorie restriction. Drugs are designed either to lower the appetite for food or inhibit the absorption of tri-acyl glycerols. After several decades of research only a few drugs have been FDA approved for treatment of obesity and its associated disorders. Treatment of obesity is highly complex because most of the targets are either undruggable or have pronounced side effects due to their function in cellular homeostasis. Most of the available appetite-suppressant drugs act on the peripheral nervous system, targeting noradrenergic receptors resulting in reduced food intake by modulating the signaling of monoamine neurotransmitters such as serotonin and norepinephrine. Sibutramine (Meridia, Abbott), an appetite suppressant, first approved in November 1997 for the

TABLE 1 | Environmental insults that can induce transgenerational inheritance of obesity and obesity associated metabolic disorders.

Environmental factor	Category	Effects	References
4,4'-dichlorodiphenyltrichloroethane (DDT) 4,4'-dichlorodiphenyldichloroethylene (DDE)	Pesticide	Weight gain, altered glucose homeostasis; increased adipogenesis and lipid accumulation in 3T3-L1 cells; F3 generation sperm epimutations and differential DNA methylation regions (DMR).	Howell and Mangum, 2011; Skinner et al., 2013; Kim et al., 2016
Methoxychlor		Increased adiposity and tumor development	Manikkam et al., 2014
Bis-phenol-A (BPA) Phthalates	Plastics	Increased adiposity and DNA methylation epimutations in sperm related to obesity genes	Manikkam et al., 2013
Cadmium Lead	Heavy metals	Increased risk of obesity in children. Increase in weight and triglycerides level, hepatic lipid accumulation, DNA hypermethylation	Green et al., 2018 Sun et al., 2017
Tributyltin (TBT)	Organotins	Increased WAT depot weights, hypertrophy, hyperplasia; hepatic lipid accumulation in three subsequent generations; transmissible changes in chromatin organization; global changes in DNA methylation; induce phenotype resembling NAFLD through atleast three subsequent generations.	Chamorro-Garcia et al., 2013; Chamorro-Garcia et al., 2017
Maternal HFD Paternal HFD	Overnutrition	Weight gain, glucose intolerance, hypertension, abnormal adipocytokine levels, epigenetic changes in adipocytokines, leptin and adiponectin genes Changes in sperm miRNA profile and methylation status of germ cell, increased adiposity in future generation.	Masuyama et al., 2015 Fullston et al., 2013
Paternal prediabetes	Metabolic defect	Alteration in methylome pattern of sperm, transgenerational inheritance of diabetes (glucose intolerance and insulin resistance in offspring).	Wei et al., 2014

long-term treatment of obesity, showed some promising results. It works by inhibiting 5-HT and norepinephrine reuptake in the hypothalamus (Astrup et al., 1998). However, in the year 2010 the drug was withdrawn from the market due to increased cardiovascular complications (James et al., 2010). Fenfluramine is another drug which targets serotonergic 5-HT2 receptor agonist and σ1 receptor antagonist. Fenfluramine and dexfenfluramine were also withdrawn from United States in the year 1997 because of heart valve damage (Connolly et al., 1997; Smith et al., 2006). Phentermine is structurally similar to amphetamine which is prescribed for short term weight loss. It stimulates the central nervous system to release norepinephrine in the hypothalamus which increases the heart rate and blood pressure and decreases appetite (Rothman et al., 2001). The combination of phentermine with fenfluramine or dexfenfluramine was once used to treat obesity. Due to their side effects and contradictions such as dizziness, insomnia, dry mouth and cardiovascular problems, it is classified as schedule IV drug and could only be prescribed for short term usage. CB1 receptor, which is widely expressed in the central nervous system, is another target for treatment of obesity. Rimonabant, an inhibitor of CB1, increases adiponectin production in adipocytes leading to increased fatty acid oxidation (Pagotto et al., 2005). Rimonabant was approved in Europe in 2006, but it was withdrawn due to its adverse effect on patients such as anxiety, depression and suicidal tendencies in the clinical trials.

Apart from appetite suppression, other strategies were derived which inhibited nutrient uptake and assimilation through suppression of gastrointestinal lipase. Orlistat is an approved drug in the United States and Europe for long term obesity treatment, targeting triacylglycerol lipase thereby reducing dietary fat uptake and weight gain. Orlistat is a safe drug, but it does have some gastrointestinal side effects such as stomach pain and uncontrolled bowel movement (Ballinger, 2000). Topiramate is a sulfamate-substituted monosaccharide generally prescribed for migraine treatment. Topiramate works by inhibiting fructose 1,6-bisphosphatase, a rate limiting enzyme for gluconeogenesis, and controls blood glucose levels. Topiramate, however, has also been shown to suppress appetite and is found to be effective in weight reduction. Although, not FDA approved for the treatment of obesity, studies have demonstrated that it helps in weight reduction in individuals affected with obesity when administered in combination with phentermine (Colman et al., 2012; Cosentino et al., 2013).

Apart from classical therapeutic approaches, targeting the epigenetic regulators and factors governing adipogenesis is becoming a new hot spot for obesity treatment. The role of PPAR, an important component of adipogenesis and fatty acid oxidation, is investigated as a drug target for obesity. PPAR agonist bezafibrate showed efficacy in adipocyte dedifferentiation to preadipocytes by regulating the metabolic flux and β-oxidation (Cabrero et al., 2001; Vázquez et al., 2001). Also, treatment of another PPAR agonist GI259578A to AKR/J (AKR) mice resulted in increased mean size of WAT in the group of mice with obese phenotype as compared to the control group. Conversely, in mice with diabetic phenotype (*db/db*), treatment of PPARγ agonist GW347845X resulted in 96.1% increased

lipid storage in BAT and 15.4% decrease in WAT indicating a more complex mechanism of adipogenesis which needs to be understood before taking this drug to the clinics (Okamoto et al., 2007). Carnitine palmitoyltransferase 1 (CPT1) is another target for treatment of obesity as it helps in the entry of long-chain fatty acids into mitochondria for β-oxidation. Etomoxir, a CPT1 inhibitor, blocks the lipid transport thereby shifting metabolism toward glycolysis and oxidative phosphorylation (Schmidt-Schweda and Holubarsch, 2000).

Identification of blood-based epigenetic markers is emerging as a promising approach in early diagnosis of obesity and metabolic diseases. Such cell-free DNA (cfDNA)-based epigenetic markers are already under clinical evaluation for early detection of cancer (Xu et al., 2017; Oussalah et al., 2018). Additionally, the analysis of placenta-specific cf-DNA/RNA during early pregnancy could also be used for detection of adverse pregnancy outcomes prior to appearance of specific clinical features (Del Vecchio et al., 2020). Recent studies suggest that obesity may influence the changes in DNA methylation (Feinberg et al., 2010; Xu et al., 2013; Dick et al., 2014) which could possibly predict the future development of metabolic diseases. A genome-wide DNA methylation study in offsprings of women with high pre-pregnancy maternal BMI and gestational diabetes mellitus (GDM) identified 76 differentially methylated CpGs including several genes which are known to be associated with metabolic diseases. The study suggested that the methylation changes in the circulating blood cells could serve as a biomarker for prediction of metabolic diseases in offsprings of women with obesity and GDM (Hjort et al., 2018). A different study identified the differential methylation status of circulating cell-free CHTOP and INS1 DNA fragments as potential biomarkers for possible islet death in youths with obesity and diabetes (Syed et al., 2020). A study by Nishimoto et al. investigated the role of cfDNA in development adipose tissue inflammation. The study demonstrated that obesity induced cfDNA release from adipocytes promoted macrophage accumulation in the adipose tissue via TLR9 (Nishimoto et al., 2016). This novel mechanism for the development of adipose tissue inflammation may provide therapeutic target for obesity related metabolic disorders. Since the cell-free epigenetic markers are non-invasive, they may consequently be of greater clinical relevance for better prediction of metabolic disorders.

Histone acetylation and methylation are two of the most important epigenetic changes that regulate gene expression. Targeting these chromatin modifiers using small molecules and inhibitors has huge potential in treating obesity. HDAC inhibitors such as sodium butyrate and Trichostatin A, significantly decreased body weight in DIO mice (Gao et al., 2009). Other inhibitors targeting DNMTs, protein arginine methyltransferases, HDMs, and HATs are widely studied and have great potential in treating obesity, if used in systemic and strategic manner. However, the side effects and collateral damages caused by them due to their involvement in other cellular processes cannot be neglected thereby making their use challenging. Drug engineering for their controlled release and to enhance their specificity, could potentially reduce the side effects and toxicity.

TABLE 2 | Drugs and their modes of action in treatment of obesity.

Drug	Mode of Action	Status	Side effects	References
Metreleptin	Activates OB receptor in peripheral tissues	Phase II	Headache, low blood sugar, abdominal pain, and dizziness	Heymsfield et al., 1999
Orlistat (Xenical®)	Pancreatic lipase inhibitor	EMA, FDA, ANVISA	Flatulence, oily stool, frequent bowel movement	Harp, 1999
Naltrexone/bupropion (Contrave®)	Opioid receptor antagonist/Noradrenaline and dopamine reuptake inhibitor	EMA, FDA	Nausea, constipation and headache	*NCT01601704
Topiramate (Topamax®)	Inhibits excitatory glutamate receptors and carbonic anhydrase	Phase II	Tiredness, drowsiness, coordination problems	*NCT01859013
Phentermine (Adipex®)	Noradrenergic sympathomimetic amine	EMA, FDA	Dizziness, dry mouth, insomnia, constipation, irritability and cardiovascular side effects	Hendricks et al., 2011
Phentermine/topiramate (Qsymia®)	Release of catecholamines and inhibits excitatory glutamate receptors and carbonic anhydrase	FDA	Paraesthesia, change in taste (dysgeusia) and metabolic acidosis	Allison et al., 2012
Sibutramine (Biomag®, Sibus®, Saciette®)	Inhibits 5-HT and norepinephrine reuptake	ANVISA	high blood pressure, shortness of breath	James et al., 2010
Rimonabant (Acomplia®, Redufast®)	Inverse agonist on the cannabinoid receptor CB1	Withdrawn after phase III	Nausea, diarrhea, and dizziness	*NCT00481975
Lorcaserin (Belviq®)	Serotonin receptor agonist	Withdrawn after phase III	Headache, dizziness, nausea, dry mouth, constipation, and increased risk of cancer	*NCT03353220
Liraglutide (Victoza Saxenda®)	GLP-1 receptor agonist	EMA, FDA, ANVISA	Nausea with vomiting are the principal adverse effects; acute pancreatitis	Gough, 2012
Empagliflozin (Jardiance®)	Sodium-glucose cotransporter 2 inhibitor	Phase I	Hypoglycemia, urinary problem	*NCT02798744
Cetilistat (Cetislim®)	Inhibits pancreatic lipase	Phase II	Loose stools, fecal incontinence and frequent bowel movements	Gras, 2013
Beloranib	Inhibitor of methionine aminopeptidase 2	Phase II and III	Diarrhea, abdominal pain	*NCT02324491

*Information retrieved from clinicaltrials.gov.

Some drugs and their modes of action in treating obesity are listed in **Table 2**.

CONCLUDING REMARKS

The past two decades of research in adipose biology made us acquainted with the fact that adipose tissue is not mere inert depot for fat storage, but is a highly complex and biologically active organ which plays vital roles in whole body energy metabolism and various physiological processes. The cooperative interplay between different transcription factors, specifically PPARγ and C/EBPα, is critical for understanding adipogenesis at molecular level. Any defects in the adipose function or adipogenesis process may result in severe metabolic abnormalities. Sometimes, genetic and acquired defects like familial lipodystrophy and diet induced obesity may also result in IR and diabetes. Therefore, understanding the heterogeneity and plasticity of adipose tissue is utmost important for targeting them to reap therapeutic benefits. Adipose tissue also serves as an endocrine organ and secretes many adipokines which associate them with different cancers. Apart from adipokines, they also secrete batokines which have been shown to improve insulin sensitivity and glucose tolerance. Thus, precise selection of batokines could serve the purpose of identifying candidates for drug development and ameliorating metabolic disorders (Villarroya et al., 2017). In recent years, there have been a number of clinical trials with anti-inflammatory agents in targeting obesity related metabolic diseases. However, none of them met the approval criteria due to small cohort size and shorter period of the trials (Mclaughlin et al., 2017). The ominous connection between epigenetic changes and environmental factors contributes largely to adult onset of obesity and metabolic disorders. Therefore, targeting epigenetic modulators using inhibitors and small molecules holds a great potential in treating obesity but their limited clinical efficacy and certain unavoidable side-effects make them difficult to use. Pharmacological therapy is used as an add-on anti-obesity therapy for the patients who fail to respond to lifestyle modifications. Some drugs, though successful, have variable response rates attributing to the individual variations. Therefore, future pharmacotherapy may include the use of personalized drugs to target obesity at individual level.

AUTHOR CONTRIBUTIONS

SC, RP, and AA contributed to conception of idea. RP, PF, VS, and AA contributed to manuscript writing. All authors contributed to manuscript editing.

ACKNOWLEDGMENTS

We are thankful to National Centre for Cell Science, Pune and Department of Biological Sciences, BITS Pilani, K. K. Birla Goa Campus for providing infrastructure, facilities and funding support. We also acknowledge the support from all the funding agencies like DBT, DST, CSIR, UGC, and ICMR.

REFERENCES

Afshin, A., Forouzanfar, M. H., Reitsma, M. B., Sur, P., Estep, K., Lee, A., et al. (2017). Health effects of overweight and obesity in 195 countries over 25 years. N. Engl. J. Med. 377, 13–27. doi: 10.1056/NEJMoa1614362

Agostini, M., Schoenmakers, E., Beig, J., Fairall, L., Szatmari, I., Rajanayagam, O., et al. (2018). A pharmacogenetic approach to the treatment of patients with PPARG mutations. Diabetes 67, 1086–1092. doi: 10.2337/db17-1236

Ahn, J., Lee, H., Jung, C. H., Jeon, T., Il, and Ha, T. Y. (2013). MicroRNA-146b promotes adipogenesis by suppressing the SIRT1-FOXO1 cascade. EMBO Mol. Med. 5, 1602–1612. doi: 10.1002/emmm.201302647

Ajluni, N., Dar, M., Xu, J., Neidert, A. H., Oral, E. A., Arbor, A., et al. (2016). Efficacy and safety of metreleptin in patients with partial lipodystrophy: lessons from an expanded access program. J Diabetes Metab. 7:659. doi: 10.4172/2155-6156. 1000659

Albuquerque, D., Nóbrega, C., Manco, L., and Padez, C. (2017). The contribution of genetics and environment to obesity. Br. Med. Bull. 123, 159–173. doi: 10. 1093/bmb/ldx022

Allison, D. B., Gadde, K. M., Garvey, W. T., Peterson, C. A., Schwiers, M. L., Najarian, T., et al. (2012). Controlled-release phentermine/topiramate in severely obese adults: a randomized controlled trial (EQUIP). Obesity 20, 330–342. doi: 10.1038/oby.2011.330

Andrew, M. S., Huffman, D. M., Rodriguez-Ayala, E., Williams, N. N., Peterson, R. M., and Bastarrachea, R. A. (2018). Mesenteric visceral lipectomy using tissue liquefaction technology reverses insulin resistance and causes weight loss in baboons. Surg. Obes. Relat. Dis. 14, 833–841. doi: 10.1016/j.soard.2018. 03.004

Anton, S., Moehl, K., Donahoo, W., Marosi, K., Lee, S., Mainous, A. III, et al. (2018). Flipping the metabolic switch: understanding and applying health. Obesity 26, 254–268. doi: 10.1002/oby.22065.Flipping

Anway, M. D., Cupp, A. S., Uzumcu, N., and Skinner, M. K. (2005). Toxicology: epigenetic transgenerational actions of endocrine disruptors and male fertility. Science 308, 1466–1469. doi: 10.1126/science.1108190

Arner, P., and Kulyté, A. (2015). MicroRNA regulatory networks in human adipose tissue and obesity. Nat. Rev. Endocrinol. 11, 276–288. doi: 10.1038/nrendo.2015. 25

Arner, P., Petrus, P., Esteve, D., Boulomié, A., Näslund, E., Thorell, A., et al. (2018). Screening of potential adipokines identifies S100A4 as a marker of pernicious adipose tissue and insulin resistance. Int. J. Obes. 42, 2047–2056. doi: 10.1038/s41366-018-0018-0

Astrup, A., Hansen, D. L., Lundsgaard, C., and Toubro, S. (1998). Sibutramine and energy balance. Int. J. Obes. Relat. Metab. Disord. 22 (Suppl. 1), S30-5; discussion S 36–37, S42.

Axelsson, A. S., Tubbs, E., Mecham, B., Chacko, S., Nenonen, H. A., Tang, Y., et al. (2017). Sulforaphane reduces hepatic glucose production and improves glucose control in patients with type 2 diabetes. Sci. Trans. Med. 9:eaah4477.

Bain, G. H., Collie-Duguid, E., Murray, G. I., Gilbert, F. J., Denison, A., McKiddie, F., et al. (2014). Tumour expression of leptin is associated with chemotherapy resistance and therapy-independent prognosis in gastro-oesophageal adenocarcinomas. Br. J. Cancer 110, 1525–1534. doi: 10.1038/bjc. 2014.45

Ballinger, A. (2000). Orlistat in the treatment of obesity. Expert Opin. Pharmacother. 1, 841–847.

Barker, D. J. P., Osmond, C., Golding, J., Kuh, D., and Wadsworth, M. E. J. (1989). Growth in utero, blood pressure in childhood and adult life, and mortality from cardiovascular disease. Br. Med. J. 298, 564–567. doi: 10.1136/bmj.298.6673.564

Baskin, A. S., Linderman, J. D., Brychta, R. J., McGehee, S., Anflick-Chames, E., Cero, C., et al. (2018). Regulation of human adipose tissue activation, gallbladder size, and bile acid metabolism by a β3-adrenergic receptor agonist. Diabetes 67, 2113–2125. doi: 10.2337/db18-0462

Bekkering, S., Saner, C., Riksen, N. P., Netea, M. G., Sabin, M. A., Saffery, R., et al. (2020). Trained immunity: linking obesity and cardiovascular disease across the life-course? *Trends Endocrinol. Metab.* 31, 378–389. doi: 10.1016/j.tem.2020.01. 008

Billon, N., Iannarelli, P., Monteiro, M. C., Glavieux-Pardanaud, C., Richardson, W. D., Kessaris, N., et al. (2007). The generation of adipocytes by the neural crest. *Development* 134, 2283–2292. doi: 10.1242/dev.002642

Birsoy, K., Chen, Z., and Friedman, J. (2008). Transcriptional regulation of adipogenesis by KLF4. *Cell Metab.* 7, 339–347. doi: 10.1016/j.cmet.2008.02.001

Blüher, M. (2010). The distinction of metabolically "healthy" from "unhealthy" obese individuals. *Curr. Opin. Lipidol.* 21, 38–43. doi: 10.1097/MOL. 0b013e3283346ccc

Blüher, M. (2013). Adipose tissue dysfunction contributes to obesity related metabolic diseases. *Best Pract. Res. Clin. Endocrinol. Metab.* 27, 163–177. doi: 10.1016/j.beem.2013.02.005

Borengasser, S. J., Zhong, Y., Kang, P., Lindsey, F., Ronis, M. J. J., Badger, T. M., et al. (2013). Maternal obesity enhances white adipose tissue differentiation and alters genome-scale DNA methylation in male rat offspring. *Endocrinology* 154, 4113–4125. doi: 10.1210/en.2012-2255

Brown, R. J., Auh, S., Gorden, P., Brown, R. J., Valencia, A., Startzell, M., et al. (2018). Metreleptin-mediated improvements in insulin sensitivity are independent of food intake in humans with lipodystrophy. *J. Clin. Invest.* 128, 3504–3516.

Bu, L., Gao, M., Qu, S., and Liu, D. (2013). Intraperitoneal injection of clodronate liposomes eliminates visceral adipose macrophages and blocks high-fat diet-induced weight gain and development of insulin resistance. *AAPS J.* 15, 1001–1011. doi: 10.1208/s12248-013-9501-7

Burýsek, L., and Houstek, J. (1997). beta-Adrenergic stimulation of interleukin-1alpha and interleukin-6 expression in mouse brown adipocytes. *FEBS Lett.* 411, 83–86. doi: 10.1016/s0014-5793(97)00671-6

Cabrero, À., Alegret, M., Sánchez, R. M., Adzet, T., Laguna, J. C., and Vázquez, M. (2001). Bezafibrate reduces mRNA levels of adipocyte markers and increases fatty acid oxidation in primary culture of adipocytes. *Diabetes* 50, 1883–1890. doi: 10.2337/diabetes.50.8.1883

Campfield, L., Smith, F., Guisez, Y., Devos, R., and Burn, P. (1995). Recombinant mouse OB protein: evidence for a peripheral signal linking adiposity and central neural networks. *Science* 269, 546–549. doi: 10.1126/science.7624778

Candelaria, P. V., Rampoldi, A., Harbuzariu, A., and Gonzalez-Perez, R. R. (2017). Leptin signaling and cancer chemoresistance: perspectives. *World J. Clin. Oncol.* 8:106. doi: 10.5306/wjco.v8.i2.106

Carmona-Vazquez, C. R., Ruiz-Garcia, M., Pena-Landin, D. M., Diaz-Garcia, L., and Greenawalt, S. R. (2015). [The prevalence of obesity and metabolic syndrome in paediatric patients with epilepsy treated in monotherapy with valproic acid]. *Rev. Neurol.* 61, 193–201.

Castellano-Castillo, D., Denechaud, P. D., Fajas, L., Moreno-Indias, I., Oliva-Olivera, W., Tinahones, F., et al. (2019a). Human adipose tissue H3K4me3 histone mark in adipogenic, lipid metabolism and inflammatory genes is positively associated with BMI and HOMA-IR. *PLoS One* 14:e0215083. doi: 10.1371/journal.pone.0215083

Castellano-Castillo, D., Moreno-Indias, I., Sanchez-Alcoholado, L., Ramos-Molina, B., Alcaide-Torres, J., Morcillo, S., et al. (2019b). Altered adipose tissue DNA methylation status in metabolic syndrome: relationships between global DNA methylation and specific methylation at adipogenic, lipid metabolism and inflammatory candidate genes and metabolic variables. *J. Clin. Med.* 8:87. doi: 10.3390/jcm8010087

Cedernaes, J., Osler, M. E., Voisin, S., Broman, J. E., Vogel, H., Dickson, S. L., et al. (2015). Acute sleep loss induces tissue-specific epigenetic and transcriptional alterations to circadian clock genes in men. *J. Clin. Endocrinol. Metab.* 100, E1255–E1261. doi: 10.1210/JC.2015-2284

Chait, A., and den Hartigh, L. J. (2020). Adipose tissue distribution, inflammation and its metabolic consequences, including diabetes and cardiovascular disease. *Front. Cardiovasc. Med.* 7:22. doi: 10.3389/fcvm.2020.00022

Chakravarthy, M. V., and Booth, F. W. (2004). Eating, exercise, and "thrifty" genotypes: connecting the dots toward an evolutionary understanding of modern chronic diseases. *J. Appl. Physiol.* 96, 3–10. doi: 10.1152/japplphysiol. 00757.2003

Chamorro-Garcia, R., Diaz-Castillo, C., Shoucri, B. M., Käch, H., Leavitt, R., Shioda, T., et al. (2017). Ancestral perinatal obesogen exposure results in a transgenerational thrifty phenotype in mice. *Nat. Commun.* 8:2012. doi: 10. 1038/s41467-017-01944-z

Chamorro-García, R., Sahu, M., Abbey, R. J., Laude, J., Pham, N., and Blumberg, B. (2013). Transgenerational inheritance of increased fat depot size, stem cell reprogramming, and hepatic steatosis elicited by prenatal exposure to the obesogen tributyltin in mice. *Environ. Health Perspect.* 121, 359–366. doi: 10. 1289/ehp.1205701

Chatterjee, T. K., Basford, J. E., Knoll, E., Tong, W. S., Blanco, V., Blomkalns, A. L., et al. (2014). HDAC9 knockout mice are protected from adipose tissue dysfunction and systemic metabolic disease during high-fat feeding. *Diabetes* 63, 176–187. doi: 10.2337/db13-1148

Chatterjee, T. K., Idelman, G., Blanco, V., Blomkalns, A. L., Piegore, M. G., Weintraub, D. S., et al. (2011). Histone deacetylase 9 is a negative regulator of adipogenic differentiation. *J. Biol. Chem.* 286, 27836–27847. doi: 10.1074/jbc. M111.262964

Chen, C., Cui, Q., Zhang, X., Luo, X., Liu, Y., Zuo, J., et al. (2018). Long non-coding RNAs regulation in adipogenesis and lipid metabolism: emerging insights in obesity. *Cell. Signal.* 51, 47–58. doi: 10.1016/j.cellsig.2018.07.012

Chen, Q., Hao, W., Xiao, C., Wang, R., Xu, X., Lu, H., et al. (2017). SIRT6 is essential for adipocyte differentiation by regulating mitotic clonal expansion. *Cell Rep.* 18, 3155–3166. doi: 10.1016/j.celrep.2017.03.006

Chen, W., Schwalie, P. C., Pankevich, E. V., Gubelmann, C., Raghav, S. K., Dainese, R., et al. (2019). ZFP30 promotes adipogenesis through the KAP1-mediated activation of a retrotransposon-derived Pparg2 enhancer. *Nat. Commun.* 10:1809. doi: 10.1038/s41467-019-09803-9

Chung, S. J., Purnachandra, G., Nagalingam, A., and Muniraj, N. (2017). ADIPOQ / adiponectin induces cytotoxic autophagy in breast cancer cells through STK11 / LKB1-mediated activation of the AMPK-ULK1 axis. *Autophagy* 13, 1386–1403.

Cioffi, M., Vallespinos-Serrano, M., Trabulo, S. M., Fernandez-Marcos, P. J., Firment, A. N., Vazquez, B. N., et al. (2015). MiR-93 controls adiposity via inhibition of Sirt7 and Tbx3. *Cell Rep.* 12, 1594–1605. doi: 10.1016/j.celrep.2015. 08.006

Cipolletta, D., Feuerer, M., Li, A., Kamei, N., Lee, J., Shoelson, S. E., et al. (2012). PPAR-γ is a major driver of the accumulation and phenotype of adipose tissue T reg cells. *Nature* 486, 549–553. doi: 10.1038/nature11132

Colman, E., Golden, J., Roberts, M., Egan, A., Weaver, J., and Rosebraugh, C. (2012). The FDA's assessment of two drugs for chronic weight management. *N. Engl. J. Med.* 367, 1577–1579. doi: 10.1056/NEJMp1211277

Connolly, H. M., Crary, J. L., McGoon, M. D., Hensrud, D. D., Edwards, B. S., Edwards, W. D., et al. (1997). Valvular heart disease associated with fenfluramine-phentermine. *N. Engl. J. Med.* 337, 581–588. doi: 10.1056/ NEJM199708283370901

Cordero, P., Gomez-Uriz, A. M., Campion, J., Milagro, F. I., and Martinez, J. A. (2013). Dietary supplementation with methyl donors reduces fatty liver and modifies the fatty acid synthase DNA methylation profile in rats fed an obesogenic diet. *Genes Nutr.* 8, 105–113. doi: 10.1007/s12263-012-0300-z

Cosentino, G., Conrad, A. O., and Uwaifo, G. I. (2013). Phentermine and topiramate for the management of obesity: a review. *Drug Des. Devel. Ther.* 7, 267–278. doi: 10.2147/DDDT.S31443

Cypess, A. M., Weiner, L. S., Roberts-Toler, C., Elía, E. F., Kessler, S. H., Kahn, P. A., et al. (2015). Activation of human brown adipose tissue by a β3-adrenergic receptor agonist. *Cell Metab.* 21, 33–38. doi: 10.1016/j.cmet.2014.12.009

Cypess, A. M., White, A. P., Vernochet, C., Schulz, T. J., Xue, R., Sass, C. A., et al. (2013). Anatomical localization, gene expression profiling and functional characterization of adult human neck brown fat. *Nat. Med.* 19, 635–639. doi: 10.1038/nm.3112

De Souza, C. T., Araujo, E. P., Bordin, S., Ashimine, R., Zollner, R. L., Boschero, A. C., et al. (2005). Consumption of a fat-rich diet activates a proinflammatory response and induces insulin resistance in the hypothalamus. *Endocrinology* 146, 4192–4199. doi: 10.1210/en.2004-1520

DeFuria, J., Belkina, A. C., Jagannathan-Bogdan, M., Snyder-Cappione, J., Carr, J. D., Nersesova, Y. R., et al. (2013). B cells promote inflammation in obesity and type 2 diabetes through regulation of T-cell function and an inflammatory cytokine profile. *Proc. Natl. Acad. Sci. U.S.A.* 110, 5133–5138. doi: 10.1073/pnas. 1215840110

Del Vecchio, G., Li, Q., Li, W., Thamotharan, S., Tosevska, A., Morselli, M., et al. (2020). Cell-free DNA methylation and transcriptomic signature prediction of pregnancies with adverse outcomes. *Epigenetics* [Epub ahead of print] doi: 10.1080/15592294.2020.1816774

Derosa, G., Catena, G., Gaudio, G., D'Angelo, A., and Maffioli, P. (2020). Adipose tissue dysfunction and metabolic disorders: is it possible to predict who will develop type 2 diabetes mellitus? Role of markErs in the progreSsion of dIabeteS in obese paTIeNts (The RESISTIN trial). *Cytokine* 127:154947. doi: 10.1016/j.cyto.2019.154947

Derosa, G., Fogari, E., D'Angelo, A., Bianchi, L., Bonaventura, A., Romano, D., et al. (2013). Adipocytokine levels in obese and non-obese subjects: an observational study. *Inflammation* 36, 914–920. doi: 10.1007/s10753-013-9620-4

Dick, K. J., Nelson, C. P., Tsaprouni, L., Sandling, J. K., Aïssi, D., Wahl, S., et al. (2014). DNA methylation and body-mass index: a genome-wide analysis. *Lancet* 383, 1990–1998. doi: 10.1016/S0140-6736(13)62674-4

Dieudonne, M. N., Bussiere, M., Dos Santos, E., Leneveu, M. C., Giudicelli, Y., and Pecquery, R. (2006). Adiponectin mediates antiproliferative and apoptotic responses in human MCF7 breast cancer cells. *Biochem. Biophys. Res. Commun.* 345, 271–279. doi: 10.1016/j.bbrc.2006.04.076

Donga, E., Van Dijk, M., Van Dijk, J. G., Biermasz, N. R., Lammers, G. J., Van Kralingen, K. W., et al. (2010). A single night of partial sleep deprivation induces insulin resistance in multiple metabolic pathways in healthy subjects. *J. Clin. Endocrinol. Metab.* 95, 2963–2968. doi: 10.1210/jc.2009-2430

Dunn, G. A., and Bale, T. L. (2011). Maternal high-fat diet effects on third-generation female body size via the paternal lineage. *Endocrinology* 152, 2228–2236. doi: 10.1210/en.2010-1461

Eaton, S. B., Konner, M., and Shostak, M. (1988). Stone agers in the fast lane: chronic degenerative diseases in evolutionary perspective. *Am. J. Med.* 84, 739–749. doi: 10.1016/0002-9343(88)90113-1

Esau, C., Kang, X., Peralta, E., Hanson, E., Marcusson, E. G., Ravichandran, L. V., et al. (2004). MicroRNA-143 regulates adipocyte differentiation. *J. Biol. Chem.* 279, 52361–52365. doi: 10.1074/jbc.C400438200

Fajas, L., Schoonjans, K., Gelman, L., Kim, J. A. E. B., Najib, J., Martin, G., et al. (1999). Regulation of peroxisome proliferator-activated receptor gamma expression by adipocyte differentiation and determination factor 1 / sterol regulatory element binding protein 1: implications for adipocyte differentiation and metabolism. *Comp. Study* 19, 5495–5503.

Fan, R., Toubal, A., Goñi, S., Drareni, K., Huang, Z., Alzaid, F., et al. (2016). Loss of the co-repressor GPS2 sensitizes macrophage activation upon metabolic stress induced by obesity and type 2 diabetes. *Nat. Med.* 22, 780–791. doi: 10.1038/nm.4114

Fang, J., Ianni, A., Smolka, C., Vakhrusheva, O., Nolte, H., Krüger, M., et al. (2017). Sirt7 promotes adipogenesis in the mouse by inhibiting autocatalytic activation of Sirt1. *Proc. Natl. Acad. Sci. U.S.A.* 114, E8352–E8361. doi: 10.1073/pnas.1706945114

Feinberg, A. P., Irizarry, R. A., Fradin, D., Aryee, M. J., Murakami, P., Aspelund, T., et al. (2010). Personalized epigenomic signatures that are stable over time and covary with body mass index. *Sci. Transl. Med.* 2:49ra67. doi: 10.1126/scitranslmed.3001262

Ferrari, A., Longo, R., Peri, C., Coppi, L., Caruso, D., Mai, A., et al. (2020). Inhibition of class I HDACs imprints adipogenesis toward oxidative and brown-like phenotype. *Biochim. Biophys. Acta Mol. Cell Biol. Lipids* 1865:158594. doi: 10.1016/j.bbalip.2019.158594

Feuerer, M., Herrero, L., Cipolletta, D., Naaz, A., Wong, J., Nayer, A., et al. (2009). Lean, but not obese, fat is enriched for a unique population of regulatory T cells that affect metabolic parameters. *Nat. Med.* 15, 930–939. doi: 10.1038/nm.2002

Finlin, B. S., Confides, A. L., Zhu, B., Boulanger, M. C., Memetimin, H., Taylor, K. W., et al. (2019). Adipose tissue mast cells promote human adipose beiging in response to cold. *Sci. Rep.* 9:8658. doi: 10.1038/s41598-019-45136-9

Foster, D. O., and Frydman, M. L. (1979). Tissue distribution of cold-induced thermogenesis in conscious warm- or cold-acclimated rats reevaluated from changes in tissue blood flow: the dominant role of brown adipose tissue in the replacement of shivering by nonshivering thermogenesis. *Can. J. Physiol. Pharmacol.* 57, 257–270. doi: 10.1139/y79-039

Fox, C. S., Massaro, J. M., Hoffmann, U., Pou, K. M., Maurovich-Horvat, P., Liu, C. Y., et al. (2007). Abdominal visceral and subcutaneous adipose tissue compartments: association with metabolic risk factors in the framingham heart study. *Circulation* 116, 39–48. doi: 10.1161/CIRCULATIONAHA.106.675355

Frühbeck, G. (2008). Overview of adipose tissue and its role. *Methods Mol. Biol.* 456, 1–22.

Fullston, T., Teague, E. M. C. O., Palmer, N. O., Deblasio, M. J., Mitchell, M., Corbett, M., et al. (2013). Paternal obesity initiates metabolic disturbances in two generations of mice with incomplete penetrance to the F2 generation and alters the transcriptional profile of testis and sperm microRNA content. *FASEB J.* 27, 4226–4243. doi: 10.1096/fj.12-224048

Gabriely, I., Ma, X. H., Yang, X. M., Atzmon, G., Rajala, M. W., Berg, A. H., et al. (2002). Removal of visceral fat prevents insulin resistance and glucose intolerance of aging: an adipokine-mediated process? *Diabetes* 51, 2951–2958. doi: 10.2337/diabetes.51.10.2951

Galic, S., Oakhill, J. S., and Steinberg, G. R. (2010). Adipose tissue as an endocrine organ. *Mol. Cell. Endocrinol.* 316, 129–139. doi: 10.1016/j.mce.2009.08.018

Gangwisch, J. E., Malaspina, D., Boden-Albala, B., and Heymsfield, S. B. (2005). Inadequate sleep as a risk factor for obesity: analyses of the NHANES I. *Sleep* 28, 1289–1296. doi: 10.1093/sleep/28.10.1289

Gao, Z., Yin, J., Zhang, J., Ward, R. E., Martin, R. J., Lefevre, M., et al. (2009). Butyrate improves insulin sensitivity and increases energy expenditure in mice. *Diabetes* 58, 1509–1517. doi: 10.2337/db08-1637

Ghasemi, A., Hashemy, S. I., Aghaei, M., and Panjehpour, M. (2018). Leptin induces matrix metalloproteinase 7 expression to promote ovarian cancer cell invasion by activating ERK and JNK pathways. *J. Cell. Biochem.* 119, 2333–2344. doi: 10.1002/jcb.26396

Gilardi, F., Winkler, C., Quignodon, L., Diserens, J. G., Toffoli, B., Schiffrin, M., et al. (2019). Systemic PPARγ deletion in mice provokes lipoatrophy, organomegaly, severe type 2 diabetes and metabolic inflexibility. *Metabolism* 95, 8–20. doi: 10.1016/j.metabol.2019.03.003

Giordano, A., Smorlesi, A., Frontini, A., Barbatelli, G., and Cint, S. (2014). White, brown and pink adipocytes: the extraordinary plasticity of the adipose organ. *Eur. J. Endocrinol.* 170, R159–R171. doi: 10.1530/EJE-13-0945

Goldsworthy, M., Absalom, N. L., Schröter, D., Matthews, H. C., Bogani, D., Moir, L., et al. (2013). Mutations in Mll2, an H3K4 methyltransferase, result in insulin resistance and impaired glucose tolerance in mice. *PLoS One* 8:e61870. doi: 10.1371/journal.pone.0061870

Gough, S. C. L. (2012). Liraglutide: from clinical trials to clinical practice. *Diabetes Obes. Metab.* 14, 33–40.

Gourdy, P., Cazals, L., Thalamas, C., Sommet, A., Calvas, F., Galitzky, M., et al. (2018). Apelin administration improves insulin sensitivity in overweight men during hyperinsulinaemic-euglycaemic clamp. *Diabetes Obes. Metab.* 20, 157–164. doi: 10.1111/dom.13055

Gras, J. (2013). Cetilistat for the treatment of obesity. *Drugs Today* 49, 755–759. doi: 10.1358/dot.2013.49.12.2099318

Green, A. J., Hoyo, C., Mattingly, C. J., Luo, Y., Tzeng, J. Y., Murphy, S. K., et al. (2018). Cadmium exposure increases the risk of juvenile obesity: a human and zebrafish comparative study. *Int. J. Obes.* 42, 1285–1295. doi: 10.1038/s41366-018-0036-y.Cadmium

Green, H., and Kehinde, O. (1975). An established preadipose cell line and its differentiation in culture II. Factors affecting the adipose conversion. *Cell* 5, 19–27. doi: 10.1016/0092-8674(75)90087-2

Green, H., and Meuth, M. (1974). An established pre-adipose cell line and its differentiation in culture. *Cell* 3, 127–133. doi: 10.1016/0092-8674(74)90116-0

Gru, F., Watanabe, H., Zamanian, Z., Maeda, L., Arima, K., Cubacha, R., et al. (2006). Endocrine-disrupting organotin compounds are potent inducers of adipogenesis in vertebrates.inol. *Mol. Endoc.* 20, 2141–2155. doi: 10.1210/me.2005-0367

Grundy, S. M., Cleeman, J. I., Daniels, S. R., Donato, K. A., Eckel, R. H., Franklin, B. A., et al. (2005). Diagnosis and management of the metabolic syndrome: an American Heart Association/National Heart, Lung, and Blood Institute scientific statement. *Circulation* 112, 2735–2752. doi: 10.1161/CIRCULATIONAHA.105.169404

Gu, L., Wang, C., DiCao, C., Cai, L. R., Li, D. H., et al. (2019). Association of serum leptin with breast cancer: a meta-analysis. *Medicine* 98:e14094. doi: 10.1097/MD.0000000000014094

Gui, Y., Pan, Q., Chen, X., Xu, S., Luo, X., and Chen, L. (2017). The association between obesity related adipokines and risk of breast cancer: a meta-analysis. *Oncotarget* 8, 75389–75399. doi: 10.18632/oncotarget.17853

Gupta, R. K., Arany, Z., Seale, P., Mepani, R. J., Ye, L., Conroe, H. M., et al. (2010). Transcriptional control of preadipocyte determination by Zfp423. *Nature* 464, 619–623. doi: 10.1038/nature08816

Halaas, J. L., Gajiwala, K. S., Maffei, M., Cohen, S. L., Chait, B. T., Rabinowitz, D., et al. (1995). Weight-reducing effects of the plasma protein encoded by the obese gene. Science 269, 543–546. doi: 10.1126/science.7624777

Han, G., Wang, L., Zhao, W., Yue, Z., Zhao, R., Li, Y., et al. (2013). High expression of leptin receptor leads to temozolomide resistance with exhibiting stem/progenitor cell features in glioblastoma. Cell Cycle 12, 3833–3840. doi: 10.4161/cc.26809

Hannibal, T. D., Schmidt-Christensen, A., Nilsson, J., Fransén-Pettersson, N., Hansen, L., and Holmberg, D. (2017). Deficiency in plasmacytoid dendritic cells and type I interferon signalling prevents diet-induced obesity and insulin resistance in mice. Diabetologia 60, 2033–2041. doi: 10.1007/s00125-017-4341-0

Harp, J. B. (1999). Orlistat for the long-term treatment of obesity. Drugs Today 35, 139–145. doi: 10.1358/dot.1999.35.2.527969

Hayashi, T., Boyko, E. J., McNeely, M. J., Leonetti, D. L., Kahn, S. E., and Fujimoto, W. Y. (2008). Visceral adiposity, not abdominal subcutaneous fat area, is associated with an increase in future insulin resistance in Japanese Americans. Diabetes 57, 1269–1275. doi: 10.2337/db07-1378

Hendricks, E. J., Greenway, F. L., Westman, E. C., and Gupta, A. K. (2011). Blood pressure and heart rate effects, weight loss and maintenance during long-term phentermine pharmacotherapy for obesity. Obesity 19, 2351–2360. doi: 10.1038/oby.2011.94

Herrera, R., Ro, H. S., Robinson, G. S., Xanthopoulos, K. G., and Spiegelman, B. M. (1989). A direct role for C/EBP and the AP-I-binding site in gene expression linked to adipocyte differentiation. Mol. Cell. Biol. 9, 5331–5339. doi: 10.1128/mcb.9.12.5331

Heymsfield, S. B., Greenberg, A. S., Fujioka, K., Dixon, R. M., Kushner, R., Hunt, T., et al. (1999). Recombinant leptin for weight loss in obese and lean adults. JAMA 282:1568. doi: 10.1001/jama.282.16.1568

Hilton, C., Neville, M. J., and Karpe, F. (2013). MicroRNAs in adipose tissue: their role in adipogenesis and obesity. Int. J. Obes. 37, 325–332. doi: 10.1038/ijo.2012.59

Hjort, L., Martino, D., Grunnet, L. G., Naeem, H., Maksimovic, J., Olsson, A. H., et al. (2018). Gestational diabetes and maternal obesity are associated with epigenome-wide methylation changes in children. JCI Insight 3:e122572. doi: 10.1172/jci.insight.122572

Hondares, E., Iglesias, R., Giralt, A., Gonzalez, F. J., Giralt, M., Mampel, T., et al. (2011). Thermogenic activation induces FGF21 expression and release in brown adipose tissue. J. Biol. Chem. 286, 12983–12990. doi: 10.1074/jbc.M110.215889

Hong, J., Hwang, E. S., Mcmanus, M. T., Amsterdam, A., Tian, Y., Kalmukova, R., et al. (2005). TAZ, a transcriptional modulator of mesenchymal stem cell differentiation. Science 309, 1074–1078.

Horie, T., Nishino, T., Baba, O., Kuwabara, Y., Nakao, T., Nishiga, M., et al. (2013). MicroRNA-33 regulates sterol regulatory element-binding protein 1 expression in mice. Nat. Commun. 4:2883. doi: 10.1038/ncomms3883

Hotamisligil, G. S., Shargill, N. S., and Spiegelman, B. M. (1993). Adipose expression of tumor necrosis factor-α: direct role in obesity-linked insulin resistance. Science 259, 87–91. doi: 10.1126/science.7678183

Hou, Y., Zhang, Z., Wang, Y., Gao, T., Liu, X., Tang, T., et al. (2020). 5mC profiling characterized TET2 as an anti-adipogenic demethylase. Gene 733:144265. doi: 10.1016/j.gene.2019.144265

Howell, G., and Mangum, L. (2011). Exposure to bioaccumulative organochlorine compounds alters adipogenesis, fatty acid uptake, and adipokine production in NIH3T3-L1 cells. Toxicol. Vitr. 25, 394–402. doi: 10.1016/j.tiv.2010.10.015

Hsieh, Y. Y., Shen, C. H., Huang, W. S., Chin, C. C., Kuo, Y. H., Hsieh, M. C., et al. (2014). Resistin-induced stromal cell-derived factor-1 expression through Toll-like receptor 4 and activation of p38 MAPK/ NFκB signaling pathway in gastric cancer cells. J. Biomed. Sci. 21:59. doi: 10.1186/1423-0127-21-59

Hu, Y. J., Belaghzal, H., Hsiao, W. Y., Qi, J., Bradner, J. E., Guertin, D. A., et al. (2015). Transcriptional and post-transcriptional control of adipocyte differentiation by Jumonji domain-containing protein 6. Nucleic Acids Res. 43, 7790–7804. doi: 10.1093/nar/gkv645

Huang, Y., Das, A. K., Yang, Q. Y., Zhu, M. J., and Du, M. (2012). Zfp423 promotes adipogenic differentiation of bovine stromal vascular cells. PLoS One 7:e47496. doi: 10.1371/journal.pone.0047496

Hwang, J. W., So, Y. S., Bae, G. U., Kim, S. N., and Kim, Y. K. (2019). Protein arginine methyltransferase 6 suppresses adipogenic differentiation by

repressing peroxisome proliferator-activated receptor γ activity. Int. J. Mol. Med. 43, 2462–2470. doi: 10.3892/ijmm.2019.4147

Imbalzano, A. N., Hu, Y. J., and Sif, S. (2013). Prmt7 is dispensable in tissue culture models for adipogenic differentiation. F1000Research 2:279. doi: 10.12688/f1000research.2-279.v1

Jack, B. H. A., and Crossley, M. (2010). GATA proteins work together with friend of GATA (FOG) and C-terminal Binding Protein (CTBP) Co-regulators to control adipogenesis. J. Biol. Chem. 285, 32405–32414. doi: 10.1074/jbc.M110.141317

James, W. P. T., Caterson, I. D., Coutinho, W., Finer, N., Van Gaal, L. F., Maggioni, A. P., et al. (2010). Effect of sibutramine on cardiovascular outcomes in overweight and obese subjects. N. Engl. J. Med. 363, 905–917. doi: 10.1056/NEJMoa1003114

Janiszewski, P. M., and Ross, R. (2010). Effects of weight loss among metabolically healthy obese men and women. Diabetes Care 33, 1957–1959. doi: 10.2337/dc10-0547

Jayashree, B., Bibin, Y. S., Prabhu, D., Shanthirani, C. S., Gokulakrishnan, K., Lakshmi, B. S., et al. (2014). Increased circulatory levels of lipopolysaccharide (LPS) and zonulin signify novel biomarkers of proinflammation in patients with type 2 diabetes. Mol. Cell. Biochem. 388, 203–210. doi: 10.1007/s11010-013-1911-4

Jufvas, Å., Sjödin, S., Lundqvist, K., Amin, R., Vener, A. V., and Strålfors, P. (2013). Global differences in specific histone H3 methylation are associated with overweight and type 2 diabetes. Clin. Epigenet. 5:15. doi: 10.1186/1868-7083-5-15

Kadoch, C., and Crabtree, G. R. (2015). Mammalian SWI/SNF chromatin remodeling complexes and cancer: mechanistic insights gained from human genomics. Sci. Adv. 1:e1500447. doi: 10.1126/sciadv.1500447

Kajimura, S. (2017). Adipose tissue in 2016: advances in the understanding of adipose tissue biology. Nat. Rev. Endocrinol. 13, 69–70. doi: 10.1038/nrendo.2016.211

Kanda, H. (2006). MCP-1 contributes to macrophage infiltration into adipose tissue, insulin resistance, and hepatic steatosis in obesity. J. Clin. Invest. 116, 1494–1505. doi: 10.1172/JCI26498

Kang, H. S., Lee, J. H., Oh, K. J., Lee, E. W., Han, B. S., Park, K. Y., et al. (2020). IDH1-dependent α-KG regulates brown fat differentiation and function by modulating histone methylation. Metabolism 105:154173. doi: 10.1016/j.metabol.2020.154173

Karelis, A. D., Faraj, M., Bastard, J. P., St-Pierre, D. H., Brochu, M., Prud'homme, D., et al. (2005). The metabolically healthy but obese individual presents a favorable inflammation profile. J. Clin. Endocrinol. Metab. 90, 4145–4150. doi: 10.1210/jc.2005-0482

Khamis, A., Boutry, R., Canouil, M., Mathew, S., Lobbens, S., Crouch, H., et al. (2020). Histone deacetylase 9 promoter hypomethylation associated with adipocyte dysfunction is a statin-related metabolic effect. Clin. Epigenet. 12:68. doi: 10.1186/s13148-020-00858-w

Khan, I. M., Dai Perrard, X.-Y., Perrard, J. L., Mansoori, A., Wayne Smith, C., Wu, H., et al. (2014). Attenuated adipose tissue and skeletal muscle inflammation in obese mice with combined CD4+ and CD8+ T cell deficiency. Atherosclerosis 233, 419–428. doi: 10.1016/j.atherosclerosis.2014.01.011

Kim, H. J., Lee, Y. S., Won, E. H., Chang, I. H., Kim, T. H., Park, E. S., et al. (2011). Expression of resistin in the prostate and its stimulatory effect on prostate cancer cell proliferation. BJU Int. 108, 77–83. doi: 10.1111/j.1464-410X.2010.09813.x

Kim, J., Sun, Q., Yue, Y., Yoon, K. S., Whang, K., Marshall Clark, J., et al. (2016). 4,4'-Dichlorodiphenyltrichloroethane (DDT) and 4,4'-dichlorodiphenyldichloroethylene (DDE) promote adipogenesis in 3T3-L1 adipocyte cell culture. Pestic. Biochem. Physiol. 131, 40–45. doi: 10.1016/j.pestbp.2016.01.005

Kurtev, M., Chung, N., Topark-ngarm, A., Senawong, T., Oliveira, R. M., De, et al. (2004). Sirt1 promotes fat mobilization in white adipocytes by repressing PPAR-g. Nature 429, 771–776.

Lai, B., Lee, J. E., Jang, Y., Lifeng, W., Peng, W., and Ge, K. (2017). MLL3/MLL4 are required for CBP/p300 binding on enhancers and super-enhancer formation in brown adipogenesis. Nucleic Acids Res. 45, 6388–6403. doi: 10.1093/nar/gkx234

le Maire, A., Grimaldi, M., Roecklin, D., Dagnino, S., Vivat-Hannah, V., Balaguer, P., et al. (2009). Activation of RXR-PPAR heterodimers by organotin environmental endocrine disruptors. Embo Rep. 10, 367–373. doi: 10.1038/embor.2009.8

LeBlanc, S. E., Konda, S., Wu, Q., Hu, Y. J., Oslowski, C. M., Sif, S., et al. (2012). Protein arginine methyltransferase 5 (Prmt5) promotes gene expression of peroxisome proliferator-activated receptor γ2 (PPARγ2) and its target genes during adipogenesis. *Mol. Endocrinol.* 26, 583–597. doi: 10.1210/me.2011-1162

Leblanc, S. E., Wu, Q., Lamba, P., Sif, S., and Imbalzano, A. N. (2016). Promoter-enhancer looping at the PPARγ locus during adipogenic differentiation requires the Prmt5 methyltransferase. *Nucleic Acids Res.* 44, 5133–5147. doi: 10.1093/nar/gkw129

Lecoutre, S., Petrus, P., Rydén, M., and Breton, C. (2018). Transgenerational epigenetic mechanisms in adipose tissue development. *Trends Endocrinol. Metab.* 29, 675–685. doi: 10.1016/j.tem.2018.07.004

Lee, E. K., Lee, M. J., Abdelmohsen, K., Kim, W., Kim, M. M., Srikantan, S., et al. (2011). miR-130 suppresses adipogenesis by inhibiting peroxisome proliferator-activated receptor expression. *Mol. Cell Biol.* 31, 626–638. doi: 10.1128/mcb.00894-10

Lee, J.-E., Schmidt, H., Lai, B., and Ge, K. (2019). Transcriptional and epigenomic regulation of adipogenesis. *Mol. Cell. Biol.* 39, e601–e618. doi: 10.1128/mcb.00601-18

Lev-Ran, A. (2001). Human obesity: an evolutionary approach. *Diabetes Metab. Res. Rev.* 17, 347–362.

Li, M., Sun, X., Cai, H., Sun, Y., Plath, M., Li, C., et al. (2016). Long non-coding RNA ADNCR suppresses adipogenic differentiation by targeting miR-204. *Biochim. Biophys. Acta Gene Regul. Mech.* 1859, 871–882. doi: 10.1016/j.bbagrm.2016.05.003

Li, P., Liu, S., Lu, M., Bandyopadhyay, G., Oh, D., Imamura, T., et al. (2016). Hematopoietic-derived Galectin-3 causes cellular and systemic insulin resistance. *Cell* 167, 973.e12–984.e12. doi: 10.1016/j.cell.2016.10.025

Li, M., Yang, S., and Björntorp, P. (1993). Metabolism of different adipose tissues in vivo in the rat. *Obes. Res.* 1, 459–468. doi: 10.1002/j.1550-8528.1993.tb00028.x

Lin, Q., Gao, Z., Alarcon, R. M., Ye, J., and Yun, Z. (2009). A role of miR-27 in the regulation of adipogenesis. *FEBS J.* 276, 2348–2358. doi: 10.1111/j.1742-4658.2009.06967.x

Linhart, H. G., Ishimura-Oka, K., Demayo, F., Kibe, T., Repka, D., Poindexter, B., et al. (2001). C/EBPα is required for differentiation of white but not brown adipose tissue. *Proc. Natl. Acad. Sci. U.S.A.* 98, 12532–12537. doi: 10.1073/pnas.211416898

Liu, J., Divoux, A., Sun, J., Zhang, J., Clément, K., Glickman, J. N., et al. (2009). Genetic deficiency and pharmacological stabilization of mast cells reduce diet-induced obesity and diabetes in mice. *Nat. Med.* 15, 940–945. doi: 10.1038/nm.1994

Liu, T., Guo, Z., Song, X., Liu, L., Dong, W., Wang, S., et al. (2020). High-fat diet-induced dysbiosis mediates MCP-1/CCR2 axis-dependent M2 macrophage polarization and promotes intestinal adenoma-adenocarcinoma sequence. *J. Cell. Mol. Med.* 24, 2648–2662. doi: 10.1111/jcmm.14984

Liu, Z., Gan, L., Xu, Y., Luo, D., Ren, Q., Wu, S., et al. (2017). Melatonin alleviates inflammasome-induced pyroptosis through inhibiting NF-κB/GSDMD signal in mice adipose tissue. *J. Pineal Res.* 63:e12414. doi: 10.1111/jpi.12414

Lizcano, F., Romero, C., and Vargas, D. (2011). Regulation of adipogenesis by nuclear receptor PPARγ is modulated by the histone demethylase JMJD2C. *Genet. Mol. Biol.* 34, 19–24. doi: 10.1590/S1415-47572010005000105

Londono Gentile, T., Lu, C., Lodato, P. M., Tse, S., Olejniczak, S. H., Witze, E. S., et al. (2013). DNMT1 is regulated by ATP-Citrate lyase and maintains methylation patterns during adipocyte differentiation. *Mol. Cell. Biol.* 33, 3864–3878. doi: 10.1128/mcb.01495-12

Long, J. Z., Svensson, K. J., Bateman, L. A., Lin, H., Kamenecka, T., Lokurkar, I. A., et al. (2016). The secreted enzyme PM20D1 regulates lipidated amino acid uncouplers of mitochondria. *Cell* 166, 424–435. doi: 10.1016/j.cell.2016.05.071

Lu, Y. P., Lou, Y. R., Bernard, J. J., Peng, Q. Y., Li, T., Lin, Y., et al. (2012). Surgical removal of the parametrial fat pads stimulates apoptosis and inhibits UVB-induced carcinogenesis in mice fed a high-fat diet. *Proc. Natl. Acad. Sci. U.S.A.* 109, 9065–9070. doi: 10.1073/pnas.1205810109

Lumeng, C. N., Bodzin, J. L., Saltiel, A. R., Lumeng, C. N., Bodzin, J. L., and Saltiel, A. R. (2007). Obesity induces a phenotypic switch in adipose tissue macrophage polarization find the latest version: obesity induces a phenotypic switch in adipose tissue macrophage polarization. *J. Clin. Invest.* 117, 175–184. doi: 10.1172/JCI29881

Lyko, F. (2018). The DNA methyltransferase family: a versatile toolkit for epigenetic regulation. *Nat. Rev. Genet.* 19, 81–92. doi: 10.1038/nrg.2017.80

Madsen, L., Petersen, R. K., and Kristiansen, K. (2005). Regulation of adipocyte differentiation and function by polyunsaturated fatty acids. *Biochim. Biophys. Acta Mol. Basis Dis.* 1740, 266–286. doi: 10.1016/j.bbadis.2005.03.001

Madsen, M. S., Siersbaek, R., Boergesen, M., Nielsen, R., and Mandrup, S. (2014). Peroxisome proliferator-activated receptor and C/EBP synergistically activate key metabolic adipocyte genes by assisted loading. *Mol. Cell. Biol.* 34, 939–954. doi: 10.1128/mcb.01344-13

Manikkam, M., Haque, M. M., Guerrero-Bosagna, C., Nilsson, E. E., and Skinner, M. K. (2014). Pesticide methoxychlor promotes the epigenetic transgenerational inheritance of adult-onset disease through the female germline. *PLoS One* 9:e102091. doi: 10.1371/journal.pone.0102091

Manikkam, M., Tracey, R., Guerrero-Bosagna, C., and Skinner, M. K. (2013). Plastics derived endocrine disruptors (BPA, DEHP and DBP) induce epigenetic transgenerational inheritance of obesity, reproductive disease and sperm epimutations. *PLoS One* 8:e55387. doi: 10.1371/journal.pone.0055387

Masuyama, H., Mitsui, T., Nobumoto, E., and Hiramatsu, Y. (2015). The effects of high-fat diet exposure in utero on the obesogenic and diabetogenic traits through epigenetic changes in Adiponectin and Leptin gene expression for multiple generations in female mice. *Endocrinology* 156, 2482–2491. doi: 10.1210/en.2014-2020

Matsubara, M., Maruoka, S., and Katayose, S. (2002). Inverse relationship between plasma adiponectin and leptin concentrations in normal-weight and obese women. *Eur. J. Endocrinol.* 147, 173–180. doi: 10.1530/eje.0.1470173

Mattos, Y., Stotz, W. B., Romero, M. S., Bravo, M., Fillmann, G., and Castro, ÍB. (2017). Butyltin contamination in Northern Chilean coast: is there a potential risk for consumers? *Sci. Total Environ.* 595, 209–217. doi: 10.1016/j.scitotenv.2017.03.264

Mayoral, R., Osborn, O., McNelis, J., Johnson, A. M., Oh, D. Y., Izquierdo, C. L., et al. (2015). Adipocyte SIRT1 knockout promotes PPARγ activity, adipogenesis and insulin sensitivity in chronic-HFD and obesity. *Mol. Metab.* 4, 378–391. doi: 10.1016/j.molmet.2015.02.007

McAllister, E. J., Dhurandhar, N. V., Keith, S. W., Aronne, L. J., Barger, J., Baskin, M., et al. (2009). Ten putative contributors to the obesity epidemic. *Crit. Rev. Food Sci. Nutr.* 49, 868–913. doi: 10.1080/10408390903372599

McKernan, K., Varghese, M., Patel, R., and Singer, K. (2020). Role of TLR4 in the induction of inflammatory changes in adipocytes and macrophages. *Adipocyte* 9, 212–222. doi: 10.1080/21623945.2020.1760674

Mclaughlin, T., Ackerman, S. E., Shen, L., and Engleman, E. (2017). Role of innate and adaptive immunity in obesity-associated metabolic disease. *J. Clin. Invest.* 127, 5–13. doi: 10.1172/JCI88876

Mercer, T. R., Dinger, M. E., and Mattick, J. S. (2009). Long non-coding RNAs: insights into functions. *Nat. Rev. Genet.* 10, 155–159. doi: 10.1038/nrg2521

Mikula, M., Majewska, A., Ledwon, J. K., Dzwonek, A., and Ostrowski, J. (2014). Obesity increases histone H3 lysine 9 and 18 acetylation at Tnfa and Ccl2 genes in mouse liver. *Int. J. Mol. Med.* 34, 1647–1654. doi: 10.3892/ijmm.2014.1958

Milagro, F. I., Mansego, M. L., De Miguel, C., and Martínez, J. A. (2013). Dietary factors, epigenetic modifications and obesity outcomes: progresses and perspectives. *Mol. Aspects Med.* 34, 782–812. doi: 10.1016/j.mam.2012.06.010

Min, S. Y., Kady, J., Nam, M., Rojas-Rodriguez, R., Berkenwald, A., Kim, J. H., et al. (2016). Human "brite/beige" adipocytes develop from capillary networks, and their implantation improves metabolic homeostasis in mice. *Nat. Med.* 22, 312–318. doi: 10.1038/nm.4031

Montes, V. N., Subramanian, S., Goodspeed, L., Wang, S. A., Omer, M., Bobik, A., et al. (2015). Anti-HMGB1 antibody reduces weight gain in mice fed a high-fat diet. *Nutr. Diabetes* 5:e161. doi: 10.1038/nutd.2015.11

Moon, Y. S., Smas, C. M., Lee, K., Villena, J. A., Kim, K., Yun, E. J., et al. (2002). Mice lacking paternally expressed Pref-1 / Dlk1 display growth retardation and accelerated adiposity. 22, 5585–5592. doi: 10.1128/MCB.22.15.5585

Morris, C. J., Purvis, T. E., Mistretta, J., and Scheer, F. A. J. L. (2016). Effects of the internal circadian system and circadian misalignment on glucose tolerance in chronic shift workers. *J. Clin. Endocrinol. Metab.* 101, 1066–1074. doi: 10.1210/jc.2015-3924

Morroni, M., Giordano, A., Zingaretti, M. C., Boiani, R., De Matteis, R., Kahn, B. B., et al. (2004). Reversible transdifferentiation of secretory epithelial cells into adipocytes in the mammary gland. *Proc. Natl. Acad. Sci. U.S.A.* 101, 16801–16806.

Muhlhausler, B., and Smith, S. R. (2009). Early-life origins of metabolic dysfunction: role of the adipocyte. *Trends Endocrinol. Metab.* 20, 51–57. doi: 10.1016/j.tem.2008.10.006

Mullen, M., and Gonzalez-Perez, R. R. (2016). Leptin-induced JAK/STAT signaling and cancer growth. *Vaccines* 4:26. doi: 10.3390/vaccines4030026

Nadal-Serrano, M., Sastre-Serra, J., Valle, A., Roca, P., and Oliver, J. (2015). Chronic-leptin attenuates cisplatin cytotoxicity in MCF-7 breast cancer cell line. *Cell. Physiol. Biochem.* 36, 221–232. doi: 10.1159/000374066

Najafi-Shoushtari, S. H., Kristo, F., Li, Y., Shioda, T., Cohen, D. E., Gerszten, R. E., et al. (2010). MicroRNA-33 and the SREBP host genes cooperate to control cholesterol homeostasis. *Science* 328, 1566–1569. doi: 10.1126/science.1189123

Nakayama, R. T., Pulice, J. L., Valencia, A. M., McBride, M. J., McKenzie, Z. M., Gillespie, M. A., et al. (2017). SMARCB1 is required for widespread BAF complex-mediated activation of enhancers and bivalent promoters. *Nat. Genet.* 49, 1613–1623. doi: 10.1038/ng.3958

Naukkarinen, J., Heinonen, S., Hakkarainen, A., Lundbom, J., Vuolteenaho, K., Saarinen, L., et al. (2014). Characterising metabolically healthy obesity in weight-discordant monozygotic twins. *Diabetologia* 57, 167–176. doi: 10.1007/s00125-013-3066-y

Nishimoto, S., Fukuda, D., Higashikuni, Y., Tanaka, K., Hirata, Y., Murata, C., et al. (2016). Obesity-induced DNA released from adipocytes stimulates chronic adipose tissue inflammation and insulin resistance. *Sci. Adv.* 2:e1501332. doi: 10.1126/sciadv.1501332

Nishimura, S., Manabe, I., Nagasaki, M., Eto, K., Yamashita, H., Ohsugi, M., et al. (2009). CD8+ effector T cells contribute to macrophage recruitment and adipose tissue inflammation in obesity. *Nat. Med.* 15, 914–920. doi: 10.1038/nm.1964

O'Brien, J., Hayder, H., Zayed, Y., and Peng, C. (2018). Overview of microRNA biogenesis, mechanisms of actions, and circulation. *Front. Endocrinol.* 9:402. doi: 10.3389/fendo.2018.00402

Oishi, Y., Manabe, I., Tobe, K., Tsushima, K., Shindo, T., Fujiu, K., et al. (2005). Krüppel-like transcription factor KLF5 is a key regulator of adipocyte differentiation. *Cell Metab.* 1, 27–39. doi: 10.1016/j.cmet.2004.11.005

Okamoto, Y., Higashiyama, H., Inoue, H., Kanematsu, M., Kinoshita, M., and Asano, S. (2007). Quantitative image analysis in adipose tissue using an automated image analysis system: differential effects of peroxisome proliferator-activated receptor- a and - g agonist on white and brown adipose tissue morphology in AKR obese and db / db diabetic mice. *Comp. Study* 57, 369–377. doi: 10.1111/j.1440-1827.2007.02109.x

Okuno, Y., Ohtake, F., Igarashi, K., Kanno, J., Matsumoto, T., Takada, I., et al. (2013). Epigenetic regulation of adipogenesis by PHF2 histone demethylase. *Diabetes* 62, 1426–1434. doi: 10.2337/db12-0628

Olea-Flores, M., Zuñiga-Eulogio, M., Tacuba-Saavedra, A., Bueno-Salgado, M., Sánchez-Carvajal, A., Vargas-Santiago, Y., et al. (2019). Leptin promotes expression of EMT-related transcription factors and invasion in a Src and FAK-dependent pathway in MCF10A mammary epithelial cells. *Cells* 8:1133. doi: 10.3390/cells8101133

Oussalah, A., Rischer, S., Bensenane, M., Conroy, G., Filhine-Tresarrieu, P., Debard, R., et al. (2018). Plasma mSEPT9: a novel circulating cell-free DNA-based epigenetic biomarker to diagnose hepatocellular carcinoma. *EBioMedicine* 30, 138–147. doi: 10.1016/j.ebiom.2018.03.029

Ouyang, D., Ye, Y., Guo, D., Yu, X., Chen, J., Qi, J., et al. (2015). MicroRNA-125b-5p inhibits proliferation and promotes adipogenic differentiation in 3T3-L1 preadipocytes. *Acta Biochim. Biophys. Sin.* 47, 355–361. doi: 10.1093/abbs/gmv024

Pagotto, U., Vicennati, V., and Pasquali, R. (2005). The endocannabinoid system and the treatment of obesity. *Ann. Med.* 37, 270–275. doi: 10.1080/07853890510037419

Pedersen, T. A., Kowenz-Leutz, E., Leutz, A., and Nerlov, C. (2001). Cooperation between C/EBPalpha TBP/TFIIB and SWI/SNF recruiting domains is required for adipocyte differentiation. *Genes Dev.* 15, 3208–3216. doi: 10.1101/gad.209901

Pei, H., Yao, Y., Yang, Y., Liao, K., and Wu, J. (2011). Kruppel-like factor KLF9 regulates PPARγ transactivation at the middle stage of adipogenesis. *Cell Death Differ.* 18, 315–327. doi: 10.1038/cdd.2010.100

Pekala, B. P., Kawakami, M., Vine, W., Lane, M. D., and Cerami, A. (1983). Studies of insulin resistance in adipocytes induced by macrophage mediator. *J. Exp. Med.* 157, 1360–1365.

Pelleymounter, M. A., Cullen, M. J., Baker, M. B., Hecht, R., Winters, D., Boone, T., et al. (1995). Effects of the obese gene product on body weight regulation in ob/ob mice. *Science* 269, 540–543. doi: 10.1126/science.7624776

Peng, Y., Xiang, H., Chen, C., Zheng, R., Chai, J., Peng, J., et al. (2013). MiR-224 impairs adipocyte early differentiation and regulatesfatty acid metabolism. *Int. J. Biochem. Cell Biol.* 45, 1585–1593. doi: 10.1016/j.biocel.2013.04.029

Perrini, S., Porro, S., Nigro, P., Cignarelli, A., Caccioppoli, C., Genchi, V. A., et al. (2020). Reduced SIRT1 and SIRT2 expression promotes adipogenesis of human visceral adipose stem cells and associates with accumulation of visceral fat in human obesity. *Int. J. Obes.* 44, 307–319. doi: 10.1038/s41366-019-0436-7

Petersen, K. F., and Shulman, G. I. (2006). Etiology of insulin resistance. *Am. J. Med.* 119, S10–S16. doi: 10.1016/j.amjmed.2006.01.009

Petkevicius, K., Virtue, S., Bidault, G., Jenkins, B., Cubuk, C., Morgantini, C., et al. (2019). Accelerated phosphatidylcholine turnover in macrophages promotes adipose tissue inflammation in obesity. *eLife* 8:e47990. doi: 10.7554/eLife.47990

Polyzos, S. A., Perakakis, N., and Mantzoros, C. S. (2019). Fatty liver in lipodystrophy: a review with a focus on therapeutic perspectives of adiponectin and/or leptin replacement. *Metabolism* 96, 66–82. doi: 10.1016/j.metabol.2019.05.001

Ravelli, A. C. J., Van Der Meulen, J. H. P., Osmond, C., Barker, D. J. P., and Bleker, O. P. (1999). Obesity at the age of 50 y in men and women exposed to famine prenatally. *Am. J. Clin. Nutr.* 70, 811–816. doi: 10.1093/ajcn/70.5.811

Rayner, K. J., Suárez, Y., Dávalos, A., Parathath, S., Fitzgerald, M. L., Tamehiro, N., et al. (2010). MiR-33 contributes to the regulation of cholesterol homeostasis. *Science* 328, 1570–1573. doi: 10.1126/science.1189862

Rehman, T., Sachan, D., and Chitkara, A. (2017). Serum insulin and leptin levels in children with epilepsy on valproate-associated obesity. *J. Pediatr. Neurosci.* 12, 135–137. doi: 10.4103/jpn.JPN_152_16

Reyes-Gutierrez, P., Carrasquillo-Rodríguez, J. W., and Imbalzano, A. N. (2019). Promotion of adipogenesis by JMJD6 requires the AT hook-like domain and is independent of its catalytic function. *bioRxiv* doi: 10.1101/609982

Romere, C., Duerrschmid, C., Bournat, J., Constable, P., Jain, M., Xia, F., et al. (2016). Asprosin, a fasting-induced glucogenic protein hormone. *Cell* 165, 566–579. doi: 10.1016/j.cell.2016.02.063

Rosen, E. D., Hsu, C., Wang, X., Sakai, S., Freeman, M. W., Gonzalez, F. J., et al. (2002). C/EBPα induces adipogenesis through PPARγ: a unified pathway. *Genes Dev.* 16, 22–26. doi: 10.1101/gad.948702.nuclear

Rosen, E. D., Sarraf, P., Troy, A. E., Bradwin, G., Moore, K., Milstone, D. S., et al. (1999). PPARγ is required for the differentiation of adipose tissue in vivo and in vitro. *Mol. Cell* 4, 611–617. doi: 10.1016/S1097-2765(00)80211-7

Rothman, R. B., Baumann, M. H., Dersch, C. M., Romero, D. V., Rice, K. C., Carroll, F. I. V. Y., et al. (2001). Amphetamine-type central nervous norepinephrine more potently than they release dopamine and serotonin. *Synapse* 39, 32–41.

Rudolph, M. C., Jackman, M. R., Presby, D. M., Houck, J. A., Webb, P. G., Johnson, G. C., et al. (2018). Low neonatal plasma n-6/n-3 PUFA ratios regulate offspring adipogenic potential and condition adult obesity resistance. *Diabetes* 67, 651–661. doi: 10.2337/db17-0890

Sakamoto, H., Kogo, Y., Ohgane, J., Hattori, N., Yagi, S., Tanaka, S., et al. (2008). Sequential changes in genome-wide DNA methylation status during adipocyte differentiation. *Biochem. Biophys. Res. Commun.* 366, 360–366. doi: 10.1016/j.bbrc.2007.11.137

Salma, N., Xiao, H., Mueller, E., and Imbalzano, A. N. (2004). Temporal recruitment of transcription factors and SWI/SNF chromatin-remodeling enzymes during adipogenic induction of the peroxisome proliferator-activated receptor γ nuclear hormone receptor. *Mol. Cell. Biol.* 24, 4651–4663. doi: 10.1128/mcb.24.11.4651-4663.2004

Saltiel, A. R. (2001). You are what you secrete. *Nat. Med.* 7, 887–888. doi: 10.1038/90911

Saxena, N. K., and Sharma, D. (2013). Multifaceted leptin network: the molecular connection between obesity and breast cancer. *J. Mammary Gland Biol. Neoplasia* 18, 309–320. doi: 10.1007/s10911-013-9308-2

Scheja, L., and Heeren, J. (2019). The endocrine function of adipose tissues in health and cardiometabolic disease. *Nat. Rev. Endocrinol.* 15, 507–524. doi: 10.1038/s41574-019-0230-6

Scherer, P. E. (2006). Adipose tissue: from lipid storage compartment to endocrine organ. *Diabetes* 55, 1537–1545. doi: 10.2337/db06-0263

Scherer, P. E., Williams, S., Fogliano, M., Baldini, G., and Lodish, H. F. (1995). A novel serum protein similar to C1q, produced exclusively in adipocytes. *J. Biol. Chem.* 270, 26746–26749. doi: 10.1074/jbc.270.45.26746

Schmidt, E., Dhaouadi, I., Gaziano, I., Oliverio, M., Klemm, P., Awazawa, M., et al. (2018). LincRNA H19 protects from dietary obesity by constraining expression of monoallelic genes in brown fat. *Nat. Commun.* 9:3622. doi: 10.1038/s41467-018-05933-8

Schmidt-Schweda, S., and Holubarsch, C. (2000). First clinical trial with etomoxir in patients with chronic congestive heart failure. *Clin. Sci.* 99, 27–35.

Sen Banerjee, S., Feinberg, M. W., Watanabe, M., Gray, S., Haspel, R. L., Denkinger, D. J., et al. (2003). The Krüppel-like factor KLF2 inhibits peroxisome proliferator-activated receptor-γ expression and adipogenesis. *J. Biol. Chem.* 278, 2581–2584. doi: 10.1074/jbc.M210859200

Shanaki, M., Omidifar, A., Shabani, P., and Toolabi, K. (2020). Association between HDACs and pro-inflammatory cytokine gene expressions in obesity. *Arch. Physiol. Biochem.* [Epub ahead of print] doi: 10.1080/13813455.2020.1734843

Shi, Y., Li, F., Wang, S., Wang, C., Xie, Y., Zhou, J., et al. (2020). miR-196b-5p controls adipocyte differentiation and lipogenesis through regulating mTORC1 and TGF-β signaling. *FASEB J.* 34, 9207–9222. doi: 10.1096/fj.201901562RR

Shoucri, B. M., Martinez, E. S., Abreo, T. J., Hung, V. T., Moosova, Z., Shioda, T., et al. (2017). Retinoid x receptor activation alters the chromatin landscape to commit mesenchymal stem cells to the adipose lineage. *Endocrinology* 158, 3109–3125. doi: 10.1210/en.2017-00348

Sinclair, K. D., Allegrucci, C., Singh, R., Gardner, D. S., Sebastian, S., Bispham, J., et al. (2007). DNA methylation, insulin resistance, and blood pressure in offspring determined by maternal periconceptional B vitamin and methionine status. *Proc. Natl. Acad. Sci. U.S.A.* 104, 19351–19356. doi: 10.1073/pnas.0707258104

Skinner, M. K., Manikkam, M., Tracey, R., Guerrero-Bosagna, C., Haque, M., and Nilsson, E. E. (2013). Ancestral dichlorodiphenyltrichloroethane (DDT) exposure promotes epigenetic transgenerational inheritance of obesity. *BMC Med.* 11:228. doi: 10.1186/1741-7015-11-228

Smith, B. M., Thomsen, W. J., and Grottick, A. J. (2006). The potential use of selective 5-HT2C agonists in treating obesity. *Expert Opin. Investig. Drugs* 15, 257–266. doi: 10.1517/13543784.15.3.257

Song, F., Del Pozo, C. H., Rosario, R., Zou, Y. S., Ananthakrishnan, R., Xu, X., et al. (2014). RAGE regulates the metabolic and inflammatory response to high-fat feeding in mice. *Diabetes* 63, 1948–1965. doi: 10.2337/db13-1636

Sonnenburg, J. L., and Bäckhed, F. (2016). Diet-microbiota interactions as moderators of human metabolism. *Nature* 535, 56–64. doi: 10.1038/nature18846

Strieder-Barboza, C., Baker, N. A., Flesher, C. G., Karmakar, M., Patel, A., Lumeng, C. N., et al. (2020). Depot-specific adipocyte-extracellular matrix metabolic crosstalk in murine obesity. *Adipocyte* 9, 189–196. doi: 10.1080/21623945.2020.1749500

Sun, H., Wang, N., Nie, X., Zhao, L., Li, Q., Cang, Z., et al. (2017). Lead exposure induces weight gain in adult rats, accompanied by DNA hypermethylation. *PLoS One* 12:e0169958. doi: 10.1371/journal.pone.0169958

Sun, L., Marin, de Evsikova, C., Bian, K., Achille, A., Telles, E., et al. (2018). Programming and regulation of metabolic homeostasis by HDAC11. *EBioMedicine* 33, 157–168. doi: 10.1016/j.ebiom.2018.06.025

Sun, Y., Jin, Z., Zhang, X., Cui, T., Zhang, W., Shao, S., et al. (2020). GATA binding protein 3 is a direct target of kruppel-like transcription factor 7 and inhibits chicken adipogenesis. *Front. Physiol.* 11:610. doi: 10.3389/fphys.2020.00610

Svensson, K. J., Long, J. Z., Jedrychowski, M. P., Cohen, P., Lo, J. C., Serag, S., et al. (2016). A secreted slit2 fragment regulates adipose tissue thermogenesis and metabolic function. *Cell Metab.* 23, 454–466. doi: 10.1016/j.cmet.2016.01.008

Syed, F., Tersey, S. A., Turatsinze, J. V., Felton, J. L., Kang, N. J., Nelson, J. B., et al. (2020). Circulating unmethylated CHTOP and INS DNA fragments provide evidence of possible islet cell death in youth with obesity and diabetes. *Clin. Epigenet.* 12:116. doi: 10.1186/s13148-020-00906-5

Takahashi, H., Alves, C. R. R., Stanford, K. I., Middelbeek, R. J. W., Nigro, P., Ryan, R. E., et al. (2019). TGF-β2 is an exercise-induced adipokine that regulates glucose and fatty acid metabolism. *Nat. Metab.* 1, 291–303. doi: 10.1038/s42255-018-0030-7

Tan, C. Y., and Vidal-Puig, A. (2008). Adipose tissue expandability: the metabolic problems of obesity may arise from the inability to become more obese. *Biochem. Soc. Trans.* 36, 935–940. doi: 10.1042/BST0360935

Tang, Q., Grønborg, M., Huang, H., Kim, J., Otto, T. C., Pandey, A., et al. (2005). Sequential phosphorylation of CCAAT enhancer-binding protein β by MAPK and glycogen synthase kinase 3 β is required for adipogenesis. *Proc. Natl. Acad. Sci. U.S.A.* 102, 9766–9771.

Tang, Q., Otto, T. C., and Lane, M. D. (2003). CCAAT/ enhancer-binding protein β is required for mitotic clonal expansion during adipogenesis. *Proc. Natl. Acad. Sci. U.S.A.* 100, 850–855.

Toffoli, B., Gilardi, F., Winkler, C., Soderberg, M., Kowalczuk, L., Arsenijevic, Y., et al. (2017). Nephropathy in Pparg-null mice highlights PPARγ systemic activities in metabolism and in the immune system. *PLoS One* 12:e0171474. doi: 10.1371/journal.pone.0171474

Tong, Q., Dalgin, G., Xu, H., Ting, C. N., Leiden, J. M., and Hotamisligil, G. S. (2000). Function of GATA transcription factors in preadipocyte-adipocyte transition. *Science* 290, 134–138. doi: 10.1126/science.290.5489.134

Tong, Q., Tsai, J., Tan, G., Dalgin, G., and Hotamisligil, G. S. (2005). Interaction between GATA and the C/EBP family of transcription factors is critical in GATA-mediated suppression of adipocyte differentiation. *Mol. Cell. Biol.* 25, 706–715. doi: 10.1128/MCB.25.2.706

Tontonoz, P., Kim, J. B., Graves, R. A., and Spiegelman, B. M. (1993). ADD1: a novel helix-loop-helix transcription factor associated with adipocyte determination and differentiation. *Mol. Cell. Biol.* 13, 4753–4759. doi: 10.1128/mcb.13.8.4753

Valdearcos, M., Robblee, M. M., Benjamin, D. I., Nomura, D. K., Xu, A. W., and Koliwad, S. K. (2014). Microglia dictate the impact of saturated fat consumption on hypothalamic inflammation and neuronal function. *Cell Rep.* 9, 2124–2138. doi: 10.1016/j.celrep.2014.11.018

Vandegehuchte, M. B., Lemière, F., Vanhaecke, L., Vanden Berghe, W., and Janssen, C. R. (2010). Direct and transgenerational impact on Daphnia magna of chemicals with a known effect on DNA methylation. *Comp. Biochem. Physiol. C Toxicol. Pharmacol.* 151, 278–285. doi: 10.1016/j.cbpc.2009.11.007

Vázquez, M., Roglans, N., Cabrero, À, Rodríguez, C., Adzet, T., Alegret, M., et al. (2001). Bezafibrate induces acyl-CoA oxidase mRNA levels and fatty acid peroxisomal β-oxidation in rat white adipose tissue. *Mol. Cell. Biochem.* 216, 71–78. doi: 10.1023/A:1011060615234

Villarroya, F., Cereijo, R., Villarroya, J., and Giralt, M. (2017). Brown adipose tissue as a secretory organ. *Nat. Rev. Endocrinol.* 13, 26–35. doi: 10.1038/nrendo.2016.136

Wan, Y., Wang, F., Yuan, J., Li, J., Jiang, D., Zhang, J., et al. (2019). Effects of dietary fat on gut microbiota and faecal metabolites, and their relationship with cardiometabolic risk factors: a 6-month randomised controlled-feeding trial. *Gut* 68, 1417–1429. doi: 10.1136/gutjnl-2018-317609

Wang, C., Lee, J. E., Lai, B., Macfarlan, T. S., Xu, S., Zhuang, L., et al. (2016). Enhancer priming by H3K4 methyltransferase MLL4 controls cell fate transition. *Proc. Natl. Acad. Sci. U.S.A.* 113, 11871–11876. doi: 10.1073/pnas.1606857113

Wang, G.-X., Zhao, X.-Y., Meng, Z.-X., Kern, M., Dietrich, A., Chen, Z., et al. (2014). The brown fat-enriched secreted factor Nrg4 preserves metabolic homeostasis through attenuation of hepatic lipogenesis. *Nat. Med.* 20, 1436–1443. doi: 10.1038/nm.3713

Wang, L., Tang, C., Cao, H., Li, K., Pang, X., Zhong, L., et al. (2015). Activation of IL-8 via PI3K/AKT-dependent pathway is involved in leptin-mediated epithelial-mesenchymal transition in human breast cancer cells. *Cancer Biol. Ther.* 16, 1220–1230. doi: 10.1080/15384047.2015.1056409

Wang, Q. A., Tao, C., Jiang, L., Shao, M., Ye, R., Zhu, Y., et al. (2015). Distinct regulatory mechanisms governing embryonic versus adult adipocyte maturation. *Nat. Cell Biol.* 17, 1099–1111. doi: 10.1038/ncb3217

Wang, Q. A., Tao, C., Gupta, R. K., and Scherer, P. E. (2013). Tracking adipogenesis during white adipose tissue development, expansion and regeneration. *Nat. Med.* 19, 1338–1344. doi: 10.1038/nm.3324

Weber, M., Hellmann, I., Stadler, M. B., Ramos, L., Pääbo, S., Rebhan, M., et al. (2007). Distribution, silencing potential and evolutionary impact of promoter DNA methylation in the human genome. *Nat. Genet.* 39, 457–466. doi: 10.1038/ng1990

Wei, L., Li, K., Pang, X., Guo, B., Su, M., Huang, Y., et al. (2016). Leptin promotes epithelial-mesenchymal transition of breast cancer via the upregulation of pyruvate kinase M2. *J. Exp. Clin. Cancer Res.* 35:166. doi: 10.1186/s13046-016-0446-4

Wei, Y., Yang, C. R., Wei, Y. P., Zhao, Z. A., Hou, Y., Schatten, H., et al. (2014). Paternally induced transgenerational inheritance of susceptibility to diabetes in mammals. *Proc. Natl. Acad. Sci. U.S.A.* 111, 1873–1878. doi: 10.1073/pnas.1321195111

Weisberg, S. P., Leibel, R. L., Anthony, W. F. Jr., Weisberg, S. P., Hunter, D., et al. (2006). CCR2 modulates inflammatory and metabolic effects of high-fat feeding find the latest version: CCR2 modulates inflammatory and metabolic effects of high-fat feeding. *J. Clin. Invest.* 1, 115–124. doi: 10.1172/JCI24335

Weisberg, S. P., McCann, D., Desai, M., Rosenbaum, M., Leibel, R. L., and Ferrante, A. W. (2003). Obesity is associated with macrophage accumulation in adipose tissue. *J. Clin. Invest.* 112, 1796–1808. doi: 10.1172/JCI200319246

Wen, H., Gris, D., Lei, Y., Jha, S., Zhang, L., Huang, M. T. H., et al. (2011). Fatty acid-induced NLRP3-ASC inflammasome activation interferes with insulin signaling. *Nat. Immunol.* 12, 408–415. doi: 10.1038/ni.2022

Whittle, A. J., Carobbio, S., Martins, L., Slawik, M., Hondares, E., Vázquez, M. J., et al. (2012). BMP8B increases brown adipose tissue thermogenesis through both central and peripheral actions. *Cell* 149, 871–885. doi: 10.1016/j.cell.2012.02.066

Wiehle, L., Raddatz, G., Musch, T., Dawlaty, M. M., Jaenisch, R., Lyko, F., et al. (2016). Tet1 and Tet2 protect DNA methylation canyons against hypermethylation. *Mol. Cell. Biol.* 36, 452–461. doi: 10.1128/mcb.00587-15

Winer, D. A., Winer, S., Shen, L., Wadia, P. P., Yantha, J., Paltser, G., et al. (2011). B cells promote insulin resistance through modulation of T cells and production of pathogenic IgG antibodies. *Nat. Med.* 17, 610–617. doi: 10.1038/nm.2353

Wu, J., Boström, P., Sparks, L. M., Ye, L., Choi, J. H., Giang, A. H., et al. (2012). Beige adipocytes are a distinct type of thermogenic fat cell in mouse and human. *Cell* 150, 366–376. doi: 10.1016/j.cell.2012.05.016

Wu, J., Dong, T., Chen, T., Sun, J., Luo, J., He, J., et al. (2020). Hepatic exosome-derived miR-130a-3p attenuates glucose intolerance via suppressing PHLPP2 gene in adipocyte. *Metabolism* 103:154006. doi: 10.1016/j.metabol.2019.154006

Wu, X., and Zhang, Y. (2017). TET-mediated active DNA demethylation: mechanism, function and beyond. *Nat. Rev. Genet.* 18, 517–534. doi: 10.1038/nrg.2017.33

Wu, Z., Rosen, E. D., Brun, R., Hauser, S., Adelmant, G., Troy, A. E., et al. (1999). Cross-regulation of C/EBPα and PPARγ controls the transcriptional pathway of adipogenesis and insulin sensitivity. *Mol. Cell* 3, 151–158. doi: 10.1016/S1097-2765(00)80306-8

Xu, R. H., Wei, W., Krawczyk, M., Wang, W., Luo, H., Flagg, K., et al. (2017). Circulating tumour DNA methylation markers for diagnosis and prognosis of hepatocellular carcinoma. *Nat. Mater.* 16, 1155–1162. doi: 10.1038/NMAT4997

Xu, X., Su, S., Barnes, V. A., De Miguel, C., Pollock, J., Ownby, D., et al. (2013). A genome-wide methylation study on obesity: differential variability and differential methylation. *Epigenetics* 8, 522–533. doi: 10.4161/epi.24506

Xu, X., Su, S., Wang, X., Barnes, V., De Miguel, C., Ownby, D., et al. (2015). Obesity is associated with more activated neutrophils in African American male youth. *Int. J. Obes.* 39, 26–32. doi: 10.1038/ijo.2014.194

Xu, Y., Takahashi, Y., Wang, Y., Hama, A., Nishio, N., Muramatsu, H., et al. (2009). Downregulation of GATA-2 and overexpression of adipogenic gene-PPARγ in mesenchymal stem cells from patients with aplastic anemia. *Exp. Hematol.* 37, 1393–1399. doi: 10.1016/j.exphem.2009.09.005

Yamauchi, N., Takazawa, Y., Maeda, D., Hibiya, T., Tanaka, M., Iwabu, M., et al. (2012). Expression levels of adiponectin receptors are decreased in human endometrial adenocarcinoma tissues. *Int. J. Gynecol. Pathol.* 31, 352–357. doi: 10.1097/PGP.0b013e3182469583

Yan, D., Avtanski, D., Saxena, N. K., and Sharma, D. (2012). Leptin-induced epithelial-mesenchymal transition in breast cancer cells requires β-catenin activation via Akt/GSK3- and MTA1/Wnt1 protein-dependent pathways. *J. Biol. Chem.* 287, 8598–8612. doi: 10.1074/jbc.M111.322800

Yang, Q. Y., Liang, J. F., Rogers, C. J., Zhao, J. X., Zhu, M. J., and Du, M. (2013). Maternal obesity induces epigenetic modifications to facilitate Zfp423 expression and enhance adipogenic differentiation in fetal mice. *Diabetes* 62, 3727–3735. doi: 10.2337/db13-0433

Yang, X., Wu, R., Shan, W., Yu, L., Xue, B., and Shi, H. (2016). DNA methylation biphasically regulates 3T3-L1 preadipocyte differentiation. *Mol. Endocrinol.* 30, 677–687. doi: 10.1210/me.2015-1135

Yap, K. L., Johnson, A. E. K., Fischer, D., Kandikatla, P., Deml, J., Nelakuditi, V., et al. (2019). Congenital hyperinsulinism as the presenting feature of Kabuki syndrome: clinical and molecular characterization of 10 affected individuals. *Genet. Med.* 21, 233–242. doi: 10.1038/s41436-018-0013-9

Yi, X., Liu, J., Wu, P., Gong, Y., Xu, X., and Li, W. (2020). The key microRNA on lipid droplet formation during adipogenesis from human mesenchymal stem cells. *J. Cell. Physiol.* 235, 328–338. doi: 10.1002/jcp.28972

Youngson, N. A., and Morris, M. J. (2013). What obesity research tells us about epigenetic mechanisms. *Philos. Trans. R. Soc. B Biol. Sci.* 368:20110337. doi: 10.1098/rstb.2011.0337

Yu, J., Kong, X., Liu, J., Lv, Y., Sheng, Y., Lv, S., et al. (2014). Expression profiling of PPARγ-regulated MicroRNAs in human subcutaneous and visceral adipogenesis in both genders. *Endocrinology* 155, 2155–2165. doi: 10.1210/en.2013-2105

Zeisel, S. H. (2009). Epigenetic mechanisms for nutrition determinants of later health outcomes. *Am. J. Clin. Nutr.* 89, 1488S–1493S. doi: 10.3945/ajcn.2009.27113B

Zhang, C., Wang, J. J., He, X., Wang, C., Zhang, B., Xu, J., et al. (2019). Characterization and beige adipogenic potential of human embryo white adipose tissue-derived stem cells. *Cell. Physiol. Biochem.* 51, 2900–2915. doi: 10.1159/000496042

Zhang, J. W., Klemm, D. J., Vinson, C., and Lane, M. D. (2004). Role of CREB in transcriptional regulation of CCAAT/enhancer-binding protein β gene during adipogenesis. *J. Biol. Chem.* 279, 4471–4478. doi: 10.1074/jbc.M311327200

Zhang, Q., Ramlee, M. K., Brunmeir, R., Villanueva, C. J., Halperin, D., and Xu, F. (2012). Dynamic and distinct histone modifications modulate the expression of key adipogenesis regulatory genes. *Cell Cycle* 11, 4310–4322. doi: 10.4161/cc.22224

Zhang, T., Liu, H., Mao, R., Yang, H., Zhang, Y., Zhang, Y., et al. (2020). The lncRNA RP11-142A22.4 promotes adipogenesis by sponging *miR-587* to modulate Wnt5β expression. *Cell Death Dis.* 11:475. doi: 10.1038/s41419-020-2550-9

Zhang, Z., Hou, Y., Wang, Y., Gao, T., Ma, Z., Yang, Y., et al. (2020). Regulation of adipocyte differentiation by METTL4, a 6 mA methylase. *Sci. Rep.* 10:8285. doi: 10.1038/s41598-020-64873-w

Zhang, Y., Proenca, R., Maffei, M., Barone, M., Leopold, L., and Friedman, J. M. (1994). Positional cloning of the mouse obese gene and its human homologue. *Nature* 372, 425–432. doi: 10.1038/372425a0

14

The mTOR–Autophagy Axis and the Control of Metabolism

Nerea Deleyto-Seldas and Alejo Efeyan*

Metabolism and Cell Signaling Laboratory, Spanish National Cancer Research Center (CNIO), Madrid, Spain

*Correspondence:
Alejo Efeyan
aefeyan@cnio.es

The mechanistic target of rapamycin (mTOR), master regulator of cellular metabolism, exists in two distinct complexes: mTOR complex 1 and mTOR complex 2 (mTORC1 and 2). MTORC1 is a master switch for most energetically onerous processes in the cell, driving cell growth and building cellular biomass in instances of nutrient sufficiency, and conversely, allowing autophagic recycling of cellular components upon nutrient limitation. The means by which the mTOR kinase blocks autophagy include direct inhibition of the early steps of the process, and the control of the lysosomal degradative capacity of the cell by inhibiting the transactivation of genes encoding structural, regulatory, and catalytic factors. Upon inhibition of mTOR, autophagic recycling of cellular components results in the reactivation of mTORC1; thus, autophagy lies both downstream and upstream of mTOR. The functional relationship between the mTOR pathway and autophagy involves complex regulatory loops that are significantly deciphered at the cellular level, but incompletely understood at the physiological level. Nevertheless, genetic evidence stemming from the use of engineered strains of mice has provided significant insight into the overlapping and complementary metabolic effects that physiological autophagy and the control of mTOR activity exert during fasting and nutrient overload.

Keywords: autophagy, mechanistic target of rapamycin, lysosome, metabolism, nutrients

THE mTOR–AUTOPHAGY AXIS

mTOR, Master Regulator of Metabolism

The mechanistic target of rapamycin (mTOR; also referred to as mammalian target of rapamycin) is an evolutionarily conserved kinase and the catalytic core of two distinct complexes: mTOR complex 1 and 2 (mTORC1 and mTORC2) defined by the presence of the key accessory proteins Raptor and Rictor, respectively. These two distinct complexes differ in substrate specificity, in their upstream regulatory cues, and in their subcellular localization. As part of mTORC1, mTOR drives most anabolic processes in the cell, including protein, lipid, cholesterol, and nucleotide synthesis, while it simultaneously boosts extracellular nutrient uptake and blocks autophagic catabolism (Buttgereit and Brand, 1995; Saxton and Sabatini, 2017; Valvezan and Manning, 2019). The coordination of such energetically onerous anabolic programs is coupled to (1) the availability of cellular nutrients and (2) the signals from the organismal nutritional state in the form of second messengers such as insulin (Efeyan et al., 2015; Shimobayashi and Hall, 2016).

Nutrients, Growth Factors, and mTORC1

The signal transduction cascade from hormones/growth factors that activates the mTOR kinase starts with the activation of a receptor tyrosine kinase at the plasma membrane that switches on the PI3K–Akt axis, which results in the inhibition of the tuberous sclerosis complex (TSC). TSC integrates inputs from cellular stress, such as hypoxia and limiting ATP levels, and is a GTPase-activating protein for the small GTPase Rheb (Garami et al., 2003; Inoki et al., 2003; Tee et al., 2003; Zhang et al., 2003). When bound to GTP, Rheb induces a conformational change in mTORC1 that results in kinase activation (Anandapadamanaban et al., 2019; Rogala et al., 2019). Importantly, Rheb is anchored at the outer surface of the lysosome, and it can only interact with and activate mTORC1 if mTORC1 is tethered to the outer lysosomal surface, a re-localization process that occurs in a cellular nutrient-dependent manner (Sancak et al., 2008; **Figure 1**).

The levels of cellular nutrients (amino acids, glucose, certain lipids, and likely other metabolites) are sensed and signaled by an expanding number of proteins (SESNs, CASTOR, KICSTOR, SAMTOR, GATOR1 and 2) (Saxton and Sabatini, 2017) that culminate in the control of the guanosine phosphate state of the members of the Rag family of GTPases, which bind mTORC1 in a nutrient-sensitive manner (**Figure 1**). In addition, Rag GTPase-independent amino acid control of mTORC1 exists (Efeyan et al., 2014; Jewell et al., 2015). The Rag GTPases operate as obligate heterodimeric partners composed of RagA or RagB plus RagC or RagD (Schurmann et al., 1995). In the presence of cellular nutrients, RagA or B are loaded with GTP, while RagC or D are loaded with GDP (Kim et al., 2008; Sancak et al., 2008). This specific nucleotide configuration allows the interaction with mTORC1 and its recruitment to the outer lysosomal surface, where the Rheb–mTORC1 interaction, and mTORC1 activation, occurs. Hence, the current paradigm of the regulation of mTORC1 states that maximal mTORC1 activity takes place when both signals are present: (1) cellular nutrients to recruit mTORC1 and (2) hormones/growth factors for kinase activation (Lawrence and Zoncu, 2019; Valvezan and Manning, 2019). This elegant mechanism of coincidence detection of inputs has been well illustrated by biochemical, cell biological, and structural approaches, but we still ignore how the convergent controls of mTORC1 activity result in the execution of a coherent, multifaceted metabolic program in real organs with physiological and pathological fluctuations in nutrients and hormones.

mTORC1, Catabolism, and Biosynthetic Capacity

At the cellular level, intense research in the last 15 years has shown that the anabolic program executed by mTORC1 is coupled to a block in catabolic processes. Otherwise, a disconnection would result in futile, cyclic synthesis and degradation of cellular components and biomass. Nonetheless, the increased demand for energy and building blocks for macromolecule synthesis upon mTORC1 activation, together with the block in autophagy, results in a biosynthetic burden that the cell alleviates with the execution of parallel programs that reinforce nutrient uptake (Park et al., 2017; Torrence et al., 2020) and synthesis (Robitaille et al., 2013; Ben-Sahra et al., 2016; Valvezan et al., 2017), and also enables the catabolic capacity

of the cells through the proteasomal degradation of proteins (Zhang et al., 2014) to remove unwanted cellular material and to boost the pool of free amino acids available for protein synthesis. Reciprocally, an increased autophagic flux and the recycling of cellular macromolecules upon extended inhibition of mTORC1 is sufficient to partially replenish intracellular or intra-lysosomal amino acid pools and to partially reactivate mTORC1 (Yu et al., 2010; **Figure 1**).

mTORC1 Governs Autophagy at the Lysosomal Surface

It is not coincidental that the subcellular location where mTORC1 activation occurs is the cytoplasmic side of the organelle responsible for internal recycling of macromolecules: the lysosome. Indeed, such spatial association has remained fixed throughout eukaryotic and metazoan evolution. The cytoplasmic side of the lysosomal membrane provides a scaffold surface for controlling mTORC1 and also enables immediate control of specific mTORC1 targets associated to the lysosome (Rabanal-Ruiz and Korolchuk, 2018). Moreover, both abundance and positioning of lysosomes are important modulators of mTORC1 and mTORC2 (Korolchuk et al., 2011; Jia and Bonifacino, 2019; Mutvei et al., 2020). Targets of mTORC1 that are transiently or permanently associated to the lysosome include ULK1, ATG13, and TFEB and its family members, but exactly how and where mTORC1 reaches and phosphorylates its targets is not clear. The coordinated control of these targets results in complementary functions that, together, tightly restrict autophagy when mTORC1 is active. On one side, the inhibitory phosphorylation of the ULK1/ATG13/FIP200 complex by mTORC1 immediately blocks the initiation of the formation of the autophagosome (Ganley et al., 2009; Hosokawa et al., 2009; Kim et al., 2011). This early block is reinforced by the inhibitory phosphorylation of TFEB and MiTF-TFE family members (Settembre et al., 2011; Roczniak-Ferguson et al., 2012; Martina and Puertollano, 2013). TFEB and family members are themselves a signaling hub that computes information from nutrient sufficiency, calcium signaling (Medina et al., 2015), and overall lysosomal stress and health (Ballabio and Bonifacino, 2020), and ultimately execute a transcriptional program that includes the synthesis of proteins that boost the degradative capacity of the cell (Napolitano and Ballabio, 2016; Ballabio and Bonifacino, 2020). The lysosomal biogenesis program encompasses lysosomal membrane proteins, lysosomal lumen enzymes that execute the catalytic degradation of cargo, and factors directly involved in the execution of autophagy (Sardiello et al., 2009; Settembre et al., 2011; **Figure 1**). Thus, the coordinated actions of mTORC1 ensure a rapid block in autophagy and a slower inhibition of this transcriptional program that ultimately restricts lysosomal biogenesis and lysosomal function (**Figure 1**).

As mentioned, phosphorylation of mTORC1 targets results in induction and in inhibition of anabolic and catabolic functions, respectively. A consensus sequence that facilitates recruitment to, and phosphorylation by mTORC1 has been inceasingly refined (Hsu et al., 2011; Yu et al., 2011; Robitaille et al., 2013). While

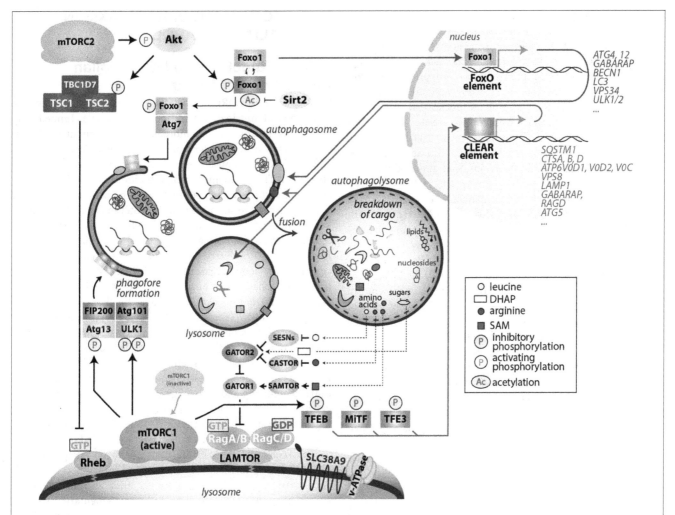

FIGURE 1 | The mTOR–autophagy axis. MTORC1 blocks the early steps in autophagy by phosphorylation-dependent inhibition of Atg13 and ULK1 and also restrains the degradative capacity of the cell by inhibiting the activity of TFEB family members. Several autophagy-related proteins and other lysosomal factors are encoded by genes that harbor a CLEAR sequence in their promoter region, and are bound and transactivated by active TFEB family members. Thus, inhibition of mTORC1 enables autophagic degradation and degradative capacity of the cell, while also suppressing anabolism and, thus, lowering the demand for energy and nutrients. In turn, lysosome-derived amino acids (leucine and arginine) and also other nutrients (glucose-DHAP, cholesterol, SAM) can partially reactivate Rag GTPase – nutrient signaling upstream of mTORC1. MTORC2 and the AGC kinases Akt and SGK1 also limit the autophagic flux and lysosomal capacity via transcription-dependent and -independent processes. The cytoplasmic sequestration of the FoxO transcription factors indirectly limits autophagic degradation, as several FoxO targets encode proteins that directly participate in different steps of autophagy and lysosomal catabolism.

for years the paradigm has stated that all mTORC1 targets interact with mTORC1 by means of the TOR signaling (TOS) motif (Schalm and Blenis, 2002), recent compelling work has demonstrated that this is not universal. In particular, TFEB family members are orphan of a TOS motif and are instead recruited to mTORC1 through a direct interaction with the RagC GTPase (Napolitano et al., 2020). Importantly, inhibition of TFEB by mTORC1 is facilitated by RagC exclusively under cellular nutrient sufficiency, thus defining an input-dependent asymmetry in the activation of different targets downstream of mTORC1 (Napolitano et al., 2020). While targets with a TOS motif result phosphorylated only if the TSC-Rheb and the Rag GTPase arms are *ON*, TFEB is sensitive to any perturbation that would result in a change in the nucleotide to which RagC is bound, such as nutrient withdrawal/replenishment, but would be

less affected by the inhibition and activation of the growth factor signaling cascade.

The physiological implications of this asymmetric control of mTORC1 targets are enormous and have been already underlined in the context of brown adipose tissue function (Wada et al., 2016), and of the Birt–Hogg–Dubé syndrome (Napolitano et al., 2020), and may underlie the occurrence of activating mutations in RagC (but not in RagA) in B-cell lymphomas (Ortega-Molina et al., 2019).

The Regulation of Autophagy by mTORC2

In addition to the suppression of autophagy when part of mTORC1, the mTOR kinase restrains autophagy when part of mTORC2. Through mechanisms that are not entirely defined, growth factor signaling activates mTORC2, and upon its activation, mTORC2 phosphorylates and activates Akt and other members of the AGC kinase family (Hoxhaj and Manning, 2020). The FoxO transcription factors are phosphorylation targets of Akt (Brunet et al., 1999), and Akt-dependent phosphorylation of FoxO1/3a results in nuclear exclusion, thus impairing the transactivation of autophagy-related factors and lysosome-tethered proteins (Mammucari et al., 2007; Zhao et al., 2007). In an interesting crosstalk between Akt and the NAD-dependent deacetylase family of Sirtuins, Sirt1 also modulates the transcriptional activity of FoxO1 (Frescas et al., 2005). Moreover, in an apparently counterintuitive manner, cytoplasmic FoxO1 can also induce the autophagic flux by its interaction with Atg7 (Zhao et al., 2010), and this cytoplasmic, transcription-independent function of FoxO1 requires its deacetylation by Sirt2, and is facilitated by nuclear exclusion of FoxO1 by Akt-dependent phosphorylation (Zhou et al., 2012). While this nucleo-cytoplasmic tug of war of FoxO1 shuttle in the control of autophagy deserves further investigation, the acetylation of FoxO1 in the cytoplasm ensures the rapid execution of autophagy even in conditions of high growth factor signaling (**Figure 1**). In addition, not all reported connections between mTORC2 and autophagy involve cytoplasmic and nuclear functions of FoxO, as Akt directly phosphorylates and inhibits ULK1 (Bach et al., 2011). Finally, transcriptional activity by FoxO includes the upregulation of Sestrins, negative regulators of the Rag-mTORC1 axis, in an additional loop of cross-regulation (Chen et al., 2010).

In addition to the functions of Akt, inhibition of another member of the AGC kinase family, SGK1, by either genetic and pharmacological means, induces autophagy *in vitro* and *in vivo* (Conza et al., 2017; Liu et al., 2018; Zuleger et al., 2018), and these effects may also be mediated by the phosphorylation of FoxO3a. In worms, suppression of the mTORC2–SGK1 axis induces autophagy in a DAF-16/FOXO-independent manner (Aspernig et al., 2019) downstream of altered mitochondrial permeability (Zhou et al., 2019), strongly suggesting that mTORC2 lies upstream of the control of autophagy by SGK1. Such control is prominent in mammalian skeletal muscle (Andres-Mateos et al., 2013; Zuleger et al., 2018). However, the fact that SGK1 knock-out mice (Wulff et al., 2002; Fejes-Tóth et al., 2008) show minimal phenotypic alterations, unlike autophagy-deficient mice (Kuma et al., 2004), may reflect the importance of SGK1 under specific stress conditions.

The enumerated multilayered, convergent, and complementary effects of mTORC1 and mTORC2 in the repression of autophagy deciphered at the molecular level point to (1) a direct, acute blockade of the phagophore–autophagosome formation, together with (2) a long-term, transcription-based limitation of the degradative machinery, but how is this complexity integrated to sustain metabolic homeostasis and how may its deregulation contribute to metabolic disease are far less understood. We next review the lessons that mouse genetic approaches have taught in the understanding of the physiology of the mTOR–autophagy axis.

THE mTORC1–AUTOPHAGY AXIS IN MAMMALIAN METABOLISM

mTOR, Autophagy and Mammalian Adaptation to Fasting

Suppression of mTORC1 activity has proven essential to endure conditions of nutrient deprivation in mammals. Immediately after birth, glucose and amino acid levels in circulation drop dramatically due to the interruption of the trans-placental supply, and mTORC1 in mouse tissues is readily inhibited within 1 h after birth. This rapid and strong inhibition is critical to unleash autophagy, which in turn boosts free amino acid levels that feed gluconeogenesis to sustain glycaemia (Efeyan et al., 2013), and is key to endure the first hours of life, before significant maternal milk supply occurs. Neonatal mice carrying a point mutation in *RagA* (RagA^{Q66L}, referred to as RagA^{GTP}) that renders mTORC1 constitutively active regardless of nutrient levels are unable to trigger autophagy after birth, suffer a profound hypoglycemic state they do not recover from, and finally succumb within 1 day after birth (Efeyan et al., 2013). A strikingly similar phenomenon was observed in mice lacking *Sestrin 1, 2* and *3*, negative regulators of the Rag GTPases (Peng et al., 2014), and in *Atg5*$^{-/-}$ (Kuma et al., 2004) and *Atg7*$^{-/-}$ mice (Komatsu et al., 2005). The phenotypic resemblance of mice with constitutive nutrient signaling and autophagy-deficient mice provides strong genetic and physiological support for the importance of the regulation of autophagy by the nutrient–mTORC1 pathway in the maintenance of metabolic homeostasis (see **Table 1**).

The sequential steps in the transition from postprandial to early and long-term fasting metabolism in adult individuals encompass a shift from glucose to lipid and ketone body metabolism, through consistent and complementary responses in the liver, skeletal muscle, and white adipose tissue (WAT), coordinated systemically by hormonal signaling. An early fasting switch involves the release of liver glycogen stores as soon as insulin levels drop. When glycogen has been entirely mobilized, gluconeogenesis occurs together with increased lipolysis from the WAT to yield circulating glycerol, a substrate for gluconeogenesis, and free fatty acids (FFA). The ATP produced by β-oxidation of FFA in the liver sustains gluconeogenesis, while acetyl-CoA is shunted to the production of ketone bodies, an essential source of energy during fasting, and particularly important for the brain.

In addition to its essentiality in neonatal mice, autophagy is required by adult mice to endure periods of fasting. Acute, full-body ablation of autophagy by tamoxifen-mediated deletion of *Atg7* impairs the survival of the mice following a 24-h fast due to severe hypoglycemia. Interestingly, amino acid levels in circulation are sustained by accelerated muscle wasting, but this increase fails to support gluconeogenesis, and decreased WAT and rapidly depleted hepatic glycogen stores compromise the endurance to long-term fasting (Karsli-Uzunbas et al., 2014).

As soon as insulin drops, autophagy is induced in the liver, and adult mice unable to trigger hepatic autophagy fail to release free amino acids and suffer from reduced blood glucose levels during fasting, an effect that can be rescued experimentally by

TABLE 1 | Metabolic phenotypes of genetically-engineered mice with increased and decreased mTORC1 activity and enhanced or suppressed autophagy.

	mTORC1 activity	Phenotype	Autophagy	Phenotype
Full body	**ON-*RagA* Q66L**	Neonatal death	**OFF-*Atg5* /*Atg7* KO**	Neonatal death
	(Efeyan et al., 2013)	Hypoglycemia	(Kuma et al., 2004)	↓Fasting circulating AA
		↓Fasting circulating AA	(Komatsu et al., 2005)	
	ON-*Sesn* 1, 2, 3 KO	Neonatal death	**OFF-*Atg7* KO 4OHT-ind**	Death—24-h fasting
	(Peng et al., 2014)		(Karsli-Uzunbas et al., 2014)	Hypoglycemia
	OFF-*Deptor* OE	↑*In vivo* adiposity	**ON-*Atg5* OE**	↓Fat mass
	(Laplante et al., 2012)	↑Body weight gain (HFD)	(Pyo et al., 2013)	↑Insulin sensitivity
				↑Glucose tolerance
Liver	**ON-*Tsc1* KO**	Defective ketogenesis	**OFF-*Atg7* KO**	Hypoglycemia
	(Kenerson et al., 2011)	Resistance to hepatic steatosis	(Ezaki et al., 2011)	Lipid droplets
	(Liko et al., 2020)	Impaired transcriptional response to fasting	(Singh et al., 2009a)	↓Fasting circulating AA
	(Sengupta et al., 2010)			
	(Yecies et al., 2011)			
	ON-*RagA* Q66L	Impaired transcriptional response to fasting		
	(de la Calle Arregui et al., 2021)	Defective ketogenesis		
	OFF-*Raptor* KO	↓Body weight gain (HFD)	**ON-*Tfeb* OE**	↑Insulin sensitivity
	(Peterson et al., 2011)	Resistance to hepatic steatosis	(Settembre et al., 2013)	↑Glucose tolerance
				↓Body weight gain (HFD)
WAT	**ON-*Tsc1* KO**	↓WAT expansion	**OFF-*Atg7* KO**	↑Mitochondrial oxidation
	(Magdalon et al., 2016)	↑Mitochondrial oxidation	(Singh et al., 2009b)	↑Fatty acid oxidation
		↑Fatty acid oxidation	(Zhang et al., 2009)	↓Body weight gain (HFD)
		↓Body weight gain (HFD)		
	OFF-*Raptor* KO	↓WAT expansion		
	(Lee et al., 2016)	Lipodystrophy		
		↓Body weight gain (HFD)		
Skeletal muscle	**ON-*Tsc1* KO**	Premature death	**OFF-*Atg7* KO**	Muscle atrophy/dystrophy
	(Bentzinger et al., 2013)	Muscle atrophy/dystrophy	(Masiero et al., 2009)	Aberrant organelles
	(Castets et al., 2019)	Aberrant organelles		
	OFF-*Raptor* KO	Premature death		
	(Bentzinger et al., 2008)	Muscle atrophy/dystrophy		

KO, knock-out; OE, overexpressor; AA, amino acids; 4OHT-ind, tamoxifen-inducible; HFD, high-fat diet; WAT, white adipose tissue.

exogenous administration of the gluconeogenic amino acid serine (Ezaki et al., 2011). It is noteworthy that in these mice, glycogen mobilization during fasting is not impaired, and neither is it in *RagA*[GTP] neonates (Efeyan et al., 2013) nor in adult *Atg7*-KO mice (Karsli-Uzunbas et al., 2014), in spite of the relevance of autophagic degradation of glycogen (glycophagy) during fasting (Schiaffino and Hanzlíková, 1972; Jiang et al., 2010). Surprisingly, mice with constitutive hepatic mTORC1 activity by means of genetic deletion of *Tsc1* (Sengupta et al., 2010; Yecies et al., 2011; Liko et al., 2020), or liver-specific activation of RagA (de la Calle Arregui et al., 2021), do not phenocopy a deficiency in autophagy and instead have an impaired transcriptional adaptation to fasting that limits ketogenesis. Thus, in adult mice undergoing fasting, mTORC1 and autophagy control complementary adaptations to nutrient limitations (see **Table 1**).

mTOR, Autophagy, and Lipid Homeostasis

In addition to supporting fasting glucose homeostasis, autophagy contributes to the hydrolysis of lipid droplets upon nutrient deprivation by the delivery of lipid droplets to lysosomes, and pharmacologic and genetic inhibition of autophagy in the liver leads to the accumulation of lipid droplets and to lower rates of β-oxidation both *in vitro* and *in vivo* (Singh et al., 2009a). *In vivo* deletion of *Atg7* specifically in WAT leads to a lean phenotype accompanied by morphological and functional changes of the WAT. Adipocytes from these animals are multilocular, with enriched content in mitochondria, and display increased rates of β-oxidation, and these mice also exhibit improved insulin sensitivity and resistance to high-fat-diet-induced obesity (Singh et al., 2009b; Zhang et al., 2009).

The phenotypes of mice with a hyper-active mTORC1 in the WAT have some features in common with those of defective autophagy. Deletion of *Tsc1* in adipocytes compromises WAT expansion, results in a higher mitochondrial oxidative activity and fatty acid oxidation and to a leaner phenotype when mice were fed a high-fat diet (Magdalon et al., 2016). While deletion of *Raptor* in WAT also results in defective WAT expansion, lipodystrophy, and resistance to diet-induced obesity (Lee et al., 2016), the overexpression of *Deptor*, a negative regulator of mTOR, promotes adipogenesis and mice gain more weight upon high-fat feeding (Laplante et al., 2012). *Deptor* overexpression decreases the negative feedback loop to Akt, while not significantly affecting other mTORC1 targets, supporting the notion that both mTORC1 and Akt activities are required for adipogenesis.

The mTORC1 target TFEB controls lipid catabolism at the transcriptional level by promoting PGC1-α-dependent PPARα activation in response to fasting (Settembre et al., 2013). An analogous process occurs in *C. elegans*, where HLH-30 (ortholog of TFEB) regulates the expression of lysosomal triglyceride lipases (O'Rourke and Ruvkun, 2013). Overexpression of *Tfeb* in mice (TFEB-Tg mice) leads to an improvement of glucose tolerance, insulin sensitivity, and weight gain in mice fed with high-fat diet and, importantly, to a lean phenotype that is abolished in an *Atg7*-deficient background, genetically demonstrating the epistasis of TFEB and autophagy (Settembre et al., 2013). This work is consistent with a report showing that autophagy is impaired in obese (ob/ob) mice, and reconstitution of autophagy in the liver by expressing *Atg7* using an adenoviral system improves their glucose tolerance and insulin sensitivity (Yang et al., 2010). Consistently, ubiquitous and moderate overexpression of *Atg5* in mice, resulting in increased autophagy, leads to a leaner phenotype, an increased glucose tolerance and insulin sensitivity, and resistance to age-induced obesity (Pyo et al., 2013).

In line with the phenotypes observed in TFEB-Tg mice and in *Atg5*-Tg mice, liver-specific *Raptor* KO mice are resistant to diet-induced obesity and to hepatic steatosis, and these effects are, at least in part, mediated by the mTORC1 target Lipin1 (Peterson et al., 2011). In an apparent contradiction, mice with hyperactive mTORC1 signaling in the liver (liver-specific *Tsc1* KO) are also resistant to age- and diet-induced hepatic steatosis (Sengupta et al., 2010), but this apparently counterintuitive finding can be explained by an indirect attenuation of Akt-SREBP1 signaling (rather by suppression of autophagy) through the induction of a negative feedback loop to the insulin receptor substrate (IRS) (Kenerson et al., 2011; Yecies et al., 2011).

Mouse genetics for the study of WAT can produce phenotypic findings of difficult interpretation. This difficulty is probably related to the strength of perturbation caused by genetic deletion, in contrast to more physiological activation or inhibition of a signaling pathway, and to the expression patterns and leakiness of Cre recombinases. Nonetheless, the *in vitro* and *in vivo* lessons together have taught us that an appropriate, dynamic, and physiological regulation of both mTORC1 activity and autophagy is necessary for adipogenesis and for maintaining the correct accumulation and mobilization of lipids and the physiological functioning of WAT (Clemente-Postigo et al., 2020) (**Table 1**).

mTOR, Autophagy, and Skeletal Muscle Homeostasis

Another tissue that exhibits a remarkable sensitivity to changes in both autophagy and mTOR activity is skeletal muscle. The muscle has the intrinsic ability to hypertrophy and atrophy by a tight balance between protein synthesis and degradation (Fry and Rasmussen, 2011). Intense research has demonstrated that, although acute activation of the Akt-mTORC1 and the mTORC2-Akt axes drive hypertrophy, both chronically aberrant

increase and decrease in mTOR activity yield muscle atrophy because dynamic synthesis–degradation oscillations are essential to maintain fiber homeostasis.

Muscle degradation occurs both in an autophagy-independent manner, by FoxO-dependent transactivation of the ubiquitin ligases Atrogin-1 and MuRF1 (Sandri et al., 2004; Stitt et al., 2004), and by autophagic degradation by FoxO-dependent transcription of many autophagy-related genes (Mammucari et al., 2007; Zhao et al., 2007). Thus, the Akt-FoxO signaling pathway coordinates the two main degradative pathways involved in atrophy: the ubiquitin–proteasome and the autophagy–lysosome.

In addition to a key role of the mTORC2–Akt–FoxO pathway in the control of muscle homeostasis, deletion of the mTORC1 component *Raptor* in the skeletal muscle results in profound atrophic and dystrophic muscles, with metabolic and structural changes incompatible with mouse survival (Bentzinger et al., 2008). While short-term genetic hyperactivation of mTORC1 in skeletal muscle by deletion of *Tsc1* results in hypertrophy, sustained mTORC1 hyperactivation eventually precipitates atrophy in most muscles and premature death (Bentzinger et al., 2013; Castets et al., 2013). The features of this myopathy are very similar to the ones developed by mice with a specific deletion of *Atg7* in the skeletal muscle, where aberrant membranous structures accumulate in muscle fibers (Masiero et al., 2009). The strong suppression of Akt through the mTORC1-mediated negative feedback loop allows the expression of Atrogin-1 and MuRF1 in young, but not in old, muscle-specific *Tsc1*-KO (sm-*Tsc1* KO) mice. Instead, the late-onset myopathy in skeletal muscle of old sm-*Tsc1* KO mice is caused by the inability to induce autophagy. Pharmacological inhibition of mTORC1 with rapamycin restores the autophagic flux and rescues the defects, pointing to pivotal and complex roles of both mTORC1 and TORC2 in the control of autophagy in the skeletal muscle from young and old individuals (Castets et al., 2013). Recent work has also shown that both the mTORC1–autophagy axis and mTORC1–Akt axis are critical for the coordination of recovery after denervation (Castets et al., 2019) (**Table 1**).

CONCLUDING REMARKS

The multilayered functional interactions of the mTOR signaling pathways and the process of autophagy are deciphered to a great extent at the cellular level, but we still have an incomplete understanding of their integration at the physiopathological level. To what extent does a blockade in autophagy explain the consequences of deregulated mTOR activity? Would the sole inhibition of mTOR unleash physiological autophagy and its benefits? Mouse genetics has contributed substantial snapshots of phenotypic similarities, epistasis, and complementary metabolic functions of mTOR inhibition and autophagy in different organs and metabolic states. A challenge for the future is to translate this body of knowledge into significant support for pharmacological manipulation of mTOR and autophagy to improve metabolism and control the pathologies associated with nutrient overload.

AUTHOR CONTRIBUTIONS

ND-S and AE conceived, wrote, and edited the text and figures. Both authors contributed to the article and approved the submitted version.

ACKNOWLEDGMENTS

AE dedicates this work to the memory of Diego Armando Maradona.

REFERENCES

Anandapadamanaban, M., Masson, G. R., Perisic, O., Berndt, A., Kaufman, J., Johnson, C. M., et al. (2019). Architecture of human Rag GTPase heterodimers and their complex with mTORC1. *Science* 366, 203–210. doi: 10.1126/science.aax3939

Andres-Mateos, E., Brinkmeier, H., Burks, T. N., Mejias, R., Files, D. C., Steinberger, M., et al. (2013). Activation of serum/glucocorticoid-induced kinase 1 (SGK1) is important to maintain skeletal muscle homeostasis and prevent atrophy. *EMBO Mol. Med.* 5, 80–91. doi: 10.1002/emmm.201201443

Aspernig, H., Heimbucher, T., Qi, W., Gangurde, D., Curic, S., Yan, Y., et al. (2019). Mitochondrial Perturbations Couple mTORC2 to Autophagy in *C. elegans*. *Cell Rep.* 29, 1399–1409.e5. doi: 10.1016/j.celrep.2019.09.072

Bach, M., Larance, M., James, D. E., and Ramm, G. (2011). The serine/threonine kinase ULK1 is a target of multiple phosphorylation events. *Biochem. J.* 440, 283–291. doi: 10.1042/BJ20101894

Ballabio, A., and Bonifacino, J. S. (2020). Lysosomes as dynamic regulators of cell and organismal homeostasis. *Nat. Rev. Mol. Cell Biol.* 21, 101–118. doi: 10.1038/s41580-019-0185-4

Ben-Sahra, I., Hoxhaj, G., Ricoult, S. J. H., Asara, J. M., and Manning, B. D. (2016). mTORC1 induces purine synthesis through control of the mitochondrial tetrahydrofolate cycle. *Science* 351, 728–733. doi: 10.1126/science.aad0489

Bentzinger, C. F., Lin, S., Romanino, K., Castets, P., Guridi, M., Summermatter, S., et al. (2013). Differential response of skeletal muscles to mTORC1 signaling during atrophy and hypertrophy. *Skelet. Muscle* 3:6. doi: 10.1186/2044-5040-3-6

Bentzinger, C. F., Romanino, K., Cloëtta, D., Lin, S., Mascarenhas, J. B., Oliveri, F., et al. (2008). Skeletal muscle-specific ablation of raptor, but not of rictor, causes metabolic changes and results in muscle dystrophy. *Cell Metab.* 8, 411–424. doi: 10.1016/j.cmet.2008.10.002

Brunet, A., Bonni, A., Zigmond, M. J., Lin, M. Z., Juo, P., Hu, L. S., et al. (1999). Akt promotes cell survival by phosphorylating and inhibiting a forkhead transcription factor. *Cell* 96, 857–868. doi: 10.1016/S0092-8674(00)80595-4

Buttgereit, F., and Brand, M. D. (1995). A hierarchy of ATP-consuming processes in mammalian cells. *Biochem. J.* 312(Pt 1)(Pt 1), 163–167. doi: 10.1042/bj3120163

Castets, P., Lin, S., Rion, N., Di Fulvio, S., Romanino, K., Guridi, M., et al. (2013). Sustained activation of mTORC1 in skeletal muscle inhibits constitutive and starvation-induced autophagy and causes a severe, late-onset myopathy. *Cell Metab.* 17, 731–744. doi: 10.1016/j.cmet.2013.03.015

Castets, P., Rion, N., Théodore, M., Falcetta, D., Lin, S., Reischl, M., et al. (2019). mTORC1 and PKB/Akt control the muscle response to denervation by regulating autophagy and HDAC4. *Nat. Commun.* 10:3187. doi: 10.1038/s41467-019-11227-4

Chen, C. C., Jeon, S. M., Bhaskar, P. T., Nogueira, V., Sundararajan, D., Tonic I., et al. (2010). FoxOs inhibit mTORC1 and activate Akt by inducing the expression of Sestrin3 and Rictor. *Dev. Cell* 18, 592–604. doi: 10.1016/j.devcel.2010.03.008

Clemente-Postigo, M., Tinahones, A., El Bekay, R., Malagón, M. M., and Tinahones, F. J. (2020). The role of autophagy in white adipose tissue function: implications for metabolic health. *Metabolites* 10:179. doi: 10.3390/metabo10050179

Conza, D., Mirra, P., Calì, G., Tortora, T., Insabato, L., Fiory, F., et al. (2017). The SGK1 inhibitor SI113 induces autophagy, apoptosis, and endoplasmic reticulum stress in endometrial cancer cells. *J. Cell. Physiol.* 232, 3735–3743. doi: 10.1002/jcp.25850

de la Calle Arregui, C., Plata-Gomez, A. B., Deleyto-Seldas, N., Garcia, F., Ortega-Molina, A., Abril-Garrido, J., et al. (2021). Limited survival and impaired hepatic fasting metabolism in mice with constitutive Rag GTPase signaling. *Nat. Commun.* doi: 10.1038/s41467-021-23857-8

Efeyan, A., Comb, W. C., and Sabatini, D. M. (2015). Nutrient-sensing mechanisms and pathways. *Nature* 517, 302–310. doi: 10.1038/nature14190

Efeyan, A., Schweitzer, L. D., Bilate, A. M., Chang, S., Kirak, O., Lamming, D. W., et al. (2014). RagA, but not RagB, is essential for embryonic development and adult mice. *Dev. Cell* 29, 321–329. doi: 10.1016/j.devcel.2014.03.017

Efeyan, A., Zoncu, R., Chang, S., Gumper, I., Snitkin, H., Wolfson, R. L., et al. (2013). Regulation of mTORC1 by the Rag GTPases is necessary for neonatal autophagy and survival. *Nature* 493, 679–683. doi: 10.1038/nature11745

Ezaki, J., Matsumoto, N., Takeda-Ezaki, M., Komatsu, M., Takahashi, K., Hiraoka, Y., et al. (2011). Liver autophagy contributes to the maintenance of blood glucose and amino acid levels. *Autophagy* 7, 727–736. doi: 10.4161/auto.7.7.15371

Fejes-Tóth, G., Frindt, G., Náray-Fejes-Tóth, A., and Palmer, L. G. (2008). Epithelial Na+ channel activation and processing in mice lacking SGK1. *Am. J. Physiol. Ren. Physiol.* 294, F1298–F1305. doi: 10.1152/ajprenal.00579.2007

Frescas, D., Valenti, L., and Accili, D. (2005). Nuclear trapping of the forkhead transcription factor FoxO1 via sirt-dependent deacetylation promotes expression of glucogenetic genes. *J. Biol. Chem.* 280, 20589–20595. doi: 10.1074/jbc.M412357200

Fry, C. S., and Rasmussen, B. B. (2011). Skeletal muscle protein balance and metabolism in the elderly. *Curr. Aging Sci.* 4, 260–268. doi: 10.2174/1874609811104030260

Ganley, I. G., Lam, D. H., Wang, J., Ding, X., Chen, S., and Jiang, X. (2009). ULK1·ATG13·FIP200 complex mediates mTOR signaling and is essential for autophagy. *J. Biol. Chem.* 284, 12297–12305. doi: 10.1074/jbc.M900573200

Garami, A., Zwartkruis, F. J., Nobukuni, T., Joaquin, M., Roccio, M., Stocker, H., et al. (2003). Insulin activation of Rheb, a mediator of mTOR/S6K/4E-BP signaling, is inhibited by TSC1 and 2. *Mol. Cell* 11, 1457–1466. doi: 10.1016/s1097-2765(03)00220-x

Hosokawa, N., Hara, T., Kaizuka, T., Kishi, C., Takamura, A., Miura, Y., et al. (2009). Nutrient-dependent mTORC1 association with the ULK1-Atg13-FIP200 complex required for autophagy. *Mol. Biol. Cell* 20, 1981–1991. doi: 10.1091/mbc.E08-12-1248

Hoxhaj, G., and Manning, B. D. (2020). The PI3K–AKT network at the interface of oncogenic signalling and cancer metabolism. *Nat. Rev. Cancer* 20, 74–88. doi: 10.1038/s41568-019-0216-7

Hsu, P. P., Kang, S. A., Rameseder, J., Zhang, Y., Ottina, K. A., Lim, D., et al. (2011). The mTOR-regulated phosphoproteome reveals a mechanism of mTORC1-mediated inhibition of growth factor signaling. *Science* 332, 1317–1322. doi: 10.1126/science.1199498

Inoki, K., Li, Y., Xu, T., and Guan, K. L. (2003). Rheb GTPase is a direct target of TSC2 GAP activity and regulates mTOR signaling. *Genes Dev.* 17, 1829–1834. doi: 10.1101/gad.1110003

Jewell, J. L., Kim, Y. C., Russell, R. C., Yu, F. X., Park, H. W., Plouffe, S. W., et al. (2015). Differential regulation of mTORC1 by leucine and glutamine. *Science* 347, 194–198. doi: 10.1126/science.1259472

Jia, R., and Bonifacino, J. S. (2019). Lysosome positioning influences mTORC2 and AKT signaling. *Mol. Cell* 75, 26-38.e3. doi: 10.1016/j.molcel.2019.05.009

Jiang, S., Heller, B., Tagliabracci, V. S., Zhai, L., Irimia, J. M., DePaoli-Roach, A. A., et al. (2010). Starch binding domain-containing protein 1/genethonin 1 is a novel participant in glycogen metabolism. *J. Biol. Chem.* 285, 34960–34971. doi: 10.1074/jbc.M110.150839

Karsli-Uzunbas, G., Guo, J. Y., Price, S., Teng, X., Laddha, S. V., Khor, S., et al. (2014). Autophagy is required for glucose homeostasis and lung tumor maintenance. *Cancer Discov.* 4, 914–927. doi: 10.1158/2159-8290.CD-14-0363

Kenerson, H. L., Yeh, M. M., and Yeung, R. S. (2011). Tuberous sclerosis complex-1 deficiency attenuates diet-induced hepatic lipid accumulation. *PLoS One* 6:e18075. doi: 10.1371/journal.pone.0018075

Kim, E., Goraksha-Hicks, P., Li, L., Neufeld, T. P., and Guan, K. L. (2008). Regulation of TORC1 by Rag GTPases in nutrient response. *Nat. Cell Biol.* 10, 935–945. doi: 10.1038/ncb1753

Kim, J., Kundu, M., Viollet, B., and Guan, K. L. (2011). AMPK and mTOR regulate autophagy through direct phosphorylation of Ulk1. *Nat. Cell Biol.* 13, 132–141. doi: 10.1038/ncb2152

Komatsu, M., Waguri, S., Ueno, T., Iwata, J., Murata, S., Tanida, I., et al. (2005). Impairment of starvation-induced and constitutive autophagy in Atg7-deficient mice. *J. Cell Biol.* 169, 425–434. doi: 10.1083/jcb.200412022

Korolchuk, V. I., Saiki, S., Lichtenberg, M., Siddiqi, F. H., Roberts, E. A., Imarisio, S., et al. (2011). Lysosomal positioning coordinates cellular nutrient responses. *Nat. Cell Biol.* 13, 453–460. doi: 10.1038/ncb2204

Kuma, A., Hatano, M., Matsui, M., Yamamoto, A., Nakaya, H., Yoshimori, T., et al. (2004). The role of autophagy during the early neonatal starvation period. *Nature* 432, 1032–1036. doi: 10.1038/nature03029

Laplante, M., Horvat, S., Festuccia, W. T., Birsoy, K., Prevorsek, Z., Efeyan, A., et al. (2012). DEPTOR Cell-autonomously promotes adipogenesis, and its expression is associated with obesity. *Cell Metab.* 16, 202–212. doi: 10.1016/j.cmet.2012.07.008

Lawrence, R. E., and Zoncu, R. (2019). The lysosome as a cellular centre for signalling, metabolism and quality control. *Nat. Cell Biol.* 21, 133–142. doi: 10.1038/s41556-018-0244-7

Lee, P. L., Tang, Y., Li, H., and Guertin, D. A. (2016). Raptor/mTORC1 loss in adipocytes causes progressive lipodystrophy and fatty liver disease. *Mol. Metab.* 5, 422–432. doi: 10.1016/j.molmet.2016.04.001

Liko, D., Rzepiela, A., Vukojevic, V., Zavolan, M., and Hall, M. N. (2020). Loss of TSC complex enhances gluconeogenesis via upregulation of Dlk1-Dio3 locus miRNAs. *Proc. Natl. Acad. Sci. U.S.A.* 117, 1524–1532. doi: 10.1073/pnas.1918931117

Liu, W., Wang, X., Wang, Y., Dai, Y., Xie, Y., Ping, Y., et al. (2018). SGK1 inhibition-induced autophagy impairs prostate cancer metastasis by reversing EMT. *J. Exp. Clin. Cancer Res.* 37:73. doi: 10.1186/s13046-018-0743-1

Magdalon, J., Chimin, P., Belchior, T., Neves, R. X., Vieira-Lara, M. A., Andrade, M. L., et al. (2016). Constitutive adipocyte mTORC1 activation enhances mitochondrial activity and reduces visceral adiposity in mice. *Biochim. Biophys. Acta Mol. Cell Biol. Lipids* 1861, 430–438. doi: 10.1016/j.bbalip.2016.02.023

Mammucari, C., Milan, G., Romanello, V., Masiero, E., Rudolf, R., Del Piccolo, P., et al. (2007). FoxO3 controls autophagy in skeletal muscle in vivo. *Cell Metab.* 6, 458–471. doi: 10.1016/j.cmet.2007.11.001

Martina, J. A., and Puertollano, R. (2013). Rag GTPases mediate amino acid-dependent recruitment of TFEB and MITF to lysosomes. *J. Cell Biol.* 200, 475–491. doi: 10.1083/jcb.201209135

Masiero, E., Agatea, L., Mammucari, C., Blaauw, B., Loro, E., Komatsu, M., et al. (2009). Autophagy is required to maintain muscle mass. *Cell Metab.* 10, 507–515. doi: 10.1016/j.cmet.2009.10.008

Medina, D. L., Di Paola, S., Peluso, I., Armani, A., De Stefani, D., Venditti, R., et al. (2015). Lysosomal calcium signalling regulates autophagy through calcineurin and TFEB. *Nat. Cell Biol.* 7, 288–299. doi: 10.1038/ncb3114

Mutvei, A. P., Nagiec, M. J., Hamann, J. C., Kim, S. G., Vincent, C. T., and Blenis, J. (2020). Rap1-GTPases control mTORC1 activity by coordinating lysosome organization with amino acid availability. *Nat. Commun.* 11:1416. doi: 10.1038/s41467-020-15156-5

Napolitano, G., and Ballabio, A. (2016). TFEB at a glance. *J. Cell Sci.* 129, 2475–2481. doi: 10.1242/jcs.146365

Napolitano, G., Di Malta, C., Esposito, A., de Araujo, M. E. G., Pece, S., Bertalot, G., et al. (2020). A substrate-specific mTORC1 pathway underlies Birt–Hogg–Dubé syndrome. *Nature* 585, 597–602. doi: 10.1038/s41586-020-2444-0

O'Rourke, E. J., and Ruvkun, G. (2013). MXL-3 and HLH-30 transcriptionally link lipolysis and autophagy to nutrient availability. *Nat. Cell Biol.* 15, 668–676. doi: 10.1038/ncb2741

Ortega-Molina, A., Deleyto-Seldas, N., Carreras, J., Sanz, A., Lebrero-Fernández, C., Menéndez, C., et al. (2019). Oncogenic Rag GTPase signalling enhances B cell activation and drives follicular lymphoma sensitive to pharmacological inhibition of mTOR. *Nat. Metab.* 1, 775–789. doi: 10.1038/s42255-019-0098-8

Park, Y., Reyna-Neyra, A., Philippe, L., and Thoreen, C. C. (2017). mTORC1 balances cellular amino acid supply with demand for protein synthesis through post-transcriptional control of ATF4. *Cell Rep.* 19, 775–789. doi: 10.1016/j.celrep.2017.04.042

Peng, M., Yin, N., and Li, M. O. (2014). Sestrins function as guanine nucleotide dissociation inhibitors for Rag GTPases to Control mTORC1 signaling. *Cell* 159, 122–133. doi: 10.1016/j.cell.2014.08.038

Peterson, T. R., Sengupta, S. S., Harris, T. E., Carmack, A. E., Kang, S. A., Balderas, E., et al. (2011). mTOR complex 1 regulates lipin 1 localization to control the srebp pathway. *Cell* 146, 408–420. doi: 10.1016/j.cell.2011.06.034

Pyo, J. O., Yoo, S. M., Ahn, H. H., Nah, J., Hong, S. H., Kam, T. I., et al. (2013). Overexpression of Atg5 in mice activates autophagy and extends lifespan. *Nat. Commun.* 4:2300. doi: 10.1038/ncomms3300

Rabanal-Ruiz, Y., and Korolchuk, V. I. (2018). mTORC1 and nutrient homeostasis: The central role of the lysosome. *Int. J. Mol. Sci.* 19, 818. doi: 10.3390/ijms19030818

Robitaille, A. M., Christen, S., Shimobayashi, M., Cornu, M., Fava, L. L., Moes, S., et al. (2013). Quantitative phosphoproteomics reveal mTORC1 activates de novo pyrimidine synthesis. *Science* 339, 1320–1323. doi: 10.1126/science.1228771

Roczniak-Ferguson, A., Petit, C. S., Froehlich, F., Qian, S., Ky, J., Angarola, B., et al. (2012). The Transcription Factor TFEB Links mTORC1 signaling to transcriptional control of lysosome homeostasis. *Sci. Signal.* 5:ra42. doi: 10.1126/scisignal.2002790

Rogala, K. B., Gu, X., Kedir, J. F., Abu-Remaileh, M., Bianchi, L. F., Bottino, A. M. S., et al. (2019). Structural basis for the docking of mTORC1 on the lysosomal surface. *Science* 366, 468–475. doi: 10.1126/science.aay0166

Sancak, Y., Peterson, T. R., Shaul, Y. D., Lindquist, R. A., Thoreen, C. C., Bar-Peled, L., et al. (2008). The Rag GTPases bind raptor and mediate amino acid signaling to mTORC1. *Science* 320, 1496–1501. doi: 10.1126/science.1157535

Sandri, M., Sandri, C., Gilbert, A., Skurk, C., Calabria, E., Picard, A., et al. (2004). Foxo transcription factors induce the atrophy-related ubiquitin ligase atrogin-1 and cause skeletal muscle atrophy. *Cell* 117, 399–412. doi: 10.1016/S0092-8674(04)00400-3

Sardiello, M., Palmieri, M., di Ronza, A., Medina, D. L., Valenza, M., Gennarino, V. A., et al. (2009). A gene network regulating lysosomal biogenesis and function. *Science* 325, 473–477. doi: 10.1126/science.1174447

Saxton, R. A., and Sabatini, D. M. (2017). mTOR signaling in growth, metabolism, and disease. *Cell* 168, 960–976. doi: 10.1016/j.cell.2017.02.004

Schalm, S. S., and Blenis, J. (2002). Identification of a conserved motif required for mTOR signaling. *Curr. Biol.* 12, 632–639. doi: 10.1016/S0960-9822(02)00762-5

Schiaffino, S., and Hanzlíková, V. (1972). Autophagic degradation of glycogen in skeletal muscles of the Newborn rat. *J. Cell Biol.* 52, 41–51. doi: 10.1083/jcb.52.1.41

Schurmann, A., Brauers, A., Massmann, S., Becker, W., and Joost, H. G. (1995). Cloning of a novel family of mammalian GTP-binding proteins (RagA, RagBs, RagB1) with remote similarity to the Ras-related GTPases. *J. Biol. Chem.* 270, 28982–28988. doi: 10.1074/jbc.270.48.28982

Sengupta, S., Peterson, T. R., Laplante, M., Oh, S., and Sabatini, D. M. (2010). mTORC1 controls fasting-induced ketogenesis and its modulation by ageing. *Nature* 468, 1100–1104. doi: 10.1038/nature09584

Settembre, C., De Cegli, R., Mansueto, G., Saha, P. K., Vetrini, F., Visvikis, O., et al. (2013). TFEB controls cellular lipid metabolism through a starvation-induced autoregulatory loop. *Nat. Cell Biol.* 15, 647–658. doi: 10.1038/ncb2718

Settembre, C., Di Malta, C., Polito, V. A., Garcia Arencibia, M., Vetrini, F., Erdin, S., et al. (2011). TFEB links autophagy to lysosomal biogenesis. *Science* 332, 1429–1433. doi: 10.1126/science.1204592

Shimobayashi, M., and Hall, M. N. (2016). Multiple amino acid sensing inputs to mTORC1. *Cell Res.* 26, 7–20. doi: 10.1038/cr.2015.146

Singh, R., Kaushik, S., Wang, Y., Xiang, Y., Novak, I., Komatsu, M., et al. (2009a). Autophagy regulates lipid metabolism. *Nature* 458, 1131–1135. doi: 10.1038/nature07976

Singh, R., Xiang, Y., Wang, Y., Baikati, K., Cuervo, A. M., Luu, Y. K., et al. (2009b). Autophagy regulates adipose mass and differentiation in mice. *J. Clin. Invest.* 119, 3329–3339. doi: 10.1172/JCI39228

Stitt, T. N., Drujan, D., Clarke, B. A., Panaro, F., Timofeyva, Y., Kline, W. O., et al. (2004). The IGF-1/PI3K/Akt pathway prevents expression of muscle atrophy-induced ubiquitin ligases by inhibiting FOXO transcription factors. *Mol. Cell* 14, 395–403. doi: 10.1016/S1097-2765(04)00211-4

Tee, A. R., Manning, B. D., Roux, P. P., Cantley, L. C., and Blenis, J. (2003). Tuberous sclerosis complex gene products, Tuberin and Hamartin, control mTOR signaling by acting as a GTPase-activating protein complex toward Rheb. *Curr. Biol.* 13, 1259–1268. doi: 10.1016/s0960-9822(03)00506-2

Torrence, M. E., MacArthur, M. R., Hosios, A. M., Asara, J. M., Mitchell, J. R., and Manning, B. D. (2020). The mTORC1-mediated activation of ATF4 promotes protein and glutathione 1 synthesis downstream of growth signals 2. *bioRxiv* [Preprint]. doi: 10.1101/2020.10.03.324186

Valvezan, A. J., and Manning, B. D. (2019). Molecular logic of mTORC1 signalling as a metabolic rheostat. *Nat. Metab.* 1, 321–333. doi: 10.1038/s42255-019-0038-7

Valvezan, A. J., Turner, M., Belaid, A., Lam, H. C., Miller, S. K., McNamara, M. C., et al. (2017). mTORC1 couples nucleotide synthesis to nucleotide demand resulting in a targetable metabolic vulnerability. *Cancer Cell* 32, 624–638.e5. doi: 10.1016/j.ccell.2017.09.013

Wada, S., Neinast, M., Jang, C., Ibrahim, Y. H., Lee, G., Babu, A., et al. (2016). The tumor suppressor FLCN mediates an alternate mTOR pathway to regulate browning of adipose tissue. *Genes Dev.* 30, 2551–2564. doi: 10.1101/gad.287953.116

Wulff, P., Vallon, V., Huang, D. Y., Völkl, H., Yu, F., Richter, K., et al. (2002). Impaired renal Na+ retention in the sgk1-knockout mouse. *J. Clin. Invest.* 110, 1263–1268. doi: 10.1172/jci15696

Yang, L., Li, P., Fu, S., Calay, E. S., and Hotamisligil, G. S. (2010). Defective hepatic autophagy in obesity promotes er stress and causes insulin resistance. *Cell Metab.* 11, 467–478. doi: 10.1016/j.cmet.2010.04.005

Yecies, J. L., Zhang, H. H., Menon, S., Liu, S., Yecies, D., Lipovsky, A. I., et al. (2011). Akt stimulates hepatic SREBP1c and lipogenesis through Parallel mTORC1-dependent and independent pathways. *Cell Metab.* 14, 21–32. doi: 10.1016/j.cmet.2011.06.002

Yu, L., McPhee, C. K., Zheng, L., Mardones, G. A., Rong, Y., Peng, J., et al. (2010). Termination of autophagy and reformation of lysosomes regulated by mTOR. *Nature* 465, 942–946. doi: 10.1038/nature09076

Yu, Y., Yoon, S.-O., Poulogiannis, G., Yang, Q., Ma, X. M., Villen, J., et al. (2011). Phosphoproteomic analysis identifies Grb10 as an mTORC1 substrate that negatively regulates insulin signaling. *Science* 332, 1322–1326. doi: 10.1126/science.1199484

Zhang, Y., Gao, X., Saucedo, L. J., Ru, B., Edgar, B. A., and Pan, D. (2003). Rheb is a direct target of the tuberous sclerosis tumour suppressor proteins. *Nat. Cell Biol.* 5, 578–581. doi: 10.1038/ncb999

Zhang, Y., Goldman, S., Baerga, R., Zhao, Y., Komatsu, M., and Jin, S. (2009). Adipose-specific deletion of autophagy-related gene 7 (atg7) in mice reveals a role in adipogenesis. *Proc. Natl. Acad. Sci. U.S.A.* 106, 19860–19865. doi: 10.1073/pnas.0906048106

Zhang, Y., Nicholatos, J., Dreier, J. R., Ricoult, S. J. H., Widenmaier, S. B., Hotamisligil, G. S., et al. (2014). Coordinated regulation of protein synthesis and degradation by mTORC1. *Nature* 513, 440–443. doi: 10.1038/nature13492

Zhao, J., Brault, J. J., Schild, A., Cao, P., Sandri, M., Schiaffino, S., et al. (2007). FoxO3 coordinately activates protein degradation by the autophagic/lysosomal and proteasomal pathways in atrophying muscle cells. *Cell Metab.* 6, 472–483. doi: 10.1016/j.cmet.2007.11.004

Zhao, Y., Yang, J., Liao, W., Liu, X., Zhang, H., Wang, S., et al. (2010). Cytosolic FoxO1 is essential for the induction of autophagy and tumour suppressor activity. *Nat. Cell Biol.* 12, 665–675. doi: 10.1038/ncb2069

Zhou, B., Kreuzer, J., Kumsta, C., Wu, L., Kamer, K. J., Cedillo, L., et al. (2019). Mitochondrial permeability uncouples elevated autophagy and lifespan extension. *Cell* 177, 299-314.e16. doi: 10.1016/j.cell.2019.02.013

Zhou, J., Liao, W., Yang, J., Ma, K., Li, X., Wang, Y., et al. (2012). FOXO3 induces FOXO1-dependent autophagy by activating the AKT1 signaling pathway. *Autophagy* 8, 1712–1723. doi: 10.4161/auto.21830

Zuleger, T., Heinzelbecker, J., Takacs, Z., Hunter, C., Voelkl, J., Lang, F., et al. (2018). SGK1 inhibits autophagy in murine muscle tissue. *Oxid. Med. Cell. Longev.* 2018:4043726. doi: 10.1155/2018/4043726

Coordinated Metabolic Changes and Modulation of Autophagy during Myogenesis

Paola Fortini[1], Egidio Iorio[2], Eugenia Dogliotti[1]* and Ciro Isidoro[3]*

[1] Department of Environment and Primary Prevention, Istituto Superiore di Sanità, Rome, Italy, [2] Department of Cell Biology and Neurosciences, Istituto Superiore di Sanità, Rome, Italy, [3] Università degli Studi del Piemonte Orientale "Amedeo Avogadro", Novara, Italy

*Correspondence:
Eugenia Dogliotti
eugenia.dogliotti@iss.it;
Ciro Isidoro
ciro.isidoro@med.uniupo.it

Autophagy undergoes a fine tuning during tissue differentiation and organ remodeling in order to meet the dynamic changes in the metabolic needs. While the involvement of autophagy in the homeostasis of mature muscle tissues has been intensively studied, no study has so far addressed the regulation of autophagy in relation to the metabolic state during the myogenic differentiation. In our recently published study (Fortini et al., 2016) we investigated the metabolic profile and regulation of autophagy that accompany the differentiation process of mouse skeletal muscle satellite cells (MSC)-derived myoblasts into myotubes. Here, we briefly present these findings also in the light of similar studies conducted by other authors. We show that during myogenic differentiation mitochondrial function and activity are greatly increased, and the activation of autophagy accompanies the transition from myoblasts to myotube. Autophagy is mTORC1 inactivation-independent and, remarkably, is required to allow the myocyte fusion process, as shown by impaired cell fusion when the autophagic flux is inhibited either by genetic or drug manipulation. Further, we found that myoblasts derived from p53 null mice show defective terminal differentiation into myotubes and reduced activation of basal autophagy. Of note, glycolysis prevails and mitochondrial biogenesis is strongly impaired in p53-null myoblasts. Thus, autophagy, mitochondrial homeostasis, and differentiation are finely tuned in a coordinate manner during muscle biogenesis.

Keywords: muscle differentiation, autophagy, metabolism, p53

Muscle cell differentiation involves significant gene reprogramming as well as cellular reshaping. The role and modulation of autophagy in muscle in several physiological and pathological conditions, including fasting, atrophy and exercise, have been deeply investigated (Vainshtein et al., 2014), but the functional relationship between autophagy and cell metabolism during muscle differentiation remains largely obscure.

Here we illustrate the main findings reported in our recently published paper (Fortini et al., 2016) where we exploited the ability of mouse skeletal Muscle Satellite Cells (MSC)-derived myoblasts to differentiate into myotubes to study the integrated network that cross-regulates autophagy metabolism reprogramming during myogenesis. The forkhead box O3 (FoxO3) transcription factor FoxO3, which is induced by oxidative stress (Li et al., 2015) and in atrophic skeletal muscle (Mammucari et al., 2007), is known to control the transcription of autophagy-related genes, including LC3. Consistently, we found that the mRNA level of FoxO3 and of LC3 increased up to three- and four-folds, respectively, during the transition from myoblast to myotube. Western blotting and immunofluorescence confirmed that autophagy was up-regulated soon after the MSC myoblasts were induced to differentiate into myocytes, and remained up-regulated during the fusion process leading to myotubes. Yet, the net production of autophagosomes slightly decreased in fully differentiated myotubes. Up-regulation of autophagy during the differentiation of myoblasts through the formation of mature myotubes has been also reported by Gottlieb and associates (Sin et al., 2016).

Macromolecular turnover is a requisite of the myogenic program. Consistent with this view, autophagy was not up-regulated in myocytes that were cultured at very low density, a condition that does not allow their fusion into myotubes. To further confirm the important role of autophagy in the myogenesis, we used two different approaches to prevent the induction of autophagy in MSC myoblasts, namely the presence of the antioxidant N-acetyl cysteine (NAC) during differentiation and the post-transcriptional silencing of Beclin 1. NAC has been shown to significantly decrease the basal autophagic flux in skeletal muscles of mice by limiting the production of reactive oxygen species (Rahman et al., 2014). Both these treatments effectively hampered the up-regulation of autophagy, and concomitantly we observed a remarkable reduction of the fusion index (by approximately two-folds).

mTORC1, a negative regulator of autophagy, plays a pivotal role in muscle biogenesis, as it controls multiple stages of the myofiber formation process (Erbay et al., 2003; Sun et al., 2010). Remarkably, mTORC1 remained active during the whole process of differentiation up to the myotube formation, and in spite of this autophagy was induced. Since the AMPk pathway was concomitantly induced along the myogenesis process, we speculate that AMPk overrides the mTOR inhibitory action gradually with time so that autophagy was modulated in a fashion compatible with the differentiation and fusion processes.

The inhibition of mTORC1 by rapamycin led to a further stimulation of autophagy, indicating that mTORC1 exerts a tonic inhibition on autophagy during the process. When the myoblasts were treated with rapamycin myotube formation was drastically impaired. The picture that emerges is that autophagy must be finely tuned and balanced in coordination with cell metabolism in order to allow the correct development of the skeletal muscle tissue.

The metabolic reprogramming during myogenesis was therefore studied in the same cell system. Interestingly, the transcription of PGC-1α, a master regulator of mitochondrial biogenesis, but not of PGC1α, was significantly up-regulated during muscle differentiation, and in parallel the number of mitochondrial DNA molecules as well as the levels of mitochondrial proteins also increased. The production of ATP+ADP, but not that of lactate, also increased during the myogenic process. These data are supportive of an increased mitochondrial activity in the passage from undifferentiated myoblasts to mature myotube. This is consistent with the recent findings reported by Sin et al. (2016) who additionally showed that a dynamic remodeling of the mitochondrial network, including mitochondrial clearance and biogenesis, is required during the myoblast/myotube transition (**Figure 1**). This mitochondrial remodeling was impaired when autophagy was blocked (Sin et al., 2016).

To get a more in depth insight into the mechanistic relationship between cell metabolism reprogramming, mitochondrial homeostasis and autophagy in the myogenic process, we performed a similar study in p53-null MSC-derived myoblasts cultivated under differentiation permissive conditions. In fact, p53 is known to affect myoblast differentiation (Porrello et al., 2000; Cam et al., 2006) and muscle metabolism (Park et al., 2009; Saleem et al., 2014), as well as autophagy (Maiuri et al., 2010; Rufini et al., 2013). Consistent with previous findings (Porrello et al., 2000; Fortini et al., 2012), the formation of myotubes was impaired in p53-null myoblasts, and in parallel we found that the induction of autophagy during the incubation in the differentiation condition was attenuated. Indeed, p53-null myoblasts showed abnormalities in the lysosomal apparatus that reflected in the reduced formation of autolysosomes. In contrast to what observed in p53-proficient myoblasts, in which the glycolytic rate did not change during myogenesis, in p53-null myoblasts an increased glycolytic flux occurred during their differentiation, as testified by the concurrent increase in lactate and in ATP+ADP. Further, in p53-null myoblasts, the mRNA level of PGC-1α remained unchanged, and the content of mtDNA, as well as the protein levels of COXIV and OXPHOS, did not increase in the course of differentiation. It is of note that p53 KO mice show greater fatigability and less locomotory endurance than wild-type animals, and this is associated with reduced expression of PGC-1α and diminished mitochondrial content and functionality in the gastrocnemius (Saleem et al., 2014) providing clear evidence that mitochondrial biogenesis and muscle performance are causally associated. We hypothesize that imperfect myogenesis in these cells could arise from impaired mitophagy. In fact, we observed that abnormal mitochondria forming aggregates accumulated in p53 null myoblasts.

In conclusion, we (Fortini et al., 2016) and others (Sin et al., 2016) demonstrated that the correct execution of the myogenesis program requires the concurrent and coordinated modulation of autophagy, cell metabolism, and mitochondrial remodeling. Further, we demonstrated that the lack of p53 attenuated autophagy and mitogenesis, caused the switch from aerobic respiration to glycolysis, and impaired myogenesis, thus highlighting the role of physiological p53 activity for muscle homeostasis (Fortini et al., 2016). The link between p53, oxidative stress, FoxO3, autophagy and mitogenesis during myogenesis clearly deserves a more in depth analysis. In this respect,

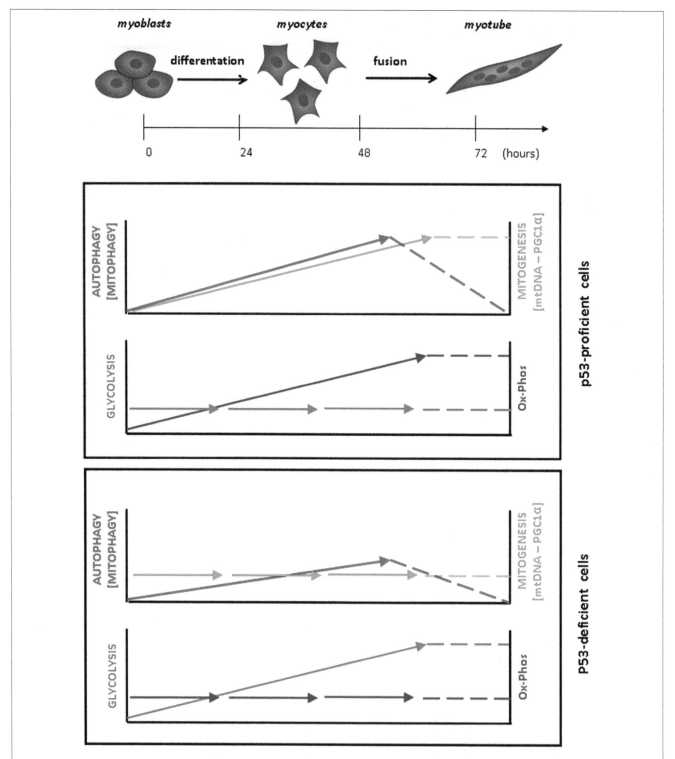

FIGURE 1 | Coordinated metabolic changes and modulation of autophagy during myoblasts differentiation and fusion into myotubes. In p53-proficient MSC-derived myoblasts, autophagy and mitophagy are activated, increase along with the differentiation of myoblasts into myocytes and continue to increase up to the step of cell-to-cell fusion. Once the myotubes have formed, autophagy and mitophagy gradually slow-down to the basal level. The remodeling of the mitochondrial asset is testified by the constant increase in the content of mitochondrial DNA and protein (associated with increased expression of the transcription factor PGC1-α) and is paralleled by the increase in the oxidative phosphorylation (Ox-Phos), while the level of glycolysis is unchanged. In p53-deficient myoblasts, by contrast, the modulation of autophagy is greatly attenuated during the myogenesis process, mitogenesis is not induced and aggregates of abnormal mitochondria accumulate in the cell. In these cells, the production of lactate and ATP increases during the differentiation of myoblasts up to the formation of myotubes, indicating that their energetic metabolism relies essentially on glycolysis.

it has been shown that, under starvation, FoxO activation, promotes the synthesis of glutamine, which in turn prevents the activation of mTOR and stimulates the autophagic flux (Van Der Vos et al., 2012). On the other hand, p53 has been shown to enhance mitochondrial respiration and ATP generation and to increase the cellular level of anti-oxidant GSH by promoting mitochondrial glutaminolysis (Hu et al., 2010).

A better understanding of the gene networks operating during muscle differentiation may open new avenues for the therapies of muscle disorders and repair.

AUTHOR CONTRIBUTIONS

The manuscript was written by ED and CI; revised by PF and EI, read and approved by all co-authors.

ACKNOWLEDGMENTS

This work was partially supported by: AIRC (grant to ED); Fondazione S Paolo (project neuroscience 2010 to CI). The fluorescence imaging facility in CI's laboratory is supported by Comoli, Ferrari and Co. SpA (Novara, Italy).

REFERENCES

Cam, H., Griesmann, H., Beitzinger, M., Hofmann, L., Beinoraviciute-Kellner, R., Sauer, M. et al. (2006). p53 family members in myogenic differentiation and rhabdomyosarcoma development. *Cancer Cell* 10, 281–293. doi: 10.1016/j.ccr.2006.08.024

Erbay, E., Park, I.-H., Nuzzi, P. D., Schoenherr, C. J., and Chen, J. (2003). IGF-II transcription in skeletal myogenesis is controlled by mTOR and nutrients *J. Cell Biol.* 163, 931–936. doi: 10.1083/jcb.200307158

Fortini, P., Ferretti, C., Iorio, E., Cagnin, M., Garribba, L., Pietraforte, D., et al. (2016). The fine tuning of metabolism, autophagy and differentiation during *in vitro* myogenesis. *Cell Death Dis.* 7, e2168. doi: 10.1038/cddis.2016.50

Fortini, P., Ferretti, C., Pascucci, B., Narciso, L., Pajalunga, D., Puggioni, E. M. R., et al. (2012). A damage response by single-strand breaks in terminally differentiated muscle cells and the control of muscle integrity. *Cell Death Diff.* 19, 1741–1749. doi: 10.1038/cdd.2012.53

Hu, W., Zhang, C., Wu, R., Sun, Y., Levine, A., and Feng, Z. (2010). Glutaminase 2, a novel p53 target gene regulating energy metabolism and antioxidant function. *Proc. Natl. Acad. Sci.* 107, 7455–7460. doi: 10.1073/pnas.1001006107

Li, L., Tan, J., Miao, Y., Lei, P., and Zhang, Q. (2015). ROS and autophagy: interactions and molecular regulatory mechanisms. *Cell. Mol. Neurobiol.* 35, 615–621. doi: 10.1007/s10571-015-0166-x

Maiuri, M. C., Galluzzi, L., Morselli, E., Kepp, O., Malik, S. A., and Kroemer, G. (2010). Autophagy regulation by p53. *Curr. Opin. Cell Biol. Cell Regul.* 22, 181–185. doi: 10.1016/j.ceb.2009.12.001

Mammucari, C., Milan, G., Romanello, V., Masiero, E., Rudolf, R., Del, P., et al. (2007). FoxO3 controls autophagy in skeletal muscle *in vivo*. *Cell Metab.* 6, 458–471. doi: 10.1016/j.cmet.2007.11.001

Park, J.-Y., Wang, P.-Y., Matsumoto, T., Sung, H. J., Ma, W., Choi, J. W., et al. (2009). p53 improves aerobic exercise capacity and augments skeletal muscle mitochondrial DNA content. *Circ. Res.* 105, 705–712. doi: 10.1161/CIRCRESAHA.109.205310

Porrello, A., Cerone, M. A., Coen, S., Gurtner, A., Fontemaggi, G., Cimino, L., et al. (2000). P53 regulates myogenesis by triggering the differentiation activity of Prb. *J. Cell Biol.* 151, 1295–1304. doi: 10.1083/jcb.151.6.1295

Rahman, M., Mofarrahi, M., Kristof, A. S., Nkengfac, B., Harel, S., and Hussain, S. N. A. (2014). Reactive oxygen species regulation of autophagy in skeletal muscles. *Antioxid. Redox Signal.* 20, 443–459. doi: 10.1089/ars.2013.5410

Rufini, A., Tucci, P., Celardo, I., and Melino, G. (2013). Senescence and aging: the critical roles of p53. *Oncogene* 32, 5129–5143. doi: 10.1038/onc.2012.640

Saleem, A., Carter, H. N., and Hood, D. A. (2014). p53 is necessary for the adaptive changes in cellular milieu subsequent to an acute bout of endurance exercise. *Am. J. Physiol. Cell Physiol.* 306, C241–C249. doi: 10.1152/ajpcell.00270.2013

Sin, J., Andres, A. M., Taylor, D. J. R., Weston, T., Hiraumi, Y., Stotland, A., et al. (2016). Mitophagy is required for mitochondrial biogenesis and myogenic differentiation of C2C12 myoblasts. *Autophagy* 12, 369–380. doi: 10.1080/15548627.2015.1115172

Sun, Y., Ge, Y., Drnevich, J., Zhao, Y., Band, M., and Chen, J. (2010). Mammalian target of rapamycin regulates miRNA-1 and follistatin in skeletal myogenesis. *J. Cell Biol.* 189, 1157–1169. doi: 10.1083/jcb.200912093

Vainshtein, A., Grumati, P., Sandri, M., and Bonaldo, P. (2014). Skeletal muscle, autophagy, and physical activity: the menage à trois of metabolic regulation in health and disease. *J. Mol. Med.* 92, 127–137. doi: 10.1007/s00109-013-1096-z

Van Der Vos, K. E., Eliasson, P., Proikas-Cezanne, T., Vervoort, S. J., Van Boxtel, R., Putker, M., et al. (2012). Modulation of glutamine metabolism by the PI(3)K-PKB-FOXO network regulates autophagy. *Nat. Cell Biol.* 14, 829–837. doi: 10.1038/ncb2536

Chaperone Mediated Autophagy in the Crosstalk of Neurodegenerative Diseases and Metabolic Disorders

Iván E. Alfaro[1]*, Amelina Albornoz[1], Alfredo Molina[2], José Moreno[2], Karina Cordero[2], Alfredo Criollo[2,3,4] and Mauricio Budini[2,3]*

[1] Fundación Ciencia & Vida, Santiago, Chile, [2] Dentistry Faculty, Institute in Dentistry Sciences, University of Chile, Santiago, Chile, [3] Autophagy Research Center (ARC), Santiago, Chile, [4] Advanced Center for Chronic Diseases (ACCDiS), University of Chile, Santiago, Chile

Correspondence:
Iván E. Alfaro
ialfaro@cienciavida.org
Mauricio Budini
mbudini@u.uchile.cl

Chaperone Mediated Autophagy (CMA) is a lysosomal-dependent protein degradation pathway. At least 30% of cytosolic proteins can be degraded by this process. The two major protein players of CMA are LAMP-2A and HSC70. While LAMP-2A works as a receptor for protein substrates at the lysosomal membrane, HSC70 specifically binds protein targets and takes them for CMA degradation. Because of the broad spectrum of proteins able to be degraded by CMA, this pathway has been involved in physiological and pathological processes such as lipid and carbohydrate metabolism, and neurodegenerative diseases, respectively. Both, CMA, and the mentioned processes, are affected by aging and by inadequate nutritional habits such as a high fat diet or a high carbohydrate diet. Little is known regarding about CMA, which is considered a common regulation factor that links metabolism with neurodegenerative disorders. This review summarizes what is known about CMA, focusing on its molecular mechanism, its role in protein, lipid and carbohydrate metabolism. In addition, the review will discuss how CMA could be linked to protein, lipids and carbohydrate metabolism within neurodegenerative diseases. Furthermore, it will be discussed how aging and inadequate nutritional habits can have an impact on both CMA activity and neurodegenerative disorders.

Keywords: CMA, neurodegeneration, lipids, carbohydrates, metabolism

INTRODUCTION

Autophagy

Autophagy is a cellular process in which proteins and organelles become degraded through lysosomes in order to maintain an adequate cellular homeostasis. In mammals, three different types of autophagy pathways have been described, (i) macroautophagy (mostly known as "autophagy"), (ii) microautophagy, and (iii) chaperone-mediated autophagy (CMA).

Macroautophagy and CMA, together with proteasome, are involved in the recycling of cellular proteins, including those that can compromise the normal physiology of the cell by adopting aberrant folded forms which are able to generate aggregates or inclusions (1). Macroautophagy is a multistep pathway that starts with the formation of an autophagosome, a double membrane vesicular structure that includes the cargo to be degraded. Autophagosome formation involves the participation of different factors like the Atg protein family, LC3-II, p62, Beclin, among others. After its formation, the autophagosome fuses to the lysosome where it releases its proteolytic material to form an autolysosome structure that finally degrades the cargo (1).

In addition to proteins, macroautophagy targets can also include damaged and/or oxidized organelles such as mitochondria (mitophagy), endoplasmic reticulum (ERphagy), peroxisomes (pexophagy), lipid droplets (lipophagy), ferritin (ferritinophagy) and zymogen granules (zymophagy) (2–5).

CMA, which will be further described below, involves the participation of HSC70 (heat shock-cognate chaperone 70 KDa) and LAMP-2A (lysosomal associated-membrane protein 2A) proteins. With respect to macro- and microautophagy, CMA has been reported only to degrade cytosolic proteins previously bound to HSC70-specific sequence (see below) (6, 7). In the case of microautophagy, it carries the degradation of proteins and organelles out, by their direct engulfment of the lysosome. In microautophagy, whereas some of the proteins can be incorporated into the lysosome through an "unspecific way", others, like those in CMA, also need the interaction with the Hsc70 chaperone. The similarities and differences between CMA and microautophagy have recently been discussed in the review of Tekiradg and Cuervo (8).

Chaperone Mediated Autophagy (CMA)
CMA Overview
Chaperone-mediated autophagy (CMA) is a specific lysosomal-dependent protein degradation pathway (9). It differs from macroautophagy because, (i) it does not involve the formation of autophagosomes and autolysosomes, (ii) its targets are cellular proteins and not organelles, (iii) the protein cargo is directly delivered into the lysosomal lumen through the interaction with HSC70 and LAMP-2A (10). HSC70 belongs to the Hsp70 protein family and it has a constitutive expression, participating principally in the CMA pathway but also in microautophagy (8). LAMP-2A protein is the A isoform of Lamp-2 (lysosome associated-membrane protein type 2) and restricts the CMA degradation process. Importantly, in CMA, selectivity resides in the fact that all CMA substrate proteins contain at least one amino acidic motif biochemically related to the penta-peptide KFERQ (11, 12). In the cell cytoplasm, HSC70 recognizes the KFERQ sequence in target proteins to form the complex HSC70-substrate. Although the temporality of this process is not well known, the complex HSC70-substrate interacts with the cytosolic tail of LAMP-2A that, in turns, drives the translocation of the target protein into the lysosome lumen (13). All cells have a basal CMA activity which helps to maintain the homeostasis of many cellular proteins. However, under certain stimulus, like nutrient starvation, serum deprivation or cellular stress (e.g., protein aggregation), CMA activity increases. This up-regulation condition can be visualized by mRNA LAMP-2A overexpression, HSC70 and LAMP-2A co-localization and LAMP-2A positive lysosomes with increased perinuclear distribution (14–16).

CMA Target Recognition
In 1985 Dice et al. found a pentapeptide in the Ribonuclease A (RNase A) which was necessary for the degradation of this protein by lysosomes in fibroblasts (11, 17–20). When different proteins were analyzed, it was found that the best aminoacidic sequence, to be present in a protein that is going to be degraded through CMA, corresponds to the pentapeptide KFERQ (11).

The general rule, is that this sequence is composed of an amino acid Glutamine (Q), that must contain in one side (right of left) a tetrapeptide, including basic-, acidic- and hydrophobic- amino acids (11). Target proteins for CMA should contain at least one KFERQ-like domain, however some of them include more than one (21). Proteins containing a KFERQ-like domain do not enter the lysosomes by themselves, they first need to be recognized and bound by the chaperone HSC70 (22). This protein, also known as HspA8, is a 73 kDa protein belonging to the Hsp70 protein family (23). Thus, HSC70 specifically recognize the KFERQ-like motive in cytosolic proteins to target them for lysosomal degradation through CMA (22). In some cases, other co-factors, or covalent modifications have been found to be necessary for the binding between the complex HSC70-protein substrate and LAMP-2A. For example, STUB1/CHIP (a ubiquitin E3 ligase) assists the degradation of HIF1A through CMA by the ubiquitination of Lysin 63 (K63) (24) and also by supporting the interaction of LAMP-2A through its chaperon binding domain (24). In addition, covalent modifications, like acetylation and phosphorylation have been described to create KFERQ-like domains capable of targeting proteins for CMA degradation (25–29).

CMA Substrate Translocation and Degradation
In the lysosome membrane, the HSC70-substrate complex interacts with the lysosome receptor LAMP-2A. The protein LAMP-2A was first described by Dr. Ana María Cuervo and Dr. J. Fred Dice (30). It was identified as the LGP96 (lysosome membrane glycoprotein 96 kDa) and it was found to be a necessary receptor for the specific degradation of GAPDH (Glyceraldehyde- 3-phosphate dehydrogenase) and RNase I (Ribonuclease I) through lysosomes (30). The authors showed that both GAPDH and RNase I, were able to bind the LGP96, which were isolated from rat liver (30). The Lysosome-associated membrane glycoprotein 2 (LAMP-2) is able to generate three variants through its pre-mRNA alternative splicing, (LAMP-2A, Lamp-2B, and Lamp-2C) but, to date, it is well established that only the variant A is responsible for the CMA activity (31). Compared to variants B and C, LAMP-2A has four positively charged residues in its C-terminal domain that specifically allow its interaction with target proteins (31). Characterization of LAMP-2A showed that multimerization of this variant (and not the others) in the lysosomal membrane is directly correlated with CMA activity (13, 31). The substrate up-take by the lysosome is a step that depends on LAMP-2A (32). Monomeric LAMP-2A is able to interact with substrates, however, substrate translocation is dependent on the formation of LAMP-2A oligomers (32). Further evidence showed that LAMP-2A arranges in a stable homotrimer, with helical transmembrane domains bound by a coiled-coil conformation, and with the cytosolic tails interacting with the complex HSC70-substrate protein (13). In addition, LAMP-2A oligomerization was shown to be regulated by different proteins. Glial fibrillary acidic protein (GFAP) helps to stabilize the translocation complex in an EF1α dependent manner. The stabilizing effect of GFAP is disrupted by the association of EF1α to GTP, which in turn is released from the translocation complex and allows the self-association between

GFAP molecules. The self-interaction between GFAP molecules have a negative impact on the stabilization of the translocation complex. Thus, GTP acts as an inhibitor of CMA activity (33). Phosphorylating and dephosphorylating signals also regulate CMA activity at the level of the translocation complex (34). For example, mTORC2 (mammalian target of rapamycin complex 2) has been shown to activate, through phosphorylation, Akt kinase, which in turn inhibits the CMA activity. The mechanism by which active Akt decreases the CMA activity is not yet well established. However, it has been postulated that active Akt phosphorylates GFAP, destabilizing its binding to the LAMP-2A translocation complex. In this scenario, both, mTORC2 and Akt act as negative regulators of CMA activity. On the contrary, Pleckstrin homology (PH) domain and leucine-rich repeat protein phosphatase 1 (PHLPP1), has been shown to be recruited to the lysosome membrane in a Rac1 dependent manner. On the lysosomal membrane, PHLPP1 induces CMA activation by dephosphorylating Akt at the same residues previously phosphorylated by mTORC2. Thus, PHLPP1 is a positive regulator of CMA activity (34). In addition, the binding and up-take of the CMA substrates through the translocation complex is assisted by HSC70 and Hsp90 (heat shock protein 90) chaperones. In the case of Hsp90, it was shown that this protein stabilizes the binding of LAMP-2A at the lysosomal membrane (32). HSC70, apart from its important role in binding to the KFERQ domain, participates in two additional steps of the CMA process. One step is related to the recycling of LAMP-2A in the absence of substrates, where HSC70 has been proposed to support the destabilization of LAMP-2A from the translocation complex (32). The other step occurs at the lumen of the lysosome, where a lysosomal HSC70 (lys-HSC70) is also involved in the up-take process of the substrate. The blockage of lys-HSC70, by a

specific antibody, has been directly correlated with an inhibition of the CMA activity (35). **Figure 1** summarizes the main aspects of the CMA mechanism.

CMA Activation
Koga et al. (36) showed that basal CMA activity is present in a variety of cell types. However, an up-regulation in this pathway can be observed under different stimulus or conditions. The most common stimulus for CMA activation is nutrient deprivation (or starvation). Starvation activates CMA both *in vitro* and *in vivo* (11, 20, 36) and, although the exact mechanism has not been described yet, at least *in vivo*, it has been proposed that it depends on the circulating ketone bodies (37). CMA over-activation has also been observed under DNA damage. Under this condition, CMA activity is up-regulated with the purpose to degrade the checkpoint protein kinase 1 (Chk1). The accelerated degradation of Chk1 by CMA reduces its nuclear entrance and consequently decreases the phosphorylation and destabilization of the MRN (Mre11–Rad50–Nbs1), a complex that participates in the early steps of particular DNA repair pathways (38). In line with this result, DNA irradiation of a hepatocellular carcinoma cell line also over-activates CMA. In this cell line, CMA up-regulation was responsible for the degradation of HMGB1 (high-mobility group box 1 protein) degradation, which in turn, provoked the down-regulation of the p53 protein and the consequent decrease in the apoptotic rate. In this case, CMA activation could be considered a mechanism by which this type of carcinoma is able to resist the irradiation treatment (39). Oxidative stress also activates CMA constitutively. Both, mRNA LAMP-2A levels and the recruitment of LAMP-2A protein to the lysosomal membrane (40, 41) were augmented under oxidative stress. The reasons by which CMA is activated under oxidative stress are unknown.

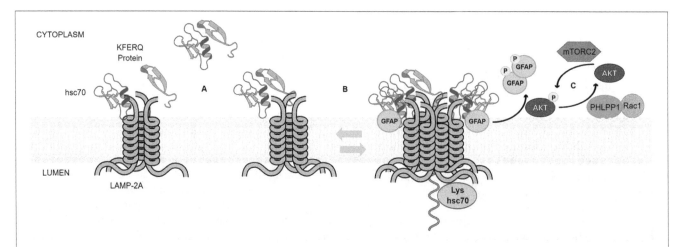

FIGURE 1 | Chaperone mediated autophagy mechanism. The scheme shows the principal events in CMA mediated translocation of proteins through the lysosomal membrane and known regulatory mechanisms. **(A)** LAMP-2A exist as an inactive oligomer at the lysosomal membrane. CMA protein substrates containing KFERQ motifs and HSC70 can bind to the cytosolic tail of LAMP-2A with similar affinity. The short C-terminal tail of LAMP-2A exposed to the cytoplasm and conformed by 12 amino acids probably binds to the chaperone and the substrate in a competitive manner. However, on the substrate, binding sites for HSC70 and LAMP-2A do not overlap allowing the HSC70-substrate complexes to interact with LAMP-2A oligomer in a substrate dependent manner. **(B)** In a dynamic fashion, GFAP favors the formation of high molecular weight aggregates of LAMP2A. Somehow, coupled and simultaneous binding of the substrate to HSC70 and LAMP-2A is sensed by the transmembrane domains of the LAMP-2A for rearrangements in the supramolecular complexes. Next, substrate unfolding and translocation to the lysosomal lumen occurs. A lysosomal-HSC70 (Lys-hsc70) collaborates in this process. **(C)** A signaling pathway involving phosphorylating and dephosphorylating signals, where AKT, MTORC2, PHLPP1, RAC1, and GFAP, regulate the stabilization of the LAMP-2A complex at lysosomal membranes.

However, a possibility could be that CMA acts as a degradative backup system for an inhibited macroautophagy pathway (42). With respect to the molecular mechanism, recent work showed that under hydrogen peroxide treatment, the transcription factor NFE2L2/NRF2 (nuclear factor, erythroid derived 2, like 2) can drive the expression of the lamp2 gene. Pharmacological activation of NFE2L2/NRF2 further supported the role of this transcription factor on lamp-2A gene overexpression (43). However, under oxidative stress, CMA up-regulation could also have a toxic effect. It was shown that CMA over-activity strongly reduces the levels of MEF2A (myocyte enhancer factor 2a), a protein necessary for the adaptive response of the cells to oxidative stress (41). Another stressor that up-regulates CMA activity is hypoxia. Over-activation of CMA was directly correlated with the survival of neuronal cells exposed to different hypoxic conditions and, on the contrary, the down-regulation of this pathway sensitized the cells to the stress (44). On the other hand, it was reported that HIF-1α, a protein that activates HIF-1 (Hypoxia-inducible factor-1) and mediates an adaptive response to hypoxia, is degraded by CMA in cells exposed to hypoxic conditions (45). Therefore, the exact mechanisms by which CMA protects cells against hypoxia, needs to be further elucidated. A constitutive activation of CMA has also been observed in different models of neurodegenerative diseases. For example, in cellular and mouse models of Huntington Disease, CMA was activated as a compensatory mechanism for the inhibition of macroautophagy. In this case, both lys-HSC70 and LAMP-2A protein levels were markedly augmented. In particular, there was an observed stability in LAMP-2A proteins at the lysosomal membrane and a transcriptional upregulation of this splice variant (46). Up-regulation of CMA was also observed in molecular mechanisms related with Parkinson's disease. For example, recent studies performed with a dopaminergic neuronal cell line, using an endoplasmic reticulum (ER) stress mouse model, showed that ER stressors are able to induce CMA activation. The mechanism for such activation involved the recruitment of MKK4 protein kinase to the lysosomal membrane and the subsequent phosphorylation of LAMP-2A by p38 MAPK protein kinase (47). This regulatory mechanism for CMA up-regulation is relevant as neurotoxins associated with PD are directly correlated with an activation of the ER-p38 MAPK–CMA response pathway (48). Additionally, in PD models, LAMP-2A and HSC70 were observed to be up-regulated when α-syn was over-expressed *in vivo*, indicating that a CMA over-activation is triggered in response to a α-syn pathological condition (49)

CMA and Metabolism
Participation of CMA in the Regulation of General Protein Metabolism

Protein homeostasis is regulated by a series of interconnected signaling pathways that sense amino acid availability, among them, the integrated signaling pathway (ISR) through the general control nonderepressible-2 protein (GCN2) and the V-ATPase/Ragulator/mTOR pathway located in lysosomes (50, 51). GCN2 is a protein kinase that is activated in the presence of accumulated deacetylated tRNAs, sensing amino acid depletion. The main target of GCN2 is the eukaryotic initiation factor 2 (eIF2), whose phosphorylation induces the inhibition of general translation and favors the synthesis of a specific set of mRNAs that regulates cell survival and promotion of macroautophagy (52). On the other hand, mTORC1 kinase is activated in response to amino acid availability, promoting translation and inhibiting macroautophagy. The mechanism of amino acid sensing, coupled with mTOR activation, involves the lysosomal amino acid transporter SLC38A9, and mTOR-binding proteins, Sestrin2 and Castor1 (50). These factors that regulate mTOR activation or inhibition, also modulate mTOR activity and thus mTOR-downstream targets involved in promotion of protein translation, cell growth and anabolism, and inhibition of macroautophagy initiation. In response to amino acid deprivation, mTOR activity is attenuated, protein translation is inhibited and macroautophagy is maximally activated to restore amino acid levels.

These non-selective mechanisms of protein homeostasis, added to a variety of mechanisms of stabilization and destabilization of protein pools, define the average life time of every protein in the cell, in nutrient rich conditions and in response to nutritional stress. Selective mechanisms of protein degradation are in contrast, generally linked to the modulation of the function of specific proteins or to the degradation of misfolded proteins that have been targeted for efficient elimination. Selective and non-selective mechanisms of proteasomal and macroautophagy protein degradation pathways have been extensively reviewed in several articles (53–56). Whereas proteins degraded by CMA need to be recognized specifically by HSC70 protein through its KFERQ domain, CMA can be considered a selective protein degradation process. An initial analysis indicated that at least 30% of cytosolic proteins contain CMA KFERQ-like motifs (7). These proteins mainly correspond to a fraction of long-lived proteins that were more rapidly degraded by lysosomes in response to serum starvation or amino acids withdrawal. Indeed, at least 90% of enhanced proteolysis observed during serum withdrawal in fibroblast cells is thought to be part of the protein pools targeted for degradation by CMA (20). In comparison to macroautophagy, the increase in degradation rates of the pool of proteins targeted to CMA is observed in response to prolonged periods of serum or nutrient deprivation (7, 12, 57). Indeed, macroautophagy activity decreases in activity after 6–12 h of nutrient removal, but CMA progressively increases in response to prolonged periods of serum or nutrient deprivation (57). Thus, CMA is a protein degradation pathway specifically activated during long term starvation. The pool of proteins degraded by CMA is very specific and different to the protein pools degraded by other protein catabolic neutral or acid proteolytic pathways. Additionally, CMA-targeted proteins accumulate in lysosomal membranes under starvation and, probably, because of this reason, this pool is excluded for degradation by proteasome or macroautophagy.

The pool of proteins targeted by CMA depends, most likely, on the periods of deprivation, type of deprivation (glucose, amino acids, serum or specific growth factors) and the cell type in the study (12). In addition, the selective pool of proteins degraded by CMA would also be associated with certain functions capable of overcoming metabolic changes in response to starvation.

This has been observed in the regulation of glycolytic flux, through the degradation of glycolytic enzymes by CMA, in order to protect cells from apoptosis (7, 21). On the other hand, proteins that do not contain KFERQ-like regions would most likely be protected against degradation, to sustain the critical functions of cells under nutritional stress. It has also been suggested that activation of non-selective macroautophagy in the first stages of starvation, help to provide metabolite building blocks (as amino acids) for the continuous synthesis of macromolecules. However, at prolonged times of starvation, a relief of macroautophagy by selective CMA-dependent protein degradation, would be necessary to avoid the elimination of essential proteins for cell survival (57). It is unknown whether nutrient deprivation directly controls the CMA activity, as with macroautophagy. The main hypothesis is that an indirect regulation of CMA by nutrient deprivation would be carried out by translational and transcriptional up-regulation of lysosomal proteins and genes involved in lysosome biogenesis (58–60). However, a recent report indicates that upregulation of CMA was responsible for mTOR activation by a mechanism that sensed the augmentation of the free amino acid content dependent on CMA activation (61). In addition, increased CMA activity, in response to LAMP2-A overexpression, was also shown to down-regulate macroautophagy through mTOR activation (62). Overall, this latter evidence reveals that CMA activation functions as a negative feedback loop for mTOR and, thus, would regulate the general amino acid and protein homeostasis signaling.

As mentioned before, basal CMA activity can be detected in different tissues, suggesting that this pathway has a constant role in the regulation of certain proteins, even under conditions of nutrient or growth factor availability (57). However, whether the degradation of these target proteins increases under CMA activation (e.g., starvation), or another specific cell response, remains to be clarified. Most likely, the latter will depend on the different affinities that these proteins would have for HSC70 and LAMP-2A, and/or on the availability of HSC70 and LAMP-2A (63).

As a consequence of its important role in controlling protein homeostasis, CMA is able to regulate metabolic pathways that are crucial to maintain balance in cellular and systemic physiology.

CMA and Regulation of Lipid Metabolism

Neutral cytosolic lipolysis and lysosome-associated acid lipolysis were classically classified in two different pathways. However, both are now recognized as synergistic, cooperative and interconnected mechanisms that contribute to lipid catabolism (64). Lysosomal lipolysis involves the degradation of lipids derived from endocytosis, as well as from cytosolic lipid stores (lipid droplets) through an autophagic process known as Lipophagy (65). Lipid droplets (LDs) are specialized organelles that store neutral lipids during fatty acid availability, mainly triglycerides (TG) and cholesterol esters, for their posterior use as energy or precursors for lipids and steroids (66). LDs consist of a core of neutral lipids separated from the aqueous cytoplasm by a phospholipid monolayer decorated by a set of proteins. These proteins are enzymes involved in lipid synthesis

and lipid hydrolysis, membrane-trafficking proteins and a set of specialized LDs-associated structural proteins called perilipins (PLINs). PLINs cover a family of 5 major proteins and some additional splice variants expressed in lower amounts. Perilipin 1 (PLIN1) and 2 (PLIN2) are exclusively associated with LDs whereas perilipins 3–5 are found in the cytoplasm, associated with LDs, as well as microdroplets and lipoprotein particles (67). Perilipins 1, 2 and 5 control, at the surface of the lipid droplets, the access of cytosolic neutral lipases. For example, phosphorylation of PLIN1 and PLIN5 by protein kinase A (PKA), in response to hormones or growth factors, trigger the recruitment of neutral lipases like hormone sensitive lipase (HSL) and triacyl-glycerol lipase (ATGL) (68, 69). In contrast to PLN1 and PLIN5, PLN2 is not phosphorylated by PKA and does not recruit lipases at LDs (67). Similar to PLIN2, PLIN3 and PLIN4 protect LDs from degradation and they seem to have a tissue-specific function in the regulation of LDs size, maturation and mitochondrial association (70–72).

The involvement of autophagy in lipid turnover was first demonstrated for macroautophagy (65). Electron-microscopy studies indicated that autophagosomes engulf LDs or small portions of large LDs for degradation, forming autolipophagosomes in a process now known as macrolipophagy. In hepatocytes, macrolipophagy and the presence of lipid-containing autophagolysosomes, is stimulated by nutrient starvation and low fatty acid treatments (65). Members of the Rab GTPase family, RAB7 and RAB10 have been involved in the early steps of autophagosome recruitment to LDs (73). Moreover, the Rab effectors, EHBP1 and EH2, have been suggested to help in the elongation of autophagosomal membranes around LDs (74, 75). Neutral lipases ATGL and HSL contain LIR motifs (LC3-interaction region) and interact with the cytosolic face of autophagosomes through LC3-II, being recruited to LDs in response to macrolipophagy activation (64, 76).

In addition to macroautophagy, CMA also plays a central role in lipid homeostasis. In a mouse model, where LAMP-2A was specifically down-regulated in liver by deleting the exon 9 of lamp2 gene, it was shown that the constitutive blockade of CMA activity induces pronounced steatosis without a substantial increase in TG synthesis (77). In addition, LAMP-2A knock-out cells were insensitive to lipolysis induced by starvation and displayed increased density, size and occupancy area of LDs (78). Interestingly, in this model, non-selective macroautophagy was intact, indicating a specific and new role of CMA in lipophagy (77). In line with this evidence, further studies found the presence of KFERQ-like motifs in PLIN2 and PLIN3 proteins, and identified these two proteins as substrates for CMA lysosomal degradation. In addition, lysosomes actives in CMA isolated from rat liver, were enriched in PLIN2 and PLIN3, supporting the fact that these proteins are CMA substrates. This evidence was further complemented by experiments indicating that PLIN2 and PLIN3 degradation was reduced in LAMP-2A knockout cells (78). With regards to the mechanism, the degradation of PLIN2 through CMA in response to nutrient starvation and lipid challenges, was correlated with an increment in the association between HSC70 and perilipins (78). Reduced degradation of PLIN2 in cells that are deficient for the CMA pathway, leads to reduced lipolysis, likely due to an impairment in the association of ATGL with LDs as well as due to the defective recruitment of autophagosomal proteins and Rab7 to LDs (25, 78). Moreover, PLIN2 phosphorylation by AMPK was found to be a necessary modification for PLIN2 association with HSC70 in a form dependent on CMA activation (25, 78). Therefore, the role of CMA in lipophagy not only relays in the regulation of the recruitment of neutral lipases to LDs trough perlipin degradation, but also in the integration of a regulatory step that involves a post-transcriptional modification guided by AMPK (25). Thus, CMA itself could be considered a nutrient sensing pathway supporting the fact that lysosomes can play a role as initial sensors and integrators of lipid homeostasis (79). Additional research, however, is needed to determine how cellular pathways involved in cellular lipid homeostasis communicate with CMA and lipophagy, and how CMA-dependent lipolysis affects different tissues.

CMA and Regulation of Carbohydrate Metabolism

As mentioned before, glycolytic enzyme glyceraldehyde 3-phosphate dehydrogenase (GAPDH) was one of the first characterized as a CMA substrate (80). Additionally, at least 8 of 10 glycolytic enzymes contain CMA-targeting motifs (77). Substrates of CMA that participate in glycolysis, validated by LAMP2-A loss of function or lysosome-transport assays, also include hexokinase-2 (HK-2) (28), the M2 isoform of pyruvate kinase (81), aldolase-A, enolase-1, 3-phosphoglyceric phosphokinase, phosphoglycerate mutase, glucose-6-phosphate-dehydrogenase and the mitochondrial proteins glutamate dehydrogenase, ornithine transcarbamoylase and malate dehydrogenase (77). Other related substrates that have been suggested to be regulated by CMA in their function include phosphofructokinase-2 (82) and aldolase B (83). Glycolytic flux regulation by CMA has been confirmed *in vivo* in a mouse model with specific down-regulation of LAMP-2A in hepatocytes (77). These mice displayed higher protein levels of glycolytic enzymes and enzymes from the tricarboxylic acid cycle (TCA), a reduction in hepatic gluconeogenesis, lower glycogen synthesis and an increase in lactate production and TCA intermediates (77). This metabolic profile suggests a switch in hepatic metabolism to carbohydrate consumption as a source of energy vs. glucose biosynthesis in response to low CMA activity (77). On the other hand, classical inhibition of hepatic glycolysis caused by serum starvation (84) was not observed in mice with liver-specific CMA down-regulation (77). These results suggest that CMA activity would be necessary for a metabolic adaptive mechanism that triggers glucose production in liver to support peripheral organs under nutritional stress conditions.

The mechanism regulating CMA in response to changes in glucose availability are not fully understood. Pointing to a central role of the lysosome in sensing glucose homeostasis, new evidence indicates that glucose starvation induces changes in lysosomal acidification in an AMPK activity dependent-manner (84, 85). The mechanisms implicated in this regulation

may involve a glucose-dependent regulation of the lysosome biogenesis through the transcription factor EB (TFEB) (86). Additional research is needed to elucidate how these lysosomal changes, induced by carbohydrate availability, regulate the CMA activity and, in turn, how this affects the cellular glycolytic flux.

CMA and Neurodegenerative Diseases

There is increasing evidence supporting the idea that dysregulation in the CMA pathway plays a crucial role in neurodegeneration.

Parkinson's Disease (PD)

Evidence indicates that a dysregulation in CMA could impact on the onset or progression of Parkinson's Disease (PD). As mentioned above, the main protein associated with this neurogenerative disorder, alpha-synuclein protein (α-syn), has been identified as a CMA substrate (87). More specifically, reduced α-syn degradation was observed when its KFERQ motif was mutated and the expression of LAMP-2A was knocked-down. The involvement of CMA in α-syn degradation was confirmed in different neuronal cell lines (PC12 and SH-SY5Y) and primary cultures of cortical and midbrain neurons (87). One of the hallmarks of PD is the neurotoxicity caused by the abnormal aggregation of α-syn. In this context, mutations in the protein impair its degradation through a CMA pathway, causing the accumulation α-syn oligomers that are unable to be degraded by the lysosome. This event blocks the entire CMA pathway, enhancing the oligomers formation and compromising the degradation of other CMA substrates (88, 89). As mentioned above, LAMP-2A and HSC70 were observed to be up-regulated when α-syn was over-expressed *in vivo* (49). In line with these results, it was shown that the down-regulation of LAMP-2A in adult rat substantia nigra, via an adeno-associated virus, induced intracellular accumulation of α-syn puncta. In addition, LAMP-2A down-regulation was also correlated with a progressive loss of dopaminergic neurons, severe reduction in striatal dopamine levels/terminals, increased astro- and microgliosis and relevant motor deficits (90). Furthermore, studies using the *Drosophila melanogaster* model, showed that the overexpression of human LAMP-2A protein protected the flies from progressive locomotor and oxidative defects induced by neuronal expression of a human pathological form of α-syn (91). Also, other PD related proteins seem to be regulated by CMA activity. This is the case of PARK7/DJ-1 and MEF2D. PARK7/DJ-1 is an autosomal recessive familial PD gene that plays a critical role in the antioxidative response and its dysfunction leads to mitochondrial defects. CMA was shown to degrade, preferentially, an oxidized and altered form of PARK7, providing protection from mitochondrial damage and impairing cell viability (92). For MEF2D (myocyte-specific enhancer factor 2D protein), it was shown that an inhibition of CMA provoked the accumulation of this protein in the cell cytoplasm (93). These results are in line with the observation that MEF2D levels are increased in brains of α-syn transgenic mice and in samples from patients with PD (93). Thus, an impairment in CMA activity, caused by the α-syn oligomers, could be the reason for MEF2D accumulation in PD. Beyond the studies performed in cell cultures and *in vivo* models, strong evidence indicates that CMA could also be dysregulated in individuals affected by PD. In this regard, LAMP-2A and HSC70 were observed to be down-regulated in PD patients, suggesting that a CMA dysregulation can occur before the appearance of α-syn aggregation and other PD associated disorders (94, 95). Although the mechanisms that lead to a reduction in LAMP-2A and HSC70 levels in PD remain unknown, some studies suggest that genetic variations in the promoter of the lamp-2A gene and the up-regulation of different microRNAs that target both LAMP-2A and HSC70, could be implicated in their down-regulation (96, 97).

Alzheimer Disease (AD)

The association between CMA and Alzheimer's Disease (AD) can be described by the degradation of the RCAN1 protein (Regulator of calcineurin 1) through this pathway. Two KFERQ-like motifs identified in RCAN1 were responsible for its degradation by the CMA pathway (98). In addition, the inhibition of CMA pathway increased RCAN1 protein levels and consequently reduced the NFAT transcription factor activity (98). Interestingly, NFAT has been involved in the transcriptional regulation of the lamp2 gene (99). Thus, inhibition of CMA activity could be further enhanced by increased levels of RCAN1, that will subsequently impair NFAT-dependent transcription of lamp2. On the other hand, the Tau protein, one of the principal factors associated with AD, has also shown to be a CMA substrate (100, 101). The Tau protein is degraded by the autophagy–lysosomal system producing different fragments that, in turn, bind to HSC70 and become CMA substrates. Although these fragments are able to reach the lysosomes, they remain bound to the lysosomal membrane, causing the formation of pathological Tau aggregates that cause lysosomal damage and block the degradation of other CMA targets (100). Additionally, the amyloid precursor protein (APP), can be processed to produce another pathogenic molecule associated with AD, the β-amyloid peptide (Aβ), which contains a KFERQ related motif (102). However, deletion of KFERQ did not affect its binding to HSC70, but did somehow keep the APP and its C-terminal fragments (CTFs) away from lysosomes. Thus, the KFERQ-like domain of APP is relevant to preclude the accumulation of APP and its CTFs but, in this case, in an CMA degradation independent manner (102).

Huntington Disease (HD)

As previously mentioned, a constitutive activation of CMA has been observed in cell lines and mouse models of HD (46, 103). In a mouse model for this disease, a strong co-localization between LAMP-2A and HSC70 was correlated with augmented lysosomal degradation of the native and aberrant huntingtin protein (Htt) (46). Furthermore, additional studies performed *in vivo* also showed that Htt aggregates could be forced to be degraded through CMA, by targeting them with a polyQ binding protein (QBP1) including a KFERQ domain in its amino acidic sequence (104). The data indicated that modulation of the CMA pathway can be a plausible strategy for HD treatment.

Amyotrophic Lateral Sclerosis (ALS) and Frontotemporal Lobar Degeneration (FTLD)

Amyotrophic Lateral Sclerosis (ALS) and Frontotemporal Lobar Degeneration (FTLD) are two important neurodegenerative diseases where the implication of CMA has been poorly studied. So far, only two studies have connected these disorders with CMA and both focus on the ribonuclear protein TDP-43. Huang et al. described an KFERQ-like domain in TDP-43 that was responsible for the interaction of this protein with HSC70 under ubiquitination condition. Mutation of the KFERQ-like domain disrupted the ubiquitin-dependent binding of TDP-43 with HSC70. In addition, the down-regulation LAMP-2A by siRNA treatment, seems to increase the level of the pathologically-related 25-KDa and 35-KDa TDP-43 C-terminal fragments, but not the full-length protein (105). On the other hand, in a recent study, Tamaki, Y., *et al* designed an antibody able to recognize abnormal (unfolded or mislocated) TDP-43. The addition of the KFERQ sequence to this antibody, was able to promote the degradation of abnormal TDP-43 through the CMA pathway. Although in this case the connection of TDP-43 with CMA was not in a physiological context, this work indicates that a forced CMA target degradation of TDP-43 can be used as a strategy to ameliorate neurodegenerative diseases associated with this protein (106).

CMA in the Crosstalk With Metabolic Disorders and Neurodegeneration
Reduced CMA Activity With Aging

Aging can be considered as a physiological process that is associated with metabolic and neurodegenerative disorders via mechanisms that in many cases are completely unknown. With regards to autophagy, it has been observed that this lysosomal degradative mechanism also declines with age (107). In the case of CMA, this was determined by isolating lysosomes from the liver of young and old rats (108). Lysosomes from old rats had reduced LAMP-2A protein levels at both, total and lysosomal levels. The decrease of the LAMP-2A protein in lysosomes is associated with changes in lipid composition of these organelles that accelerate the degradation rate of the protein (108). With respect to the HSC70 protein, although the total protein levels remained unchanged, lysosomal HSC70 levels were augmented, probably to compensate the decline observed in the CMA activity (108). Further experiments demonstrated that, although the levels of Lamp2A mRNA were unchanged, there was a problem in the localization of LAMP-2A at the lysosomal membrane in old rats, consequently reducing the CMA activity (109). Furthermore, by using an animal model with specific down-regulation of CMA in the liver, it was possible to demonstrate that reduced CMA activity in old animals had an impact on the ability to overcome proteostasis induced by different stressors like oxidative stress, lipid challenging and aging (110). The mentioned evidences clearly demonstrate that CMA activity is reduced in older individuals and that this protein degradative pathway helps to stabilize the different disorders associated with aging.

Thus, considering that CMA activity is reduced with age, it is possible to argue that a decline in CMA activity during aging can be a risk factor for the development of neurodegenerative disorders associated with adult and senior people. In fact, beyond of what it can be concluded from *in vitro* and *in vivo* models, more evidence is coming out revealing that a dysregulation in CMA activity can be present in human neurodegeneration. Most

of the evidence is a result of studies on PD. For example, a study performed with peripheral blood mononuclear cells from PD patients, showed that affected people had reduced HSC70 protein levels (111). Another study, analyzing CSF (cerebrospinal fluid) of PD patients with mutations in the repeat kinase 2 (LRRK2) gene, confirmed that LAMP-2A protein levels were reduced in affected females, compared to healthy people (112).

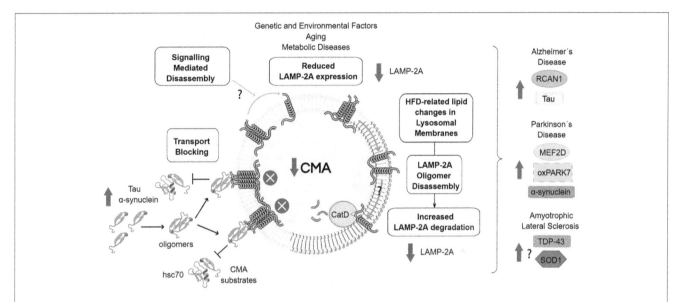

FIGURE 2 | Consequences of downregulated CMA activity. The scheme shows the principal mechanisms of CMA downregulation. Reduced expression of the lamp2 gene has been related with genetic polymorphisms (96), aging (108) and metabolic disorders (132). In relation to the latter situation, HFD has been shown to modify the lipid composition of lysosomal membranes, including increased levels of cholesterol and ceramide (132). These modifications induces the formation of organized lipid microdomains, which prevent LAMP-2A multimerization and stimulate subsequent degradation through proteolysis by Cathepsin D (CatD) (133). Independently of the mechanism, a reduction in CMA activity can induce an increase in the levels of some proteins related with the development of neurodegenerative diseases. In the case of tau, α-synuclein or other less characterized CMA protein substrates that are able to aggregate, increases the total mass that these proteins would contribute to protein oligomerization, an event associated with a blockade of CMA transport. In addition, oxidative damage, would enhance the aggregation process. Additionally, changes in signaling pathways that control LAMP2A oligomerization and membrane stabilization can alter LAMP-2A membrane dynamics and CMA activity. Finally, CMA down-regulation can alter a series of other specific proteins related with neuronal survival or neuroinflammation, that participate in the development of neurodegenerative diseases.

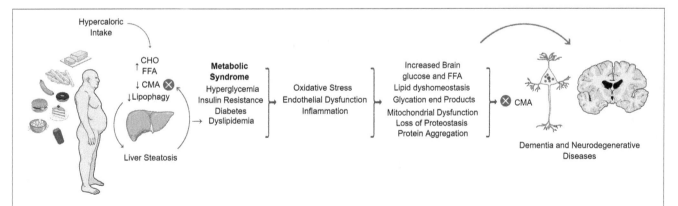

FIGURE 3 | CMA in the crosstalk of metabolic dysfunction and neurodegenerative diseases. Increased caloric intake in humans produces elevated circulating levels of carbohydrates (CHO) and free fatty acids (FFA). In the liver, FFAs accumulate in lipid droplets leading to hepatic steatosis. FFAs also inhibit CMA and lipophagy. The latter contributes to hepatic fat accumulation and systemic dyslipidemia that, together with increased levels of glucose, leads to metabolic syndrome characterized by insulin resistance and diabetes. Metabolic syndrome is a general status also characterized by oxidative stress, inflammation and endothelial dysfunction. This condition is present throughout the body and is also capable of affecting the nervous system, resulting in lipid dyshomeostasis, mitochondrial dysfunction, loss of proteostasis and protein aggregation in the brain. All of these processes have been shown to alter proteostatic mechanisms, including CMA. Loss of neuronal proteostasis finally alters neuronal function which leads to dementia or the development of neurodegenerative diseases.

However, studies focused on analyzing the levels of LAMP-2A and HSC70 in healthy people during normal aging, failed to find any positive association (113). Thus, future studies need to focus on whether changes in CMA activity (or CMA protein players) are altered during normal aging in healthy people, or if they are only associated with patients affected by neurodegeneration. The latter will help to elucidate whether observed changes in CMA protein players are a cause or a consequence of these disorders.

CMA Activity, Metabolic Disorders and Neurodegenerative Diseases

In vivo models strongly support the hypothesis that CMA activity decreases with aging. Considering this evidence, which of these could be the consequence of CMA activity in people with a high fat diet (HFD)? Rodriguez-Navarro et al. showed that chronic exposure of rats to an HFD or cholesterol-enriched diet, provoked a decrease in CMA activity (114). Further characterization of these animals showed that isolated lysosomes from liver have reduced LAMP-2A protein at lysosomal membranes. The latter was triggered by an accelerated degradation of lysosomal LAMP-2A, something also observed in older animals. Interestingly, authors also found that lysosomal membranes from animals with a HFD presented changes in lipid composition, in a similar way than that was observed with age (114). Thus, a dysregulation of CMA activity produced by aging, could impact on the LDs composition, affecting the aggregation of some proteins involved in neurodegenerative diseases.

In addition, a systemic decrease in CMA activity, and the onset or progression of neurodegenerative disorders, could be enhanced by an HFD. Different works demonstrate that a HFD can be a risk factor for the development of neurodegenerative diseases. For example, in a mouse model of PD, it was observed that HFD provoked a reduction in Parkin protein levels (115). In addition, similar results were obtained with a α-syn transgenic mouse model of PD. Compared with wild type mice, an HFD causes obesity and glucose intolerance in transgenic mice. Furthermore, transgenic mice also had an accelerated onset of PD disease and premature movement phenotype and death (116). The same situation was observed in transgenic mice models for AD. The model with an HFD, presented exacerbated neuropathology, defects in synaptic stability/plasticity, apoptotic neuronal cell death (117) and increased levels of insoluble amyloid-β (AB) and Tau (118). On the other hand, LDs have been found to play a role in neurodegenerative diseases. For example, as reviewed by Pennetta et al. LDs seem to be important for the progression of motor neuron diseases (MND) (119). The mechanisms by which LDs are affecting neurodegeneration processes are unknown, however it has been observed that they can affect protein aggregation. For example, in cells treated with an HFD, α-syn accumulated in triglyceride-riche LDs (120). In a similar way, amyloidal fibrils from amyloidotic polyneuropathy (FAP), were observed to be colocalizing with a high density lipoprotein (HDL) (121). Altogether, these data support the idea that LDs could be involved with the aggregation process of neurodegenerative disease associated proteins.

On the other hand, there is increasing evidence which now supports the idea that a high carbohydrate diet (HCD) is a risk factor for certain neurodegenerative diseases (122). Probably, because of a dysregulation in protein glycation, which can control the balance between protein solubility and aggregation (123, 124). Moreover, many reports indicate that there is a strong association between diabetes and people affected by AD (125, 126), suggesting that a dysregulation in glucose metabolism could impact on the onset of this and other neurodegenerative diseases (127). Although the mechanisms are not clear, evidence has shown that there is an increase in the activity of glycolytic enzymes in AD patients (128). In addition, α-syn was observed to bind GAPDH, increasing the activity of this enzyme (129). Also, analyses performed with postmortem human brain tissue, reported a reduction of glucose-6-phosphate dehydrogenase and 6-phosphogluconate dehydrogenase in AD and PD (127).

Carbohydrate metabolism dysregulation has also been found in different models of HD. Gouarné et al. found that a rat model of HD had a deficit in glycolysis in striatal neurons (130). In a mouse model of HD, it was observed that glycolysis inhibition decreases the levels of glutamate transport and provoked neurotoxicity (131). On the contrary, in two different models of HD, it was found that the activity of some glycolytic enzymes was higher. The latter results were not correlated with the enhanced conversion of glucose to lactate and increased ATP in the brain and tissue, respectively. Altogether, this evidence indicates that in neurodegenerative diseases, an imbalance in a glycolytic pathway could play an important role in the onset or progression of the disease. Considering that CMA regulates the homeostasis of glycolytic enzymes, changes in the activity of this pathway along with aging could strongly impact on the risk to develop a neurodegenerative disease. In addition, the risk can also be augmented by aging and by a continuous intake of a high carbohydrate diet. **Figure 2** shows the main mechanisms that can influence CMA down-regulation and its impact in neurodegenerative diseases.

CONCLUDING REMARKS

As part of the autophagic pathways, CMA has been involved in regulating the metabolism of different proteins. Many of these proteins are strongly associated with neurodegenerative diseases affecting humans, while others are involved in the regulation of metabolic pathways such as lipids and carbohydrate metabolism. In addition, neurodegenerative diseases and metabolic disorders are common features of aged humans and many reports associate the dysregulation in lipids or carbohydrate metabolism, with the risk of developing some type of neurodegenerative disease. It has also been reported that a high fat, or high carbohydrate diet (or glucose reach diet), can also increase neurodegeneration prevalence or progression. On the other hand, CMA activity, has been observed to decline with age and with a non-balanced dietary intake such as a high fat diet. Overall, CMA can be considered a common factor in the regulation of metabolic and neurodegenerative pathways and a dysregulation in CMA, provoked by normal aging, or by metabolic disorders induced by deficient nutritional habits, which could tilt the balance toward a pathological situation. **Figure 3** shows an overview of how CMA could be connected with metabolic dysfunctions and neurodegenerative disorders.

AUTHOR CONTRIBUTIONS

AA and MB wrote the article. IEA wrote the article and created the figures. AM, JM, KC, and AC made important contributions, participated in discussions and provided corrections to the manuscript.

REFERENCES

Kaushik S, Cuervo AM. The coming of age of chaperone- mediated autophagy. *Nat Rev Mol Cell Biol.* (2018) 19:365–81. doi:10.1038/s41580-018-0001-6

Iwata J, Ezaki J, Komatsu M, Yokota S, Ueno T, Tanida I, et al. Excess peroxisomes are degraded by autophagic machinery in mammals. *J Biol Chem.* (2006) 281:4035–41. doi: 10.1074/jbc.M512283200

Lamb CA, Yoshimori T, Tooze SA. The autophagosome: origins unknown, biogenesis complex. *Nat Rev Mol Cell Biol.* (2013) 14:759–74. doi: 10.1038/nrm3696

Narendra D, Tanaka A, Suen DF, Youle RJ. Parkin is recruited selectively to impaired mitochondria and promotes their autophagy. *J Cell Biol.* (2008) 183:795–803. doi:10.1083/jcb.200809125

Grasso D, Ropolo A, Lo Re A, Boggio V, Molejon MI, Iovanna JL, et al. Zymophagy, a novel selective autophagy pathway mediated by VMP1-USP9x-p62, prevents pancreatic cell death. *J Biol Chem.* (2011) 286:8308–24. doi: 10.1074/jbc.M110.197301

Agarraberes FA, Dice JF. A molecular chaperone complex at the lysosomal membrane is required for protein translocation. *J Cell Sci.* (2001) 114:2491–9.

Cuervo AM, Knecht E, Terlecky SR, Dice JF. Activation of a selective pathway of lysosomal proteolysis in rat liver by prolonged starvation. *Am J Physiol.* (1995) 269:C1200–8. doi:10.1152/ajpcell.1995.269.5.C1200

Tekirdag K, Cuervo AM. Chaperone-mediated autophagy and endosomal microautophagy: joint by a chaperone. *J Biol Chem.* (2018) 293:5414–24. doi: 10.1074/jbc.R117.818237

Isenman LD, Dice JF. Secretion of intact proteins and peptide fragments by lysosomal pathways of protein degradation. *J Biol Chem.* (1989) 264:21591–6.

Arias E, Cuervo AM. Chaperone-mediated autophagy in protein quality control. *Curr Opin Cell Biol.* (2011) 23:184–9. doi: 10.1016/j.ceb.2010.10.009

Dice JF. Peptide sequences that target cytosolic proteins for lysosomal proteolysis. *Trends Biochem Sci.* (1990) 15:305–9. doi:10.1016/0968-0004(90)90019-8

Wing SS, Chiang HL, Goldberg AL, Dice JF. Proteins containing peptide sequences related to Lys-Phe-Glu-Arg-Gln are selectively depleted in liver and heart, but not skeletal muscle, of fasted rats. *Biochem J.* (1991) 275(Pt 1):165–9. doi: 10.1042/bj27 50165

Rout AK, Strub MP, Piszczek G, Tjandra N. Structure of transmembrane domain of lysosome-associated membrane protein type 2a (LAMP- 2A) reveals key features for substrate specificity in chaperone-mediated autophagy. *J Biol Chem.* (2014) 289:35111–23. doi: 10.1074/jbc.M114.609446

Arias E. Methods to study chaperone-mediated autophagy. *Methods Enzymol.* (2017) 588:283–305. doi: 10.1016/bs.mie.2016.10.009

Kaushik S, Cuervo AM. Chaperone-mediated autophagy. *Methods Mol Biol.* (2008) 445:227–44. doi:10.1007/978-1-59745-157-4_15

Patel B, Cuervo AM. Methods to study chaperone-mediated autophagy. *Methods* (2015) 75:133–40. doi:10.1016/j.ymeth.2015.01.003

McElligott MA, Miao P, Dice JF. Lysosomal degradation of ribonuclease A and ribonuclease S-protein microinjected into the cytosol of human fibroblasts. *J Biol Chem.* (1985) 260:11986–93.

McElligott MA, Dice JF. Degradation of microinjected ribonuclease A and ribonuclease S-protein by lysosomal pathways. *Prog Clin Biol Res.* (1985) 180:471–3.

Dice JF, Backer JM, Miao P, Bourret L, McElligott MA. Regulation of catabolism of ribonuclease A microinjected into human fibroblasts. *Prog Clin Biol Res.* (1985) 180:385–94.

Chiang HL, Dice JF. Peptide sequences that target proteins for enhanced degradation during serum withdrawal. *J Biol Chem.* (1988) 263:6797–805.

Cuervo AM, Gomes AV, Barnes JA, Dice JF. Selective degradation of annexins by chaperone-mediated autophagy. *J Biol Chem.* (2000) 275:33329– 35. doi: 10.1074/jbc.M005655200

Chiang HL, Terlecky SR, Plant CP, Dice JF. A role for a 70-kilodalton heat shock protein in lysosomal degradation of intracellular proteins. *Science* (1989) 246:382–5. doi:10.1126/science.2799391

Stricher F, Macri C, Ruff M, Muller S. HSPA8/HSC70 chaperone protein: structure, function, and chemical targeting. *Autophagy* (2013) 9:1937–54. doi: 10.4161/auto.26448

Ferreira JV, Soares AR, Ramalho JS, Pereira P, Girao H. K63 linked ubiquitin chain formation is a signal for HIF1A degradation by Chaperone-Mediated Autophagy. *Sci Rep.* (2015) 5:10210. doi: 10.1038/srep10210

Kaushik S, Cuervo AM. AMPK-dependent phosphorylation of lipid droplet protein PLIN2 triggers its degradation by CMA. *Autophagy* (2016) 12:432–8. doi: 10.1080/15548627.2015.1124226

Quintavalle C, Di Costanzo S, Zanca C, Tasset I, Fraldi A, Incoronato M, et al. Phosphorylation-regulated degradation of the tumor-suppressor form of PED by chaperone-mediated autophagy in lung cancer cells. *J Cell Physiol.* (2014) 229:1359–68. doi: 10.1002/jcp.24569

Bonhoure A, Vallentin A, Martin M, Senff-Ribeiro A, Amson R, Telerman A, et al. Acetylation of translationally controlled tumor protein promotes its degradation through chaperone-mediated autophagy. *Eur J Cell Biol* (2017) 96:83–98. doi: 10.1016/j.ejcb.2016.12.002

Lv L, Li D, Zhao D, Lin R, Chu Y, Zhang H, et al. Acetylation targets the M2 isoform of pyruvate kinase for degradation through chaperone- mediated autophagy and promotes tumor growth. *Mol Cell* (2011) 42:719– 30. doi: 10.1016/j.molcel.2011.04.025

Thompson LM, Aiken CT, Kaltenbach LS, Agrawal N, Illes K, Khoshnan A, et al. IKK phosphorylates Huntingtin and targets it for degradation by the proteasome and lysosome. *J Cell Biol.* (2009) 187:1083–99. doi: 10.1083/jcb.200909067

Cuervo AM, Dice JF. A receptor for the selective uptake and degradation of proteins by lysosomes. *Science* (1996) 273:501–3. doi:10.1126/science.273.5274.501

Cuervo AM, Dice JF. Unique properties of lamp2a compared to other lamp2 isoforms. *J Cell Sci.* (2000) 113(Pt 24):4441–50.

Bandyopadhyay U, Kaushik S, Varticovski L, Cuervo AM. The chaperone-mediated autophagy receptor organizes in dynamic protein complexes at the lysosomal membrane. *Mol Cell Biol.* (2008) 28:5747–63. doi: 10.1128/MCB.02070-07

Bandyopadhyay U, Sridhar S, Kaushik S, Kiffin R, Cuervo AM. Identification of regulators of chaperone-mediated autophagy. *Mol Cell* (2010) 39:535–47. doi: 10.1016/j.molcel.2010.08.004

Arias E, Koga H, Diaz A, Mocholi E, Patel B, Cuervo AM. Lysosomal mTORC2/PHLPP1/Akt Regulate Chaperone-Mediated Autophagy. *Mol Cell* (2015) 59:270–84. doi: 10.1016/j.molcel.2015.05.030

Agarraberes FA, Terlecky SR, Dice JF. An intralysosomal hsp70 is required for a selective pathway of lysosomal protein degradation. *J Cell Biol.* (1997) 137:825–34. doi:10.1083/jcb.137.4.825

Koga H, Martinez-Vicente M, Macian F, Verkhusha VV, Cuervo AM. A photoconvertible fluorescent reporter to track chaperone-mediated autophagy. *Nat Commun.* (2011) 2:386. doi: 10.1038/ncomms1393

Finn PF, Dice JF. Ketone bodies stimulate chaperone-mediated autophagy. *J Biol Chem.* (2005) 280:25864–70. doi: 10.1074/jbc.M502456200

Park C, Suh Y, Cuervo AM. Regulated degradation of Chk1 by chaperone-mediated autophagy in response to DNA damage. *Nat Commun.* (2015) 6:6823. doi: 10.1038/ncomms7823

Wu JH, Guo JP, Shi J, Wang H, Li LL, Guo B, et al. CMA down-regulates p53 expression through degradation of HMGB1 protein to inhibit irradiation-triggered apoptosis in hepatocellular carcinoma. *World J Gastroenterol.* (2017) 23:2308–17. doi: 10.3748/wjg.v23.i13.2308

Kiffin R, Christian C, Knecht E, Cuervo AM. Activation of chaperone-mediated autophagy during oxidative stress. *Mol Biol Cell* (2004) 15:4829–40. doi: 10.1091/mbc.e04-06-0477

Zhang L, Sun Y, Fei M, Tan C, Wu J, Zheng J, et al. Disruption of chaperone-mediated autophagy-dependent degradation of MEF2A by oxidative stress-induced lysosome destabilization. *Autophagy* (2014) 10:1015–35. doi: 10.4161/auto.28477

Wang Y, Singh R, Xiang Y, Czaja MJ. Macroautophagy and chaperone- mediated autophagy are required for hepatocyte resistance to oxidant stress. *Hepatology* (2010) 52:266–77. doi: 10.1002/hep.23645

Pajares M, Rojo AI, Arias E, Diaz-Carretero A, Cuervo AM, Cuadrado A. Transcription factor NFE2L2/NRF2 modulates chaperone-mediated autophagy through the regulation of LAMP2A. *Autophagy* (2018) 14:1310–22. doi: 10.1080/15548627.2018.1474992

Dohi E, Tanaka S, Seki T, Miyagi T, Hide I, Takahashi T, et al. Hypoxic stress activates chaperone-mediated autophagy and modulates neuronal cell survival. *Neurochem Int.* (2012) 60:431–42. doi: 10.1016/j.neuint.2012.01.020

Hubbi ME, Hu H, Kshitiz, Ahmed I, Levchenko A, Semenza GL. Chaperone-mediated autophagy targets hypoxia-inducible factor-1alpha (HIF-1alpha) for lysosomal degradation. *J Biol Chem.* (2013) 288:10703–14. doi: 10.1074/jbc.M112.414771

Koga H, Martinez-Vicente M, Arias E, Kaushik S, Sulzer D, Cuervo AM. Constitutive upregulation of chaperone-mediated autophagy in Huntington's disease. *J Neurosci.* (2011) 31:18492–505. doi: 10.1523/JNEUROSCI.3219-11.2011

Li W, Yang Q, Mao Z. Signaling and induction of chaperone-mediated autophagy by the endoplasmic reticulum under stress conditions. *Autophagy* (2018) 14:1094–96. doi: 10.1080/15548627.2018.1444314

Li W, Zhu J, Dou J, She H, Tao K, Xu H, et al. Phosphorylation of LAMP2A by p38 MAPK couples ER stress to chaperone-mediated autophagy. *Nat Commun.* (2017) 8:1763. doi: 10.1038/s41467-017-01609-x

Mak SK, McCormack AL, Manning-Bog AB, Cuervo AM, Di Monte DA. Lysosomal degradation of alpha-synuclein *in vivo. J Biol Chem.* (2010) 285:13621–9. doi: 10.1074/jbc.M109.074617

Wolfson RL, Sabatini DM. The dawn of the age of amino acid sensors for the mTORC1 pathway. *Cell Metab.* (2017) 26:301–9. doi: 10.1016/j.cmet.2017.07.001

Anthony TG. Homeostatic responses to amino acid insufficiency. *Anim Nutr.* (2015) 1:135–7. doi: 10.1016/j.aninu.2015.10.001

Castilho BA, Shanmugam R, Silva RC, Ramesh R, Himme BM, Sattlegger E. Keeping the eIF2 alpha kinase Gcn2 in check. *Biochim Biophys Acta* (2014) 1843:1948–68. doi: 10.1016/j.bbamcr.2014.04.006

Dikic I. Proteasomal and autophagic degradation systems. *Annu Rev Biochem.* (2017) 86:193–224. doi: 10.1146/annurev-biochem-061516-044908

Sorokin AV, Kim ER, Ovchinnikov LP. Proteasome system of protein degradation and processing. *Biochemistry* (2009) 74:1411–42. doi: 10.1134/S000629790913001X

Feng Y, He D, Yao Z, Klionsky DJ. The machinery of macroautophagy. *Cell Res.* (2014) 24:24–41. doi: 10.1038/cr.2013.168

Gatica D, Lahiri V, Klionsky DJ. Cargo recognition and degradation by selective autophagy. *Nat Cell Biol.* (2018) 20:233–242. doi: 10.1038/s41556-018-0037-z

Massey A, Kiffin R, Cuervo AM. Pathophysiology of chaperone- mediated autophagy. *Int J Biochem Cell Biol.* (2004) 36:2420–34. doi: 10.1016/j.biocel.2004.04.010

Lai MC, Chang CM, Sun HS. Hypoxia induces autophagy through translational up-regulation of lysosomal proteins in human colon cancer cells. *PLoS ONE* (2016) 11:e0153627. doi: 10.1371/journal.pone.0153627

Puertollano R, Ferguson SM, Brugarolas J, Ballabio A. The complex relationship between TFEB transcription factor phosphorylation and subcellular localization. *EMBO J.* (2018) 37:e98804. doi: 10.15252/embj.201798804

Martina JA, Puertollano R. TFEB and TFE3: the art of multi- tasking under stress conditions. *Transcription* (2017) 8:48–54. doi: 10.1080/21541264.2016.1264353

Le Y, Zhang S, Ni J, You Y, Luo K, Yu Y, et al. Sorting nexin (2018) 10 controls mTOR activation through regulating amino-acid metabolism in colorectal cancer. *Cell Death Dis.* 9:666. doi: 10.1038/s41419-018-0719-2

Han Q, Deng Y, Chen S, Chen R, Yang M, Zhang Z, et al. Downregulation of ATG5-dependent macroautophagy by chaperone-mediated autophagy promotes breast cancer cell metastasis. *Sci Rep.* (2017) 7:4759. doi: 10.1038/s41598-017-04994-x

Cuervo AM, Terlecky SR, Dice JF, Knecht E. Selective binding and uptake of ribonuclease A and glyceraldehyde-3-phosphate dehydrogenase by isolated rat liver lysosomes. *J Biol Chem.* (1994) 269:26374–80.

Zechner R, Madeo F, Kratky D. Cytosolic lipolysis and lipophagy: two sides of the same coin. *Nat Rev Mol Cell Biol.* (2017) 18:671–84. doi: 10.1038/nrm.2017.76

Singh R, Kaushik S, Wang Y, Xiang Y, Novak I, Komatsu M, et al. Autophagy regulates lipid metabolism. *Nature* (2009) 458:1131–5. doi: 10.1038/nature07976

Guo Y, Cordes KR, Farese RV Jr, Walther TC. Lipid droplets at a glance. *J Cell Sci.* (2009) 122:749–52. doi: 10.1242/jcs.037630

Sztalryd C, Brasaemle DL. The perilipin family of lipid droplet proteins: gatekeepers of intracellular lipolysis. *Biochim Biophys Acta* (2017) 1862:1221–32. doi: 10.1016/j.bbalip.2017.07.009

Cuervo AM, Mann L, Bonten EJ, A. d'Azzo, Dice JF. Cathepsin A regulates chaperone-mediated autophagy through cleavage of the lysosomal receptor. *EMBO J.* (2003) 22:47–59. doi: 10.1093/emboj/cdg002

Wang H, Sreenivasan U, Hu H, Saladino A, Polster BM, Lund LM, et al. Perilipin 5, a lipid droplet-associated protein, provides physical and metabolic linkage to mitochondria. *J Lipid Res.* (2011) 52:2159–68. doi: 10.1194/jlr.M017939

Ramos SV, Turnbull PC, MacPherson RE, LeBlanc PJ, Ward WE, Peters SJ. Changes in mitochondrial perilipin 3 and perilipin 5 protein content in rat skeletal muscle following endurance training and acute stimulated contraction. *Exp Physiol.* (2015) 100:450–62. doi: 10.1113/expphysiol.2014.084434

Bell M, Wang H, Chen H, McLenithan JC, Gong DW, Yang RZ, et al. Consequences of lipid droplet coat protein downregulation in liver cells: abnormal lipid droplet metabolism and induction of insulin resistance. *Diabetes* (2008) 57:2037–45. doi: 10.2337/db07-1383

Chen W, Chang B, Wu X, Li L, Sleeman M, Chan L. Inactivation of Plin4 downregulates Plin5 and reduces cardiac lipid accumulation in mice. *Am J Physiol Endocrinol Metab.* (2013) 304:E770–9. doi: 10.1152/ajpendo.00523.2012

Li Z, Schulze RJ, Weller SG, Krueger EW, Schott MB, Zhang X, et al. A novel Rab10-EHBP1-EHD2 complex essential for the autophagic engulfment of lipid droplets. *Sci Adv.* (2016) 2:e1601470. doi: 10.1126/sciadv.1601470

Wang P, Liu H, Wang Y, Liu O, Zhang J, Gleason A, et al. RAB-10 Promotes EHBP-1 bridging of filamentous actin and tubular recycling endosomes. *PLoS Genet.* (2016) 12:e1006093. doi: 10.1371/journal.pgen.1006093

Cai B, Giridharan SS, Zhang J, Saxena S, Bahl K, Schmidt JA, et al. Differential roles of C-terminal Eps15 homology domain proteins as vesiculators and tubulators of recycling endosomes. *J Biol Chem.* (2013) 288:30172–80. doi: 10.1074/jbc.M113.488627

Martinez-Lopez N, Garcia-Macia M, Sahu S, Athonvarangkul D, Liebling E, Merlo P, et al. Autophagy in the CNS and periphery coordinate lipophagy and lipolysis in the brown adipose tissue and liver. *Cell Metab.* (2016) 23:113–27. doi: 10.1016/j.cmet.2015.10.008

Schneider JL, Suh Y, Cuervo AM. Deficient chaperone-mediated autophagy in liver leads to metabolic dysregulation. *Cell Metab.* (2014) 20:417–32. doi: 10.1016/j.cmet.2014.06.009

Kaushik S, Cuervo AM. Degradation of lipid droplet-associated proteins by chaperone-mediated autophagy facilitates lipolysis. *Nat Cell Biol.* (2015) 17:759–70. doi: 10.1038/ncb3166

Mony VK, Benjamin S, O'Rourke EJ. A lysosome-centered view of nutrient homeostasis. *Autophagy* (2016) 12:619–31. doi: 10.1080/15548627.2016.1147671

Aniento F, Roche E, Cuervo AM, Knecht E. Uptake and degradation of glyceraldehyde-3-phosphate dehydrogenase by rat liver lysosomes. *J Biol Chem.* (1993) 268:10463–70.

Xia HG, Najafov A, Geng J, Galan-Acosta L, Han X, Guo Y, et al. Degradation of HK2 by chaperone-mediated autophagy promotes metabolic catastrophe and cell death. *J Cell Biol.* (2015) 210:705–16. doi: 10.1083/jcb.201503044

Bockus LB, Matsuzaki S, Vadvalkar SS, Young ZT, Giorgione JR, Newhardt MF, et al. Cardiac insulin signaling regulates glycolysis through phosphofructokinase 2 Content and Activity. *J Am Heart Assoc.* (2017) 6:e007159. doi: 10.1161/JAHA.117.007159

Susan PP, Dunn WA Jr. Starvation-induced lysosomal degradation of aldolase B requires glutamine 111 in a signal sequence for chaperone-mediated transport. *J Cell Physiol.* (2001) 187:48–58. doi: 10.1002/1097-4652(2001)9999:9999<00::AID-JCP1050>3.0.CO;2-I

McGuire CM, Forgac M. Glucose starvation increases V-ATPase assembly and activity in mammalian cells through AMP kinase and phosphatidylinositide 3-kinase/Akt signaling. *J Biol Chem.* (2018) 293:9113–23. doi: 10.1074/jbc.RA117.001327

Nwadike C, Williamson LE, Gallagher LE, Guan JL, Chan EYW. AMPK inhibits ULK1-dependent autophagosome formation and lysosomal acidification via distinct mechanisms. *Mol Cell Biol.* (2018) 38:e00023-18. doi: 10.1128/MCB.00023-18

Li L, Friedrichsen HJ, Andrews S, Picaud S, Volpon L, Ngeow K, et al. A TFEB nuclear export signal integrates amino acid supply and glucose availability. *Nat Commun.* (2018) 9:2685. doi: 10.1038/s41467-018-04849-7

Vogiatzi T, Xilouri M, Vekrellis K, Stefanis L. Wild type alpha- synuclein is degraded by chaperone-mediated autophagy and macroautophagy in neuronal cells. *J Biol Chem.* (2008) 283:23542–56. doi: 10.1074/jbc.M801992200

Martinez-Vicente M, Talloczy Z, Kaushik S, Massey AC, Mazzulli J, Mosharov EV, et al. Dopamine-modified alpha-synuclein blocks chaperone- mediated autophagy. *J Clin Invest*. (2008) 118:777–88. doi: 10.1172/JCI32806

Xilouri M, Vogiatzi T, Vekrellis K, Park D, Stefanis L. Abberant alpha- synuclein confers toxicity to neurons in part through inhibition of chaperone-mediated autophagy. *PLoS ONE* (2009) 4:e5515. doi:10.1371/journal.pone.0005515

Xilouri M, Brekk OR, Polissidis A, Chrysanthou-Piterou M, Kloukina I, Stefanis L. Impairment of chaperone-mediated autophagy induces dopaminergic neurodegeneration in rats. *Autophagy* (2016) 12:2230–47. doi: 10.1080/15548627.2016.1214777

Issa AR, Sun J, Petitgas C, Mesquita A, Dulac A, Robin M, et al. The lysosomal membrane protein LAMP2A promotes autophagic flux and prevents SNCA-induced Parkinson disease-like symptoms in the Drosophila brain. *Autophagy* (2018) 14:1898–910. doi: 10.1080/15548627.2018.1491489

Wang B, Cai Z, Tao K, Zeng W, Lu F, Yang R, et al. Essential control of mitochondrial morphology and function by chaperone-mediated autophagy through degradation of PARK7. *Autophagy* (2016) 12:1215–28. doi: 10.1080/15548627.2016.1179401

Yang Q, She H, Gearing M, Colla E, Lee M, Shacka JJ, et al. Regulation of neuronal survival factor MEF2D by chaperone-mediated autophagy. *Science* (2009) 323:124–7. doi: 10.1126/science.1166088

Murphy KE, Gysbers AM, Abbott SK, Spiro AS, Furuta A, Cooper A, et al. Lysosomal-associated membrane protein 2 isoforms are differentially affected in early Parkinson's disease. *Move Disord*. (2015) 30:1639–47. doi: 10.1002/mds.26141

Sala G, Stefanoni G, Arosio A, Riva C, Melchionda L, Saracchi E, et al. Reduced expression of the chaperone-mediated autophagy carrier hsc70 protein in lymphomonocytes of patients with Parkinson's disease. *Brain Res*. (2014) 1546:46–52. doi: 10.1016/j.brainres.2013.12.017

Pang S, Chen D, Zhang A, Qin X, Yan B. Genetic analysis of the LAMP-2 gene promoter in patients with sporadic Parkinson's disease. *Neurosci Lett*. (2012) 526:63–7. doi: 10.1016/j.neulet.2012.07.044

Alvarez-Erviti L, Seow Y, Schapira AH, Rodriguez-Oroz MC, Obeso JA, Cooper JM. Influence of microRNA deregulation on chaperone-mediated autophagy and alpha-synuclein pathology in Parkinson's disease. *Cell Death Dis*. (2013) 4:e545. doi: 10.1038/cddis.2013.73

Liu H, Wang P, Song W, Sun X. Degradation of regulator of calcineurin 1 (RCAN1) is mediated by both chaperone-mediated autophagy and ubiquitin proteasome pathways. *FASEB J*. (2009) 23:3383–92. doi: 10.1096/fj.09-134296

Valdor R, Mocholi E, Botbol Y, Guerrero-Ros I, Chandra D, Koga H,., et al. Chaperone-mediated autophagy regulates T cell responses through targeted degradation of negative regulators of T cell activation. *Nat Immunol*. (2014) 15:1046–54. doi: 10.1038/ni.3003

Wang Y, Martinez-Vicente M, Kruger U, Kaushik S, Cuervo M, Wong E, et al. Tau fragmentation, aggregation and clearance: the dual role of lysosomal processing. *Hum Mol Genet*. (2009) 18:4153–70. doi: 10.1093/hmg/ddp367

Wang Y, Martinez-Vicente M, Kruger U, Kaushik S, Wong E, Mandelkow EM, et al. Synergy and antagonism of macroautophagy and chaperone- mediated autophagy in a cell model of pathological tau aggregation. *Autophagy* (2010) 6:182–3. doi: 10.4161/auto.6.1.10815

Park JS, Kim DH, Yoon SY. Regulation of amyloid precursor protein processing by its KFERQ motif. *BMB Rep*. (2016) 49:337–42. doi: 10.5483/BMBRep.2016.49.6.212

Qi L, Zhang XD, Wu JC, Lin F, Wang J, DiFiglia M, et al. The role of chaperone-mediated autophagy in huntingtin degradation. *PLoS ONE* (2012) 7:e46834. doi: 10.1371/journal.pone.0046834

Bauer PO, Goswami A, Wong HK, Okuno M, Kurosawa M, Yamada M, et al. Harnessing chaperone-mediated autophagy for the selective degradation of mutant huntingtin protein. *Nat Biotechnol*. (2010) 28:256–63. doi: 10.1038/nbt.1608

Huang CC, Bose JK, Majumder P, Lee KH, Huang JT, Huang JK, et al. Metabolism and mis-metabolism of the neuropathological signature protein TDP-43. *J Cell Sci*. (2014) 127:3024–38. doi: 10.1242/jcs.136150

Tamaki Y, Shodai A, Morimura T, Hikiami R, Minamiyama S, Ayaki T, et al. Elimination of TDP-43 inclusions linked to amyotrophic lateral sclerosis by a misfolding-specific intrabody with dual proteolytic signals. *Sci Rep*. (2018) 8:6030. doi: 10.1038/s41598-018-24463-3

Marino G, Fernandez AF, Lopez-Otin C. Autophagy and aging: lessons from progeria models. *Adv Exp Med Biol*. (2010) 694:61–8. doi:10.1007/978-1-4419-7002-2_6

Cuervo AM, Dice JF. Age-related decline in chaperone-mediated autophagy. *J Biol Chem*. (2000) 275:31505–13. doi: 10.1074/jbc.M002102200

Kiffin R, Kaushik S, Zeng M, Bandyopadhyay U, Zhang C, Massey AC, et al. Altered dynamics of the lysosomal receptor for chaperone- mediated autophagy with age. *J Cell Sci*. (2007) 120:782–91. doi: 10.1242/jcs. 001073

Schneider JL, Villarroya J, Diaz-Carretero A, Patel B, Urbanska AM, Thi M. M, et al. Loss of hepatic chaperone-mediated autophagy accelerates proteostasis failure in aging. *Aging Cell* (2015) 14:249–64. doi: 10.1111/acel.12310

Papagiannakis N, Xilouri M, Koros C, Stamelou M, Antonelou R, Maniati M, et al. Lysosomal alterations in peripheral blood mononuclear cells of Parkinson's disease patients. *Mov Disord*. (2015) 30:1830–4. doi: 10.1002/mds.26433

Klaver AC, Coffey MP, Aasly JO, Loeffler DA. CSF lamp2 concentrations are decreased in female Parkinson's disease patients with LRRK2 mutations. *Brain Res*. (2018) 1683:12–16. doi: 10.1016/j.brainres.2018. 01.016

Loeffler DA, Klaver AC, Coffey MP, Aasly JO. Cerebrospinal fluid concentration of key autophagy protein lamp2 changes little during normal aging. *Front Aging Neurosci*. (2018) 10:130. doi: 10.3389/fnagi.2018. 00130

Rodriguez-Navarro JA, Kaushik S, Koga H, Dall'Armi C, Shui G, Wenk MR, et al. Inhibitory effect of dietary lipids on chaperone-mediated autophagy. *Proc Natl Acad Sci USA* (2012) 109:E705–14. doi: 10.1073/pnas.11130 36109

Khang R, Park C, Shin JH. Dysregulation of parkin in the substantia nigra of db/db and high-fat diet mice. *Neuroscience* (2015) 294:182–92. doi: 10.1016/j.neuroscience.2015.03.017

Rotermund C, Truckenmuller FM, Schell H, Kahle PJ. Diet-induced obesity accelerates the onset of terminal phenotypes in alpha-synuclein transgenic mice. *J Neurochem*. (2014) 131:848–58. doi: 10.1111/jnc.12813

Kim D, Cho J, Lee I, Jin Y, Kang H. Exercise attenuates high- fat diet-induced disease progression in 3xTg-AD Mice. *Med Sci Sports Exerc*. (2017) 49:676–86. doi: 10.1249/MSS.0000000000 001166

Julien C, Tremblay C, Phivilay A, Berthiaume L, Emond V, Julien P, et al. High-fat diet aggravates amyloid-beta and tau pathologies in the (2010) 3xTg-AD mouse model. *Neurobiol Aging* 31:1516–31. doi: 10.1016/j.neurobiolaging.2008.08.022

Pennetta G, Welte MA. Emerging links between lipid droplets and motor neuron diseases. *Dev Cell* (2018) 45:427–32. doi: 10.1016/j.devcel.2018.05.002

Cole NB, Murphy DD, Grider T, Rueter S, Brasaemle D, Nussbaum RL. Lipid droplet binding and oligomerization properties of the Parkinson's disease protein alpha-synuclein. *J Biol Chem*. (2002) 277:6344–52. doi: 10.1074/jbc. M108414200

Sun X, Ueda M, Yamashita T, Nakamura M, Bergstrom J, Zeledon Ramirez ME, et al. Lipid droplets are present in amyloid deposits in familial amyloidotic polyneuropathy and dialysis related amyloidosis. *Amyloid* (2006) 13:20–3. doi: 10.1080/13506120500537137

Taylor MK, Sullivan DK, Swerdlow RH, Vidoni ED, Morris JK, Mahnken JD, et al. A high-glycemic diet is associated with cerebral amyloid burden in cognitively normal older adults. *Am J Clin Nutr*. (2017) 106:1463–70. doi: 10.3945/ajcn.117.162263

Vicente Miranda H, Outeiro TF. The sour side of neurodegenerative disorders: the effects of protein glycation. *J Pathol*. (2010) 221:13–25. doi: 10.1002/path.2682

Liu F, Zaidi T, Iqbal K, Grundke-Iqbal I, Gong CX. Aberrant glycosylation modulates phosphorylation of tau by protein kinase A and dephosphorylation of tau by protein phosphatase 2A and 5. *Neuroscience* (2002) 115:829–37. doi: 10.1016/S0306-4522(02)00510-9

Valente T, Gella A, Fernandez-Busquets X, Unzeta M, Durany N. Immunohistochemical analysis of human brain suggests pathological synergism of Alzheimer's disease and diabetes mellitus. *Neurobiol Dis*. (2010) 37:67–76. doi: 10.1016/j.nbd.2009.09.008

Seneff S, Wainwright G, Mascitelli L. Nutrition and Alzheimer's disease: the detrimental role of a high carbohydrate diet. *Eur J Intern Med*. (2011) 22:134–40. doi: 10.1016/j.ejim.2010.12.017

Dunn L, Allen GF, Mamais A, Ling H, Li A, Duberley KE, et al. Dysregulation of glucose metabolism is an early event in sporadic Parkinson's disease. *Neurobiol Aging* (2014) 35:1111–5. doi: 10.1016/j.neurobiolaging.2013.11.001

Bigl M, Bruckner MK, Arendt T, Bigl V, Eschrich K. Activities of key glycolytic enzymes in the brains of patients with Alzheimer's disease. *J Neural Transm (Vienna)* (1999) 106:499–511. doi: 10.1007/s007020050174

Barinova K, Khomyakova E, Semenyuk P, Schmalhausen E, Muronetz V. Binding of alpha-synuclein to partially oxidized glyceraldehyde-3-phosphate dehydrogenase induces subsequent inactivation of the enzyme. *Arch Biochem Biophys*. (2018) 642:10–22. doi: 10.1016/j.abb.2018.02.002

Gouarne C, Tardif G, Tracz J, Latyszenok V, Michaud M, Clemens LE, et al. Early deficits in glycolysis are specific to striatal neurons from a rat model of huntington disease. *PLoS ONE* (2013) 8:e81528. doi: 10.1371/journal.pone.0081528

Estrada-Sanchez AM, Montiel T, Massieu L. Glycolysis inhibition decreases the levels of glutamate transporters and enhances glutamate neurotoxicity in the R6/2 Huntington's disease mice. *Neurochem Res*. (2010) 35:1156–63. doi: 10.1007/s11064-010-0168-5

Rodriguez-Navarro JA, Cuervo AM. Dietary lipids and aging compromise chaperone-mediated autophagy by similar mechanisms. *Autophagy* (2012) 8:1152–4. doi: 10.4161/auto.20649

Kaushik S, Massey AC, Cuervo AM. Lysosome membrane lipid microdomains: novel regulators of chaperone-mediated autophagy. *EMBO J.* (2006) 25:3921–33. doi: 10.1038/sj.emboj.7601283

Permissions

The contributors of this book come from diverse backgrounds, making this book a truly international effort. This book will bring forth new frontiers with its revolutionizing research information and detailed analysis of the nascent developments around the world.

We would like to thank all the contributing authors for lending their expertise to make the book truly unique. They have played a crucial role in the development of this book. Without their invaluable contributions this book wouldn't have been possible. They have made vital efforts to compile up to date information on the varied aspects of this subject to make this book a valuable addition to the collection of many professionals and students.

This book was conceptualized with the vision of imparting up-to-date information and advanced data in this field. To ensure the same, a matchless editorial board was set up. Every individual on the board went through rigorous rounds of assessment to prove their worth. After which they invested a large part of their time researching and compiling the most relevant data for our readers.

The editorial board has been involved in producing this book since its inception. They have spent rigorous hours researching and exploring the diverse topics which have resulted in the successful publishing of this book. They have passed on their knowledge of decades through this book. To expedite this challenging task, the publisher supported the team at every step. A small team of assistant editors was also appointed to further simplify the editing procedure and attain best results for the readers.

Apart from the editorial board, the designing team has also invested a significant amount of their time in understanding the subject and creating the most relevant covers. They scrutinized every image to scout for the most suitable representation of the subject and create an appropriate cover for the book.

The publishing team has been an ardent support to the editorial, designing and production team. Their endless efforts to recruit the best for this project, has resulted in the accomplishment of this book. They are a veteran in the field of academics and their pool of knowledge is as vast as their experience in printing. Their expertise and guidance has proved useful at every step. Their uncompromising quality standards have made this book an exceptional effort. Their encouragement from time to time has been an inspiration for everyone.

The publisher and the editorial board hope that this book will prove to be a valuable piece of knowledge for researchers, students, practitioners and scholars across the globe.

List of Contributors

Zuqing Su, Bing Feng, Lipeng Tang, Guangjuan Zheng and Ying Zhu
Guangdong Provincial Hospital of Chinese Medicine, The Second Clinical College of Guangzhou University of Chinese Medicine, Guangzhou, China

Yanru Guo
Guangdong Provincial Hospital of Chinese Medicine, The Second Clinical College of Guangzhou University of Chinese Medicine, Guangzhou, China

Xiufang Huang
Guangdong Provincial Hospital of Chinese Medicine, The Second Clinical College of Guangzhou University of Chinese Medicine, Guangzhou, China
The First Affiliated Hospital of Guangzhou University of Chinese Medicine, Guangzhou, China

Ana Isabel Álvarez-Mercado
Department of Biochemistry and Molecular Biology II, School of Pharmacy, Granada, Spain
Institute of Nutrition and Food Technology "José Mataix", Biomedical Research Center, Parque Tecnológico Ciencias de la Salud, Granada, Spain
Instituto de Investigación Biosanitaria ibs. GRANADA, Complejo Hospitalario Universitario de Granada, Granada, Spain

Carlos Rojano-Alfonso, Marc Micó-Carnero, Albert Caballeria-Casals and Carmen Peralta
Institut d'Investigacions Biomèdiques August Pi i Sunyer (IDIBAPS), Barcelona, Spain

Araní Casillas-Ramírez
Hospital Regional de Alta Especialidad de Ciudad Victoria "Bicentenario 2010", Ciudad Victoria, Mexico
Facultad de Medicina e Ingeniería en Sistemas Computacionales de Matamoros, Universidad Autónoma de Tamaulipas, Matamoros, Mexico

Nerea Deleyto-Seldas and Alejo Efeyan
Metabolism and Cell Signaling Laboratory, Spanish National Cancer Research Center (CNIO), Madrid, Spain

Jing Xu
Department of Diabetology and Endocrinology, Kanazawa Medical University, Uchinada, Japan

Department of Endocrinology and Metabolism, The Affiliated Hospital of Guizhou Medical University, Guiyang, China

Munehiro Kitada and Daisuke Koya
Department of Diabetology and Endocrinology, Kanazawa Medical University, Uchinada, Japan
Division of Anticipatory Molecular Food Science and Technology, Medical Research Institute, Kanazawa Medical University, Uchinada, Japan

Yoshio Ogura
Department of Diabetology and Endocrinology, Kanazawa Medical University, Uchinada, Japan

Vincenza Frisardi
Clinical and Nutritional Laboratory, Department of Geriatric and NeuroRehabilitation, Arcispedale Santa Maria Nuova (AUSL-IRCCS), Reggio Emilia, Italy

Carmela Matrone
Division of Pharmacology, Department of Neuroscience, School of Medicine, University of Naples Federico II, Naples, Italy

Maria Elisabeth Street
Division of Paediatric Endocrinology and Diabetology, Paediatrics, Department of Mother and Child, Arcispedale Santa Maria Nuova (AUSL-IRCCS), Reggio Emilia, Italy

Ezekiel Uba Nwose
School of Community Health, Charles Sturt University, Orange, NSW, Australia
Department of Public and Community Health, Novena University, Kwale, Nigeria

Phillip Taderera Bwititi
School of Biomedical Sciences, Charles Sturt University, Wagga Wagga, NSW, Australia

Scott Frendo-Cumbo and Victoria L. Tokarz
Cell Biology Program, Hospital for Sick Children, Toronto, ON, Canada
Department of Physiology, University of Toronto, Toronto, ON, Canada

Philip J. Bilan
Cell Biology Program, Hospital for Sick Children, Toronto, ON, Canada

John H. Brumell
Cell Biology Program, Hospital for Sick Children, Toronto, ON, Canada
Department of Molecular Genetics, University of Toronto, Toronto, ON, Canada
Institute of Medical Science, University of Toronto, Toronto, ON, Canada
SickKids Inflammatory Bowel Disease (IBD) Centre, Hospital for Sick Children, Toronto, ON, Canada

Amira Klip
Cell Biology Program, Hospital for Sick Children, Toronto, ON, Canada
Department of Physiology, University of Toronto, Toronto, ON, Canada
Department of Biochemistry, University of Toronto, Toronto, ON, Canada

Yunyun Fang, Linlin Ji, Chaoyu Zhu, Yuanyuan Xiao, Junxi Lu and Li Wei
Shanghai Key Laboratory of Diabetes Mellitus, Department of Endocrinology and Metabolism, Shanghai Diabetes Institute, Shanghai Clinical Center for Diabetes, Shanghai Key Clinical Center for Metabolic Disease, Shanghai Jiao Tong University Affiliated Sixth People's Hospital, Shanghai, China

Jingjing Zhang
National Demonstration Center for Experimental Fisheries Science Education, Shanghai Ocean University, Shanghai, China

Jun Yin
Shanghai Key Laboratory of Diabetes Mellitus, Department of Endocrinology and Metabolism, Shanghai Diabetes Institute, Shanghai Clinical Center for Diabetes, Shanghai Key Clinical Center for Metabolic Disease, Shanghai Jiao Tong University Affiliated Sixth People's Hospital, Shanghai, China
Department of Endocrinology and Metabolism, Shanghai Eighth People's Hospital, Shanghai, China

Seung-Hyun Ro, Julianne Fay, Cesar I. Cyuzuzo and Edward N. Harris
Department of Biochemistry, University of Nebraska-Lincoln, Lincoln, NE, United States

Yura Jang
Department of Biochemistry, University of Nebraska-Lincoln, Lincoln, NE, United States
Department of Neurology, Institute for Cell Engineering, Johns Hopkins University School of Medicine, Baltimore, MD, United States

Naeun Lee
Department of Biological Systems Engineering, University of Nebraska-Lincoln, Lincoln, NE, United States

Hyun-Seob Song
Department of Biological Systems Engineering, University of Nebraska-Lincoln, Lincoln, NE, United States
Department of Food Science and Technology, Nebraska Food for Health Center, University of Nebraska-Lincoln, Lincoln, NE, United States

Richa Pant, Priyanka Firmal and Vibhuti Kumar Shah
National Centre for Cell Science, SP Pune University Campus, Pune, India

Aftab Alam
Roswell Park Comprehensive Cancer Center, Buffalo, NY, United States

Samit Chattopadhyay
National Centre for Cell Science, SP Pune University Campus, Pune, India
Department of Biological Sciences, BITS Pilani, Goa, India

Shuangyu Lv, Honggang Wang and Xiaotian Li
Institute of Biomedical Informatics, Bioinformatics Center, School of Basic Medical Sciences, Henan University, Kaifeng, China

Jessica Maiuolo, Micaela Gliozzi, Vincenzo Musolino, Cristina Carresi, Federica Scarano, Saverio Nucera, Miriam Scicchitano, Francesca Bosco, Stefano Ruga, Maria Caterina Zito, Roberta Macri and Rosamaria Bulotta
IRC-FSH Department of Health Sciences, University "Magna Graecia" of Catanzaro, Catanzaro, Italy

Carolina Muscoli and Vincenzo Mollace
IRC-FSH Department of Health Sciences, University "Magna Graecia" of Catanzaro, Catanzaro, Italy
IRCCS San Raffaele, Rome, Italy

Vitor de Miranda Ramos, Alicia J. Kowaltowski and Pamela A. Kakimoto
Departamento de Bioquímica, Instituto de Química, Universidade de São Paulo, São Paulo, Brazil

María C. Paz, Pablo F. Barcelona, Paula V. Subirada, Magali E. Ridano, Gustavo A. Chiabrando and María C. Sánchez
Departamento de Bioquímica Clínica, Facultad de Ciencias Químicas, Universidad Nacional de Córdoba, Córdoba, Argentina
Centro de Investigaciones en Bioquímica Clínica e Inmunología, Consejo Nacional de Investigaciones Científicas y Técnicas, Córdoba, Argentina

Claudia Castro
Instituto de Medicina y Biología Experimental de Cuyo, Consejo Nacional de Investigaciones Científicas y Técnicas, Facultad de Ciencias Médicas, Universidad Nacional de Cuyo, Mendoza, Argentina

Paola Fortini and Eugenia Dogliotti
Department of Environment and Primary Prevention, Istituto Superiore di Sanità, Rome, Italy

Egidio Iorio
Department of Cell Biology and Neurosciences, Istituto Superiore di Sanità, Rome, Italy

Ciro Isidoro
Università degli Studi del Piemonte Orientale "Amedeo Avogadro", Novara, Italy

Iván E. Alfaro and Amelina Albornoz
Fundación Ciencia & Vida, Santiago, Chile

Alfredo Molina, José Moreno and Karina Cordero
Dentistry Faculty, Institute in Dentistry Sciences, University of Chile, Santiago, Chile

Alfredo Criollo
Dentistry Faculty, Institute in Dentistry Sciences, University of Chile, Santiago, Chile
Autophagy Research Center (ARC), Santiago, Chile
Advanced Center for Chronic Diseases (ACCDiS), University of Chile, Santiago, Chile

Mauricio Budini
Dentistry Faculty, Institute in Dentistry Sciences, University of Chile, Santiago, Chile
Autophagy Research Center (ARC), Santiago, Chile

Index

Printed in the USA
CPSIA information can be obtained
at www.ICGtesting.com
JSHW051405091023
49903JS00006B/285